Hospital Infections

Hospital Infections

Edited by

John V. Bennett, M.D.

Director, Bacterial Diseases Division, Bureau
of Epidemiology, Center for Disease Control,
U.S. Public Health Service, Atlanta

Philip S. Brachman, M.D.

Director, Bureau of Epidemiology,
Center for Disease Control,
U.S. Public Health Service; Clinical Associate
Professor of Preventive Medicine and
Community Health, Emory University
School of Medicine, Atlanta

Foreword by Maxwell Finland, M.D.
Hospital Epidemiologist, Boston City Hospital,
Boston

Little, Brown and Company, Boston

Contents

Foreword by Maxwell Finland   ix
Preface   xv
Contributing Authors   xvii

I: Basic Considerations of Hospital Infections

1. **Introduction**   3
   Philip S. Brachman

2. **Epidemiology of Nosocomial Infections**   9
   Philip S. Brachman

3. **Hospital Personnel**   27
   Richard A. Kaslow and Julia S. Garner

4. **Surveillance of Nosocomial Infections**   53
   Robert C. Aber and John V. Bennett

5. **Investigation of Endemic and Epidemic Infections**   63
   Richard E. Dixon

6. **The Inanimate Environment**   81
   George F. Mallison

7. **Areas of Special Concern**   93

   A. The Hemodialysis Unit   93
   John A. Bryan

   B. The Intensive Care Unit   99
   Alfred E. Buxton

   C. The Newborn Nursery   104
   James R. Allen and
   Thomas K. Oliver, Jr.

   D. The Pharmacy   115
   Stephen R. Zellner and
   Leighton E. Cluff

   E. Food Services   117
   Eugene J. Gangarosa

F. *Central Service*   123
George F. Mallison

G. *Linens and Laundry*   126
George F. Mallison

H. *The Operating Room*   129
Harold Laufman

I. *The Admitting and Outpatient
Departments*   137
Kathryn S. Wenzel Owens

J. *The Clinical Laboratory*   139
Marie B. Coyle and John C. Sherris

8. **The Microbiology Laboratory: Its Role
in Surveillance, Investigation, and
Control**   147
Raymond C. Bartlett, John V. Bennett,
Robert A. Weinstein, and
George F. Mallison

9. **Isolation Policies and
Procedures**   169
Julia S. Garner and
Philip S. Brachman

10. **Legal Aspects of Nosocomial
Infections**   181
R. Crawford Morris

11. **Antibiotics and Nosocomial
Infections**   195
Theodore C. Eickhoff

12. **The Relationship Between the Hospital
and the Community**   223
William Schaffner

II: *Endemic and Epidemic Hospital Infections*

13. **Incidence and Nature of Endemic and
Epidemic Nosocomial Infections**   233
John V. Bennett

14. **Urinary Tract Infections**   239
Calvin M. Kunin

15. **Lower Respiratory Tract Infections** 255
    Jay P. Sanford and Alan K. Pierce

16. **Surgical Infections: Incisional Wounds** 287
    William A. Altemeier

17. **Infections of Cardiac and Vascular Prostheses** 307
    John P. Burke

18. **Infections of Skeletal Prostheses** 321
    Jorge A. Franco and
    William F. Enneking

19. **Infections of Burn Wounds** 335
    J. Wesley Alexander and
    Bruce G. MacMillan

20. **Selected Infections of the Skin and Eye** 355
    Walter E. Stamm, Allen C. Steere,
    and Richard E. Dixon

21. **Infectious Gastroenteritis** 381
    Herbert L. DuPont

22. **Puerperal Endometritis** 395
    William J. Ledger

23. **The Central Nervous System: Meningitis** 409
    Harry N. Beaty

24. **Selected Viral Infections of Nosocomial Importance** 419
    Paul F. Wehrle

25. **Intravenous Cannula–Associated Infections** 433
    Frank S. Rhame, Dennis G. Maki,
    and John V. Bennett

26. **Intravenous Infusion–Associated Infections** 443
    Donald A. Goldmann,
    Dennis G. Maki, and John V. Bennett

27. **Transplant-Associated
Infections**   453
John E. Swartzberg and
Jack S. Remington

28. **Other Procedure-Related
Infections**   489
Robert A. Weinstein and
Lowell S. Young

29. **Gram-Negative Rod Bacteremia**   507
Allen C. Steere, Walter E. Stamm,
Stanley M. Martin, and
John V. Bennett

Index   519

Foreword

Maxwell Finland

In the introduction to their book *The Control of Infections in Hospitals* (1966), LeRiche and co-workers date the beginnings of hospitals, as an expression of charity, to AD 325 when the bishops at the Council of Nicaea were instructed to provide a hospital in every cathedral city. For more than half a millennium, hospitals mixed all patients within their wards, including those convalescing from, or still ill with, active and terminal infections. Thus, the prevalent plagues—cholera, smallpox, typhoid fever, and others—were introduced and spread to those not already dying of surgical and other causes. Infections of surgical wounds were almost inevitable, and most of them were fatal. In the middle of the nineteenth century, the mortality rate following amputations was found to be four times as high in those who were hospitalized as in those who remained at home.

In 1843, Oliver Wendell Holmes, in his classic paper *On the Contagiousness of Childbed Fever,* postulated that puerperal infections were spread physically to parturient women by physicians from infected materials in autopsies they had performed or from infected women they had attended. A few years later, Semmelweis published his epochal findings on puerperal fever, which showed that women delivered by physicians were infected four times as often as those delivered at home by midwives, and that hospitals without students had better results, except in Paris where midwives did their own autopsies. He effected a marked reduction in maternal mortality through the practice of proper hand-washing by attending physicians. In the decades that followed, Lister introduced the principles of antisepsis in surgery, which were followed by those of asepsis during the early years of the era of bacteriology.

The beginnings of epidemiology were traced by Leslie T. Webster to the Books of Hippocrates in the fifth century BC. Those works contained observations on different types of sickness and on fluctuations in their prevalence, from which Hippocrates concluded that individuals and populations differ among themselves and undergo changes in resistance to various sicknesses. Webster also mentions the treatise on contagion published by Franciscatus in 1576.

Webster's own studies were focused on the role of susceptibility and immunity of individuals within a population in the origins, spread, course, and termination of epidemics of infection; he used a single strain of organism in closed and controlled populations of experimental animals for his model. Similar studies had been reported earlier by Topley and Greenwood in England as well as by Harold Amos at the Rockefeller Institute, where Webster worked.

The principles derived from experimental epidemiology are clearly applicable to hospital infections. In the experimental model, however, a single virulent strain of organism is used to infect one or more susceptible animals that are then introduced into closed populations of other susceptible animals of the same breed. The organism spreads to some of the uninfected susceptible animals, and it produces infections from which some die while others survive. Those that survive either clear their organisms or become carriers, with or without residual infected focuses. New groups of susceptible animals introduced into this residual population have the same fate as the original population, and the infection can be perpetuated by continuous introduction of new susceptible individuals, with the earlier survivors generally being spared.

Needless to say, humans—particularly hospitalized patients—are far more complex with respect to their susceptibility or resistance to infection than are the purebred stocks of laboratory animals used in experimental epidemiology. Also, the hospital is a far more complex environment than the carefully arranged cages in the animal quarters that house the colony used in the model. Moreover, instead of the single strain of infecting organism that is introduced from outside of the animal colony, we have a variable number of virulent pathogens being brought in constantly from the community by new patients admitted with infections, in addition to those already in the patient population and in the complex environment to which those patients are exposed, including the hospital staff. The hospitalized patients can be expected to be more susceptible than healthy individuals in the community due to their underlying disease, or their tissues may be rendered more susceptible to infections by injuries acquired outside the hospital or inflicted on them by the surgical procedures and instrumentations to which they are subjected during their hospitalization.

The present volume deals with the many facets of the complex environment of the hospital and with the numerous problems affecting the patients who acquire infections while there, either as a result of exposure to elements of that environment or as a result of decreased resistance to their own endogenous microbial flora. The large number of chapters and the size of the volume attest to the magnitude and complexity of such problems and to the large amount of accumulated information already available about them. This material is based on extensive investigations throughout the country, and it is reinforced by the experiences of those within the Bureau of Epidemiology and of others at the U.S. Public Health Service Center for Disease Control (CDC). The effects of the extensive usage of antimicrobial agents in hospitalized patients on the occurrence and character of nosocomial infections are included among the discussions in this book.

Interest in nosocomial infections has grown at a very rapid rate since the early 1960s, when it was stimulated by the alarming increase in the numbers of serious staphylococcal infections with their high mortality rate that were being encountered in hospitals throughout the United States and in many other countries. More recently, serious infections with gram-negative rods and outbreaks of such infections with organisms resistant to most of the available antibiotics have been increasing steadily in large hospitals, where they have superceded in importance those infections due to staphylococci, except perhaps in newborn nurseries. Partly as a result of experiences with such outbreaks, several important conferences and symposia dealing with nosocomial infections and their control were convened, particularly in the United States and the United Kingdom. The transactions of those assemblies have been published and contain many important contributions. Other textbooks and monographs dealing with this subject have also been published during this time, in addition to the increased attention being given to such problems in the annual (or periodic) publications dealing with infectious diseases published in this country by such national organizations as the American Public Health Association, American Hospital Association, American Academy of Pediatrics, American College of Surgeons, and by CDC itself.

Why, then, publish another book at this time? Many reasons may be cited. First is the rapidly changing character and increasing seriousness of the infections being encountered and the increasing difficulty of controlling them. Then there is the rapidly changing character of the hospitals and the increasing number and complexity of the services they provide. The latter have involved the performance of a great many new and extensive surgical procedures, particularly those involving the transplantation of organs and the implantation of foreign bodies in the repair or replacement of defective organs and tissues. Such procedures have also involved extensive and intensive use of immunosuppressive agents, which are also applied in the management of neoplastic diseases and other chronic disorders. There have also been marked increases in the use of invasive and noninvasive instruments and appliances and the multiplication and increased utilization of intensive-care units. Increasing and more intensive uses of antimicrobial agents have permitted many patients with immunologic defects— whether indigenous or produced by the new therapies—to survive infections and to become susceptible again to infection with other organisms or even the same ones that are now resistant to the actions of such antibiotics. Also, there has been an increase in our knowledge of and ability to control and prevent certain nosocomial infections.

As a result, interest has rapidly grown in the subject, and there has been a correspondingly rapid increase in the numbers of hospital personnel involved in the early recognition of nosocomial infections, in attempts to control them, and in efforts to reduce the enormous amount of illness, disability, mortality, and economic burden they entail. Thus, over the past decade a marked increase has occurred in the number of physicians, nurses, and others, including administrators, who are interested in infectious diseases and hospital epidemiology. The nurses have been known as "infection control nurses." Over the past several years, a variety of hospital personnel other than nurses (e.g., public health officers, physicians, and microbiologists) have successfully performed the same functions. Accordingly, a new title, "practitioners of infection control," is used by some to designate people who perform this function, and they have organized as a society, the Association for Practitioners in Infection Control (APIC). There have also been greater emphasis and increasing activity on the part of Infection Control Committees within hospitals. The use of periodic or continuous surveillance of infections is being introduced in more and more hospitals, and many of them are making increasing use of computers to compile, store, retrieve, analyze, and compare the information thus acquired.

This volume also differs from others in that it covers—in a broader, more complete, and better documented manner—each aspect of the various problems. It does more than merely provide a syllabus or systematic guide to the procedures involved in the recognition of infections and in their control, such as is provided in some of the handbooks issued by the various national societies, although such material is also included here.

The editors of this volume are therefore to be commended for undertaking and bringing to fruition this much needed, new, and authoritative source book of information on the increasingly important subject of hospital infections. It should be most valuable for reference and guidance to all students and practitioners in the fields of infectious diseases, epidemiology, and hospital management, as well as being of value to all physicians caring for hospitalized patients who may acquire infections during their hospitalization.

Preface

The importance of nosocomial infections can be put into perspective by noting that about 5 percent of patients admitted to acute care hospitals develop a nosocomial infection, the majority of which are endemic infections; however, epidemics of nosocomial infections are always a threat. The estimated direct annual cost of those infections is in excess of $1 billion. The indirect costs could double this figure. Additionally, 3 percent of nosocomial infections probably result directly in the death of the patient. Nosocomial infections may affect not only the patient who develops the infection but other patients, the hospital staff, the patient's family, and the community as well. Data accumulated over past years indicate that under certain conditions as much as half of all nosocomial infections may be preventable.

This book was written because of our concern that despite the significance of the problem today and the increasing complexity of factors related to its development, no single reference existed that clearly discussed nosocomial infections in detail from an epidemiologic perspective and included practical and effective means of control and prevention. Thorough understanding of the latter depends on epidemiologic knowledge. Also, there are sometimes substantial clinical, laboratory, and epidemiologic differences between nosocomial and community-acquired infections; yet these distinctions are seldom treated adequately in existing texts. Their importance is highlighted by the fact that about one-third of all infections seen in hospital practice are nosocomial in origin.

Much has been written in the scientific literature concerning nosocomial infections, and this book attempts to consolidate the pertinent, informative data available on a comprehensive range of topics. The authors have direct personal and professional experience relevant to their subjects and are recognized authorities in the field. The book not only provides useful information for controlling and preventing hospital infections but also comprehensively discusses each problem and its solution, incorporating epidemiologic, clinical, and laboratory aspects of nosocomial infections, with emphasis on the former.

Part I defines the overall problem, discusses the impact of contributing factors, identifies and describes areas of special concern, and sets forth general concepts of control and prevention. Part II includes comprehensive discussions of specific infection problems related to different organ systems and procedures.

This book is directed toward all interested persons as well as those with responsibility for controlling and preventing nosocomial infections. It should be useful for the in-depth study of particular nosocomial infections. Those who master its contents should be able to organize and implement surveillance, investigations, and control and preventive measures for both endemic and epidemic nosocomial infection problems. Although all nosocomial infections cannot be prevented, implementation of the approaches discussed in this textbook could go a long way toward reducing the impact that nosocomial infections have on the health of hospitalized patients and on the economics of health care delivery.

The editors express their appreciation to the authors, the publisher, and many other persons for their patience, skills, and assistance without which this book could not have been written. Also, we gratefully acknowledge the insights and perspectives of hospital personnel of all disciplines in many hospitals throughout the country whose interests, concerns, and cooperative interactions with the editors and authors have been of prime importance in expanding our collective knowledge and understanding of nosocomial infections and their control.

J. V. B.
P. S. B.

Contributing Authors

Robert C. Aber, M.D.

Assistant Professor of Medicine, Division of Infectious Diseases, Pennsylvania State University College of Medicine, Hershey

J. Wesley Alexander, M.D., Sc.D.

Professor of Surgery, University of Cincinnati College of Medicine; Attending Surgeon and Director, Transplantation Division, Cincinnati General Hospital; Active Staff and Associate Director of Research, Shriners Burns Hospital, Cincinnati

James R. Allen, M.D., M.P.H.

Chief, National Nosocomial Infections Study, Hospital Infections Branch, Bacterial Diseases Division, Bureau of Epidemiology, Center for Disease Control, U.S. Public Health Service, Atlanta

William A. Altemeier, M.S., M.D.

Professor and Chairman, Department of Surgery, University of Cincinnati College of Medicine; Chairman, Departments of Surgery, Cincinnati General Hospital, Children's Hospital, and Holmes Hospital, Cincinnati

Raymond C. Bartlett, M.D.

Director, Division of Microbiology, Department of Pathology, Hartford Hospital, Hartford, Connecticut

Harry N. Beaty, M.D.

Professor and Chairman, Department of Medicine, The University of Vermont College of Medicine, Burlington

John V. Bennett, M.D.

Director, Bacterial Diseases Division, Bureau of Epidemiology, Center for Disease Control, U.S. Public Health Service, Atlanta

Philip S. Brachman, M.D.

Director, Bureau of Epidemiology, Center for Disease Control, U.S. Public Health Service; Clinical Associate Professor of Preventive Medicine and Community Health, Emory University School of Medicine, Atlanta

John A. Bryan, M.D.

Director, Viral Diseases Division, Bureau of Epidemiology, Center for Disease Control, U.S. Public Health Service, Atlanta

John P. Burke, M.D.

Associate Professor of Medicine, University of Utah College of Medicine; Chief, Infectious Diseases, LDS Hospital, Salt Lake City

Alfred E. Buxton, M.D.

Postdoctoral Fellow, Cardiovascular Section, Department of Medicine, University of Pennsylvania School of Medicine; Fellow in Cardiology, Hospital of the University of Pennsylvania, Philadelphia

Leighton E. Cluff, M.D.

Vice President, The Robert Wood Johnson Foundation, Princeton, New Jersey; Adjunct Professor of Medicine, University of Pennsylvania School of Medicine, Philadelphia

Marie B. Coyle, Ph.D.

Assistant Professor, Departments of Microbiology and Immunology and of Laboratory Medicine, University of Washington School of Medicine; Director, Clinical Microbiology, Harborview Medical Center, Seattle

Richard E. Dixon, M.D.

Chief, Hospital Infections Branch, Bacterial Diseases Division, Bureau of Epidemiology, Center for Disease Control, U.S. Public Health Service; Assistant Clinical Professor of Medicine, Emory University School of Medicine, Atlanta

Herbert L. DuPont, M.D.

Professor and Director, Program in Infectious Diseases and Clinical Microbiology, The University of Texas Medical School at Houston; Professor of Medicine, Hermann Hospital, Houston

Theodore C. Eickhoff, M.D.

Professor of Medicine and Head, Division of Infectious Disease, University of Colorado School of Medicine, Denver; Director, Department of Medicine, Denver General Hospital

William F. Enneking, M.D.

Professor and Chairman, Department of Orthopaedic Surgery, University of Florida College of Medicine, Gainesville

Jorge A. Franco, Ph.D.

Visiting Assistant Professor, Department of Microbiology and Immunology, The Hahneman Medical College and Hospital of Philadelphia; Director of Clinical Microbiology and Immunology, Laboratory Procedures East, Subsidiary of The Upjohn Company, King of Prussia, Pennsylvania

Eugene J. Gangarosa, M.D.

Dean, Faculty of Health Sciences, American University of Beirut, Beirut, Lebanon

Julia S. Garner, R.N., M.N.

Nurse-Epidemiologist, Hospital Infections Branch, Bacterial Diseases Division, Bureau of Epidemiology, Center for Disease Control, U.S. Public Health Service, Atlanta

Donald A. Goldmann, M.D.

Assistant Professor of Pediatrics, Harvard Medical School; Hospital Epidemiologist and Director, Bacteriology Laboratory, Children's Hospital, Boston

Richard A. Kaslow, M.D.

Epidemiologist, Arthritis and Immunologic Diseases Activity, Chronic Diseases Division, Bureau of Epidemiology, Center for Disease Control, U.S. Public Health Service, Atlanta

Calvin M. Kunin, M.D.

Professor of Medicine, University of Wisconsin Medical School; Chief, Medical Service, William S. Middleton Veterans Administration Hospital, Madison

Harold Laufman, M.D., Ph.D.

Professor of Surgery, Albert Einstein College of Medicine of Yeshiva University; Director, Institute for Surgical Studies, Division of the Department of Surgery, Montefiore Hospital and Medical Center, New York

William J. Ledger, M.D.

Professor and Chairman, Department of Obstetrics and Gynecology, Cornell University Medical College; Physician in Charge, Lying In Hospital, New York Hospital, Cornell Medical Center, New York

Bruce G. MacMillan, M.D.

Shrine Professor of Surgery, University of Cincinnati College of Medicine; Chief of Staff, Shriners Burns Institute, Cincinnati

Dennis G. Maki, M.D.

Associate Professor of Medicine, University of Wisconsin Medical School; Chief, Infectious Disease Section, University of Wisconsin Hospitals, Madison

George F. Mallison, M.P.H.

Assistant Director, Bacterial Diseases Division, Bureau of Epidemiology, Center for Disease Control, U.S. Public Health Service, Atlanta

Stanley M. Martin, M.S.

Chief, Statistical Services Branch, Bacterial Diseases Division, Bureau of Epidemiology, Center for Disease Control, U.S. Public Health Service, Atlanta

R. Crawford Morris, LL.B.

Defense Trial Counsel, University Hospital and Mt. Sinai Hospital; General Counsel, Fairview General Hospital; Counsel, Marymount Hospital; A Senior Partner, Arter and Hadden, Attorneys, Cleveland; Member, American Society of Hospital Attorneys, American Medical Association

Thomas K. Oliver, Jr., M.D.

Professor and Chairman, Department of Pediatrics, University of Pittsburgh School of Medicine; Pediatrician-in-Chief, Children's Hospital, Pittsburgh

Kathryn S. Wenzel Owens, R.N.

Former Infection Control Nurse, Stanford University Hospital, Stanford, California

Alan K. Pierce, M.D.

Professor of Medicine, The University of Texas Southwestern Medical School at Dallas; Chief, Pulmonary Disease Division, Parkland Memorial Hospital, Dallas

Jack S. Remington, M.D.

Professor of Medicine, Division of Infectious Diseases, Department of Medicine, Stanford University School of Medicine, Stanford; Chief, Division of Allergy, Immunology, and Infectious Diseases, Palo Alto Medical Research Foundation, Palo Alto, California

Frank S. Rhame, M.D.

Assistant Professor of Medicine and Laboratory Medicine, University of Minnesota School of Medicine; Hospital Epidemiologist, University of Minnesota Hospitals and Clinics, Minneapolis

Jay P. Sanford, M.D.

Dean, School of Medicine, and Professor of Medicine, Uniformed Services University of Health Sciences, Bethesda, Maryland; Attending Physician, Department of Medicine, Walter Reed Army Medical Center and National Naval Medical Center, Washington, D.C.

William Schaffner, M.D.

Associate Professor of Medicine and Preventive Medicine, Vanderbilt University School of Medicine; Hospital Epidemiologist and Director, Clinical Microbiology Laboratory, Vanderbilt University Medical Center, Nashville

John C. Sherris, M.D.

Professor and Chairman, Department of Microbiology and Immunology, University of Washington School of Medicine; Consultant, University Hospital, Seattle

Walter E. Stamm, M.D.

Assistant Professor, Division of Infectious Diseases, Department of Medicine, University of Washington School of Medicine, Harborview Medical Center, Seattle

Allen C. Steere, M.D.

Assistant Professor of Medicine and Epidemiology, Yale University School of Medicine; Hospital Epidemiologist, Yale-New Haven Hospital, New Haven

John E. Swartzberg, M.D.

Assistant Clinical Professor, Department of Medicine, University of California, San Francisco, School of Medicine; Director of Microbiology Control, Alta Bates Hospital, Berkeley

Paul F. Wehrle, M.D.

Hastings Professor of Pediatrics, University of Southern California School of Medicine; Director of Pediatrics, Los Angeles County–USC Medical Center, Los Angeles

Robert A. Weinstein, M.D.

Assistant Professor of Medicine, University of Chicago–Pritzker School of Medicine; Hospital Epidemiologist and Associate Attending Physician, Department of Medicine, Michael Reese Hospital and Medical Center, Chicago

Lowell S. Young, M.D.

Associate Professor of Medicine, University of California School of Medicine, Los Angeles; Associate Attending Physician, U.C.L.A. Center for the Health Sciences, Los Angeles

Stephen R. Zellner, M.D.

Private Practice, Internal Medicine and Infectious Diseases, Fort Myers, Florida

Notice

The indications and dosages of all drugs in this book have been recommended in the medical literature and conform to the practices of the general medical community. The medications described do not necessarily have specific approval by the Food and Drug Administration for use in the diseases and dosages for which they are recommended. The package insert for each drug should be consulted for use and dosage as approved by the FDA. Because standards for usage change, it is advisable to keep abreast of revised recommendations, particularly those concerning new drugs.

I

Basic Considerations of Hospital Infections

1

Introduction
Philip S. Brachman

Nosocomial infections are a major public health problem today not only for patients, but also for each patient's family, community, and state. Indeed, they present a problem for the entire country, because the occurrence of nosocomial infections makes a significant intrusion upon the health dollar, whether from the private or public sector. Estimates based on surveillance and prevalence data are that approximately 5 percent of all patients admitted to hospitals in the United States contract an infection while hospitalized. Since this is an average figure, there are some hospitals with a lower rate, but others have a more serious problem, which can be defined only through an active surveillance program. If a hospital indicates that it has no problem, it is almost a certainty that the staff is not conducting surveillance, and thus they do not have an appreciation of their own nosocomial infection situation. As will be emphasized in this book, some areas of a hospital have more serious problems than other areas, and some patients are at greater risk than others. Nosocomial infections are not limited to the United States; they occur in hospitals throughout the world and would appear to be more prevalent and serious in developing countries. Some countries are actively pursuing a solution to the problem, while others have not yet developed a systematic approach.

The major problem with nosocomial infections is the occurrence of sporadic cases as distinct from epidemics of disease. Epidemics do occur, but it is the endemic cases that reflect the ongoing, day-to-day problems. Not all nosocomial infections are preventable. It is estimated that approximately half of them are infections that will occur despite precautions.

In addition, hospitals should be aware of patients being admitted with community-acquired infections. There are two important points to consider in this regard. First, these cases must be noted upon admission and placed under the appropriate isolation precautions, since they may become the source of transmission of infectious agents, resulting in a nosocomial infection. Second, community-acquired infections can serve as a sentinel surveillance system concerning the occurrence of infections in the community.

In both Part I and Part II of this book, the reader should be aware of the changing nature of nosocomial infections, which reflects changing relationships among the agent, the modes of transmission, and the compromised host. These factors are discussed throughout this book and indicate the dynamic nature of nosocomial infections.

Part I includes discussions of the general background and basic techniques of nosocomial infection control, special problem areas within the hospital, the role of the community, and legal aspects of nosocomial infections. The material covered should help anyone desiring to develop an effective, meaningful, and sensitive nosocomial infection control program in any health-care facility. The authors have been selected because of their personal involvement in infection control programs and their expertise in the subject about which they have written.

Readers are encouraged to consider each of the subjects carefully and adapt the recommendations to meet the needs and specifications of their own nosocomial infection control program. The components of the nosocomial infection control program will be dependent upon the specific needs of the hospital as dictated by its own nosocomial infection problems, the size of the institution, the type of patients admitted, and the number of hospital personnel assigned to the program, as well as the availability of other supporting resources.

Chapter 2 covers the general subject of epidemiology as related to nosocomial infections. Three basic epidemiologic methods are discussed, and their applicability to both surveillance and investigations of nosocomial infections is emphasized. The relationships among the agent, mode of transmission, and the host in the milieu of the hospital environment are outlined; these are the links in the chain of infection.

Hospital employees are constantly—whether knowingly or unknowingly—exposed to infectious agents while working in the hospital. Accordingly, a program designed to provide appropriate protection for them must be enforced. In addition to providing facilities for good personal hygiene, hospitals must develop an effective vaccination program. Another aspect of employee health concerns the employee himself serving as a reservoir or source of infection for the susceptible host. It is important that each employee be reminded of this aspect of nosocomial infections. Employees should be encouraged to report their own illnesses to the hospital personnel health service; thus, if they are a hazard to patients, appropriate measures can be taken to prevent the transmission of infection. The treatment program for such infections must not penalize the employee in any way if it is to be effective.

A hospital's infection control program should be the responsibility of an Infection Control Committee that operates under a mandate from the highest administrative authority in the hospital. Two positions that are critical to this committee's effectively discharging its responsibilities are those of the hospital epidemiologist and the infection control nurse. The latter has the daily responsibility for maintenance of the program.

Probably the single most important aspect of the nosocomial infection control program is surveillance. Without an active and sensitive surveillance program, it is not possible to appreciate fully what the problems are or to develop and maintain appropriate control measures. An active surveillance program must be a cooperative effort among all hospital personnel with the strong backing of the hospital's administration. The amount of time necessary to devote to the infection control program is basically determined by the number of hospital beds. One infection control nurse would be necessary for approximately 250 beds.

Chapter 5 on the investigation of endemic and epidemic infections is a practical summary of the specific activities that need to be carried out in endemic and epidemic investigations. Investigations can be conducted by the infection control nurse with assistance and supervision from the hospital epidemiologist. Additionally, assistance can be requested from local public health authorities. Laboratory support must be available, preferably within the hospital; if such support is not possible, then a local public health laboratory should be contacted. The extent to which nosocomial infections are investigated will depend on the sensitivity of the surveillance system, the concern of the staff, and the resources available. Certainly any unusual occurrence of disease—whether of an unusual type or an unusual number of cases—should be promptly investigated.

In Chapter 6, the attention that should be paid the inanimate environment is stressed. The inanimate environment is involved in nosocomial infections primarily because of its relationship to transmission; however, the environment also influences the agent and the host. Methods of disinfection and sterilization of objects are summarized, and the pros and cons of various methods are discussed. A useful table provides recommended methods of disinfection and sterilization for various objects and materials. Other control measures related to the inanimate environment are summarized. Also discussed are (1) the importance of hospital design, engineering, and maintenance; (2) housekeeping, including sanitation, ventilation, and the critical areas of food handling; and (3) the laundry. Hospitals need to have the services of an engineer and a sanitarian, either full-time or on a consulting basis. The significance of hands in the transmission of infectious agents is discussed, and the need for proper hand-washing is stressed: overall, no single preventive action is as important as proper hand-washing. The concepts of environmental surveillance are placed in the proper perspective. Inappropriate stress is frequently placed on the environment in hospitals, and an excessively elaborate, routine surveillance program may be established; this drains valuable resources from other, more meaningful, nosocomial infection control activities. There are some routine environmental surveillance activities that should be part of the regular program; other activities need to be considered as dictated by the occurrence of nosocomial infections.

The chapter on areas of special concern (Chapter 7) deals with geographic areas within the hospital that demand special attention. Some patient-care areas and some specific service areas play a direct role in the transmission of disease. The hemodialysis unit exposes susceptible patients and personnel to complex equipment that frequently is difficult to decontaminate. The major problem is the transmission of hepatitis B, although outbreaks of hepatitis A and bacterial septicemia also have been reported from this source. Another important area, the intensive-care unit, houses critically ill patients who, by the nature of their underlying disease, are highly susceptible to infection. Additionally, because of the proximity of the patients to one another, the complexity of the equipment, and the need for rapid action related to medical emergencies, aseptic technique recommendations and isolation precautions are frequently abridged. Control of these problems can be approached by considering the physical or structural aspects of the area and the behavioral patterns of the hospital staff working in this area.

The nursery is another area where highly susceptible patients are housed closely together, which increases the ease of transmission of infection. Because of the closeness of bassinets and the need for frequent contact with newborn infants, it is not uncommon for personnel to fail to wash their hands between patient contacts. This creates a mechanism for transmission of infection, which is the main method by which nosocomial infections are transmitted in the newborn nursery. In addition, there have been problems with epidemics of salmonellosis caused by contaminated formula.

Contaminated food can cause nosocomial infections either in susceptible patients or in employees who then may transmit infection to hospitalized patients. The problems related to hospital food services are similar to those found in community food services. The major difference is that the hospitalized susceptible patient is more likely to develop infection following contact with contaminated food than the non-hospitalized individual in contact with the same contaminated food. Preventive measures are directed toward improvements in food-handling techniques. Furthermore, disease surveillance of kitchen personnel is important in order to identify problems at a time when preventive action can be taken.

The central supply department and the laundry are two areas that prepare and handle equipment and supplies, which, if not properly handled, may be contaminated with pathogens that can cause disease when they come in contact with highly susceptible patients. Materials that come from the central supply are assumed to be sterile or disinfected and thus are not further treated. Although linens are usually not sterilized, they should be free of pathogens, which should be removed by the normal laundering process. Additionally, personnel who work in the laundry and handle the dirty laundry must do so with care in order to avoid infecting themselves from the dirty linens.

The pharmacy plays an important role in the prevention of nosocomial infections since the products from the pharmacy are considered to be free of pathogens and are not further processed on the wards. Of special concern are intravenous fluids, especially those that contain additives, which, if not added with care, may allow contamination to enter the fluid. It has been shown that certain organisms, especially gram-negative organisms, may multiply in such fluids to infectious doses. Also, the pharmacy can help the infection committee monitor the use of antimicrobial drugs and should provide pertinent drug information to the hospital staff.

The operating room admits patients who are highly susceptible to infections and who are further compromised by surgery. Because of the nature of surgical procedures and the susceptibility of the surgical patient, environmental factors play a more important role in the surgical suite than in many other areas of the hospital. Personnel activities are also important areas for concern, however, and techniques for hand-washing and patient preparation must be carefully established and monitored.

The outpatient department and admitting department are areas of the hospital not frequently associated with nosocomial infections, but they, too, can be the site of significant problems. Patients who acquire pathogenic organisms while in the hospital but who do not develop overt infection until after discharge may return later to the outpatient department for therapy. Surveillance must be maintained in the outpatient department for such infections, which

should be classified as nosocomial infections. Outpatient infections may also be community-acquired; however, they deserve the same degree of concern as inpatient infections because outpatient infections can be transmitted to other patients and to hospital personnel in the outpatient department. Physicians must be aware that when they have patients who may have a communicable disease, they should notify the admitting department so the patient can immediately be admitted and isolated in order to minimize the potential spread of infection.

The clinical laboratory plays an important role in the control of nosocomial infections by being responsible for identifying pathogens. Such pathogens are primarily from human specimens but at times are from inanimate specimens. Clinical laboratory personnel should be made aware of the risk of becoming infected from the specimens they process, and they should be warned to always use the very best hygienic measures. The clinical laboratory must be informed of the most recent methods of isolating microorganisms and performing diagnostic studies, and it must be able to handle an extra number of specimens related to investigations. If they are unable to perform certain necessary studies, the laboratory personnel must be ready to contact another laboratory to perform them. The clinical laboratory will also be a source of surveillance information; thus, their records must be kept in such a way as to be useful in the surveillance program.

Isolation procedures are frequently the most misunderstood activities in the nosocomial infection control program. In some hospitals, personnel associate isolation with excessively restrictive measures concerning the handling of patients and thus underutilize many isolation procedures. In other institutions, isolation is overemphasized and this is responsible for excessive restriction; in still other hospitals, the manual of isolation is exceedingly complex, and almost every disease has a different set of isolation requirements. Because of these problems, a practical and effective system of isolation has been developed that categorizes diseases in order to limit the number of different types of isolation precautions hospitals need to establish. The system, outlined in Chapter 9, can be adapted to meet the individual needs of any hospital.

The development of a nosocomial infection may trigger legal action against the hospital and its associated medical and nonmedical personnel. Since many such legal actions are settled out of court, there is no accurate accounting of nosocomial infections in which legal action is considered. Enough cases have been reported, however, for guidelines to be set, and these are discussed in Chapter 10.

Overuse of antibiotics is a continuing problem; 25 to 35 percent of hospitalized patients receive systemic antibiotic therapy on any single day. Such treatment not only is expensive, but it may also subject the patient to unnecessary risk. The pressure of excessive use of an antibiotic may be demonstrated by the appearance of bacterial strains resistant to that antibiotic, which may result in specific therapeutic problems. A discussion of some of the general principles of chemotherapy, especially as they relate to nosocomial infections, is included in Chapter 11.

Hospitals are part of the community in which they are located, and thus they need to develop and maintain close relationships with the local public health department. Infections spread from hospital to community as well as from community to hospital. When either event occurs, close cooperation between the two groups is needed. Hospitals do not need to maintain a full staff of all disciplines necessary to fully investigate all epidemics thoroughly. The local, state, or federal health department can provide assistance in the investigation, and should be involved in investigations where commercially distributed foods, drugs, and medical devices are suspect vehicles. One other important area of hospital-community contact is the system of reporting disease. The hospital administration needs to know what diseases are reportable and the mechanism for reporting them. As has been stated, surveillance is the backbone of an effective infection control program; hospital personnel need to support surveillance and report all cases of reportable diseases to the appropriate local authorities.

2

Epidemiology of Nosocomial Infections

Philip S. Brachman

Basic Considerations

This chapter is a review of the basic principles of epidemiology as they relate to nosocomial infections. An understanding of the epidemiology of nosocomial infections is necessary for effective control and prevention measures. One uses epidemiologic methods to define all the factors related to the occurrence of disease, including the relationships among the agent, its reservoir and source, the environment, the route of transmission, and the host. Once all these relationships have been defined for a specific disease, the most appropriate and effective means of control and prevention should become apparent. Without defining each of these relationships, control and prevention efforts are, at best, a gamble. Defining the epidemiologic relationships introduces science into control and prevention and leads to more effective and economical utilization of all resources.

Definitions

EPIDEMIOLOGY. The term *epidemiology* is derived from the Greek *epi* (on or upon), *demos* (people or population), and *logos* (word or reason). Literally, it means the study of things that happen to people; historically, it has involved the study of epidemics. Epidemiology is the dynamic study of the determinants, occurrence, and distribution of health and disease in a population, which—for nosocomial infections—is the hospital population. Epidemiology defines the relationship of disease to the population at risk and involves the determination, analysis, and interpretation of rates. There are many different rates used by epidemiologists; the most common is the attack rate, which is the number of cases of the disease divided by the population at risk. Calculation of other rates helps define the outbreak, for example, calculation of rates among a selected contact group in order to compare with the group in which cases occurred.

INFECTION. *Infection* entails the replication of organisms in the tissues of a host; if this results in overt clinical manifestations, the state is known as *disease;* however, if the infection only provokes an immune response without overt clinical disease, it is referred to as an inapparent or subclinical infection. *Colonization* implies the presence of a microorganism in or on a host with growth and multiplication of the microorganism, but without any overt clinical expression or detected immune reaction at the time it is isolated. *Subclinical* (or *inapparent*) *infection* refers to a relationship between the host and the microorganism in which the microorganism is present; there is no overt expression of the presence of the microorganism, but there is interaction between the host and the microorganism that results in a detectable immune response, such as a serologic reaction. Therefore, special serologic tests may be needed to differentiate colonization from subclinical infection. In the absence of such information, it is customary to employ the term colonization. A *carrier* (or colonized person) is an individual colonized with a specific microorganism and from whom the organism can be recovered (i.e., cultured) but who shows no overt expression of the presence of the microorganism at the time it is isolated; a carrier can have a history of previous disease, such as typhoid. The carrier state may be *transient* (or short-term), *intermittent* (or occasional), or *chronic* (long-term, persistent, or permanent). We have found, for example, in culture studies of hospital staff for nasal carriage of *Staphylococcus aureus,* approximately 15 to 20 percent are noncarriers, 60 to 70 percent are intermittent carriers, and 10 to 15 percent are persistent carriers. Epidemiologically, the important consideration is whether the carrier is the source of the infection for another individual; any carrier who is disseminating or shedding the organism may subsequently infect another person. Also, the carrier may develop disease with the source of the organism being him- or herself.

DISSEMINATION. *Dissemination* or shedding of microorganisms refers to the movement of organisms from an individual carrying the organism into the immediate environment. To show this, one samples and cultures samples of air or surfaces and objects onto which microorganisms from the carrier may have been deposited. Shedding studies may be conducted in specially constructed chambers designed to quantitate dissemination. While shedding studies have occasionally been useful to document unusual dissemination, they have not been useful in identifying carriers whose dissemination has resulted in infection in other individuals. In the hospital setting, dissemination is most efficiently identified by noting the occurrence of infection among previous contacts as compared to new contacts. When infection is shown to result from dissemination of organisms from a person, the latter is known as a "dangerous disseminator."

The demonstration by culturing techniques that an individual is carrying a certain organism defines a potential problem, whereas epidemiologic demonstration by surveillance and investigative techniques defines the real problem. In some hospitals, routine culture surveys of all or selected asymptomatic staff may be conducted in an attempt to identify carriers of certain organisms, but such surveys lack practical relevance unless the results are related to specific cases or an outbreak of disease. This practice only identifies those who are culture-positive and does not in itself reliably separate colonized persons into disseminators as distinct from other colonized persons. Usually only a fraction of colonized persons are actually disseminating, and thus they are not associated with the actual spread of disease. Furthermore, dissemination may occur without disease developing in the contacts. If disease transmission has occurred and a human source of infection is suspected, culture surveys in conjunction with epidemiologic investigation to identify the potential source are realistic, and further laboratory study to confirm the presence of a dangerous disseminator may then be undertaken. Thus, culture surveys and microbiologic studies of dissemination in the absence of disease problems are usually inappropriate and wasteful of resources.

In some instances, dissemination from a carrier has been reported to be influenced by the occurrence of an unrelated disease such as a second infection. One report, for example, suggested that infants carrying staphylococci in their nares disseminate staphylococci only after the onset of a viral respiratory infection. Such infants are called "cloud babies" (see Part I, Chapter 5). In another instance, a physician disseminated staphylococci from his skin because of a reactivation of chronic dermatitis. Desquamation of his skin led to the transmission of staphylococci to patients with whom he had contact. Dissemination has been reported of tetracycline-resistant *Staphylococcus aureus* from individuals carrying this organism who were treated with tetracycline. Dissemination may be constant or sporadic. If sporadic, it may result from the intermittent occurrence of some precipitating event, such as a second infection, or it may be due to other, unknown factors. The risk of dissemination is generally greater from individuals with disease caused by that organism than from individuals with subclinical infection or who are colonized with the organism.

Contamination refers to microorganisms that are transiently present on a body surface (such as hands) without tissue invasion or physiologic reaction. Contamination also refers to the presence of microorganisms on or in an inanimate object.

NOSOCOMIAL INFECTIONS. *Nosocomial infections* are those infections that develop within a hospital or are produced by microorganisms acquired during hospitalization (e.g., serum hepatitis). Nosocomial infections may involve not only patients, but also anyone else who has contact with a hospital, including members of the staff, volunteers, visitors, workmen, salesmen, and delivery personnel. The majority of nosocomial infections in patients become clinically apparent while they are still hospitalized; however, the onset of disease can occur after a patient has been discharged. As many as 25 percent of postoperative wound infections, for example, begin to show symptoms after the patient has been discharged. In these cases, the patient became colonized or infected while in the hospital, but the incubation period was longer than the patient's hospital stay. This is seen in some infections of newborns and in most breast abscesses of new mothers. Hepatitis B is another example of a nosocomial disease with a long incubation period; its clinical onset usually occurs long after the patient is discharged from the hospital.

Infections incubating at the time of the patient's admission to the hospital are not nosocomial; they are community-acquired, unless, of course, they resulted from a previous hospitalization. Community-acquired infections can serve as a ready source of infection for other patients or personnel and thus must be considered in the total scope of nosocomial infections.

The term *preventable infection* implies that some event related to the infection could have been altered (given the present state of the preventive arts), and such alteration would have prevented the infection from occurring. A medical attendant who does not wash his or her hands between contacts with the urinary collection equipment of two patients, for example, may transmit gram-negative organisms from the first patient to the second patient, which may result in a urinary tract infection. Handwashing might have prevented this infection from occurring. The identification of such an event in retrospect, however, is likely to be impossible and, at best, difficult to distinguish from circumstances where both patients developed infections from their own autogenous flora (e.g., from *Escherichia coli*). It is often impossible to identify the precise mode of acquisition of individual nosocomial infections. More than one mode may contribute to the development of the same infection, and not all modes may be preventable.

A *nonpreventable infection* will occur despite all possible precautions; for example, infection in an immunosuppressed patient due to his or her own flora may not be preventable, no matter what precautions are taken. It has been estimated that as many as half of all reported nosocomial infections are preventable. Common-source outbreaks are potentially preventable, and, given ideal circumstances, many infections caused by flora acquired during hospitalization are preventable by prevention of nosocomial acquisition or avoidance of predisposing procedures in those who have acquired nosocomial strains. Prompt investigation and the institution of rational control measures should reduce the number of cases involved in outbreaks. The consistent application of recognized, effective control measures for endemic infections is probably the single most important factor at present in reducing the overall level of nosocomial infections.

SOURCE: ENDOGENOUS (OR AUTOGENOUS), EXOGENOUS. Organisms that cause nosocomial infections come from either endogenous (autogenous) or exogenous sources. *Endogenous* infections are caused by the patient's own flora; *exogenous* infections result from transmission of organisms from a source other than the patient. Either endogenous organisms are brought into the hospital by a patient (this represents colonization outside the hospital), or the patient becomes colonized after being admitted to the hospital. In either instance, the organisms colonizing the patient may become the cause of a nosocomial infection. It may not always be possible to determine whether a particular organism isolated from the patient with an infection caused by that organism is exogenous or endogenous, and the term "autogenous" should be used in this situation. *Autogenous* infection indicates that the infection was derived from the flora of the patient, whether or not the infecting organism became part of the patient's flora subsequent to admission. Information about current disease problems in the community or in hospital contacts may be useful in differentiating the two sources. Microbiologic determinations of the characteristics of the organism—such as phage typing, antibiograms, or biochemical reactions—may help identify strains of nosocomial origin.

SPECTRUM OF OCCURRENCE OF CASES. To determine whether a nosocomial infection problem exists in a particular hospital, one must relate the current frequency of cases to the past history of the disease in that institution. To characterize a disease's frequency as sporadic, endemic, or epidemic, investigators must know something of the past occurrence of that disease in relation to time, place, and person. *Sporadic* means that cases occur occasionally and irregularly, without any specific pattern. *Endemic* means that the disease occurs with ongoing frequency in a specific geographic area in a finite population and a defined time period. *Hyperendemic* refers to what appears to be a gradual increase in the occurrence of a disease in a defined area beyond the expected number

of cases; however, it may not be certain whether the disease will occur at epidemic proportions. An *epidemic* is a definite increase in the incidence of a disease above its expected endemic occurrence. *Outbreak* is used interchangeably with epidemic; however, some people use outbreak to mean an increased rate of occurrence, but not at levels as serious as an epidemic (see Part I, Chapter 4).

An occasional gas gangrene infection among postoperative patients is an example of a sporadic infection. An endemic nosocomial infection is represented by the regular occurrence of infections—either in a particular site or at different sites—which are due to the same organism, occur at a nearly constant rate, and are generally considered by the hospital to be within "expected and acceptable" limits. Surgical wound infections due to a single organism that follow operations classified as "contaminated surgery," for example, could represent the endemic level of postoperative wound infections.

An epidemic classically begins with a sudden increase in the occurrence of disease among susceptible individuals who have had contact with a contaminated source, but the onset of disease occurs at an unusually high frequency relative to that expected. On the other hand, an epidemic may also result from prolonged exposure to the source of the organism. Cases of salmonellosis, for example, may result from contact with a contaminated food that patients and staff are exposed to over a long period of time, possibly months before it is identified. Only an occasional case of salmonellosis may result from this exposure, but, depending on the past history of salmonellosis in this institution, these cases may represent "epidemic" salmonellosis. The prolonged epidemic pattern may represent intermittent exposure or variable host susceptibility, with only an occasional host becoming infected.

A characteristic sharp and abrupt increase in the number of cases may fail to occur with diseases having a long and variable incubation period. Many people may be exposed to hepatitis B, for example, at one particular time, but the appearance of the resulting disease may be spread out over several weeks, thereby obscuring the presence of an epidemic.

INCIDENCE AND PREVALENCE. Occurrence of infection is quantified by calculating its incidence and prevalence. *Incidence* is the number of new cases in a specific population in a defined time period. In order to determine the true incidence of a disease, culture or serologic surveys may be necessary. *Prevalence* is the total number of current cases of an infection in a defined population at one point in time (point prevalence) or over a longer period of time (period prevalence). The prevalence rate will include cases of recent onset as well as those cases of earlier onset that are still clinically apparent (see Part I, Chapter 4).

Epidemiologic Methods

There are generally three techniques used in epidemiologic studies—descriptive, analytic, and experimental—all of which may be used in investigating nosocomial infections. Additionally, the principles involved in these methods have application to surveillance; surveillance data are commonly analyzed by the descriptive method, and such analysis may suggest the need for analytic studies to identify certain features of a disease. Furthermore, analysis of surveillance data may lead to the development of experimental studies to deal with a specific disease.

Descriptive Epidemiology

The basic epidemiologic method, descriptive epidemiology, is used in most investigations. Once the initial problem has been defined, however, additional studies using one of the other two methods can be conducted in order to develop more information about the occurrence of the epidemic, to confirm initial impressions, to prove and disprove hypotheses, and to evaluate the effectiveness of control measures, prevention measures, or both.

Descriptive epidemiology describes the occurrence of disease in terms of time, place, and person; each case of a disease is first characterized by describing these three attibutes (see Part I, Chapter 5). When data from the individual cases are combined and analyzed, the parameters of the epidemic or disease problem should be characterized.

TIME. There are four time trends to consider: secular, periodic, seasonal, and acute. *Secular* trends are long-term trends in the occurrence of a disease, that is, variations that occur over a period of years. The gradual but steady reduction in the incidence of diphtheria in the United States over the past 50 years, for example, is the secular trend of that disease. This downward trend generally reflects the rising immunity and improved socioeconomic and nutritional levels of the overall population. *Periodic* trends are temporal interruptions of the general secular trend. The upsurge in influenza A activity every two to three years, for instance, portrays the periodic trend of this disease and is generally the result of antigenic drift.

Seasonal trends are the annual variations in disease incidence that are related in part to seasons. In general, the occurrence of a particular communicable disease increases when the circumstances that influence its transmission are favorable. The seasonal pattern of both community-acquired and nosocomial respiratory disease, for example, is high in the fall and winter months, when transmission is enhanced because people are together in rooms with closed windows and are breathing unfiltered, recirculating air. Thus, they have greater contact with each other and with droplets as well as with droplet nuclei. There may also be agent and host factors that influence the seasonal trends. The seasonal trend of foodborne disease is manifested by its higher incidence in the summer months when ambient temperatures are elevated. Foods contaminated with non-disease-producing levels of microorganisms may be allowed to incubate, resulting in the attainment of infectious doses. There are undoubtedly other influencing factors, such as the increased frequency of picnics, the greater need for refrigeration (which is not always adequate to keep foods at the proper temperature), and the like.

The fourth type of time variation is the *acute* or epidemic occurrence of a disease with its characteristic upsurge in incidence. The overall shape of the epidemic curve depends on the interaction of many factors: the characteristics of the specific agent; its pathogenicity, concentration, and incubation period; the mode and ease of its transmission; host factors, including the susceptibility and concentration of susceptible individuals; and environmental factors, such as temperature, humidity, movement of air, and general housekeeping.

An epidemic can be portrayed by an *epidemic curve,* that is, a graphic representation of the occurrence of the number of cases of the disease plotted against time. The time scale will vary according to the incubation or latency period, ranging from minutes, as in an outbreak of disease following exposure to a toxin or a chemical, to months, as in a nosocomial epidemic of hepatitis B. The time scale (abscissa or horizontal scale) should be selected with three facts in mind: (1) The unit time interval should be equal to or less than the average incubation period so the true epidemic curve will be apparent (i.e., so all the cases will not be bunched together); (2) the scale should be carried out far enough in time to allow all cases to be plotted; and (3) any cases that occurred before the epidemic should be plotted in order to give a basis for comparison with the epidemic experience.

If the epidemic curve starts with the *index case* (i.e., the first case in the outbreak), the time between the index case and onset of the next case is the *incubation period* if transmission was from the index case directly to the next case, that is, from person to person. The upslope in the curve is determined by the incubation period, the number and concentration of exposed susceptible persons, and the ease of transmission. The height of the peak of the curve is influenced by the total number of cases. The downslope of the curve is usually more gradual than the upslope; its gradual change reflects cases with longer incubation periods and the decreasing number of susceptible individuals. Cases resulting from *secondary transmission*—that is, resulting from contact with earlier cases in the epidemic—will also be represented on the downslope of the epidemic curve or, occasionally, by a second upswing, which reflects a second, distinct, and usually smaller "wave" of disease following the main outbreak. Consecutive waves of disease may represent ongoing transmission from new fo-

cuses or from one focus that is intermittently or periodically infective or from which organisms are periodically disseminated. In a common-vehicle epidemic, the epidemic curve usually rises rather sharply and then gradually falls off. In a contact-spread epidemic (person-to-person), the epidemic curve usually rises gradually, has a flatter peak than the common-vehicle curve, and then falls off.

The components of descriptive epidemiology (time, place, and person) may obviously be related to disease because of the influence or association with other factors. It is important to remember that disease causation is multifactorial.

PLACE. The second feature of descriptive epidemiology is place, that is, the geographic area where contact between the agent and the susceptible host occurs. In the hospital setting, "place" refers to the ward, surgical-care unit, operating room, or other area where the infection occurred. In an outbreak of postoperative wound infections due to the same organism, for example, a common source of infection would be suspected. A careful review of each involved patient's hospital location during the proposed incubation period should result in identifying the place where the infection occurred. Knowing something about the place may help determine where control measures can be applied most effectively. If one is dealing with a food-borne disease outbreak in a hospital, for instance, knowing where the food became contaminated—whether it was contaminated before being brought into the hospital, in the hospital kitchen, or on a ward before being served—is of prime importance in developing appropriate control measures. If the source of contamination is in the kitchen, changing the supply of the food for the hospital will not control subsequent outbreaks due to the same source.

In an epidemiologic investigation, the place of actual contact between the patient and the microorganism is the important geographic factor; of secondary importance (though important for control purposes) is where the patient is when the infection becomes clinically apparent. This point is emphasized in considering the frequent movement of patients between services and clinics. Thus, the location of the patient at the time of onset of disease may be different from the place where the infection was acquired. A careful chronologic tabulation of the location(s) of cases within the hospital is necessary for a successful investigation. In one outbreak of salmonellosis among hospitalized patients, the source of infection was the radiology department, where barium used for gastrointestinal tract roentgenographic examinations was contaminated with *Salmonella*. The patients infected by having contact with the barium were scattered throughout the hospital at the time of onset of the gastroenteritis and could have served as separate focuses for additional cases. The place of acquisition of the initial infection provided the important descriptive epidemiologic information necessary for establishing control of this outbreak.

Another aspect of place relates to the location where a common vehicle became contaminated. In an outbreak of septicemia associated with intravenous fluid, for example, it is important to determine whether the fluid became contaminated in the process of manufacture (*intrinsic* contamination) or after the fluid had been bottled (*extrinsic* contamination). Extrinsic contamination can occur during shipment to the hospital, after being brought into the hospital, while being prepared for use, or during actual use.

PERSON. The third major component of descriptive epidemiology is the persons involved. Careful evaluation of host factors related to the individual person includes consideration of age, sex, race, immunization status, and presence of underlying disease that may influence susceptibility (acute or chronic), therapeutic or diagnostic procedures, medications, and nutritional status (see Part I, Chapter 5). In essence, all host factors that can influence the development of the disease being investigated must be considered and described.

Age sometimes influences the occurrence of diseases and also provides a clue regarding the cause of an outbreak. Persons at either end of the age spectrum—the young and the elderly—are generally more susceptible to disease. Such susceptibility may reflect levels of immunity, both active and passive, as well as the level of less specific personal factors of protection

against development of disease. Age can also be an important clue to the source of an outbreak of disease. If, in an apparent common-source outbreak, for example, all ages from infancy to old age are involved, then the source of the outbreak must have been available to patients scattered through at least several wards. On the other hand, if all the patients involved in an epidemic are women in the childbearing ages, then in attempting to identify the place where the exposure took place, the investigation can be narrowed to the obstetric ward, though it may also be necessary to consider the gynecologic ward.

Consideration of therapeutic procedures is of similar importance. If all patients who developed bacteremia due to the same organism have received intravenous-fluid therapy, then a common source of intravenous fluids would be suspected as the cause of the outbreak.

Thus, the description of individual host factors among the involved patients may point to important information that may lead to a solution of the epidemic problem.

Analytic Epidemiology
The second method of epidemiologic investigation is *analytic epidemiology,* in which the determinants of disease distribution are evaluated in terms of possible causal relationships. Two basic methods are used: case-control and cohort studies. In both instances, relationships between cause and effect are analyzed: the *case-control* method starts with the effect and searches for the cause; the *cohort* method starts with the cause and evaluates the effect. The case-control and cohort methods have also been referred to as retrospective and prospective studies, respectively; both methods, however, can be either retrospective or prospective. These terms indicate the temporal frame of reference for the collection of specific data: in a *retrospective* study, data is collected after the event has occurred; in a *prospective* study, the data is collected as the event occurs.

CASE-CONTROL STUDY. The case-control method starts with an allocation of persons between a study group (those already affected with the disease) and a comparison-control group or groups (see Part I, Chapter 5). Any differences between these groups are then determined. In an outbreak of nosocomial urinary tract infections due to *Proteus rettgeri,* for example, a group of patients with this infection was compared to a group that did not have urinary tract infection due to *P. rettgeri.* It was shown that the infected patients were more likely than the comparison group to have had indwelling urinary tract catheters, to have been located in the same area of the hospital, and to have previously received systemic antibiotic therapy. Thus, it was concluded that in this epidemic, indwelling urethral catheters, proximity of patients to one another, and previous systemic antibiotic therapy were directly related to the subsequent development of urinary tract infections due to *P. rettgeri.*

The case-control approach has the advantages of being inexpensive, relatively quick, and easily reproducible. It is used most often in acute disease investigations, since the epidemiologist arrives after a problem is recognized and often after the peak of the epidemic has passed. This approach, however, may introduce bias into the selection of the control group since it may be difficult to retrospectively reconstruct the involved and noninvolved populations. In selecting a comparison-control group, bias may be introduced if one is unable to exclude patients who are asymptomatically infected with the causative agent being studied. A lesser problem but a real one is ascertaining in retrospect that a patient actually had disease, rather than was asymptomatically infected or colonized. This latter circumstance presents considerable difficulty in categorizing critically ill patients with manifestations that resemble those of infection but that stem from other causes. Fortunately, the search for sources can be pursued by including all culture-positive persons in the case definition, and thus it need not be restricted to those with clinical disease. This approach does, however, jeopardize the search for important host factors related to disease occurrence. Another limitation is the memory of the involved patients for past events, the specification of which may be important to the investigation. Also, the hospital records may lack documentation of events important to the investigation. These limitations derive from the

retrospective approach rather than deficiencies in the case-control approach per se. Indeed, prospective case-control studies can be implemented, but usually they have little utility in outbreak investigations.

COHORT STUDY. In the cohort method, patients exposed to a "cause" are compared with a group not exposed to the cause to see what the effect will be. In the above outbreak of *P. rettgeri* urinary tract infections, for example, the importance of the proximity of patients with catheters—an infectious risk—was prospectively analyzed by scattering certain patients with urethral catheters throughout the hospital. Inhibition of the nosocomial spread of infection was demonstrated by this cohort approach.

The advantage of the cohort study is that it provides a direct estimate of the risk of a particular factor on disease occurrence, and this is relatively easy to accomplish when the incubation period is short. Although bias may still be a problem, it is less likely to be introduced in this type of a study which usually is conducted prospectively. The cohort study, however, is usually more difficult, more expensive, and more time-consuming than retrospective studies. For diseases with long incubation periods, the difficulties may be insurmountable. An example of a prospective cohort study is one in which a cohort of patients who received blood transfusions over a specific period of time is followed to see which ones develop hepatitis B. A retrospective cohort study would involve studying a cohort of patients who developed hepatitis to see which ones received blood transfusions within the past six months.

Experimental Epidemiology

The third method of epidemiologic investigation is the experimental method, which is used to test hypotheses and is a definitive method of proving or disproving a hypothesis. The *experimental* method assumes that causes are followed by effects and that a deliberate manipulation of the cause is predictably followed by an alteration in the effect that could rarely be explained by chance alteration of the effect. The two groups selected for study are similar in all respects except for the presence of the study factor in one group. Either the case-control or the cohort method is used to evaluate the interaction between the cause and the effect.

An example of the experimental method is the evaluation of a new drug as treatment for a disease: a group of patients with the disease is randomly divided into two subgroups that are equal in all respects, except one of the subgroups is treated with the drug and the other subgroup (the control group) is given a placebo. If there were no other variation between the two groups, then any difference in the course of the disease in the treated group compared with the control group would be ascribed to the use of the drug.

The experimental method has less direct use in the investigation of outbreaks of nosocomial disease today than the other two methods. This method, however, does have usefulness in assessing general patient-care practices and in evaluating new methods to control and prevent epidemics as long as the patient is not at any increased health risk. It has less use in therapeutic studies, because of the need for informed consent and the need to prevent placing the patient at an unjustified or greater risk in attempting to conduct a specific study.

Chain of Infection

General Aspects

Infection results from the interaction between an infectious agent and a susceptible host. This interaction—called *transmission*—occurs by means of contact between the agent and the host. Three interrelated factors—the agent, transmission, and the host—represent the *chain of infection.*

The links interrelate in the milieu of and are affected by the environment; this relationship is referred to as the *ecology of infection,* that is, the relationship of microorganisms to disease as affected by the factors of their environment. In attempting to control nosocomial infections, an attack upon the chain of infection at its weakest link is generally the most effective procedure. With knowledge of the links in the chain of infection for each nosocomial infection, future trends of the disease should be predictable, and it should be possible to develop the most

effective control and prevention techniques. Defining the chain of infection leads to specific action, in contrast to the incorporation of nonspecific actions in an attempt to control a nosocomial infection problem.

Agent

The first link in the chain of infection is the microbial agent, whether it be a bacterium, virus, fungus, parasite, or rickettsia. The majority of nosocomial infection problems are caused by bacteria and viruses; funguses occasionally and parasites rarely cause nosocomial infections.

PATHOGENICITY. The measure of the ability of microorganisms to induce disease is referred to as *pathogenicity,* and it may be assessed by disease–colonization ratios. One organism with high pathogenicity is *Yersinia pestis;* it almost always causes clinical disease in a host. An organism with low pathogenicity is α-hemolytic streptococcus; it commonly colonizes in humans but only rarely causes clinical disease. The pathogenicity of an organism is further described by characterizing the organism's virulence and invasiveness.

Virulence is the measure of the severity of the disease. In epidemiologic studies, virulence is defined more specifically by assessing morbidity and mortality rates and the degree of communicability. The virulence of organisms ranges from slight to highly virulent. Although some organisms are described as avirulent, it appears that any organism can cause disease in a highly susceptible host. It may be possible to reduce virulence by a deliberate manipulation of the organism, for example, by repeated subculturing on a specific medium or by exposure to a certain drug or to radiation. Purposeful attempts to develop "avirulent" strains have been related to efforts to develop a microbial strain for vaccination purposes, such as the attenuated poliomyelitis virus used for oral vaccination. Under certain host-factor conditions, however, clinical poliomyelitis can result from oral "vaccination" with the attenuated strain. Some naturally occurring organisms have been considered avirulent or of low virulence; however, under certain conditions—such as high doses, reduced or defective host resistance, or both—

disease has resulted from contact with these organisms. For years, *Serratia marcescens,* for example, was considered to be an avirulent organism; because of this and because certain strains have easily recognizable red pigment, these organisms were used for environmental studies in hospitals. As more and more nosocomial disease due to *S. marcescens* organisms subsequently became recognized and reported, however, it became apparent that this organism could cause disease in individuals with compromised defense systems as well as in other patients. Thus, avirulence is a relative term; whether an organism is "avirulent" depends upon host factors such as susceptibility, agent factors such as dose, and other characteristics of the agent that influence the occurrence of disease.

Invasiveness describes the ability of microorganisms to invade tissues. Some organisms can penetrate the intact integument, whereas other microorganisms can enter only through a break in the skin or mucous membranes. An example of the former is *Leptospira* and of the latter *Clostridium tetani. Vibrio cholerae* organisms are noninvasive; once in the gastrointestinal tract, they do not invade the endothelium; rather, they elaborate a toxin that reacts with the mucosal tissue and causes diarrhea. *Shigella* organisms are highly invasive and cause a symptomatic response by invading the submucosal tissue.

DOSE. Another important "agent" factor in the chain of infection is *dose:* that is, the number of organisms available to cause infection. The *infective dose* of an agent is that quantity of the agent necessary to cause infection. The number of organisms necessary to cause infection varies from organism to organism and from host to host, and it will be influenced by the mode of transmission. The relationship of dose to the onset of typhoid fever, for example, was shown in volunteer studies by Hornick [2], who demonstrated that with an inoculum of 10^3 *Salmonella typhosa,* no clinical disease developed in normal volunteers. However, when the inoculum was increased to 10^7 salmonellae, there was a 50 percent attack rate among the volunteers, and with an inoculum of 10^9 organisms, there was a 95 percent attack rate.

SPECIFICITY. Microorganisms may be specific with respect to their range of hosts. St. Louis encephalitis virus, for example, has a broad range of hosts, including many avian species, mammals, and mosquitoes. On the other hand, *Rickettsia prowazekii,* the species that causes typhus, has a very narrow host range, involving body lice and man. *Brucella abortus* is highly communicable in cattle but not in man. Some *Salmonella* species, such as *S. typhimurium,* are common to both animals and man, but others have a narrow range of specificity; for example, *S. dublin* primarily infects bovines, and *S. typhosa* is known to infect only man.

OTHER AGENT FACTORS. Other characteristics of the organism, such as the production of enzymes, are directed toward overcoming the defense mechanisms of the host. The streptococci, for example, produce leukocidin, hemolysin, and proteinase, all of which are directed toward overcoming humoral and tissue defense mechanisms of the host.

Certain antigenic variations within species of microorganisms influence the disease-producing potential of the organism. Of the 83 different pneumococcal serotypes, for instance, 14 cause over 80 percent of human pneumococcal pneumonia infections. Among streptococci, group A organisms are associated with infections of the pharynx, whereas group B organisms are primarily associated with infections of the genitourinary tract.

The antigenic makeup of an organism may change, allowing a new variant to spread through a population because of the lack of host resistance to the new variant. This is seen with influenza A; every two to three years, a modified variant becomes prevalent and spreads throughout the country. This phenomenon is known as *antigenic drift.* More significant changes in influenza A occur every seven to ten years (e.g., Asian strain, 1958–59; Hong Kong strain, 1968–69; Victoria strain, 1975–76); these changes are known as *major antigenic shifts.*

Resistance-transfer plasmids also influence the occurrence of nosocomial disease. The transfer of R plasmids from one enteric organism to another has occurred in hospital outbreaks and may account for a change in the antibiotic sensitivity of a strain. The antibiotic sensitivity of "hospital organisms" is also influenced by the use of antibiotics in the hospital; more resistant strains are selected as a result of the increased use of a particular antibiotic (or antibiotics) against which specific resistance plasmids are commonly carried by prevalent nosocomial strains. If a common R-plasmid-mediated resistance pattern of *Escherichia coli* in a hospital is ampicillin, tetracycline, sulfonamide, for example, then the pressures deriving from the use of any one of these drugs will concurrently select for strains with the other two resistances as well. This change in antibiotic sensitivity may make therapy difficult; it can result in an increasing prevalence of the resistant strain, reduce the infecting or colonizing doses of the organism in those receiving drugs to which these strains are resistant, increase the numbers of organisms disseminated from persons colonized with these strains, and subsequently cause a greater frequency of nosocomial infections due to this more resistant strain.

Other organism factors, some plasmid-mediated, include the ability to adhere to intestinal mucosa, to resist gastric acid and disinfectants, and to produce bacteriocins active against endogenous flora.

RESERVOIR AND SOURCE. All organisms have a reservoir and a source; these may be the same or different, and both are important to identify if an organism is associated with an actual or a potential nosocomial infection problem. The *reservoir* is where the organism maintains its presence, metabolizes, and replicates. Viruses generally survive better in human reservoirs; the reservoir of gram-positive bacteria is usually a human, whereas gram-negative bacteria may have either a human reservoir (or animal, e.g., in the case of *Salmonella*) or an inanimate reservoir (e.g., *Pseudomonas* in water). The reservoir may be quite specific: for poliomyelitis virus, for example, the reservoir is always human. On the other hand, *Pseudomonas* species may be found in either an animate or an inanimate reservoir.

The *source* is the place from which the infectious agent passes to the host, either by direct contact or by indirect contact through a vehicle as the means of transmission. The reservoir and the source may be the same location, or the source may become contaminated from the reservoir; either may be animate or inanimate. For example, a reservoir for *Pseudomonas* organisms may be the tap water in a hospital; however, the source from which it is transmitted to the patient may be a humidifier that has been filled directly with the contaminated tap water. In a common-source outbreak of measles, the reservoir and the source may be the same individual.

The source may be mobile or fixed. A susceptible patient may be brought to a fixed source (e.g., a patient who comes to use a contaminated whirlpool bath), or the source may be mobile and brought to the patient (e.g., contaminated food brought from the kitchen to the patient's bedside).

PERIOD OF INFECTIVITY. *Infectivity* refers to the ability of an organism to spread from a source to a host. An infected human may be infective during the incubation period, the clinical disease state, or convalescence. Additionally, an asymptomatic carrier may be infective but not show evidence of clinical disease at the time. Colonized persons may also be infectious for others. An example of a disease that is primarily infectious during the incubation period is hepatitis A: the infected individual is infective during the latter half of the incubation period and during the first several days of clinical disease. In measles, the patient is infective during the prodromal stage to approximately four days after the onset of the rash. In chickenpox, the individual is infective from approximately five days prior to the skin eruption to not more than six days after the appearance of the eruption. A disease in which the individual is infective primarily during the initial clinical-disease phase is exemplified by influenza, where the individual is infective for a period of several days after the onset of symptoms. In cases of tuberculosis and typhoid fever, the individual may be infective for essentially the entire pretreatment clinical phase, with infectivity usually significantly decreasing when there is clinical evidence of successful chemotherapy. Examples of diseases that are infectious into the convalescent period are salmonellosis, shigellosis, and diphtheria. In some diseases, such as typhoid fever and hepatitis B, a chronic carrier state may develop in which the individual may be infective for a long time, possibly years, while showing no symptoms of illness. In spite of these examples, the microorganisms that most commonly cause nosocomial infections—such as *E. coli, Klebsiella, Enterobacter,* and *Pseudomonas*—do not demonstrate the same patterns of infectivity or evoke the protective immune responses that the diseases mentioned above do (i.e., typhoid fever and hepatitis B).

Asymptomatic or subclinical carriers may also be infective for brief periods and continue to be the source of infection for susceptible individuals for long periods. This is seen, for example, in poliomyelitis and hepatitis A. In poliomyelitis, the ratio is approximately 100 carriers to one clinical case, and in hepatitis, ten to one. In spite of not showing clinical evidence of infection, the person with a subclinical infection may be an active transmitter of infection, and clinical disease may result from such transmission. Dissemination from an asymptomatic carrier may be related to a specific event, such as the occurrence of a second disease process (see previous discussion). However, dissemination may also occur that is unrelated to any definable event. The staphylococcus carrier provides a classic example of the asymptomatic dissemination of infectious organisms; in this case, the site of dissemination may be the anterior nares or, at times, the skin. Similarly, the site of asymptomatic streptococcal carriage may be in the pharynx, perianal area, or vagina.

The source of an infection may be an atypical case of a specific disease whose clinical course has been modified either by therapy, by vaccine (as in measles), or by prophylaxis (such as the use of immune serum globulin in hepatitis A). Also, the source may be an abortive case of disease in which the typical expression of the disease has been modified by treatment with antibiotics.

Animals may also provide a source of infection, although this is of less concern in the hospital setting.

EXIT. The portal of exit for organisms from humans is usually single, though it may be multiple. It may not always be the obvious portal of exit; in smallpox, where the crusts are the most visible concern, exit from the oral cavity by the airborne route is also of great importance in the transmission of the virus. The major portals of exit are the respiratory, gastrointestinal, and genitourinary tracts as well as the skin and wounds. Blood may also be the portal of exit, as in hepatitis B infections.

Transmission
Transmission, the second link in the chain of infection, describes the movement of organisms from the source to the host. Spread may occur through one or more of four different routes: contact, common-vehicle, airborne, or vectorborne. An organism may have a single route of transmission, or it may be transmissible by two or more routes. Tuberculosis, for example, is almost always transmitted by the airborne route; measles is primarily a contact-spread disease but may also be transmitted through the air; salmonellae may be transmitted by contact or by the common-vehicle or airborne routes. Thus, in defining the route of transmission, although one route may be the obvious one involved in a nosocomial infection problem, another route may also be operative. Knowledge regarding the route of transmission for a specific disease can be very helpful in the investigation of a nosocomial infection problem. Such information can point to the source and may allow control measures to be introduced more rapidly.

CONTACT SPREAD. In contact-spread disease, the victim has contact with the source, and that contact is either direct, indirect, or by droplets. *Direct contact,* of which person-to-person spread is an example, occurs when there is actual physical contact between the source and the victim, such as in the fecal-oral spread of hepatitis A virus. Infections resulting from organisms within the patient may be referred to as *autogenous infections;* that is, the mode of acquisition is autogenous, even though transmission occurred earlier, namely, at the time when the host became colonized with the organism. A postoperative cholecystectomy wound infection due to coliform organisms from the patient's own gallbladder, for instance, would represent an autogenous contact infection.

Indirect contact refers to a situation in which the victim comes in contact with a contaminated intermediate object (usually inanimate) from which there is transfer of an infectious agent that results in an infection. The intermediate object may become contaminated from an animate or an inanimate source. Indirect-contact transmission is distinguished from direct-contact transmission by the participation of an intermediate object that is passively involved in the transmission of the infectious agent from the source to the victim. An example is the transfer to susceptible hosts of enteric organisms on an endoscope that initially became contaminated when brought in contact with one patient (the index patient) who was infected with the organism.

Droplet spread refers to the brief passage of the infectious agent through the air when the source and the victim are relatively near each other, usually within several feet, such as when there is transmission by talking or sneezing. Droplets are large particles that rapidly settle out on horizontal surfaces; thus they are not transmitted beyond a radius of several feet from the source. Examples of droplet-spread infections include measles and streptococcal pharyngitis.

COMMON-VEHICLE SPREAD. In *common-vehicle* spread infection, a contaminated inanimate vehicle serves as the vector for transmission of the agent to multiple persons. The victims become infected after contact with the common vehicle. This contact may be direct or indirect. Direct-contact spread is exemplified by salmonellosis when the organism actually replicates in the food. Indirect-contact spread is exemplified by hepatitis A transmission through infected food when the organism did not replicate in the food but replicated in the human who infected the food. Other types of common vehicles include blood and blood products (hepatitis B), intravenous fluids (gram-negative septicemia), and drugs (salmonellosis) where units or batches of a product become contaminated from a common source and serve as a common vehicle for multiple infections. Thus, multiple vehicles may all become contaminated from a single, common source. Even though there are multiple vehicles involved, these infections may be considered as all being transmitted by a common vehicle because the epidemiologic principles are the same. It should be noted that "common source" and "common vehicle" are not interchangeable terms. A common source is just that: a source common to multiple vehicles from which the vehicles become infected. A common vehicle, on the other hand, is a vehicle of infection associated with two or more cases of a disease. If only a single infection results, the designation of direct-contact or indirect-contact spread, whichever is appropriate for the circumstances, should be used.

AIRBORNE SPREAD. *Airborne* transmission describes organisms that have a true airborne phase in their route of dissemination, which usually involves a distance of more than several feet between the source and the victim. The organisms are contained within droplet nuclei or dust particles; the former are airborne particles that result from the evaporation of droplets, are 5 μ or smaller in size, and may remain suspended in air for prolonged periods of time. Dust is material that has settled on surfaces, becomes resuspended by physical action, and may also remain airborne for a prolonged time. Skin squamae may become airborne and provide a mechanism for the airborne transmission of organisms such as staphylococci. Airborne particles may remain suspended for hours or possibly days, depending upon environmental factors. Movement may be within a room, or—again depending upon environmental factors, especially air currents—transmission may be over a longer distance. The size and density of the airborne particle will also influence the distance it moves.

Airborne spread by means of droplet nuclei is exemplified in the transmission of tuberculosis and, in some instances, staphylococcal infections. The classic experiments of Riley [3] demonstrated the airborne route of infection for tubercle bacilli, where the source of the organisms was disseminating patients with active, sputum-positive, cavitary disease. Some nosocomial staphylococcal disease has been shown to be transmitted by the airborne route. In one report [4], several postoperative wound infections were said to have resulted from the airborne spread of staphylococci from a staff member who remained at the periphery of the operating room throughout the surgical procedure; the only route for transmission of the organisms was through the air, there being no opportunity in this case for contact or common-vehicle spread.

Organisms may be transmitted in dust, as was seen, for example, in an outbreak of salmonellosis where the transmission occurred by means of contaminated dust contained in a vacuum cleaner bag; the dust became resuspended each time the vacuum cleaner was used [1].

VECTORBORNE SPREAD. Vectorborne-spread nosocomial disease, though unreported in the United States, could occur; it includes external and internal vector transmission. *External vectorborne transmission* refers to the mechanical transfer of microorganisms on the body or appendages of the vector; shigellae and salmonellae are transferred in this way by flies, for example. *Internal vectorborne transmission* includes harborage and biologic transmission. In *harborage* transmission, there is no biologic action between the vector and the agent; this is seen with *Yersinia pestis* organisms in the gastrointestinal tract of the flea. *Biologic* transmission occurs when the agent (e.g., a parasite) goes through biologic changes within the vector, as malaria parasites do within the mosquito.

Host

The third link in the chain of transmission is the host or victim. Disease does not always follow upon the transmission of infectious agents to a host. As previously discussed, various agent factors play a part; similarly, a variety of host factors must also be surmounted before infection occurs and disease develops. Host factors that influence the development of infections are the site of deposition of the agent and the host's defense mechanisms, both specific and non-specific.

ENTRANCE. Sites of deposition include the skin, mucous membranes, or the respiratory, gastrointestinal, or urinary tracts. Organisms such as leptospires can gain entrance through normal skin. Other organisms, such as staphylococci, need a minute breech in the integrity of the skin to gain entrance to the body. There may be mechanical transmission through the normal skin, as with hepatitis B virus on a contaminated needle. Abnormal skin, such as a preexisting wound, may be the site of deposition of organisms such as *Pseudomonas aeruginosa*. Mucous membranes may be the site of entrance, as the conjunctiva is for adenovirus type 8.

Another site of deposition is the respiratory tract. The exact area of deposition will depend on the size of the airborne particle and the aerodynamics at the time of transmission. Generally, particles 5 μ or larger in diameter will be deposited in the upper respiratory tract, whereas those less than 5 μ in diameter will be deposited in the lower respiratory tract.

Infectious agents may gain entrance to the body through the intestinal tract by means of ingestion of contaminated foods or liquids, through contaminated supplemental feedings, or through contaminated equipment, such as endoscopes inserted into the intestinal tract. Within the gastrointestinal tract, some organisms cause disease by secreting a toxin that is absorbed through the mucosa (enterotoxigenic *E. coli*), while others invade the wall of the intestinal tract (*Shigella*). Some microorganisms involve primarily the upper part of the gastrointestinal tract (*Staphylococci*), and others, the lower part of the tract (*Shigella*). The urinary tract may become infected from contaminated foreign objects such as catheters or cystoscopes inserted into the urethra, or by the retrograde movement of organisms on the external surface of a catheter inserted into the bladder.

Organisms may gain entrance into the host via the placenta, as occurs in rubella and toxoplasmosis. Transplantation is another method by which microorganisms enter the host; infection may follow renal transplantation if the donated kidney is infected with cytomegalovirus.

An organism may colonize one site and cause no disease, but the same organism at another site may result in clinical disease. *E. coli,* for example, routinely colonizes the gastrointestinal tract and under normal circumstances does not cause disease; however, the same organism in the urinary tract may very well cause infection. *S. aureus* may be carried in the external nares without any evidence of disease, but when the same organism colonizes a fresh surgical wound, a postoperative wound infection may develop.

DEFENSE MECHANISMS: NONSPECIFIC. A host's defense mechanisms may be nonspecific or specific; the quantity and quality of these mechanisms will vary from person to person (see Part II, Chapter 15). Nonspecific defense mechanisms include the skin, mucous membranes, and certain bodily secretions. The skin forms the first barrier against infection; it is a mechanical barrier and contains secretions that have an antibacterial action. Tears, a form of epithelial secretions, have an antibacterial action (due to lysozyme), and they also mechanically remove entrapped organisms. The gastrointestinal tract secretes acid that acts as a barrier against enteric organisms. Other secretions, such as mucus and enzymes, bolster the defense mechanisms. The muscular contractions of the intestinal tract act to move the contents through the tract and thus reduce the available time for organisms to invade the mucosa. Within the nose and upper respiratory tract, the cilia act to remove organisms that impinge on them. The blanket of mucus serves to entrap and remove infectious agents. The lower respiratory tract is protected by secretions and macrophages that ingest microorganisms and carry them to regional lymph nodes.

The local inflammatory response provides another nonspecific host defense mechanism. Other nonspecific protective mechanisms include genetic, hormonal, and nutritional factors, as well as behavioral patterns and personal hygiene. Age, as influenced by these nonspecific factors, is associated with decreased resistance at either end of the spectrum; the very young and the very old frequently are more susceptible to infection. Surgery and the presence of chronic diseases—such as diabetes, blood disorders, certain lymphomas, and collagen diseases—alter host resistance, which again reflects the influence of the above nonspecific factors.

DEFENSE MECHANISMS: SPECIFIC. Specific immunity results from either natural events or artificially induced events. *Natural immunity* results from having certain diseases—such as rubella and poliomyelitis (type-specific)—and usually persists for the life of the host. With other diseases, there is a latent stage following clinical illness in which immunity is imperfect; the agent will remain in the latent stage until some triggering mechanism initiates disease. Such latency is shown in infection with herpes simplex virus. Immunity may also develop after inapparent infection, such as in diphtheria or poliomyelitis.

Artificial immunity can be either active or passive. *Active* artificial immunity follows the use of vaccines. There are attenuated vaccines, such as those used against poliomyelitis, yellow fever, and tuberculosis; killed vaccines, used against such diseases as typhoid fever and pertussis; and toxoids, which are used against diphtheria and tetanus. *Passive* immunity results from the use of immune serum globulin (i.e., serum that contains antibody); this is employed, for example, in prophylaxis against hepatitis A infections. Transplacental antibodies, such as measles antibodies, also provide an example of passive antibody protection. Passive antibody protects the individual from disease, but it neither protects against infection nor prevents subsequent spread of the agent to others. Passive protection is of relatively short duration, usually at most several months.

HOST RESPONSE. The spectrum of the host's response to a microorganism may range from a subclinical (or inapparent) infection to a clinically apparent illness, the extreme being death.

The clinical spectrum of disease varies from mild, to a "typical" course (though a certain disease may typically be mild), to severe disease and possible death. The degree of host response is determined by both agent and host factors and includes the dose of the infecting organism, its organ specificity, the pathogenicity of the infecting organism, its virulence and invasiveness, and its portal of entry. Host factors include the quantitative and qualitative level of the specific and nonspecific immunologic factors previously discussed.

The same organism infecting different hosts

can result in a clinical spectrum of disease that is the same, similar, or different in various individuals. In an epidemic, for example, many cases of what appears to be the epidemic disease may meet the clinical case definition, while other cases that epidemiologically are related to the same outbreak may not meet the same case definition. They may, in fact, be cases of the epidemic disease, but with a different clinical spectrum (as can occasionally be demonstrated by serologic tests). They may also be cases of another disease(s) occurring concurrently with the epidemic.

Environment

The environment significantly influences the multiple factors in the chain of infection. The transmission of the agent from its source to the host occurs in an "environment" that represents the summation of many individual factors; changes in any of these can have an impact on any link in the chain of infection. Some environmental factors are under strict control, such as the air in an operating room, whereas other environmental factors are not.

At times, too much emphasis is placed on the role of the environment; for example, it is inappropriate to take environmental cultures routinely throughout a hospital (see Part I, Chapters 6 and 8). In other instances, not enough attention is paid to the environment. There needs to be a healthy respect for the environment, with maintenance that does not deliberately promote the transmission of disease-causing agents to hosts, but without excessive control measures that impose unnecessary and ineffective actions on the hospital staff and a consequent loss of efficiency, effectiveness, and money. Knowledge of environmental factors and their influence on the chain of infection and an awareness of adverse changes in the environment should be sufficient to alert one to the need to investigate these environmental factors in order to ascertain their role in a nosocomial infection problem.

Some environmental factors can influence all the links in the chain of infection, while others are more limited in their range of action. Humidity, for example, can influence a multiplicity of factors; it can affect the persistence of an agent at its source, its transmission through the air, and the effectiveness of a host's mucous membranes in resisting infection. Other environmental factors, however, have a more limited effect on the occurrence of infection; for example, the temperature-pressure relationship in a specific autoclave affects sterilization within that autoclave, but it has no direct effect on the host.

Certain environmental factors directly affect the agent. Replication of the agent at its reservoir may depend on certain substances in the environment. The agent's survival is influenced by the temperature, humidity, and radiation at its reservoir or source; its survival is even influenced by such factors during its transmission. There may also be toxic substances in the environment that are lethal for the agent.

The transmission of agents will be affected by environmental factors such as temperature and humidity, as mentioned above. Airborne transmission is influenced by air velocity and the direction of its movement. The stability and concentration of an aerosol is directly related to environmental factors. In winter, people tend to be indoors with closed windows and reduced air circulation, and this increases the risk of airborne disease in winter compared with summer, when room air is air-conditioned or diluted with outside air. In outbreaks associated with common-vehicle transmission, the temperature of the environment will influence the level of contamination in the vehicle. The spread of vectorborne disease also reflects favorable conditions in the environment for the survival and movement of the vector.

The host's resistance mechanisms are affected by environmental factors; for example, in an excessively dry atmosphere, mucous membranes become dry and are less able to protect against microbial invasion. Also, the host's behavioral patterns are influenced by heat and cold.

References

1. Bate, J., and James, U. *Salmonella typhimurium* infection dust-borne in a children's ward. *Lancet* 2:713, 1958.

2. Hornick, R. B., Greisman, S. E., and Woodward, T. E. Typhoid fever: Pathogenesis and immunologic control. *N. Engl. J. Med.* 283:686, 1970.

3. Riley, R. L., et al. Aerial dissemination of pulmonary tuberculosis: A two-year study of contagion in tuberculosis ward. *Am. J. Hyg.* 70:2, 1959.

4. Waller, C. W., Kuntsin, R. B., and Brubaker, M. M. The incidence of airborne wound infections during operation. *J.A.M.A.* 186:908, 1963.

3

Hospital Personnel

Richard A. Kaslow and Julia S. Garner

Ages ago, Hippocrates exhorted his followers first to do no harm. Nowhere does this charge to the practitioner of medical art seem more relevant today than in institutions devoted to medical care, and in few other areas of institutional medicine does the fulfillment of that cardinal principle seem more attainable than in practitioners' efforts to control nosocomial infection. All hospital personnel from the administrator to the part-time volunteer are part of that effort. This chapter outlines the infection control responsibilities of and for hospital personnel, the approaches to major risks of nosocomial infection to and from hospital personnel, and the possible contribution of a hospital personnel health service to infection control.

Responsibilities in Infection Control

Infection Control Committee

A multidisciplinary committee with responsibility for the control of infection within the hospital is a requirement of the Joint Commission on Accreditation of Hospitals [21]. An Infection Control Committee that is responsive and competent is an important aspect of a program for the control of nosocomial infections. The purpose of the committee should be the prevention of nosocomial infection and of secondary spread to the community. In large measure, the composition of the committee will determine its success.

COMPOSITION. For the committee to achieve its purpose of preventing nosocomial infections, special consideration should be given to selecting the Infection Control Committee members. A primary consideration in choosing committee members is their interest and personal commitment to the prevention of nosocomial infections. In addition, committee members should acquire and maintain thorough knowledge of their discipline, and they should be respected among their peers. When possible, they should also have the authority to speak for the department they represent in matters concerning policy without clearance from a supervisor or department chief. They should maintain communication with the department members whom they represent by encouraging input from their department associates and sharing committee ideas and decisions.

Committee members can be appointed either permanently or for a specified term. Interested and experienced members may serve better on a relatively permanent basis. If members must be chosen without regard to interest and experience, temporary appointment may be more appropriate. If members serve temporarily, it seems sensible to stagger the terms of service for continuity.

The Infection Control Committee should have a permanent or temporary chairman who is a physician, preferably with demonstrated knowledge of and commitment to infection control. The same advantages and disadvantages of temporary and permanent appointment apply to the chairman that apply to other committee members. Because a new chairman usually requires several months to become confident and capable of fulfilling the responsibilities of the position, a rotating chairman should hold the position for at least two years.

The members of the Infection Control Committee should include representatives from the major medical departments, the nursing service, the clinical microbiology laboratory, and the hospital administration, as well as the hospital epidemiologist and the infection control nurse. If a hospital has a house staff, then their representative, preferably an interested chief or senior resident, should also be a member.

In addition to regular members, representatives from other hospital departments should serve as ex officio or ad hoc members and attend meetings only as necessary. Such members from the hospital can include representatives from the admitting department, central service, data processing, dental services, dietary department, engineering and maintenance, housekeeping, inhalation therapy, laundry, personnel health, pharmacy, operating room, x-ray, and others as appropriate. The Infection Control Committee might well include representatives from the local or state health department.

ACTIVITIES AND FUNCTIONS. The Infection Control Committee should have the ultimate responsibility for developing the policies and procedures for hospital infection control. The decisions of the Infection Control Committee should receive serious attention through deliberation or approval by other hospital committee(s) or the Board of Trustees. New policies may necessitate changes in hospital bylaws or other measures to assure rapid translation of Infection Control Committee decisions into hospital policy.

A principal responsibility of the committee is to establish policies and mechanisms for the surveillance of nosocomial infections. Certain details should be settled before surveillance is initiated; these include (1) definitions of infections for all sites, (2) methods for case finding, (3) methods for tabulating and analyzing data, and (4) methods for reporting these data to Infection Control Committee members, other hospital personnel, and local and state health authorities if the diseases are reportable (see Part I, Chapter 4, Surveillance).

Another committee responsibility is to develop procedures to prevent nosocomial infections that are based on sound epidemiologic principles. Standard patient-care procedures should be followed for the use and care of equipment (e.g., intravenous catheters or urinary catheters), as well as for inhalation therapy, tracheostomies, dressing changes, and other aseptic techniques. After approval, the procedures should be circulated in writing to all departments of the hospital. The procedures should be written clearly and concisely. The following is an example of pertinent considerations in the prevention of intravenous therapy-associated infections that should be included in the procedure for the use and care of intravenous therapy:

1. recommendations for general use, including suggestions for alternative therapy;
2. types of hospital personnel responsible for the insertion of cannulas;
3. aseptic techniques to be used by hospital personnel who insert intravenous cannulas;
4. skin preparation for site chosen for cannula placement;
5. daily care and maintenance of the cannula site;

6. frequency of changing administration sets and indwelling cannulas; and
7. protocol for evaluation of suspect intravenous system (see Part II, Chapters 25 and 26).

The committee also has the responsibility for formulating the policy and procedures for appropriate isolation of patients with communicable infections and of uninfected patients who have seriously impaired resistance. In addition to the pertinent considerations in isolation techniques and specific precautions stated in a later chapter (Part I, Chapter 9), the Infection Control Committee should specify:

1. the person(s) responsible for ordering isolation,
2. a procedure to follow if isolation is indicated but not ordered by the person(s) responsible, and
3. the person(s) responsible for the ultimate decision regarding isolation if conflicts of opinion arise.

The Infection Control Committee in cooperation with the appropriate chiefs or directors has the responsibility for specifying the infection control policies and procedures that shall be used in special care areas and supportive areas of the hospital. Such special patient-care areas include the cardiac catheterization laboratory, emergency department, endoscopy rooms, hemodialysis unit, intensive-care unit(s), nursery, obstetric department, operating room, outpatient department, and x-ray department. Sensitive support areas of the hospital include the blood bank, central supply, engineering and maintenance, food-handling services, housekeeping, laundry, and the pharmacy (see Part I, Chapter 7).

The Infection Control Committee has the responsibility for certain aspects of the clinical microbiology laboratory that relate to infection control. The committee should help ensure that:

1. specimens are adequately collected and handled,
2. species of organisms are determined,
3. antibiotic sensitivity testing is done using the Kirby-Bauer or equivalent method,
4. assessable, relevant, adequate, and easy-to-use records are kept that allow for rapid retrieval of data on isolates of major organisms by major sites and by patient identification number and date,
5. tabulations of antimicrobial susceptibility patterns for pathogens identified in the hospital laboratory are distributed to the medical staff at least twice yearly,
6. a quality control system is utilized, and
7. appropriate environmental sampling and personnel culturing can be undertaken when epidemiologically indicated (see Part I, Chapter 7, The Clinical Laboratory, and Chapter 8).

In addition to considering policies and procedures for surveillance, patient care, and the clinical microbiology laboratory, the Infection Control Committee is responsible for the infection control aspects of personnel health, continuing education, and environmental control. Not only does the Infection Control Committee devise the infection control program, policy, and procedures for the hospital, but it also has the responsibility for meaningful implementation by relating the policies and procedures to those responsible. The committee should also have the means to assess the implementation of policies and procedures and to alter them as necessary.

METHODS TO ACCOMPLISH OBJECTIVES. A monthly meeting of the Infection Control Committee is desirable, but meetings may be necessary more often as problems arise. All members whose comments would be desirable should attend the meetings.

The planned agenda should include a review of the important portions of a monthly infection report prepared by the infection control nurse and hospital epidemiologist. Committee members should receive the agenda and a synopsis of the monthly infection report (see The Infection Control Nurse, Duties and Activities, below) several days before the committee meeting. In addition, a review of at least one major control policy or procedure each month may be useful for updating hospital practice. Situations such as the sudden withdrawal of a drug from the market by the Food and Drug Administration and the discovery of potentially harmful or contaminated products of certain manufacturers exemplify the need for the most current information; the Infection Control Committee must be able to decide promptly on alternative therapies or products. Because of rapid advances in the approaches to nosocomial infection, all major policies and procedures relating to infection control should be reviewed at least yearly by the Infection Control Committee.

In the Infection Control Committee meeting, the members must share pertinent information and use their expertise to make decisions aimed at controlling nosocomial infections. Minutes of each meeting should be taken and circulated appropriately.

The following shortcomings and pitfalls are to be avoided:

1. *Committee has no authority.* In some hospitals, the policies and practices developed by the committee require protracted deliberation and approval by administrative authority. The hospital should strive to develop an organizational structure that permits the Infection Control Committee to work autonomously toward the prevention of nosocomial infection. Where further discussion by the medical board or Board of Trustees is necessary, the committee should provide their recommendations, the alternatives, and their assessment of the consequences.
2. *Committee lacks knowledge.* Some Infection Control Committee members may have limited knowledge or understanding of the purposes and details of nosocomial infection control. Recommendations for surveillance methods, patient-care procedures, and other areas for which the Infection Control Committee has responsibility are available from the Center for Disease Control (CDC), The American Hospital Association, and state health departments.
3. *Committee is too large.* In some hospitals, the Infection Control Committee is so large that it is ineffective. Business can usually be conducted most effectively when no more then ten persons are participating. Only those ex officio members who can contribute

meaningfully to the discussion need attend. Using subcommittees or working groups can prevent the committee from becoming unwieldy.
4. *Committee members are not interested.* Disinterest in the committee may be a result of the three previously listed pitfalls. If disinterest persists after these pitfalls are alleviated, the tasks at hand may be best accomplished by replacing disinterested members with new, more committed members.
5. *Committee wastes time on surveillance activities.* Review of patient charts to determine the presence of a nosocomial infection is a surveillance function; it should be performed by the infection control nurse and the hospital epidemiologist before the meeting. They should adhere to the definitions for nosocomial infections previously developed by the Infection Control Committee. The committee meetings can then be devoted to developing policies and procedures for infection control.

The Infection Control Nurse

The infection control nurse (nurse epidemiologist, infection control practitioner, or whatever) is usually the only hospital employee whose primary and full-time responsibility is infection control. This person is the central figure in the infection control program and is responsible for the day-to-day activities of the program. Because of these key responsibilities, special attention should be given to selection of this person.

QUALIFICATIONS. The infection control nurse should be intelligent and experienced in clinical nursing. The infection control nurse should know, practice, and demonstrate aseptic techniques and methods for preventing cross-infection, including isolation techniques and precautions. The infection control nurse should develop experience in evaluating the proper aseptic use of procedures and equipment.

Personal characteristics of the infection control nurse are important, because she or he must influence diverse groups toward infection control. The ability to communicate well with all disciplines in a tactful and nonthreatening manner is essential.

In addition to the personal characteristics and nursing qualifications and experience, the infection control nurse needs a reasonable working knowledge of the basic principles of epidemiology. Also, the infection control nurse must be familiar with the agents that cause disease; the reservoirs of these agents, including their natural and usual habitats; the spectrum of disease, particularly with reference to the concepts of colonization, infection, disease, and the carrier state; modes of transmission; host factors that enhance susceptibility to disease; and the various approaches to the control of infectious disease in hospitals.

The infection control nurse also needs at least a rudimentary understanding of microbiology and biostatistics. His or her knowledge should include the general characteristics of microorganisms and their usual antimicrobial sensitivity patterns as well as methods for taking specimens and for isolation and identification of important hospital pathogens. It should also include the ability to calculate rates of infection, to use appropriate control groups of uninfected patients for assessment of important risk factors, to investigate an epidemic, and to use simple tests of statistical significance.

It may be impossible for a hospital to attract a nurse from elsewhere with all these qualifications and experience. The alternative is to select an experienced nurse from the staff. The nurse selected should be well respected by the nursing and medical staff for his or her knowledge and skills in nursing and interpersonal relationships, and the individual should have as many of the previously mentioned qualifications as possible. The infection control nurse should then be given formal and informal training to obtain the skills needed.

Few formal programs leading to an advanced degree in hospital infection control presently exist in the United States; therefore, the infection control nurse must obtain the majority of training from short-term courses. Short-term training courses in infection control are given by universities, local and state health departments, the Center for Disease Control, and associations such as the Association for Practitioners in Infection Control (APIC). These training courses are particularly beneficial to the novice, but they may also be useful to the experienced infection control nurse who wants to keep up with developments or expand his or her expertise in infection control problems and solutions. In addition, a number of local infection control groups composed primarily of infection control nurses have been created to share experiences and common problems; these may also be helpful to the infection control nurse. Moreover, meetings of the APIC are devoted exclusively to nosocomial infection control, with sessions for both the experienced worker and beginner.

DUTIES AND ACTIVITIES. Major responsibilities of the infection control nurse are to detect and record nosocomial infections on a systematic and current basis, analyze such infections with the help of the hospital epidemiologist, and prepare a monthly infection report for the Infection Control Committee (for further details, see Part I, Chapter 4). In some hospitals, the infection control nurse also has the responsibility for detecting and recording community-acquired infections that represent cross-infection hazards as well as for reporting reportable diseases to the local and state health department. Whether the infection control nurse will assume these latter responsibilities should be determined by the Infection Control Committee.

The infection control nurse, together with the hospital epidemiologist, should be responsible for the epidemiologic investigation of all significant infection problems (see Part I, Chapter 5).

Another important responsibility of the infection control nurse is to interpret hospital policy on the isolation and disposition of patients who have community-acquired or nosocomial infections that require such special care. The infection control nurse can also assist ward personnel in determining where, from an infection control standpoint, to place an infected patient who requires precautions but who does not require a private room so there is the least possible chance for cross-infection.

The infection control nurse should also be responsible for assisting in the development, implementation, or both of any improved infection control measures, whether or not these are involved in direct patient care. The nurse may serve on or consult with the committees charged with evaluating procedures and proposed new patient equipment.

The infection control nurse may assist with employee orientation and in-service training programs related to infection prevention and control. New patient-care employees should be introduced to the overall infection control program of the hospital. Depending upon the structure of the hospital, the infection control nurse might share the responsibility for formal or informal in-service education in infection control. If a formal in-service education program exists in the hospital, the infection control nurse can indicate to the in-service department which particular areas or personnel may need instructions. Analysis of nosocomial infection data will often delineate these needs.

The infection control nurse is in an excellent position to influence the quality of patient care by being available to the medical and nursing staff to help them implement the infection control program. Tangible improvement will depend on the nurse's awareness of the problems with implementation of the program and his or her eagerness to report these to the Infection Control Committee and others who need to know of them.

METHODS TO ACCOMPLISH OBJECTIVES. The infection control nurse should have enough working time to carry out the surveillance and reporting activities as well as to fulfill prevention and control responsibilities. All time and energy should not be directed exclusively toward one responsibility at the expense of the others, except in an emergency or epidemic situation. One infection control nurse working full time with the responsibilities previously listed can be expected to cover approximately 250 beds and associated personnel. Larger hospitals will need supplementary personnel. In addition, secretarial or clerical support will be needed to assist in preparation of monthly infection control reports.

Administratively, the infection control nurse can report to the infectious disease or infection control department, hospital administration, nursing service, or the clinical laboratory ser-

vice. There are advantages and disadvantages to being responsible to any one of these departments. Regardless of the department or organizational structure, the infection control nurse should have a specified person as a supervisor, preferably the hospital epidemiologist, not a committee or a group of supervisors. Above all, assignment of the infection control nurse to any particular department in the hospital should provide maximal flexibility and facilitate crossing of departmental lines.

Some individuals who are not nurses have carried out many of the activities of the infection control nurse discussed above. Persons conducting surveillance and control activities cannot be effective, however, unless they are able to communicate adequately with patient-care personnel and are knowledgeable about patient-care activities.

The Hospital Epidemiologist

The hospital epidemiologist position usually involves part-time duties for a physician on the hospital staff. Most hospitals with an active infection control program have such a person who fulfills the responsibilities. In small community hospitals, the chairman of the Infection Control Committee may serve as hospital epidemiologist, whereas in large community or university hospitals, the position of hospital epidemiologist may be separate. The duties ordinarily require only a few hours per week, depending on the size of the hospital. In some larger hospitals, however, the position has become full time, with opportunities for research and teaching in addition to infection control responsibilities. The hospital epidemiologist has both responsibility to and authority delegated by the Infection Control Committee and the hospital administration.

QUALIFICATIONS. Ideally, the hospital epidemiologist should be a physician with some training in infectious disease, epidemiology, and biostatistics. If such a person is unavailable to the hospital, a physician who is well respected in the hospital for his or her knowledge of and interest in the prevention and control of nosocomial infections is recommended. Usually, this person is appointed from the existing hospital staff, although in some communities, one trained person may serve as hospital epidemiologist for several hospitals.

RESPONSIBILITIES. A primary responsibility of the hospital epidemiologist is to advise and direct the infection control nurse. The hospital epidemiologist should supervise the accurate collection and analysis of data on nosocomial infections and assist in determining whether those nosocomial infections meet the accepted hospital definitions, particularly in complicated cases.

The hospital epidemiologist should be responsible for instituting emergency infection control measures when a problem arises in the hospital. The hospital epidemiologist also should be responsible for initiating studies to define a suspected or apparent problem. Likewise, the hospital epidemiologist should be responsible for recommending general control measures to the committee for endemic problems.

The qualified hospital epidemiologist may also serve as an expert infectious disease consultant to the Infection Control Committee on infection control measures.

METHODS FOR FULFILLING RESPONSIBILITIES. The hospital epidemiologist should be readily accessible to the infection control nurse when questions or problems arise. The hospital epidemiologist and infection control nurse should plan to discuss at least weekly the infections detected by the surveillance mechanisms and any infection control problems in the hospital. They should also meet prior to the monthly Infection Control Committee meeting to analyze the monthly infection data and prepare a monthly infection control report.

Experience has shown an infection control program will flounder unless the hospital epidemiologist and infection control nurse are interested in infection control, fulfill the designated responsibilities, and interact well with each other.

The Hospital Administrator

The hospital administrator, as the agent of the Board of Trustees of the hospital, has the responsibility for seeing that the Infection Control Committee is discharging its responsibility of developing and implementing infection control policies and procedures for the hospital. The administrator should maintain an organizational framework that readily permits translation of the decisions of the Infection Control Committee into the policy of the hospital. When disputes arise between departments and the Infection Control Committee, the administrator should serve as the mediator.

The administrator should see that funds are appropriated for the infection control program, including those needed for special studies. The administrator may also take responsibility for approving and releasing publicity concerning the infection control program and infection problems associated with the hospital.

Other Hospital Staff

PHYSICIANS. Each practicing physician has a responsibility to alert the hospital staff regarding infections in his currently hospitalized patients and possible nosocomial infections in those who have been hospitalized recently. Communication between the hospital and physicians is particularly important regarding surgical and newborn patients, who are more likely than other patients to develop nosocomial infections following discharge. The physician has the responsibility to ensure that suspected and confirmed infections are cultured to treat the infections appropriately, and to prescribe the use of proper isolation techniques where indicated. The physician has the responsibility of conforming to the policy and procedures outlined by the Infection Control Committee. Physicians must wash their hands between patient contacts; they *must* set a positive example for other hospital personnel to follow.

NURSES. Each practicing nurse has a responsibility to report signs and symptoms of infection to the attending physicians and the infection control nurse. The nurse should conform to the policy and procedures established by the Infection Control Committee. The responsibility for maintaining asepsis, particularly for washing hands between patient contacts, and for exemplary professional practice falls on the nurse as well as on the physician.

OTHER PERSONNEL. All other hospital personnel—auxilliary nursing personnel; students from the various professional schools; laboratory, radiology, laundry, housekeeping, and kitchen personnel; volunteers; and others—have the responsibility of conducting their work in a manner that minimizes cross-infection hazards. They should be expected to follow infection control policy and procedures pertinent to their work. Personnel have the responsibility of reporting suspected or confirmed infection problems to their supervisors who, in turn, should report such problems to the Personnel Health Service, the infection control nurse, or the hospital epidemiologist.

Control of Infections in and by Personnel

The hazard of nosocomial spread of infection from hospital personnel to patients emerged during the last century at the time Semmelweis and his contemporaries enunciated the concept of hospital-acquired infection. Patient-care personnel have long since been implicated both as reservoirs and as vectors of institutional outbreaks. On the other hand—except for smallpox, tuberculosis, and hepatitis—the occupational risks of infection transmitted from patients to personnel have received relatively scant attention.

This section has two purposes. The first is to discuss the major hazards of infection transmitted to and from hospital personnel. Such infection signals a warning that the mechanisms usually available for prevention may not be operating optimally. It calls for a review of the epidemiology and microbiology most relevant to the involved hospital personnel and high-risk personnel groups, as well as for an outline of preventive measures applicable to personnel health.

Certain institutional infections that required considerable attention in the past have received only brief comment or none at all. Typhoid fever and puerperal streptococcal disease involving hospital personnel are relatively unusual occurrences, and, at the time of writing of this chapter, all indications are that smallpox is virtually extinct. Conversely, epidemics of Lassa fever and other hemorrhagic fevers have taken dreadful tolls of patients and health workers in hospitals in Africa, but the geographic remoteness and our ignorance of the nosocomial epidemiology of these diseases seem to justify including only this reminder of their existence. Finally, no more than passing reference is made here to the possibly infectious and peculiarly nosocomial entities: epidemic neuromyasthenia and epidemic phlebodynia.

The second purpose of this section is to encompass the elements and goals of an occupational health service with regard only to infection control in a hospital. The program outlined makes no pretense of considering the peculiarities of hospital character, size, or geography or of providing a blueprint for comprehensive health care; rather, it presents a general viewpoint regarding what a hospital employee health service might do to support the infection control activities.

Cytomegalovirus

Cytomegalovirus (CMV) infection produces a spectrum of disease. In adults, it can present as a mild, nonspecific, self-limiting illness, a mononucleosis-like syndrome, hepatitis, or interstitial pneumonia (see Part II, Chapter 24). As in rubella, the real and devastating risk is to the fetus of a woman infected in the early months of pregnancy.

Congenital CMV infection also displays a spectrum ranging from inapparent acquisition and excretion to gross congenital malformation. Although no direct evidence has come from studies of hospital personnel, infected infants pose a serious potential risk to pregnant women working in close contact with these infants. A less frequent but no less serious risk is exposure of pregnant personnel to adults with CMV infection.

Serologic screening for immunity is not sufficiently well developed or widely available to be recommended for routinely identifying susceptible persons. Currently, the only practical means of protecting against nosocomial congenital CMV infection is to inform women of childbearing age of the risk they may incur through contact during early pregnancy with infected patients. No woman in the early stages of pregnancy should have contact with a patient with CMV infection. Serial serology may help determine whether recent infection has occurred as a result of exposure during pregnancy.

Diphtheria

About 200 to 300 cases of diphtheria have been reported annually in the United States over the past decade, and about one-third of the cases occur in adults. Infection generally develops from very close contact with a case or a carrier of *Corynebacterium diphtheriae*. Hospital personnel caring for patients, especially in pediatrics, may have such contact. Clinical infection of personnel is apparently quite rare following the routine care of infected patients; no cases were observed in unprotected personnel with ordinary patient contact during one reported outbreak.

No more than half of the institutional personnel or medical students sampled in published surveys were considered to be adequately protected against diphtheria, despite the recommendation that everyone should be immunized. All persons—and certainly hospital personnel who may be at higher risk of developing diphtheria than other adults—should be immunized regularly. Those not previously immunized should be given primary immunization; booster toxoid (generally together with tetanus toxoid) should be given to all persons every ten years after primary immunization. Toxoid should be given to susceptible hospital personnel who have had respiratory contact with patients with diphtheria. Such personnel also should have nose and throat cultures taken; those with positive cultures should be removed from patient-care duties, treated, and allowed to resume their duties when the cultures are negative.

Hepatitis

Recognized and unrecognized cases of hepatitis A (infectious hepatitis) may enter health-care facilities; they provide a source for both sporadic hospital acquisition (see Part II, Chapter 24) and outbreaks. Although parenteral spread is possible, most nosocomial cases of hepatitis A appear to be attributable to lapses in practice of enteric asepsis and the result of fecal-oral spread. Of course, occasional unrecognized

cases may escape the most effective enteric precautions and result in nosocomial transmission.

Delay in diagnosis has actually led to outbreaks among pediatric patient-care staff in two hospitals. Personnel in dialysis units have also been involved in outbreaks of hepatitis A. Currently available data do not clearly establish a higher risk of hepatitis A for other hospital personnel than for the general population.

Good hygiene practiced routinely and the enforcement of optimal precautions in suspected cases should minimize any occupational risk. Personnel who will have or have had intimate exposure (i.e., close contact with patients' excreta or accidental parenteral inoculation with infective blood components) to hepatitis A or hepatitis of unknown etiology should be offered standard immune serum globulin (ISG) for passive protection against intense clinical manifestations. The appropriate dose is most effective before or for one to two weeks after exposure and declines thereafter. The disease is communicable in the preclinical and early clinical phases. Although the infection may remain communicable for up to ten days before serum hepatic transaminase levels reach a peak, recent data on the intensity of virus shedding have suggested that communicability may already be waning as the enzyme levels first rise. In practice, the diagnosis is often suspected when the serum transaminase levels rise, and employees could be relieved of duty at that time or immediately upon the onset of jaundice when it is the first manifestation of the disease. Resumption of duties depends on the decline in communicability and would vary according to individual circumstances.*

Hepatitis B (serum hepatitis) virology and epidemiology have been advancing rapidly. The infection has been directly associated with the appearance of hepatitis B antigen (HB_sAg) in blood and other body fluids and less closely with a specific antibody to that antigen (anti-HB_s). Much of the discussion that follows draws heavily on studies of HB_sAg, for which

---

* Visualization by electron microscopy of hepatitis A virus and the development of immunologic techniques for studying infection and immunity should lead to a better understanding of the role of hospital personnel in nosocomial hepatitis A infections.

immunologic tests have been widely available. Characterization of the virus with core and surface antigenic markers and the correlation of antigenic characteristics with corresponding antibodies provide additional powerful tools for the study of the infectivity, transmission, and prevention of hepatitis B involving hospital personnel.

Certain personnel working in dialysis units, hematology-oncology units, operating rooms, hematology laboratories, and other areas of hospitals where blood products from HB$_s$Ag-positive patients are handled intensively have higher rates of clinical and subclinical infection (i.e., HB$_s$Ag carriage) than their counterparts with less intensive exposure. The numerous reports of dialysis-associated hepatitis B in patients with renal failure as well as in the personnel caring for them (see Part I, Chapter 7, The Hemodialysis Unit) exemplify this problem. Dentists, dental surgeons, and other personnel giving oral care also pose special risks [38]. Staff as well as patients may be at increased risk of hepatitis in institutions for the mentally retarded. Concern has also been expressed that still other surgical and medical-care personnel may contract and transmit hepatitis B in the course of their work [17]. Finally, one well-studied instance of the probable transmission of hepatitis B from a hospital worker to patients involved direct contact (parenteral injections) by an infected nurse [6].

In contrast to the clear danger of overt hepatitis B in hospital patients and personnel, the significance of carriage of HB$_s$Ag and anti-HB$_s$ is less well understood. Different prevalence surveys conducted among health-care personnel have produced estimates of HB$_s$Ag carriage rates of 0.8 to 1.7 percent [24]. One survey of personnel in 15 dialysis centers detected a mean antigen carriage rate of 2.4 percent. In a retrospective analysis of an outbreak, laboratory personnel with the greatest exposure to blood from an affected dialysis unit experienced both the highest rates of clinical infection and the highest rates of anti-HB$_s$ seropositivity [41].

Personnel in high-risk areas such as hemodialysis units should be screened prior to employment and regularly thereafter for HB$_s$Ag and anti-HB$_s$ on a schedule adjusted to the findings [10]. Because knowledge about antigen or antibody carriage can be important both for individual clinical assessments and for controlling the spread of hepatitis B, some hospitals may choose to have serologic testing performed periodically on other personnel who appear to be at greater risk of infection with hepatitis. Although HB$_s$Ag testing does provide some reflection of the exposure to and activity of hepatitis B virus, the detection of antigens such as hepatitis B "core" (HB$_c$Ag) and "e" (HB$_e$Ag) and their antibodies may provide firmer handles on its epidemiology. Further understanding of the risk conferred by carriage of surface and core antigens, perfection of hepatitis B immunoglobulin, or the development of an active vaccine may eventually mandate wide serologic surveillance. At present, hospitals can decide individually whether personnel risks beyond those cited justify devoting resources to more extensive screening. In addition to its usual purposes, properly performed screening may also provide valuable specific epidemiologic insight into patterns of transmission and preventive measures in the immediate environment.

Regardless of how widely serologic testing is performed, a surveillance system for identifying and following presumptive hepatitis B cases and carriers falls within the responsibilities of all infection control and personnel health units. In addition, personnel should be instructed on the risks peculiar to their assignments and on the precautionary measures against avoidable oral and parenteral contact. In this regard, since maternal infection in the latter stages of pregnancy may produce significant illness in the newborn, pregnant personnel should avoid unnecessary intensive or regular contact with cases and carriers. Details of prevention are elaborated in another chapter (Part II, Chapter 24) as well as in other sources [34].

For a susceptible worker who has had hazardous contact with hepatitis B, it is expected that specific hepatitis B immunoglobulin will provide effective passive prophylaxis. Current lots of standard immune serum globulin do contain some specific antibody, and their use has been advocated.

Clinical hepatitis B in personnel requires removing them from service, at least during the acute phase of the disease. It is not clear at what point the health worker convalescing from HB$_s$Ag-positive hepatitis is no longer more likely to communicate the disease than the clinically well HB$_s$Ag carrier, and there is no firm rule for deciding when duties may be resumed. The decision will depend in part on the individual's duties and conscientiousness about personal hygiene. Close clinical observation of such asymptomatic carriers of HB$_s$Ag (whose carriage is confirmed by repeated testing) is advisable. Retesting of seropositive personnel three and six months after the initial positive test may help distinguish those who have returned to the antigenically negative state from the 5 to 10 percent who may become persistent carriers [10].

Normally, the incidental asymptomatic carrier of HB$_s$Ag does not appear to endanger susceptible seronegative persons except through direct inoculation or ingestion of the carrier's blood or other secretions in the susceptible person. As noted, on occasion, infected healthcare workers have probably transmitted hepatitis B to persons whom they have contacted; careful surveillance for hepatitis B could help determine whether a specific staff member represents a source of infection for other people. However, unless he or she is implicated in transmission by epidemiologic search, the incidental asymptomatic carrier need not be restricted with regard to patient-care responsibilities. At this time, it appears both sensible and sufficient to urge personnel who carry HB$_s$Ag without evidence of transmission to exercise proper caution against direct contact between their bodily fluids and the patients under their care.

Herpes
Mild vesiculopustular herpetic lesions ("cold sores" or "fever blisters") undoubtedly go unrecognized in many children and adults in the hospital. For certain groups of patients, infection with herpesvirus may lead to serious illness [27]. Those at particularly high risk are neonates, patients with severe malnutrition, and patients in immunodeficient states, particularly those with hematologic malignancies affecting cellular immunity and those on immunosup-

pressive agents such as corticosteroids. The fetus is at greatest risk of congenital anomalies due to herpesvirus infection during the first trimester, but it may be vulnerable to infection later in pregnancy as well.

Personnel who develop lesions on their hands are presumably most likely to transmit infection by contact and could reasonably be asked to refrain from caring for high-risk patients during the contagious vesicular stage. Those with herpetic lesions on their hands who continue to work outside high-risk patient areas should wash their hands and use gloves to prevent nosocomial spread.

There is insufficient evidence that oral or genital infections among personnel represent excessive risk. Asymptomatic oral colonization is quite common and does not seem to justify special preventive measures. The large numbers of virus particles usually present in moist, focal lesions, coupled with frequent hand-to-mouth contact, may facilitate spread, however. By wearing an appropriate barrier—such as a mask or gauze dressing (see Part II, Chapter 20)—those with fluid-filled lesions around the nose and mouth or in the genital area may minimize whatever respiratory or contact spread can occur. Patients inadvertently exposed to personnel with transmissible herpes infection may benefit from administration of ISG.

Several reports suggest that hospital personnel, especially those who have direct manual contact with respiratory tract secretions, acquire herpesvirus from patients with occult infection [28,31]. One survey of a neurosurgical service [31] indicated that one-third of the nurses without antibody developed skin lesions —herpetic paronychia or whitlow—during the study period. These lesions may be painful and unsightly, but there is no evidence that the lesions are of any danger to otherwise healthy personnel. The risks to patients and the proper management are outlined above. Hand-washing and wearing gloves for contact with suspected cases should help prevent this hazard.

The serious effects of congenital infection were mentioned above. Women in their reproductive years should be instructed to avoid unnecessary exposure to suspected herpesvirus infection. Whenever possible, pregnant personnel should not work in areas where such cases are usually hospitalized.

Influenza

During the influenza season, a proportion of hospital patients and personnel who have acquired influenza in the community will inevitably introduce the virus into the hospital environment. Personnel who experience benign influenza infection may transmit virus to patients who are at high risk of more serious influenzal illness or complications (i.e., elderly patients; those with underlying cardiovascular, pulmonary, metabolic, or other chronic diseases; or those under immunosuppressive therapy). Conversely, hospitalized cases may subject personnel to greater contact or contact with a greater diversity of strains than they might have without occupational exposure. Although spread of nosocomial influenza between patients and personnel has not been carefully documented, the problem seems to be a real one [7,9]. Visitors represent still another, though relatively small, mobile reservoir of influenza viruses.

Some latitude exists in the management of cases of influenza. Certain cases, such as those properly diagnosed early in their communicable stage, may warrant respiratory isolation. When relatively low diagnostic suspicion or a short duration of illness does not justify isolation, the patient with possible influenza infection may at least be so located as to minimize contact with especially vulnerable patients. Removing personnel with symptoms from direct contact with high-risk patients and immunizing certain groups of personnel prior to the influenza season would also help prevent serious nosocomial influenza. Assignment of recovered or immunized personnel to patients who are at high risk or in the most contagious stages could presumably further reduce hospital spread.

According to U.S. Public Health Service recommendations for the general population [12], personnel whose age or chronic disease renders them likely to tolerate influenza poorly should be immunized. A hospital should consider immunization for any personnel whose mild infection may jeopardize groups of high-risk patients not currently singled out for advance im-

munization (e.g., some patients in respiratory-care or other intensive-care units, obstetric units, and nurseries). Some authorities have also encouraged immunization of personnel whose absence in the midst of community-wide illness would impair provision of essential patient services. Changing influenza patterns and other local factors should guide each hospital's immunization policy.

During the influenza season, hospitals should make their own policies concerning visitors, using as their guides previous experience, current conditions in the community, and the physical and psychologic status of the intended patient contacts.

Measles

Measles has increasingly become a disease of late childhood and early adulthood, and severe disease occasionally occurs in these age groups. There has been a report noting an apparent excess in abortion and prematurity following measles during pregnancy [13]. These findings have gained support from more recent work, which also identified congenital malformations as possible consequences of measles infection during pregnancy.

Estimates based on cases of measles reported in 1977 indicate that over one quarter were in persons 15 years old or older, but fewer than five percent were in those 20 years old or older. Recent serologic surveys demonstrate immunity in over 95 percent of young adults tested. Thus, although measles shares features with rubella (see p. 40), the relatively small proportion of susceptible adults has made nosocomial transmission involving personnel seem less urgent.

The costs and benefits of a routine measles screening and immunization program for personnel should be examined individually. Priorities in each hospital may differ. Susceptible female personnel of childbearing age would seem to represent a hazard to themselves, to their possible pregnancy, and to susceptible patients. Susceptible men and women who care for older children and adolescents or for prenatal patients are another group to consider.

History of measles is generally unreliable, so susceptibility should be established by appropriate serologic testing. Persons found susceptible should be vaccinated. Women should not be vaccinated during pregnancy and should be advised not to become pregnant for at least three months after vaccination. Contraindications to vaccination with the live, attenuated vaccine include leukemia, lymphomas, and other generalized malignancies and disorders of the immune system; therapy that depresses resistance, such as irradiation and steroids, alkylating agents or antimetabolite therapy; severe febrile illness; immune serum globulin (ISG) administration within eight to twelve weeks; and severe egg sensitivity.

Susceptible personnel exposed to measles may be afforded some protection by live measles vaccine given shortly after exposure or by ISG (0.25 mg./kg.) given within six days after exposure (see Part II, Chapter 24). Their contact with immunosuppressed patients should be restricted for the duration of their communicable stage (from about eight days after exposure until about four days after the rash appears). If ISG is given more than three days after exposure, communicability may be sufficient to justify avoidance of contact with any susceptible person during the communicable period. Live measles vaccine should be given at least three months after ISG administration to avoid interference with the vaccine effect by residual immunoglobulin.

Meningococci
Clinically severe meningococcal infection invariably requires hospitalization and intensive medical and nursing care. There appears to be a negligible risk of disease in personnel following casual contact with sporadic meningococcal infection. Reports of apparent nosocomial transmission of meningococcal disease to personnel are rare and poorly documented [37]. No outbreaks of meningococcal disease in hospital personnel have ever been described, and there is no documentation of an increased risk of meningococcal carriage among hospital personnel who have been exposed to meningococcal disease.

In short, current understanding of meningococcal epidemiology suggests that the concern about risk to personnel from casual contact with patients has been excessive. Nasopharyngeal culture and chemoprophylaxis can be safely limited to instances of inadvertent intensive personnel contact with a patient with meningococcal disease, as that which would occur, for example, in giving mouth-to-mouth respiration. Rifampin administration is currently recommended for initial prophylaxis, although it would be reasonable to substitute a sulfonamide if the strain from the index case proves sensitive.

Mumps
Mumps is a childhood disease, but about 6 percent of reported cases occur in adults over 19 years old. As many as 20 percent of adult males with mumps may experience orchitis, and adults occasionally develop central nervous system infection. Since few infected adults require hospitalization, however, hospitalized cases of mumps would most likely be found on the pediatric service, where the risk to susceptible personnel would probably be increased. One outbreak of mumps in interns has been reported from a department of pediatrics [32]; however, an outbreak among infants in a newborn nursery elsewhere did not extend to personnel who were considered susceptible [20].

The personnel health service can explain the risk and offer mumps vaccine to pediatric patient-care and other personnel who are not presumed to be immune by history of disease or immunization. Immune status can also be determined by serology and, less reliably, by skin testing. Women should not be vaccinated if they are pregnant or likely to become pregnant within three months after vaccination.

Pertussis
Pertussis is highly communicable among unvaccinated children and is often severe or fatal in infants. Infection and morbidity are less common in adults and are usually limited to a mild respiratory illness. Outbreaks have suggested that unprotected personnel, primarily those with pediatric patient contact, may be at somewhat higher risk of infection than the general population [25].

Vaccination of persons over the age of six years has generally not been recommended, because morbidity in that age group is minimal, and febrile and neurologic complications have occurred with the standard vaccine dose. The risk of pertussis infection in any hospital personnel group, particularly pediatric staff, should be recognized, but it is probably not serious enough to warrant routine vaccination, at least until an immunizing regimen with negligible untoward reactions is available. Personnel with symptoms of infection should be restricted from duties that may pose a hazard to patients, at least until treatment is begun with erythromycin. Asymptomatic personnel who have had contact with patients presumed to have pertussis can be observed and treated if symptoms develop within the incubation period (up to 21 days). An outbreak in the hospital might dictate a more extensive screening program for carriers that employs fluorescent-antibody or culture techniques.

Plague
In recent years, sporadic human infection with *Yersinia pestis* has occurred in the southwestern United States, usually through contact with rodents and their fleas. Hospitalized patients most frequently have buboes. An accepted approach to protect personnel from spread involves the use of wound and skin precautions for suspected *Y. pestis* wound infection and the clinical observation of any person who has contact with the lesion. The temperature of the personnel in contact with plague patients should be recorded twice daily for at least a week.

Pneumonic plague is seen in a small proportion of cases. The pneumonic form is usually highly contagious, requiring strict isolation. Personnel having close respiratory contact with these patients could develop infection by the respiratory route. Personnel with such contact should have a nasopharyngeal culture specimen taken and should immediately be given tetracycline as prophylaxis for at least one week; close monitoring for the development of illness is imperative.

Routine immunization is not advised for any hospital personnel, because the frequency of intra-hospital spread is extremely low and the vaccine is too reactogenic.

Poliomyelitis
Morbidity and mortality from poliomyelitis in the United States remain quite low. Although the overall incidence of infection has been higher in children, nearly half of the paralytic cases have occurred in persons over 20 years of age. More serious cases usually enter hospitals and may expose personnel to infection. Prior to the widespread availability of effective vaccine, three isolated outbreaks of poliomyelitis among hospital personnel had been described [39]. In a more recent survey of personnel, no nosocomial secondary cases of poliomyelitis were detected, and no significant difference in serologic response was found between personnel caring for 128 patients with poliomyelitis and those caring for other patients during a one-year period.

The risk of poliomyelitis for hospital personnel may currently be no greater than for the general population. Nevertheless, at least in circumstances where the disease may still occur, it would be quite important to ensure vaccination of those few personnel who are likely to have contact with recognized or unrecognized cases. Either oral or killed vaccine can be used. When an unvaccinated person will be clearly exposed to a known case, ISG may be protective. That person should be vaccinated about three months later for more durable protection.

Rubella (German Measles)
Rubella is a rather mild exanthem seen increasingly in older children and young adults. Although the illness is unpleasant and often interferes briefly with regular activity, concern over rubella and vigorous public health efforts are directed at serious congenital rubella infection transmitted from mother to fetus early in pregnancy.

In recent years both the proportion of cases and the incidence rates have increased in persons 15 years of age and older. Approximately 20 percent of unvaccinated adults, including female nursing personnel, remain susceptible according to serologic testing [22].

Rubella, frequently unrecognized, is constantly imported into the hospital. The problem was highlighted by a recent outbreak of disease in hospital personnel, some of whom had contact with a large number of women receiving prenatal care at the hospital. In other circumstances, nosocomial transmission has occurred [8]. Exposure of pregnant employees is also a potential hazard: in another outbreak affecting hospital personnel the highest attack rates were among females of childbearing age. There has also been a study suggesting that pregnant women working with infants with congenital anomalies may themselves have been at excessive risk of bearing infants with congenital defects.

Until women who enter childbearing years are reliably rendered immune by natural infection or immunization, the need to protect susceptible women in the hospital environment will exist. Proper serologic screening of all female hospital personnel of childbearing age and vaccination of all susceptible women should ensure that no female personnel will be responsible for transmitting congenital rubella. Conversely, no susceptible pregnant woman should work in an area where contact with rubella is likely. Male personnel are equally likely to develop and transmit infection by respiratory contact and may thereby endanger pregnant women in the hospital who may be inadvertently susceptible. Consideration must also be given to vaccinating males, at least those shown to be susceptible by serology. Whereas men can be vaccinated with only notification of the relatively minor rheumatic and neurologic sequelae, women must be advised not to be vaccinated if they are pregnant and also to prevent pregnancy for at least three months after vaccination. See Part II, Chapter 24.

Any person who has an illness compatible with rubella should be excluded from the hospital environment until communicability has ceased. Paired sera can be obtained from exposed susceptible persons to determine whether infection has occurred.

Salmonellosis and Shigellosis

The problem of enteric disease in health-care institutions due to *Salmonella* and *Shigella* infection has been addressed in Part I, Chapter 7 (Food Service) and Part II, Chapter 21. However, the involvement of personnel in the acquisition and spread of these organisms deserves special attention here [5,15,33]. Data are sparse on the prevalence of asymptomatic carriers of enteric pathogens among hospital personnel and on the risks engendered by such carriage. Where infected personnel have appeared to present a risk to patients, the danger has come from those who are or have recently been ill with gastroenteritis. Even in conjunction with nosocomial outbreaks of salmonellosis [15,33], the role of the asymptomatic carrier who is frequently discovered during broad culture surveys is unclear. Regarding the risk to personnel, infectious gastroenteritis has rarely been as serious as it is for those patients whose defenses are reduced, such as the splenectomized individual.

Instruction and continued reinforcement in hygienic measures such as hand-washing and the proper handling and storage of prepared foods are of paramount importance. Screening asymptomatic personnel through periodic, routine stool cultures would be expected to detect only a small proportion of the transient carriers of enteropathogens. The detection and management of such carriage would appear to be an expensive and inefficient preventive approach; it is not recommended. Although local health regulation may require screening for carriage of *Salmonella typhosa* or other enteric pathogens among hospital food-service personnel, even this is likely to be of only marginal value.

The approach to the prevention of spread when illness does occur in the hospital should depend largely on rapidly identifying patients and personnel with gastrointestinal illness and separating them from uninfected persons by mechanical barriers (e.g., gowns and gloves for common contacts) or distance. Rectal swabs (or, preferably, stool specimens) should be taken for culture at least once from all potentially involved personnel. Repeated sampling of an individual may improve the detection of carriers. When nosocomial illness seems to be occurring among personnel, restriction of infected individuals or carriers from close interpersonal contact with others in the hospital or their temporary removal from service until culture determinations revert to negative is a reasonable means of preventing spread.

Staphylococci

Staphylococcal infection is ubiquitous and protean in its manifestations. While the involvement of personnel in relatively uncommon, coagulase-negative staphylococcal disease has not been examined in depth, the role of personnel in the spread of coagulase-positive staphylococci has received exhaustive attention. Fortunately, serious staphylococcal disease is probably no more common among hospital personnel than it is among other persons, but minor or entirely inapparent infections in personnel may represent a prime hazard to patients, and these often frustrate even the most conscientious preventive efforts.

The possibility that the patient-care worker with rather insignificant staphylococcal infection can theoretically be responsible for devastating disease has led to an emphasis in the past on the routine screening of hospital personnel for staphylococcal carriage. Epidemiologic studies, however, challenge the rationale of this approach. Up to 70 percent of adults are intermittent carriers of coagulase-positive staphylococci, and 15 percent may harbor these organisms as more-or-less continuous carriers. The intensity of individual colonization may vary. The relatively small proportion of carriers who are intermittent or persistent heavy shedders of high numbers of organisms, especially in conjunction with any overt staphylococcal disease, appear to pose the greatest threat to susceptible patients. Desquamating skin disease in a carrier may also represent a special hazard. Routine surveys of large groups of personnel are therefore usually irrelevant to immediate staphylococcal problems and inordinately inefficient (see Part II, Chapter 20).

A colonization survey would be more legitimately undertaken in response to an increased carriage rate or an unusual cluster of infections. Common sites of carriage include any draining or crusted lesion, the anterior nares, the nasopharynx and oropharynx, and the skin of the axilla, fingers, and perineum. Initially, culture specimens are taken from lesions and from both anterior nares. This survey would be directed at identifying all persons carrying a strain identical to that isolated from clinically infected patients. Antimicrobial sensitivity testing and phage typing usually narrow the potentially involved personnel to a small number, who can be related or excluded on the basis of epidemiologic information. Perineal carriage should be specifically sought when an obvious common source has eluded detection through routine culture determinations.

Implication of a hospital worker as a source of staphylococcal disease is a matter of some gravity that will demand considerable attention to that individual over time. The implicated worker cannot justifiably continue to be a member of a surgical or obstetric team or to have direct contact with high-risk patients such as premature neonates. The temporary elimination or suppression of staphylococci with topical antibacterial therapy would permit the individual to return to duties with proper arrangements for follow-up evaluation; systemic antimicrobial therapy by itself will not reliably eliminate nasal staphylococci. Recurrent or persistent carriage in such personnel may require retreatment, modifications in personal hygiene (e.g., frequent bathing with soap containing hexachlorophene or another antimicrobial), or other techniques to characterize and interrupt dissemination. Details of these approaches can be found in other publications [19,40].

Streptococci

Streptococcal infections are as ubiquitous and variable as those produced by staphylococci (see previous section). In terms of hospital epidemiology, the two classes of infection also have many analogous features. While strains from all streptococcal serologic groups may cause infection from time to time, strains from groups A and B are the more important pathogens that potentially involve hospital personnel. Streptococci are carried principally on the superficial epithelial tissues in a large proportion of health persons and would not be expected to cause more than minor inflammatory disease in those so colonized. These minor infections can, however, be transmitted to patients and result in more serious disease. Sporadic outbreaks of nosocomial streptococcal infection have been traced to carriers among personnel and have stimulated extensive routine microbiologic screening. Such routine screening is not recommended, however, just as it is not recommended in searching for staphylococcal carriage. Epidemiologic investigation should focus attention on the small number of personnel who are likely to be related to clinical infection. If signs of significant skin, nasal, or pharyngeal carriage are absent and if circumstances point to a common source, then vaginal, perineal, and rectal carriage must be sought.

Concern has grown over the possibility of nosocomial spread of serious group B streptococcal infections in neonates [16,26]. Active study of the epidemiology of these infections to date has suggested that maternal colonization is a significant source. Another sizable proportion of infections may well follow passive spread from infant to infant. A carrier state in patients and personnel has been documented. Nevertheless, an increased risk for neonates from prolonged carriage among personnel has not been established. Preventive efforts should focus on physical measures to interrupt transmission, unless a single worker draws suspicion as a result of epidemiologic investigation. A worker implicated because of a lesion or as a disseminator should receive antimicrobial therapy that is effective against streptococcal colonization during his or her temporary removal from patient-care duties. Careful follow-up of such a carrier also is recommended.

Tetanus

Most of the nearly 200 cases of tetanus in the United States each year occur in persons who do not have a clear history of recent immunization. Because the disease is often severe or fatal, virtually all affected persons in this country are hospitalized. Outside the United States, nosocomial acquisition has been encountered. Nevertheless, there are no documented instances of person-to-person transmission, nor is there reason to suspect there is a risk to hospital personnel beyond that of self-infection, as in other persons.

Surveys have disclosed inadequate protection against tetanus in more than one-third of the hospital personnel sampled. As with diphtheria, it is well accepted that hospital personnel along with all other persons should be fully immunized through primary immunization when there

is no history of previous disease or immunization, and booster doses of toxoid, usually in combination with diphtheria toxoid, are recommended for all persons not immunized within the preceding ten years. Tetanus toxoid should also be given to anyone who incurs more than a clean, minor wound five or more years beyond the last booster dose.

Tuberculosis

The incidence of tuberculosis has declined steadily over the years in the United States; in 1977 approximately 30,000 new active and reactive cases were reported. Manifestations can vary from inapparent infection to aggressive pulmonary or systemic illness. Known cases often require hospitalization; others enter hospitals for different reasons, the tuberculous infection remaining unidentified or unexpressed clinically. These potentially communicable tuberculous infections constitute a hazard for hospital personnel as well as for other patients (see Part II, Chapter 15).

Surveys of risk to hospital personnel have generally focused on tuberculosis and tuberculin reactivity in house staff, nursing personnel, and medical and nursing students, for whom the risk is presumably the greatest.

Few published surveys of annual skin-test conversion rates in hospital personnel have been rigorous enough in their design or representative enough in their selection of populations to be generally applicable. Conversion rates have varied from less than 1 percent to 5 percent or higher [3,4,23,29]. Furthermore, it is difficult to determine from published studies just how much of the risk is due solely to occupational exposure. One noncontrolled study [4] indicated that a proportion of new tuberculosis cases in personnel developed from infection acquired prior to the inception of the study and probably outside the hospital environment. On the other hand, a recent report from another institution [14] illustrated well the value of thorough surveillance. Although the overall annual conversion rate in this institution was only about 0.5 percent for all hospital personnel and students, those who had contact with patients with tuberculosis were clearly identified as a high-risk group by a conversion rate that was more than six times that found in personnel and students with no known contact. The tuberculosis control program described in this report included elements for confirming a suspected high-risk situation and for initiating prompt and effective preventive measures.

The most widely accepted approach to the care of personnel in health-care facilities follows the recommendations for surveillance and control in the general population issued jointly by the American Thoracic Society, the American Lung Association, and CDC [2], and those of the *Guidelines for Prevention of TB Transmission in Hospitals* [36]. These published resources should be consulted along with standard references for details regarding the evaluation and management of persons at risk for tuberculosis. Skin testing with tuberculin to determine whether infection has occurred at some time in the past should be performed on every employee prior to assumption of duties. The interpretation of skin-test results should take into account factors that may influence reactivity, such as the possibility of a "booster" effect from recent tuberculin testing or cross-reactivity due to atypical mycobacterial infection.

Personnel who are reactive at the time of their preemployment examination or following the assumption of duties should be evaluated medically and epidemiologically and managed according to the guidelines summarized below. Tuberculin-positive personnel should have a chest roentgenogram to determine the presence, extent, and activity of pulmonary tuberculosis.

Personnel discovered to have active tuberculosis should be isolated until effective treatment has diminished their infectivity, and they should be managed just as other persons with active disease. Careful culture documentation of noncommunicability should precede their return to patient contact if conscientious compliance with the chemotherapeutic regimen is in doubt.

Isoniazid (INH) should be given in the following priority to personnel with:

1. recent intimate or extensive contact with untreated tuberculous disease;
2. new positive skin test, positive roentgenogram, negative sputum bacteriologic examination, and no history of adequate treatment;
3. new infection (tuberculin reaction increased by at least 6 mm. from less than 10 mm. to greater than 10 mm. induration within the past two years);
4. high risk because of immunosuppressive or prolonged corticosteroid therapy, reticuloendothelial neoplasm, diabetes, silicosis, or gastrectomy; or
5. positive skin tests if they are under 35 years of age and previously untreated.

The duration of INH use will vary according to individual circumstances. The need to continue prophylaxis in personnel with close contact with tuberculous patients can be determined with a tuberculin test about 10 to 12 weeks after such hazardous contact is broken. Regularly scheduled skin testing can then be resumed for the individual whose tuberculin tests remain negative, although occasionally a late converter may still require preventive therapy.

In addition, if personnel are in continued close contact with children, immunodeficient patients, or others whose susceptibility to more serious tuberculous infection is great, then standard preventive therapy might be justified for previously untreated tuberculin reactors over 35 years of age who would not otherwise be given therapy. Reactors who are not given chemotherapy should be followed with roentgenograms every 6 to 12 months and monitored closely for symptoms of tuberculosis.

In the absence of unusually high risk, personnel who are nonreactive to tuberculin should be retested regularly at an interval appropriate to their risk of infection (e.g., 12 months, or even longer in institutions where active pulmonary tuberculosis is encountered infrequently). Some effort can also be made to reduce contact. Whenever it is consistent with good medical care, hospitals can avoid assignment of tuberculin-negative personnel to areas where exposure to communicable tuberculosis is highly likely.

Authoritative opinion divides [1,2,11,30, 35,36] over advocacy of immunoprophylaxis for hospital personnel with the attenuated mycobacterial strain, BCG (bacillus Calmette-

Guerin). The controversy centers around the efficacy of vaccination versus other modes of prevention and the uncertain cost-efficiency of administering the alternative control programs. The joint recommendations on tuberculosis in the United States by the American Thoracic Society, the American Lung Association, and CDC do not endorse BCG vaccination of any hospital personnel [11]. The American Hospital Association has recently designated a 1 percent annual conversion rate as a signal for a given hospital to contemplate vaccinating personnel [1]. However, familiarity with the use of BCG, thorough knowledge of recent community and hospital experience with tuberculous infection, clear delineation of high-risk subgroups among personnel, and firmly established mechanisms for surveillance during and even beyond employment in the hospital must precede consideration of BCG vaccination. For the vast majority of hospitals in the United States, the current frequency of tuberculous infection in personnel seldom, if ever, calls for immunization. In the end, whatever approach is taken, compulsive attention to the details of surveillance and administration is probably the primary determinant of success.

Varicella-Zoster

Varicella-zoster (V-Z) virus is highly communicable, leading to high attack rates of exanthematous chickenpox among healthy, susceptible children. A small proportion of adults have escaped even asymptomatic childhood varicella and remain susceptible. A reliable serologic test to identify susceptible individuals is not widely available; immunity is usually presumed to be present when there is a clear history of chickenpox or of intensive household contact with chickenpox. Complications such as pneumonia and encephalitis are probably more frequent in adults. More serious infection also occurs in patients whose susceptibility is enhanced by immunosuppression due to reticuloendothelial malignancy or chemotherapy.

Patients with such enhanced susceptibility and, less frequently, healthy adults may develop zosteriform infection that is presumably due to reactivation of latent virus but perhaps occasionally to exogenous infection. Thus, certain patients and personnel who are present in the hospital (usually for other reasons) may harbor communicable V-Z virus or may be at increased risk of new infection. It is worth stressing here that no person who may have or may be incubating V-Z virus infection should enter a hospital unnecessarily.

Susceptible patient-care personnel may acquire or transmit infection through patient contact. The appearance of an exanthem compatible with V-Z virus infection in any person in the hospital environment should activate an established mechanism for locating and protecting susceptible patients and personnel who have had close contact with the affected person. Additionally, the original affected person should immediately be isolated or be removed from the hospital environment when possible. Optimally executed isolation of known cases in the hospital should minimize direct person-to-person spread (Part I, Chapter 9). Since the virus may be shed as early as the seventh day of the incubation period, healthy susceptible personnel with known exposure who may be incubating V-Z virus infection should subsequently abstain from patient contact, at least with those who would be expected to tolerate V-Z infection poorly. They can return to duties after clinical varicella has subsided or the maximum incubation period (at least 21 days) has elapsed without sign of illness.

Susceptible personnel caring for known cases have transmitted their nosocomial infection to their susceptible family contacts. When possible, healthy personnel whose history indicates susceptibility should probably avoid contact with even well-isolated cases of varicella. Susceptible personnel at high risk because of predisposing conditions would wisely exclude themselves from the care of pediatric patients in general, as well as of other patients likely to carry communicable V-Z virus.

Standard human immune serum globulin may attenuate illness in healthy susceptible personnel who are accidentally exposed, but its use is not strongly recommended. High-risk, susceptible personnel who are accidentally exposed should receive zoster immune plasma or zoster immunoglobulin, should the latter become more widely available (Table 3-1).

Table 3-1. Guidelines for Immunizations[a]

Disease or agent	Immunization guideline[b]	Other recommendations for management of personnel
Diphtheria	All personnel should be immunized with diphtheria toxoid, primary or booster, depending on history.	Culture tests should be done on case contacts; those with positive tests should be relieved of duty and treated until throat culture is negative.
Hepatitis A	Persons with direct oral or parenteral contact should receive ISG.	Personnel with suspected disease should be relieved from duty at the time of rising and peak hepatic enzyme levels, development of jaundice, or both and for up to 2 or 3 weeks thereafter, although communicability may wane earlier.
Hepatitis B	Persons with parenteral contact and inadvertent oral contact with infected secretions or excretions should receive hepatitis B immunoglobulin.[c] Administration of standard ISG is currently advocated by some.	(See text.)
Influenza	Personnel in high-risk categories, those exposed to high-risk patients, and those whose unexpected absence would affect the quality of service significantly should be considered for vaccination. Each hospital can formulate a policy individually.	Appropriate precautions against spread of respiratory infection may include restriction of personnel with symptoms from patient-care responsibilities.
Measles	All personnel susceptible by history or serology, especially pediatric personnel and women of childbearing age, should be protected.[d] Susceptible individuals with case contact can be given standard ISG (see text).	None
Meningococcal infection	None	Chemoprophylaxis should be reserved for personnel with intensive respiratory contact, e.g., as in mouth-to-mouth resuscitation of a patient presumed to have disease.
Mumps	All pediatric-care personnel susceptible by history should be offered mumps vaccine.[d]	None
Pertussis	None[e]	Asymptomatic case contacts should be observed during the incubation period and treated if symptoms develop; personnel with symptoms should be relieved from duty, at least in pediatric-care areas, until effective treatment is underway.
Poliomyelitis	At least those personnel likely to have contact with poliomyelitis patients should receive polio vaccine.[b] Susceptible individuals with case contact can be given standard ISG (see text).	None

Table 3-1 (Continued)

Disease or agent	Immunization guideline[b]	Other recommendations for management of personnel
Rubella	Women of childbearing age susceptible by hemagglutination inhibition antibody determination should be given rubella vaccine.[d] Susceptibility and vaccination of male personnel who have frequent contact with women in early pregnancy should be considered.	Contact between cases and potentially pregnant women should be prevented; paired sera should be taken from exposed, susceptible pregnant women and implications of seroconversion should be reviewed with them. A single preexposure or early postexposure specimen may be useful.
Tetanus	All personnel should be immunized with tetanus toxoid, primary or booster, depending on history.	None
Tuberculosis	BCG is not recommended for use under current conditions among hospital personnel in the United States.	A detailed control program is advised (see text).
Varicella-zoster	Exposed personnel in high-risk categories should receive zoster immunoglobulin[c] or zoster immune plasma.	Susceptible personnel should avoid contact with even well-isolated cases; susceptible individuals with case contact should suspend patient-care duties after the seventh day of the incubation period. Susceptible persons should also be advised of the continuing hazard to them from pediatric patient care.

[a] See text for detailed discussions.
[b] Current Advisory Committee on Immunization Practices recommendations should be consulted.
[c] As effective agent becomes available.
[d] Pregnancy is a contraindication and must be prevented for at least 3 months after vaccination.
[e] Infrequency and mildness of pertussis in adults makes currently available vaccine unnecessary.

Personnel Health Services

Nosocomial infection should represent a major concern of comprehensive occupational health services for hospital personnel. Personnel health services should reflect that concern in a clear definition of purposes and functions, in professional staffing, and in administrative relationships with other units and services.*

* Risks involving persons with casual or intermittent contact with the hospital are generally difficult to establish. Insofar as volunteers and visitors in hospitals have exposure to patients comparable in quality, intensity, and duration to that of hospital personnel, reasonable efforts should be made to apprise them of their responsibilities in the area of infection control and to protect them appropriately from nosocomial hazards. Women who may be in the early months of pregnancy, for example, can be warned of the hazards of CMV, herpesvirus, rubella, and other congenital infections (see previous sections). Adherence to isolation procedures and proper hand-washing are important factors in reducing transmission.

Purposes

In the realm of nosocomial infection control, the general purposes of personnel health services include:

1. evaluation of the health of new personnel as it might relate to them, to their work, and to patients;
2. periodic reevaluation of the health of active-duty personnel as it relates to their work, as well as evaluation as required by their symptoms or exposure to an infectious hazard;
3. recommendation and provision of appropriate immunizations, chemotherapy, or both;
4. maintenance of immunization and other records pertinent to occupational health of current and former personnel;
5. education and reeducation of prospective and active-duty personnel in recognizing

and protecting against potential occupational hazards to patients, to the other personnel, to themselves, and to their families;

6. assurance that personnel receive adequate medical care for health problems resulting from occupational hazards; and

7. contribution of facilities, records, and staff to investigations of health problems resulting from occupational hazards.

Staffing

The professional staff and the medical and administrative machinery needed to perform health-service functions will obviously vary from one hospital to another. Health services should be accessible. A hospital health service organized to fulfill infection control functions (detailed below) as part of a more comprehensive occupational health-care program should consider employing one physician working regularly at least part-time and one registered nurse working full-time during routine business hours. In addition, one or more knowledgeable physicians or nurses could be designated to be available at all other times for consultation and to arrange provision of essential services in specific situations. The number of personnel served and the extent of the services offered would determine the additional staffing needs. Where a hospital is committing significant resources to personnel health, physicians and nurses with some demonstrated interest—if not background and experience in occupational or preventive medicine—and those familiar with the problems of the hospital and its workers would obviously be the most appropriate candidates for staff. The often casual, occasionally disinterested attitude traditionally held by medical personnel toward prevention of infection and even toward their own health [18] makes paramount the appointment of individuals firmly oriented to the kind of preventive health care outlined in this chapter.

Policies

Probably more crucial than the orientation or training of those appointed to operate the health service is the development of relevant personnel health policies and procedures. Their successful institution depends on coordinating representatives of the Infection Control Committee, the personnel health service, the hospital administration, patient-care staff, and other employees. These representatives should be encouraged to recommend policy and to offer criticism, suggestions, and regular reassessment of policies. It is worth reemphasizing the importance of integrating overlapping infection control and personnel health activities.

Codification of personnel health routines should minimize the confusion and disagreement likely to result from unfamiliarity with health service functions. Naturally, not all problems can be anticipated. Many essential screening and preventive measures can be enumerated explicitly, however, and simple standards can be formulated for the management of potential occupational hazards. As long as the policies in force are subject to timely reevaluation and revision, the disadvantage of such standardization should be outweighed by the efficient, consistent performance of personnel health service functions.

Policies should cover at least the functions discussed below:

1. preemployment medical evaluation,
2. medical reevaluation and health maintenance,
3. immunizations,
4. intercurrent illness,
5. investigation, and
6. education and reeducation.

It is obvious that certain infectious risks are more frequent or more serious than others and that surveillance and preventive techniques for some infections are safer, more effective, easier, or less expensive than they are for others. Each hospital should take these factors into account when establishing priorities for its own personnel health service. However, principles in two policy areas are worth mentioning explicitly. First, since women of childbearing age constitute a significant segment of the patient-care and other personnel in hospitals, the general hazards of infection and of immunization with live virus vaccines during pregnancy should be recognized and discussed prior to employment. Second, it should be appreciated that personnel represent a "vehicle" between the hospital and the community. Relatively insignificant infections—such as those of the respiratory tract or the skin acquired inside or outside of the hospital—may have consequences of far greater magnitude for patients whose defenses are impaired as well as for other personnel whose duties may have to be interrupted. Conversely, personnel may carry infections such as tuberculosis, hepatitis, or varicella-zoster out of the hospital and into their immediate community environment. The decision to restrict or remove a worker from patient-care activities should, in the end, be based not simply on the worker's own state of health, but also on the potential effects of the specific infection in the worker's particular hospital or community setting. These principles relate to an even more fundamental one: some consideration can and should be given to known risks and to individual susceptibility when personnel are being assigned to areas where such risks prevail.

Preemployment Medical Evaluation
Detailed recommendations for general preventive health care are beyond the scope of this discussion. For the purposes of infection control, each prospective worker would be evaluated according to the duties to be assumed. Certain procedures—tuberculin testing or rubella antibody screening, for example—may be desirable for certain large groups of patient-care personnel in all classes of work (and even volunteers) whose duties involve frequent and direct patient contact. The tasks of the health service can be simplified if applicants provide all current and future information, directly or through records from a personal physician, regarding:

1. personal and family history relevant to significant past and current infections, to conditions predisposing to infection, and to their management;
2. previous or current physical findings relevant to those infections or predisposing conditions;
3. previous relevant diagnostic studies, prophylaxis, or therapy for particular infections; and
4. immunizations.

Attention should be directed specifically toward acute or chronic cutaneous, gastrointestinal, cardiovascular, and respiratory infections; hepatitis; tuberculosis; diabetes; and malignancy and other immunodeficient states.

The hospital health service can usually complete the history and physical examination and obtain laboratory studies on personnel for whom reliable results are not available from another physician. A tuberculin skin test, a chest roentgenogram, and, in appropriate circumstances, serologic tests for syphilis, rubella, measles, and hepatitis B should be included unless obviated by carefully documented records or previous studies. Appropriate immunizations are discussed in the previous sections on the individual diseases. Current knowledge dictates that applicants for work in hemodialysis, oral and other surgery, blood banks, hematology laboratories, and other positions involving frequent contact with blood products be considered for serologic testing for HB_sAg and anti-HB_s. Routine preemployment culture determinations for dietary or patient-care personnel are not recommended. The personnel health service can comply with local or state health department requirements for screening for enteric pathogens, without allowing extensive screening to divert attention from the more important aspects of preemployment evaluation.

Medical Reevaluation and Health Maintenance
A brief reevaluation by a personal physician or the personnel health service at appropriately frequent intervals should assure that any new finding potentially pertinent to the transmission of nosocomial infection will become part of the employee's health record. It may also be used to remind the employee that the prompt reporting of illness and of certain exposures may help protect both patients and personnel.

More specifically, the status of certain personnel should be reassessed with regard to the following:

1. tuberculin sensitivity (see previous section on tuberculosis),
2. hepatitis B antigen (or antibody) carriage (see section on hepatitis B), and
3. Immunizations (see sections on individual diseases).

It may simplify the hospital's preventive efforts to make pregnancy testing of female personnel available upon request.

Intercurrent Personnel Illness
Early detection and reporting of infectious disease in personnel as well as in patients are at the foundation of nosocomial infection control. A well-planned and executed policy would both motivate and require workers in designated positions to report even minor symptoms of infection to the personnel health service as early as possible. Making services available to personnel from any work shift is one example of means to that end. Motivation and requirements should be especially strong for personnel caring for newborns, obstetric and intensive-care patients, and other patients with impaired host defenses.

Optimal safeguard of patients and personnel calls for prompt evaluation and administrative action for recent or current (1) fever or chills; (2) acute skin eruption; (3) purulent drainage; (4) jaundice; (5) sore throat; (6) productive cough; (7) "flu" syndrome; (8) diarrhea; (9) exposure of a susceptible individual to designated infection such as rubella, chickenpox, hepatitis, or tuberculosis; and (10) immunization with live virus vaccine such as vaccinia or oral poliovirus vaccine.

When the presence of infection is suspected or established, it may be important to consider the possibility of nosocomial acquisition and its implications. Depending on the clinical evaluation and the duties of the person involved, the health service can recommend his or her removal from service, judicious restriction of his or her activity, or the imposition of extra precautions as may be necessary to minimize the risk.

Personnel with relatively mild infections (e.g., herpesvirus, influenza, certain bacterial infections, or hepatitis) who continue working during the communicable stages may represent a double hazard. They may transmit infection to their co-workers, thereby potentially extending illness and absenteeism among "essential" personnel, or they may expose susceptible high-risk patients to more severe illness. Sound epidemiologic and clinical judgment of the risk should prevail over arbitrary administrative and minor financial deterrents. Mandatory reporting of symptoms and interruption of duties for any legitimate occupational health problem, as in other industries, should be accompanied by a guarantee against penalties imposed by means of loss of wages, benefits, and job status. Notification of the return of personnel to duties could be helpful when the resumption of duties was not prearranged with the health service, for example, when it depends on a private physician's examination or laboratory report.

Management of personnel illness will depend in large part on the precise arrangements the individual worker may have for his medical care. Where the hospital assumes responsibility, arrangements for group coverage through the hospital should be simple enough that personnel will seek desirable care, particularly for commonly acquired infections.

Immunization
General immunization recommendations are made officially by the U.S. Public Health Service Advisory Committee on Immunization Practices and are published periodically in the *Morbidity and Mortality Weekly Report.* Table 3-1 (see p. 46) summarizes guidelines for immunizations that should be considered for certain hospital patient-care personnel. In each case, specific guidelines and the rationale for active or passive immunizations of hospital personnel other than laboratory personnel have been presented in detail earlier in the separate sections on each disease. Immunizations for laboratory personnel are considered later (see Part I, Chapter 7, The Clinical Laboratory).

Investigations
In hospitals with active infection control and personnel health programs, the health service should have the administrative authority and the logistic capability to contribute to the investigation of suspected problems of employee nosocomial infections. Although the hospital epidemiologist or infection control officer would normally direct the investigation, assistance from the health service may take such forms as providing selective record reviews, determining the location of exposed, susceptible persons,

communicating with personnel and their physicians, performing diagnostic screening procedures, coordinating prophylactic intervention, and preparing prospective surveys. As with intercurrent illness, any interruption of duties necessitated by a risk from or to personnel that is discovered in the course of any screening program or investigation should be accompanied by a guarantee against loss of wages, benefits, or job status.

Education

Practical instruction in infection control for employees depends on motivation, repetition, and reinforcement. The personnel health service has a unique opportunity to initiate these processes even before the employee's hospital duties are assumed. The preemployment evaluation can be used in part to provide personnel with both oral and written guidance about their role in the prevention of nosocomial infections. Advantage can likewise be taken of the continued periodic contact that personnel should automatically have with the health service. Advice, instruction, and constructive criticism in the context of concern about the worker's own health may be received more positively than that given by a supervisor to a subordinate. Helpful suggestions by the health service about avoiding illness or bringing it promptly to medical attention could also be presented to personnel privately, if appropriate, as an effort to avert any embarrassing publicity about personal health and hygiene that might be prompted by the belated discovery of an infection.

References

1. American Hospital Association. Guidelines on tuberculosis control programs for hospital employees. *Hospitals* 44:57, 1975.
2. American Thoracic Society. Preventive therapy of tuberculous infection. *Am. Rev. Respir. Dis.* 110:371, 1974.
3. Ashley, M. J., and Wigle, W. D. The epidemiology of active tuberculosis in hospital employees in Ontario, 1966–69. *Am. Rev. Respir. Dis.* 104:851, 1971.
4. Atuk, N., and Hunt, E. H. Serial tuberculin testing and isoniazid therapy in general hospital employees. *J.A.M.A.* 218:1795, 1971.
5. Baine, W. B., and Gangarosa, E. J. Institu-

tional salmonellosis. *J. Infect. Dis.* 128:357, 1973.
6. Bryan, J. A., Carr, H. E., and Gregg, M. B. An outbreak of non-parenterally transmitted hepatitis B. *J.A.M.A.* 223:279, 1973.
7. Burk, R. D., Schaffner, W., and Koenig, M. G. Severe influenza virus pneumonia in the pandemic of 1968–69. *Arch. Intern. Med.* 127:1122, 1971.
8. Carne, S., Dewhurst, C. J., and Hurley, R. Rubella epidemic in a maternity unit. *Br. Med. J.* 1:444, 1973.
9. Center for Disease Control. Influenza—Arizona, New York City, Ohio. *Morbid. Mortal. Weekly Rep.* 24:40, 1975.
10. Center for Disease Control. Perspectives on the control of viral hepatitis, type B. *Morbid. Mortal. Weekly Rep.* 25 (Suppl.):1, 1976.
11. Center for Disease Control. Recommendation of the Public Health Service Advisory Committee on Immunization Practices. BCG vaccines. *Morbid. Mortal. Weekly Rep.* 24:69, 1975.
12. Center for Disease Control. Recommendation of the Public Health Service Advisory Committee on Immunization Practices: influenza vaccine. *Morbid. Mortal. Weekly Rep.* 27:285, 1978.
13. Christensen, P. E., Schmidt, H., Bang, H. O., Anderson, V., Jordal, B., and Jensen, O. An epidemic of measles in southern Greenland, 1951: measles in virgin soil. II. *Acta Med. Scand.* 144:430, 1953.
14. Craven, R. B., Wenzel, R. P., and Atuk, N. O. Minimizing tuberculosis risk to hospital personnel and students exposed to unsuspected disease. *Ann. Intern. Med.* 82:628, 1975.
15. Datta, N., and Pridie, R. B. An outbreak of infection with *Salmonella typhimurium* in a general hospital. *J. Hyg.* (London) 58:229, 1958.
16. Franciosa, R. A., Knostman, J. D., and Zimmerman, R. A. Group B streptococcal neonatal and infant infections. *J. Pediatr.* 82:707, 1973.
17. Grob, P. J., and Moeschlin, P. Risk to contacts of a medical practitioner carrying HS$_s$Ag. *N. Engl. J. Med.* 293:197, 1975.
18. Heller, R. J., Robertson, L. S., and Alpert, J. J. Health care of house officers: a comparative study. *N. Engl. J. Med.* 277:907, 1967.
19. Herbiter, D. T., and Baker, C. E. Control of staphylococcal carriers in the hospital. *Public Health Rep.* 82:329, 1967.
20. Ikeda, S., Chiba, S., Chiba, Y., and Nakao, T. Epidemiological, clinical, and serological studies on epidemic of mumps in an infant nursery. *Tohoku J. Exp. Med.* 105:327, 1971.
21. Joint Commission on Accreditation of Hos-

pitals. *Accreditation Manual for Hospitals.* Chicago: Joint Commission on Accreditation of Hospitals, 1976.

22. Lerman, S. J., Lerman, L. M., Nankervis, G. A., and Gold, E. Accuracy of rubella history. *Ann. Intern. Med.* 74:97, 1971.

23. Levine, I. Tuberculosis risk in students of nursing. *Arch. Intern. Med.* 121:545, 1968.

24. Lewis, T. L., Alter, J. H., Chalmers, T. C., Holland, P. V., Purcell, R. H., Alling, D. W., Young, D., Frenkel, L. D., Lee, S. L., and Lamson, M. E. A comparison of the frequency of hepatitis B antigen and antibody in hospital and non-hospital personnel. *N. Engl. J. Med.* 289:647, 1973.

25. Linnemann, C. C., Jr., Ramundo, N., Perlstein, P. H., Minton, S. D., and Englender, G. .S. Use of pertussis vaccine in an outbreak involving hospital staff. *Lancet* 2:540, 1975.

26. MacKnight, J. E., Ellis, P. J., Jensen, K. A., and Franz, B. Group B streptococci in neonatal deaths. *Appl. Microbiol.* 17:926, 1969.

27. Nahmias, A. J., and Roizman, B. Infection with herpes-simplex viruses 1 and 2. *N. Engl. J. Med.* 289:667, 719, and 781, 1973.

28. Rosato, F. E., Rosato, E. F., and Plotkin, S. A. Herpetic paronychia—An occupational hazard of medical personnel. *N. Engl. J. Med.* 283:804, 1970.

29. Sartwell, P. E. Tuberculin sensitivity of physicians. *Am. Rev. Respir. Dis.* 82:731, 1960.

30. Smith, D. T. Isoniazid prophylaxis and BCG vaccination in the control of tuberculosis: high risk groups. *Arch. Environ. Health* 23:235, 1971.

31. Stern, H., Elek, S. D., Millar, D. M., and Anderson, H. F. Herpetic whitlow: a form of cross-infection in hospitals. *Lancet* 2:871, 1959.

32. St. Geme, J. W., Jr. Susceptibility of medical students to mumps: dubious value of currently available skin test antigens. *Pediatrics* 49:314, 1972.

33. Sweeney, F. J., Jr., and Randall, E. L. Clinical and Epidemiological Studies of *Salmonella derby* Infections in a General Hospital. In *Proceedings of National Conference on Salmonellosis: March 11–13, 1964.* U.S. Department of Health, Education, and Welfare, Public Health Service. Washington, D.C.: U.S. Government Printing Office (Publ. No. 1262), 1965, pp. 130–139.

34. Syndman, D. R., Bryan, J. A., and Dixon, R. E. Prevention of nosocomial viral hepatitis, type B (hepatitis B). *Ann. Intern. Med.* 83:838, 1975.

35. Tuberculin testing in hospital staff (editorial). *Br. Med. J.* 3:592, 1977.

36. U.S. Department of Health, Education, and Welfare, Public Health Service, Center for Disease Control, Atlanta, Georgia. *Guidelines for Prevention of TB Transmission in Hospitals.* 1975.

37. U.S. Department of Health, Education, and Welfare, Public Health Service, Center for Disease Control, Atlanta, Georgia. *National Nosocomial Infections Study, Fourth Quarter 1971.* 1972, pp. 19–23.

38. Vaisrub, S. Hepatitis B—Traffic in the dentist's office. *J.A.M.A.* 232:1270, 1975.

39. Wehrle, P. F. The risk of poliomyelitis infection among exposed hospital personnel. *Pediatrics* 17:237, 1956.

40. Williams, J. D., Waltho, C. A., Ayliffe, G. A. J., and Lowbury, E. J. L. Trials of five antibacterial creams in the control of nasal carriage of *Staphylococcus aureus.* *Lancet* 2:390, 1967.

41. Williams, S. V., Huff, J. C., Feinglass, E. J., Gregg, M. B., Hatch, M. H., and Matsen, J. M. Epidemic viral hepatitis, type B, in hospital personnel. *Am. J. Med.* 57:904, 1974.

4

Surveillance of Nosocomial Infections

Robert C. Aber and John V. Bennett

Surveillance

Surveillance, when applied to disease, may be defined as the systematic, active, ongoing observation of the occurrence and distribution of disease within a population and of the events or conditions that increase or decrease the risk of such disease occurrence. The term implies that the observational data are regularly analyzed and disseminated to those individuals who need to know them in order to take appropriate actions.

Surveillance of disease should be a continuous process that consists of the following elements: (1) defining the events to be surveyed as concisely and precisely as possible, (2) collecting the relevant data in a systematic way, (3) consolidating or tabulating the data collected into meaningful arrangements, (4) analyzing and interpreting the data, and (5) disseminating the data and interpretations to those who need to know them.

Some individuals would argue that surveillance implies more than the monitoring of infections and that taking appropriate actions based upon analysis and interpretation of the data is also entailed in the concept. We prefer that such actions be considered "infection control efforts" rather than surveillance activities.

Uses of Surveillance

INHERENT SCIENTIFIC VALUE. Surveillance may be of purely scientific value in the absence of planned actions for infection control. Systematic observation of natural phenomena is the foundation of the inductive process that is responsible for many scientific breakthroughs in describing fundamental natural relationships. Although surveillance simply for the sake of surveillance may be useful, we feel it is essential that the surveillance of infection in the hospital be used to control infections within individual hospitals and, by sharing surveillance information, within all hospitals.

AUGMENTING CONTROL EFFORTS. A program of infection control that does not incorporate surveillance (i.e., control without surveillance) is difficult to defend. One might argue that as long as the control program has incorporated the most up-to-date information available about infection control, surveillance is unnecessary, since nothing more can be done anyway. The opportunity for early detection of outbreaks, however, especially when an unrecognized common source is at fault, would be greatly compromised in the absence of baseline surveillance data. Furthermore, such programs are poorly equipped to assess the effectiveness of old control measures and to develop and establish the effectiveness of new measures; they are dependent upon those hospitals that conduct surveillance for up-to-date information on infection control.

IDENTIFYING PROBLEMS. A hospital infection surveillance program, then, provides a mechanism to collect and analyze hospital infection information in an orderly manner, primarily for the use of those individuals charged with the prevention and control of such infections. Surveillance is required for determining baseline information about the frequency and type of endemic infections occurring in a hospital so endemic problems and upward deviations from this baseline (i.e., hyperendemic or epidemic problems) can be recognized and investigated. Appropriate control measures may then be instituted with minimal morbidity to both patients and hospital personnel and with minimal time delay. Furthermore, significant changes in the baseline rates can be used in evaluating the effects of new control measures or patient-care practices.

REINFORCING PREVENTION PRACTICES. Surveillance data can also be utilized as a continuing reminder to medical and nursing personnel of the importance of adhering to the details of good infection control practices that are often deleted or diluted in the drudgery of daily routine. Washing one's hands is a good example of such a practice, and evidence of an increasing incidence of cross-infection may provide the motivation necessary to encourage optimal hand-washing techniques.

SATISFYING STANDARDS. The Joint Committee of Accreditation of Hospitals [2] has recently revised its interpretation of Standards dealing with the infection control program, and

it currently directs each Infection Control Committee to develop a practical surveillance system for reporting, evaluating, and keeping records of infections among patients and hospital personnel in order to provide an indication of the endemic level of all nosocomial infections, to identify the sources of infections, and to determine epidemic or potentially epidemic situations. The implications of this statement should be clear.

Elements of Surveillance
Collecting the Data

DEFINING EVENTS TO BE SURVEYED. It is of utmost importance in developing a surveillance system to define carefully those events to be surveyed and then to apply the accepted definitions systematically in the data-collecting process. In attempting to understand the relationship between urinary tract infection and urinary catheterization, for example, it is necessary first to define or establish criteria to decide what will be called a "urinary tract infection" and what will be considered "urinary catheterization." Once the event to be surveyed has been defined as concisely and precisely as possible and the criteria for determining its presence or absence have been established, then it is imperative that these definitions and criteria be applied systematically and uniformly henceforth. Ideally, all members of the population judged at risk for the occurrence of the event would be systematically and continuously assessed for the presence or absence of the properties specified by the criteria that define the event or the infection being sought.

The Center for Disease Control (CDC) has published guidelines for determining the presence and classification of infection [1]. These guidelines are not rigorous definitions of disease, but rather they serve as practical, operational guidelines for most hospitals, regardless of their size or medical sophistication.

It is also important that consistent criteria be used in determining the service to which a patient belongs. The service to which the patient was assigned at the time of acquisition of the infection should be used. If this determination is not possible, then the patient should be assigned to the service on which he or she resided at the time of onset of the infection.

ROLE OF THE INFECTION CONTROL NURSE. A number of methods of collecting infection data have been described in the literature. In general, the most satisfactory and practical method at present employs a person (or persons), often called the infection control officers (ICO) or infection control nurses (ICN), who are hired specifically to collect surveillance data as part of their duties. Details of the qualifications, functions, and responsibilities of the ICN were given previously (Part I, Chapter 3). The ICN is responsible to the Infection Control Committee and should be under the immediate supervision of the hospital epidemiologist. The choice of a nurse to fill this position has been primarily based upon her or his professional training and ability to interact primarily with other nursing personnel in the data-collection process, but experience has shown that persons other than nurses can also function well in this capacity. One ICN can conduct surveillance of about 250 acute-disease hospital beds and have sufficient remaining time for other duties and responsibilities.

MINIMAL DATA TO COLLECT ABOUT INFECTIONS. The precise information collected in conjunction with each infection may vary according to the institution, service, site of infection, or causative agent. Certain essential identifying data, however, can be recommended: the names, ages, sex, hospital identification numbers, ward or location within the hospital and service, and dates of admission of the infected patients; the date of onset of the infection; the site of infection; the organism or organisms isolated in culture studies; and the antimicrobial susceptibility pattern of the organisms isolated. Additional information should be collected only if it will be analyzed and used by the hospital. Some institutions may wish to include the primary diagnoses of the infected patients, an assessment of the severity of underlying illness [3], the name(s) of the attending physician(s), whether exposure occurred before the onset of infection to therapies that may predispose to infection (e.g., surgery; antibiotic, steroid, or immunosuppressive therapy; or instrumentation), what anti-microbial agents were used to treat the infection, and some assessment of the mortality related to the infection. Infection-specific determination of the presence or absence of particular exposure factors may be useful for urinary tract infections and catheterization; respiratory infections and respiratory therapy equipment; and primary bacteremia and the use of intravenous catheters.

This information may be recorded on a file card or a sheet by the ICN, and it may subsequently be transferred to a computer for analysis if such is available. It is important to update the infection file—whether it be on cards, sheets, or computer tape—as new information becomes available.

DENOMINATORS. Denominator information for calculating rates can usually be obtained from Medical Records. The number of admissions or discharges by ward and by service for a specified period of time (usually a month or longer) should be obtained. The number of admissions is theoretically superior to the number of discharges in reflecting the number of patients at risk, since patients who die may not be included in discharges. Practically, however, these differences do not significantly affect the rates of infection, and the choice between them is decided on the basis of the ease with which they can be obtained. Also, the census of hospitalized patients at the start of the surveillance interval theoretically needs to be added to the number of admissions to yield the precise number of patients at risk during the surveillance interval, which is usually one month. This correction is customarily ignored, since this census is small in comparison to the total number of admissions to an acute-care hospital over a period of a month or longer. This correction, however, can become highly important when the surveillance intervals are short (e.g., one week or less) or when the average duration of hospital stay is excessively long (e.g., in a chronic-care facility).

Special denominators—such as the number of intensive-care unit admissions or discharges or the number of patients undergoing a surgical procedure—must sometimes be obtained from special log books maintained within the appropriate hospital area. Such denominators as the number of patients receiving indwelling urinary catheters, intravenous catheters, or other predisposing factors by service or hospital location are often more difficult to obtain. Central supply and pharmacy records may be useful, and, in some hospitals, such data may be retrieved from the computer files of the hospital's business office.

Sources of Infection Data

THE MICROBIOLOGY LABORATORY. The effective infection control nurse must utilize a wide variety of sources of infection information, both from within and outside the hospital, to insure maximal characterization of the infection.

Sources of nosocomial infection information include the following:

1. microbiology laboratory reports,
2. ward rounds (special attention is given to patients with fever, on antibiotic therapy, in isolation, or having high-risk procedures or serious underlying disease),
3. the admissions office,
4. the pharmacy (e.g., the distribution of antibiotics),
5. x-ray reports (e.g., of pneumonias),
6. autopsy reports (e.g., of undetected infections),
7. the employee health clinic,
8. the outpatient clinic,
9. postdischarge follow-up of selected patients (e.g., surgical or newborn patients),
10. local public health officials (e.g., regarding community outbreaks), and
11. verbal or other reports by physicians and nurses.

Of the sources of infection information listed above, one of the most useful is the periodic (usually daily) review of microbiology laboratory reports. This may be performed each morning prior to making ward rounds, so any new or potential infections can be inspected during ward rounds. Such review implies an understanding by the ICN of the infections and epidemiologic potential of various microorganisms; such knowledge might be achieved in a laboratory training period at the time of employment and reinforced by periodic, in-service, review sessions. It must be stressed that a review of the microbiology laboratory reports alone is not sufficient for the identification of nosocomial infections, because not all infections are given culture studies and not all infectious agents (e.g., viruses) will be identified in a particular hospital laboratory. Furthermore, the identification of a potentially pathogenic organism from a culture specimen does not mean that infection is present; the latter requires clinical verification.

WARD ROUNDS. Periodic (preferably daily) ward rounds by the ICN should be included as an integral part of an effective surveillance program. The purposes of such rounds are to identify new infections, to follow up previously identified infections, and to consult with the nursing staff about infection control policies and practices. New infections may be identified outright by physicians or nurses working in the area visited, by review of temperature records, by follow-up of suspicious microbiology laboratory reports, by review of patients having high-risk procedures (such as surgery, urinary tract instrumentation, or indwelling urinary or intravenous catheters), and by review of patients in isolation or receiving antimicrobial therapy. Ward visitation also allows direct inspection and documentation of visible infections, which increase the validity of the data collected.

OTHER SOURCES. Additional infection information may be obtained through a periodic review of x-ray laboratory reports, records of personnel health clinic visits, and autopsy reports. The surveillance of infection in discharged patients (though often neglected) may be of particular value in newborn infants and postoperative patients. These patients are often discharged within the incubation period of the infections characteristic for each group. Telephone surveys or reports from the patients' private physicians may be of assistance in detecting such infections.

The exclusive use of alternative methods of infection data collection—such as the review of postdischarge medical records or the use of infection report sheets filled out by attending physicians or floor nurses—is less satisfactory from the standpoint of infection control. The former method suffers from its ex post facto nature. Valuable time may be lost between the onset of the infection and its discovery by this method, and such delay may result in excessive morbidity or mortality among patients or hospital personnel. The latter method mentioned above has been utilized in a number of hospitals, but it suffers from the lack of systematic application of standard definitions and criteria for detecting infection, as well as from great variation from person to person in the completeness of reporting infection.

Consolidating and Tabulating Data

It is difficult to recognize potentially important relationships or patterns of infection from the raw data on the file cards, worksheets, or line listing forms, so it is necessary to consolidate the data in preparation for determining specific infection rates for analysis. This step simply involves counting and listing the number of infections by (1) single tabulations (e.g., ward or hospital location, service, site, and pathogen) and (2) two-way tabulations (e.g., site and hospital location, pathogen and hospital location, site and service, site and pathogen, and service and pathogen). A separate table should be prepared for each of these tallies. In addition, the antimicrobial susceptibility patterns should be tallied by site and by pathogen.

It is usually practical to perform the single and two-way tabulations referred to by hand, but three-way (e.g., service-site-pathogen), four-way (e.g., pathogen-susceptibility-hospital location-site), and more complex tabulations usually require mechanical or computer assistance.

Calculating Rates

DEFINITION OF RATE. After these tabulations are complete, tables with rates of infection should be calculated for each of the tallied tables containing numerator data. A *rate* is an expression of the probability of occurrence of some particular event, and it has the form $k(x/y)$, where x, the numerator, equals the number of times an event has occurred during a specific time interval; y, the denominator, equals a population from which those experiencing the event were derived during the same time interval; and k equals a round number (100, 1000, 10,000, 100,000, and so on), or a base. The *base* that is used depends upon the relative magnitude of x and y, and it is selected to permit the rate to be expressed as a convenient whole number. It is important to emphasize that in determining a rate, both the time interval and the population must be specified, and these must apply to both the numerator (x) and the denominator (y) of the rate expression.

TYPES OF RATES. Three specific kinds of rates—prevalence, incidence, and attack—are fundamental tools of epidemiology and, as such, must be familiar to infection control personnel. *Prevalence* is the total frequency of the disease within a defined population either during a specific period of time or at a specific point in time (point prevalence); these concepts are discussed in a later section of this chapter. *Incidence* measures the frequency of addition of *new* cases of disease within a specified population at risk during a specified interval of time. In Figure 4-1, which portrays the infection status of ten hospitalized patients, the incidence of infection during either time period A or B, for example, would be 3/10, or 30 percent, since three infections began among the ten patients during each time interval.

An *attack rate* is a special kind of incidence: it is usually expressed as a percentage (i.e., $k = 100$ in the rate expression), and it is used for particular populations having a limited period at risk (e.g., in common-source exposure), which frequently occurs in an epidemic. If 100 infants in a newborn nursery, for example, were exposed to a contaminated lot of infant formula over a three-week period, and if 14 of the infants developed a characteristic illness thought to be caused by the contaminated formula, then the attack rate for those infants exposed to the formula would be 14 percent. This would also represent the incidence of such infant illness during the specified time interval.

CHOICE OF NUMERATOR AND DENOMINATOR. Multiple infections occasionally occur in single patients. However, we have found rates based on the number of infections to be far easier to

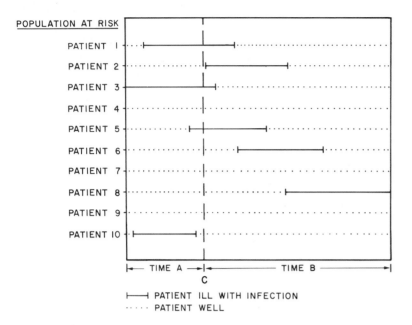

Figure 4-1. Infection status of ten hospitalized patients. *Incidence* of infection during either time period A or B is 30 percent (three new cases were added during each time period); *prevalence* of infection during time period A is 40 percent and during B, 60 percent (four cases and six cases, respectively, occur in each period of time); and *point prevalence* of infection at time C is 30 percent (three cases exist at that point in time).

obtain than, and equally as useful as, rates based on the number of patients with infection. For assessing mortality, the number of deaths per infection episode and the number of deaths per persons with such episodes are both useful.

We have also found that rates of infection using a denominator based on the number of patients at risk are adequate for the comparison of infection experiences among acute-care hospitals. We prefer these to rates based on patient-days of stay. The latter method produces rates whose implications are less obvious and more difficult to comprehend. Institutions with average durations of hospitalization that are unusually long or short, however, should probably base their rates on patient-days of stay.

It is especially important that the denominator reflect the appropriate population at risk as precisely as possible. In determining the attack rate of surgical wound infection among pa-

tients on the urology service, for example, only those urology patients who actually undergo a surgical procedure that results in a wound capable of being infected would ideally be included in the denominator. Practical difficulties in obtaining such refined denominators, however, often dictate the use of a less precise denominator, such as the total number of admissions or discharges from the urology service during the appropriate interval of time.

Calculated rates may be displayed in graphic form to facilitate visual assimilation of the data.

Analysis

COMPARING PATIENT GROUPS. Analysis implies careful examination of the body of tabulated data in an attempt to determine the nature and relationship of its component parts. This includes comparison of current infection rates to determine whether significant differences exist among different groups of patients. Suppose, for instance, that both the gynecology and general surgery services have had eight catheter-associated urinary tract infections during a given month; however, during the same month there were 20 patients discharged from the gynecology service and 100 patients discharged from the general surgery service who had indwelling catheters. Thus, the respective rates for gynecology and general surgery patients were 40 percent and 8 percent. Determination of whether the difference observed between these infection rates is significant (i.e., greater than what we would expect by random or chance occurrence alone if indeed no real difference exists) requires the use of a statistical process known as *significance testing.*

Several tests of significance—such as the chi-square test, Fisher's Exact test, and Student's *t* test for comparison of sample means—should be familiar to epidemiologists and to the ICN, but their description is beyond the scope of this chapter. Recent technologic advances have produced programmable calculators that are compact and simple to operate; these can be programmed to perform a variety of significance tests rapidly and accurately. In the preceding example, the difference between the observed infection rates (40 percent versus 8 percent) is highly significant at $p < .001$ according to the chi-square test (two-tailed), which means that assuming no real difference exists between the catheter-associated urinary tract infection rates on the gynecology and general surgery services, a difference as large as or larger than that observed (40 percent versus 8 percent) would be expected to occur by chance alone less than one time in 1000. Thus, it is more likely that there is a real difference between the infection rates on the two services, and further investigation is indicated to explain why such a difference exists.

COMPARING RATES IN TIME. Another type of analysis involves the comparison of current infection rates with those established in the past to determine whether significant changes have occurred over time. Rate tables for the present month and each of several preceding months can be visually inspected or rates can be plotted on graph paper to detect changes of potential importance. Potentially important deviations from baseline rates should then be subjected to tests of statistical significance, and further investigation (see Part I, Chapter 5) undertaken if indicated. Epidemic threshold analysis can be of definite value in the detection of outbreaks within individual hospitals, but, without computer assistance, this method cannot be thoroughly applied to each cell of

each specific rate table for each of several months. This type of analysis uses previous experience as a baseline and statistically compares the current infection rates (e.g., by service, ward, site, site-pathogen, and so on) with those baseline rates. The current rates whose probability of occurrence exceeds a predetermined threshold (e.g., $p < .05$ or $p < .01$) may be considered potential outbreaks that deserve further investigation.

CLUSTERS. Screening for clustering of specific patterns of antimicrobial susceptibility of organisms is another potentially valuable analytic tool for detecting outbreaks, especially when it is applied to particular pathogens on specific wards or in particular geographic areas.

Interpretation
Interpretation of the data is considered by many as the final step in analysis; it is simply an intellectual process by which some meaning is ascribed to the tabulated and analyzed body of information. The interpretation may vary from no significant change in the current infection rates to the detection of a possible outbreak in the hospital. Often, however, more information—particularly that obtained through further investigation directed specifically at problem areas identified by means of the analysis of the surveillance data—will be necessary for final interpretation of the data. Additional uses of other information collected through surveillance, such as the time of onset of infection, are described in Part I, Chapter 5.

Reporting the Data
It is essential that the tabulated data—or at least the analyses and interpretations of the data—get to those people in the hospital who need to know them in order to take appropriate actions. A monthly report containing the tabulated data and the analyses and interpretation of the data should routinely be submitted to the Infection Control Committee and maintained on record in the hospital. Of course, weekly or even daily reports may be necessary during epidemics or unusual situations. It is not necessary—in fact, it is often very inefficient—to include a line listing of infections in

this report. Also, the analysis of a single month of infection data may yield some tables that contain insufficient data to justify inclusion in the report. These tables should be retained and a summary table released whenever sufficient monthly data have accumulated.

Summary reports or graphic representations of the data should also be widely distributed to the professional staff of the hospital. Summary data may also be placed on bulletin boards and sent to local or state health departments, to other local hospitals, or elsewhere as judged necessary or desirable by the Infection Control Committee.

Prevalence

Definition

Prevalence measures the frequency of all current cases of active disease (new and old) within a specified population at risk during a specified interval of time. In Figure 4-1, the prevalence of infection during time period A would be 4/10, or 40 percent, and during time period B, 6/10, or 60 percent. (The *incidence* of infection during each time period, as mentioned previously, is 3/10, or 30 percent.) *Point prevalence* measures the frequency of all current cases of disease (old and new) at a given instant in time; for example, the point prevalence of infection at point C in Figure 4-1 would be 3/10, or 30 percent. *Period prevalence,* on the other hand, measures the frequency of all current cases of disease (old and new) during a specified period of time, as in the example above. It should be apparent that the difference between point and period prevalence is arbitrary; an interval that is considered a "point" on one time scale may become a "period" on a different time scale.

The Prevalence Survey

The *prevalence survey,* as it is applied to nosocomial infections, consists of a systematic scrutiny of a defined population for evidence of infection at a given point in time, that is, the point prevalence is determined for such a population. The prevalence survey cannot distinguish between new and old infections with the same accuracy as continuing surveillance un-

less it is performed so frequently that it approximates a continuous process. The terms "incidence" and "prevalence" are often confused in the literature, but an important distinction lies in whether one is measuring *all* the active cases (new and old) of a disease in a population or just the *new* cases occurring during a specified time interval. In a hospital population, prevalence rates almost always exceed incidence rates, since the infection is often responsible for a prolonged hospital stay.

Uses of Prevalence Data

SECULAR TRENDS. Repeated prevalence surveys in the same institution have been used to document secular trends in the epidemiology of nosocomial infections. Such studies have demonstrated a shift in the predominant pathogens associated with nosocomial infections, for example, as well as having documented the patterns of antimicrobial use in hospitalized patients. The number of infections detected among patients hospitalized at the time of a point prevalence study may be insufficient, especially in small hospitals, to permit reliable comparisons with past data. Surveillance data are much better suited for detecting and examining secular trends.

EFFICIENCY OF SURVEILLANCE. Prevalence surveys may be used to determine the efficiency of the hospital's surveillance system. The survey team should apply standard criteria, identical to those used for routine surveillance by the ICN, for determining and classifying infection. For this purpose, it must be assumed that the survey team is 100 percent complete and accurate in detecting infections actually present at the time of the survey. By comparing the number of individual infections identified by the survey team during the prevalence survey with that detected by the surveillance system, an *efficiency factor* can be derived that can be used to adjust monthly infection rates. Past experience indicates that 80 percent or greater efficiency is often possible.

ESTIMATING INCIDENCE. Modified prevalence surveys can be used to determine approximate data regarding the incidence of infection that are comparable to those derived from continuous surveillance [4]. Surveys are performed at regular intervals (e.g., weekly) that must be considerably less than the average duration of stay of infected patients. Only infections that began since the preceding survey are tabulated. Rates should probably be based on the number of admissions during the interval plus the census at the start of the period. Some loss in completeness, accuracy, and timeliness in detecting infections—as compared to the results of surveillance studies—must be accepted by persons who choose to employ such modified prevalence surveys.

OTHER USES. Prevalence studies may prove useful to individual hospital Infection Control Committees not only to adjust infection rates and possibly as an educational device, but also to provide valuable information about antimicrobial drug usage, the need for isolation rooms, the frequency of use of intravenous and indwelling urinary catheters, and so on.

Prevalence surveys have also been useful for increasing the awareness of nosocomial infection problems in those hospitals without surveillance programs. Indeed, the results of such surveys have often been important in a hospital's decision to institute a surveillance system.

References

1. Garner, J. S., Bennett, J. V., Scheckler, W. E., Maki, D. G., and Brachman, P. S. Surveillance of Nosocomial Infections. In P. S. Brachman and T. C. Eickhoff (Eds.), *Proceedings of the International Conference on Nosocomial Infections.* Chicago: American Hospital Association, 1971.
2. Joint Commission on Accreditation of Hospitals. Infection Control. In *Accreditation Manual for Hospitals.* Chicago: Joint Commission on Accreditation of Hospitals, 1976.
3. McCabe, W. R., and Jackson, G. G. Gram-negative bacteremia. *Arch. Intern. Med.* 110: 847, 1962.
4. Wenzel, R. P., Osterman, C. A., Hunting, K. J., and Gwaltney, J. M., Jr. Hospital-acquired infections. I. Surveillance in a university hospital. *J. Epidemiol.* 103:251, 1976.

5

Investigation of Endemic and Epidemic Infections

Richard E. Dixon

Effective routine infection control practices do much to reduce the incidence of nosocomial infections. Nosocomial infections continue to occur, however, even in hospitals with very effective infection control programs. Although some of these infections can be prevented with techniques now available, many cannot be. In order to reduce the occurrence of preventable infections, the goals of a hospital infection control program should be to identify those infections that are avoidable, determine their causes, and institute measures to correct those causes. This chapter describes methods for approaching these goals, although it seems impractical to expect at this time that any hospital can realize the ultimate goal of preventing all avoidable nosocomial infections.

Infection control resources should be used to investigate and control preventable infections rather than be invested heavily in evaluating those that are unavoidable. Often, however, it is impossible to know whether a patient's infection is preventable. Furthermore, no maximum acceptable infection rates are yet available that may serve as a norm against which a hospital's experience can be judged. In practice, the hospital epidemiologist judges that infections are potentially preventable—and thereby worthy of attention—if they occur in relation to an epidemic or if they seem to occur more frequently in one hospital than in other, comparable hospitals.

A classic epidemic is marked by an unusual, statistically significant increase in the incidence of a particular disease, it usually occurs during a brief interval in a single patient population, and it is caused by a single microbial strain. This broad definition is useful, but one often finds that for a specific problem, there are no guidelines to define how large the increased incidence must be or over what time period infections must occur before an epidemic is considered to be present. Furthermore, an epidemic may involve several different strains, and the unique host population is often not obvious until after an investigation is completed. As a result, the presence of an epidemic is often arbitrarily defined, and the decision to investigate a potential epidemic is frequently based on intuition.

Center for Disease Control (CDC) epidemiologists have formally investigated approximately 20 to 25 hospital outbreaks and have consulted on approximately 120 additional ones each year in the early 1970s. Several trends in the types of epidemics investigated are apparent (see Part II, Chapter 13). In the late 1950s, outbreaks due to gram-positive bacteria predominated. By the mid-1960s, outbreaks due to gram-negative bacteria were being investigated more frequently than ones due to gram-positive strains. In the past decade, increasing numbers of nonbacterial outbreaks have been investigated; in 1976 through 1977, only 54 percent of formally investigated outbreaks were caused by bacteria. The rest have been due to viruses (primarily hepatitis and herpesviruses), funguses, mycobacteria, and parasites. Of course, the epidemics investigated by CDC are not representative of the broad range of problems seen in hospitals. Neonatal staphylococcal outbreaks still occur commonly, for example, but increasingly sophisticated infection control personnel in hospitals often conduct epidemiologic investigations of those outbreaks without requiring outside consultation.

From 1973 to 1974, the CDC studied infection clusters occurring in six hospitals that were part of the Comprehensive Hospital Infections Project, a closely monitored study of nosocomial infections in selected community hospitals. Any cluster of infections (caused by the same pathogen and occurring at the same anatomic site) that occurred at a statistically significant higher frequency than in a baseline period was identified as a possible outbreak cluster, and a portion of these clusters were investigated on the site by CDC epidemiologists. Approximately 9.2 percent of the nearly 3500 patients with nosocomial infections in these hospitals were part of such a cluster, and study hospitals had an average of six clusters for every 10,000 patients discharged. Some true epidemics were undoubtedly excluded by the methods used to define

potential outbreaks, and some clusters observed were probably not outbreaks of preventable infection. It is clear, however, that community hospitals have frequent episodes that potentially require epidemiologic assessment. In university, municipal, and other referral hospitals, such outbreak clusters almost certainly occur even more frequently.

Preventable infections also occur sporadically. Indeed, sporadic (endemic) infections probably represent the bulk of nosocomial infections that can be prevented. Some of these endemic infections are also investigated profitably, since correctable host or exposure factors can be identified and their influences on infection risk altered. There are no good criteria for determining when endemic infections are worthy of study. A decision to launch an investigation is most often made when the hospital epidemiologist suspects that a group of infections have occurred more frequently than they should and that some common, correctable risk factor underlies them. Such suspicion may be based on intuition, on recognizing that less than optimal patient-care practices exist, or on comparing a hospital's infection rates with the rates observed previously in the same institution or in comparable patient populations in other institutions.

It is clear that infection rates differ regularly and substantially between hospitals, even when adjustments are made for factors such as patient characteristics, types of treatment provided, and hospital characteristics. These differences in infection rates presumably result in part from preventable nosocomial infections. Thus high endemic infection rates (i.e., hyperendemic infection rates) may also be worthy of epidemiologic investigation.

Epidemic and hyperendemic infection problems may be caused by a variety of factors; these include the breakdown of recommended practices by patient-care personnel, the development of new therapeutic maneuvers with unrecognized infection hazards, the introduction of an especially virulent microbial strain, or the introduction of a contaminated common vehicle into the hospital. General attempts to improve standard infection control practices may fail to correct a problem unless the cause of that problem is identified and specific corrective actions are undertaken. Thus, each hospital must have the resources for prompt and skilled evaluation of such problems.

Principles of Epidemiologic Investigation

For an infection to occur, a sufficient number of pathogenic microorganisms (the agent) must be present, an individual (the host) must be susceptible to infection, and a means (the mode of transmission) for the agent to have appropriate contact with the host must be present. An infection may be prevented by altering any one of these factors, that is, by eradicating the source or reservoir of the agent, by increasing host resistance, or by interrupting the mode of transmission. The goal of an epidemiologic investigation is to determine which of these factors may be most easily altered in order to prevent disease.

Usually at the outset of an investigation, there are many factors that seem important. There may be, for example, many potential reservoirs of the agent. Numerous host susceptibility factors may be present, and various modes of transmission may be reasonably considered. Which of these is related to the disease is unknown, and it is therefore difficult to know how to control the problem. The task, then, of the epidemiologic investigation is to direct control measures efficiently and to minimize concerns about the potentially large number of unrelated reservoirs of the agent, the unimportant susceptibility factors of the host, and the potential modes of transmission that are not responsible for disease. This is accomplished by comparing the characteristics of the affected individuals (the case population) with those of a similar population of unaffected persons (the control population). The major differences between the case and the control populations are assumed to play a role in determining the occurrence of disease.

Before describing the steps used in a typical epidemiologic investigation, we must consider several fundamental assumptions made by epidemiologists. To show a relationship between cigarette smoking and the development of lung cancer, for example, the epidemiologist does not insist that every smoker acquires cancer or that all persons with cancer will have smoked. Instead, a causal association is presumed to exist if cancer occurs at a statistically significant higher incidence among cigarette smokers than among a comparable population of nonsmokers. As a result, the epidemiologist is able to show a higher risk of disease for a defined population but is usually unable to prove that a specific exposure caused disease in a particular patient.

The epidemiologist may also be willing to use less precise data than would be required by a clinician treating an individual patient. If a nursing mother has a breast abscess, her physician would prefer microbiologic proof before making the diagnosis of staphylococcal infection. However, if the same patient's records were reviewed by an epidemiologist during the investigation of a nursery staphylococcal outbreak and if the woman's infant had staphylococcal disease, the epidemiologist should reasonably assume that she, too, had a staphylococcal infection, whether a culture was obtained or not.

Protocol for Epidemiologic Investigation in a Hospital

There can be no rigid approach to epidemiologic investigations; not only will each epidemiologist approach a problem somewhat differently, but the relative importance and sequence of steps will also differ according to the nature of the problem. The majority of epidemiologic investigations of nosocomial infections do not require unusual resources. Some investigations, however, are so complex that an individual formally trained in epidemiology, statistical consultation, or sophisticated manipulation of data may be necessary. The steps summarized below have proved to be practical and effective when employed by CDC epidemiologists in investigating nosocomial infections.

1. Perform a preliminary evaluation of available information to establish
   A. the nature of the infection problem,
   B. the magnitude and gravity of the problem,

C. the control measures that should be immediately instituted,
D. the actions required to insure the availability of adequate data, and
E. the need to notify or consult others.
2. Seek additional cases of the disease.
3. Characterize the cases of disease according to time, place, and person.
4. Formulate tentative hypotheses.
5. Refine these hypotheses to identify causal factors through
A. a retrospective case-control study,
B. a cohort study,
C. a prospective intervention study, or
D. a microbiologic study.
6. Institute and evaluate control measures.
7. Evaluate other hospital practices.

Assessing Initially Available Information
When a potential problem is recognized, the epidemiologist must first quickly review the available data to provide a basis for several important decisions. The review includes (1) a preliminary assessment of the nature or type of disease present, (2) an estimate of the magnitude of the problem, (3) a determination of the control measures that should be implemented before the investigation begins, (4) a judgment about the actions required to insure that the data to be used in the investigation are adequate, and (5) a decision about obtaining outside consultation.

Recognizing that these decisions are usually based on inadequate information, the epidemiologist often refers to this as the "quick and dirty" phase of the investigation: the available data are of uncertain quality and the resulting decisions are tentative.

ESTABLISHING THE NATURE OF THE INFECTION PROBLEM. The first task is to identify the potential problem. What clinical sites of infection are involved? Is the illness nosocomial, community-acquired, or a combination of the two? Is a single microorganism responsible? If so, is it unique in any way, such as in having an unusual antimicrobial susceptibility pattern or biochemical characteristic? What are the general characteristics of the patient population affected? When did the problem begin? As a rule, the full extent of the problem is not rec-

ognized at the start of an investigation, perhaps only the more obvious or dramatic illnesses have been recognized, and, on occasion, surveillance data may be incomplete. The epidemiologist should complete these tasks promptly by conducting a survey of the surveillance data as well as the microbiologic or other laboratory summary logs and by quickly reviewing a sample of patient records. From that survey, a tentative case definition can be established; the case definition sets up the criteria that must be satisfied for a patient to be included in the group of cases. Where there is uncertainty, it is wise to use a broad case definition at this stage; the case definition can be sharpened as the investigation progresses, and patients can be removed from the case group later if need be. If the original case definition is too restrictive initially, true cases of disease may never be evaluated.

The case definition may stipulate that a specific microorganism be isolated. This is useful when a definite epidemic strain is known to be responsible for an outbreak. If the isolation of a specific strain is the sole criterion for the case definition, the resulting case population may include both colonized and diseased patients. Such a population is valuable in order to define the distribution of a pathogen, its virulence, and the spectrum of disease that it causes. Alternatively, the case definition may emphasize the clinical features of the disease, and it may not require the isolation of a pathogen. Here, the case category may include those patients infected with a variety of microorganisms, but the role of asymptomatic infection will be deemphasized. Yet another patient population will be selected if the case definition includes particular patient characteristics. An investigation of surgical wound infections, for example, might restrict study patients to those having clean surgical procedures [1] in order to decrease the contribution of autogenous sources of infection. The case definitions selected in most investigations combine these factors by including criteria about the sites of infection, the pathogens involved, and the affected host population.

ESTABLISHING THE MAGNITUDE OF THE PROBLEM. Using the tentative case definition, a rapid review of the readily available data should provide a rough estimate of the magnitude of the problem. When the case definition requires the isolation of a particular microbial strain, a rapid enumeration of the microbiology laboratory isolates, tabulated by time period, provides a crude estimate of the size of the problem as well as its course over time. As another example, walking through patient wards to learn the prevalence of diarrhea will suffice to establish the preliminary magnitude of an acute gastroenteritis outbreak.

INSTITUTING CONTROL MEASURES. It is sometimes impossible to implement any reasonable control measure until the epidemiologic investigation has identified the cause of the problem. The problem may have many potential causes, and it is often impractical to implement measures to control each. On occasion, especially with unusual problems, no cause is initially obvious. Nonetheless, the epidemiologist must often institute changes in an attempt to prevent the occurrence of additional disease, especially if serious infections are seen. These changes may be patterned after measures used to control similar problems in the past.

The institution of control measures may be followed by an apparent resolution of the problem, and the epidemiologist must then decide whether to pursue a thorough investigation. Further assessment is generally indicated because, without an investigation, it will remain uncertain which measures were beneficial. Since changes introduced to control a problem may be inconvenient and expensive, hospital personnel often desire to return to the use of previously routine practices. No control measure can be relaxed, however, without risking a recurrence of the disease. Furthermore, the control measures may have had no effect, and a temporary reduction in disease occurrence may have occurred fortuitously. In such circumstances, a recurrence of the problem is highly probable.

INSURING THE ADEQUACY OF AVAILABLE DATA. In the initial phase of an investigation, the epidemiologist must insure that the recognition of the problem does not paradoxically impair the chances that it can be investigated successfully. Hospital practices prevalent during the problem period must be documented, potential microbial reservoirs and sources evaluated, and microbial isolates saved.

Widespread changes in hospital practices usually occur when a problem is recognized. Some changes result from well-documented measures that are introduced by infection control personnel, but others are undocumented because they result from the natural tendency of personnel to reevaluate and change their individual practices upon learning about an infection problem. As a result, the epidemiologist must take steps to document as completely as possible the practices actually prevalent during the problem period.

Potential sources of the infectious agent may be eradicated during the initial flurry of hospital changes. Commercially supplied materials used in treatment of affected patients are often discarded or returned to the manufacturer, thereby making them unavailable for subsequent independent testing if they are epidemiologically implicated. Thus, the epidemiologist must assure that these materials are placed in quarantine and saved for public health authorities, such as those of the Food and Drug Administration (FDA). Other potential reservoirs of the infecting strain may be cleaned. As a result, selected specimens of materials likely to be epidemiologically relevant should be collected for testing. While it is quite uneconomical and generally unrewarding to initiate widespread, indiscriminate culturing of specimens from patients, personnel, or the inanimate environment, the epidemiologist must judiciously select for sampling those sources that are highly suspect on the basis of past experience.

Finally, subcultures of the microorganisms isolated from affected patients should be saved, since it is often necessary to compare these strains with one another, with other strains obtained in the investigation, and with strains that may be unrelated to the problem.

DETERMINING WHETHER CONSULTATION IS REQUIRED. Some infection problems should be reported immediately to local and state health departments or to other public health agencies. A large number of infections or one associated with very serious disease may call for outside consultation if hospital infection control personnel have little experience in epidemic investigation, if they have insufficient time to conduct a prompt full-scale investigation, or if hospital facilities such as the clinical laboratory cannot provide adequate support for the investigation. Because of the widespread changes that occur in a hospital after a problem is recognized, consultation is most likely to be useful if obtained promptly. State and many local health departments are generally able to advise hospitals regarding epidemiologic investigations and can often assist in arranging epidemiologic and laboratory support when indicated.

When contamination of a commercially supplied medication or device is suspected, public health authorities should be notified immediately. Since other hospitals are also likely to be affected, the FDA and CDC have the responsibility to control such problems and should be notified by the state health department or by the hospital.

Seeking Additional Cases
All affected patients should next be identified. Case-finding methods are determined by the problem being investigated. Carefully collected surveillance data are a prime resource; however, case finding should not be limited to a review of these data, since even in hospitals with excellent surveillance for nosocomial infections, not all nosocomial infections are recognized. Microbiology records may be reviewed to find other patients with isolates similar to the epidemic strain. A questionnaire or telephone survey (depending on the urgency) of hospitalized and discharged patients may be useful if a characteristic clinical syndrome is being investigated. Clinical examination and culture studies, skin tests, or serologic surveys of high-risk patients may identify previously unrecognized cases of infection. If the onset of a disease may occur after hospital discharge (as may be seen with hepatitis, surgical wound infections, nursery staphylococcal disease, and other diseases), inquiries to other hospitals and community physicians may be useful. Employees, visitors, and outpatients may be evaluated in some investigations.

As noted previously, it is important that a broad case definition be used for case finding

in the initial phases of the investigation so important instances of infection will not be ignored. Neonatal staphylococcal infection, for example, has an average seven-day incubation period. As a result, such disease in term infants often begins after hospital discharge, and disease with onset during hospitalization occurs more often in infants with prolonged stay. Thus, a nursery staphylococcal problem may initially seem to be limited to premature infants or those born by cesarean section. If additional cases were sought only in these populations and a community inquiry about disease were not undertaken, an unrepresentative sample of affected infants would be identified.

Case finding should extend sufficiently into previous periods to identify when the first case of disease occurred, because the most recently occurring cases may have different epidemiologic characteristics from those of cases occurring earlier. A hypothetical group-A streptococcal surgical wound infection outbreak will serve to illustrate this point. The epidemic strain may first be introduced by a surgeon who carries and disseminates the epidemic strain. After several hospitalized patients are infected, they provide another source for the organism. If only those infections that occur late in the outbreak are evaluated, the patient-to-patient component of the outbreak may be identified, but the association with the carrier (i.e., the surgeon) may not be apparent. Control measures that are limited to preventing spread between patients will fail to prevent a recurrence of the epidemic streptococcal infection, since the original source will remain untreated.

Characterizing Cases of Disease by Time,
Place, and Person
The characteristics of each patient identified by active case finding should next be systematically reviewed. During this review, the tentative case definition should be refined; it may be necessary to place patients into several groups, such as definite, probable, or possible cases.

Basic patient identifying information should be recorded that will allow subsequent retrieval of clinical records, and selected clinical data should be abstracted. The data to be ab-

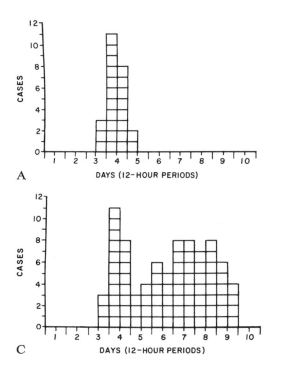

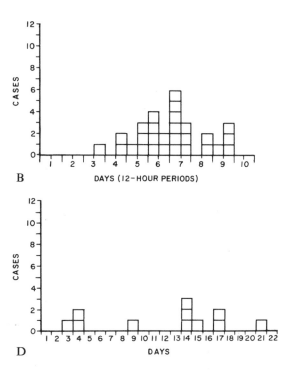

Figure 5-1. Sample epidemic curves depicting commonly observed temporal characteristics of outbreaks in hospitals.

A. A common-source outbreak of a disease with an incubation period of 18 to 36 hours. Disease occurrence reaches its peak rapidly.

B. Person-to-person transmission of a disease with a similar incubation period. The first case of disease (index case) is followed by increasing numbers of cases as the disease spreads.

C. Mixed common-source and person-to-person transmission of the same disease. The initial peak represents those patients exposed to the contaminated common source, and the later, broader peak represents secondary spread of the disease.

D. Intermittent exposure to a common-source is represented by an indeterminate pattern. This pattern is also consistent with that of a common-source outbreak of a disease with a variable incubation period, that of spread from asymptomatic carriers, or that of spread from infected persons who have prolonged carriage.

stracted fall into several categories that are considered epidemiologically in terms of time, place, and person (see also Part I, Chapter 2).

TIME. The time course of an infection problem provides valuable epidemiologic information. An *epidemic curve*—that is, a graph showing the number of cases of disease according to time of onset—should be plotted. This curve allows ready comparison of an epidemic period with a preepidemic, or baseline, period, and, in addition, it may allow identification of temporal clusters of cases of disease. The characteristics of the epidemic curve often suggest how disease is spread. An abrupt increase in the number of cases suggests a single exposure to a point source of contamination, as is shown in Figure 5-1A. A more protracted course may be compatible with person-to-person spread (Fig. 5-1B). Mixed modes of transmission may be implied by curves such as that shown in Figure 5-1C. As in Figure 5-1D, the epidemic curve is occasionally consistent with several different modes of spread.

When the epidemic curve is drawn, the time-scale intervals should be shorter than the presumed incubation period of the disease, since person-to-person spread may appear to be common-source spread if longer intervals are used (Fig. 5-2).

Similar plots showing dates of exposure to potential sources of disease, rather than dates of clinical onset, may be especially useful when the disease has a long or variable incubation period. Such plots may suggest common exposures that are not apparent in curves showing the dates of disease onset.

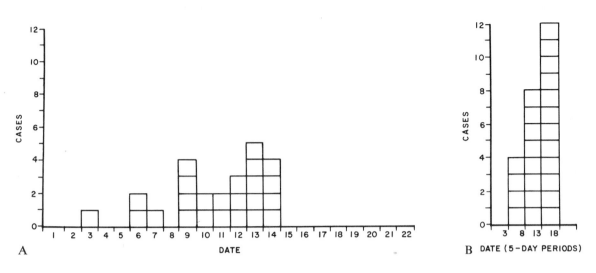

A

B DATE (5-DAY PERIODS)

Figure 5-2. Effects of the time-scale upon the appearance of the epidemic curve. The epidemic curves represent the same outbreak caused by a pathogen with a two-day incubation period.
A. The curve can correctly suggest person-to-person spread if the time scale has intervals slightly shorter than the incubation period.
B. When long intervals are used, the curve incorrectly suggests a common-source exposure.

PLACE. Geographic clustering should also be evaluated. Pictorial representation in the form of *spot maps,* where each case of disease is located by its point of onset or acquisition, is most useful. This simple technique often makes prominent otherwise inapparent clustering and may also suggest the mode of spread. Clustering in a single ward implies a common source or person-to-person spread. Hospital airflow patterns may explain the spatial clustering of disease, as is shown in Figure 5-3 [2]. This spot map shows the distribution of cases of smallpox in a German hospital (see also Part II, Chapter 24). The index case (patient 1) had no direct or indirect contact with any of the other cases (secondary and tertiary cases). All secondary and tertiary cases, however, occurred in rooms that received air exhausted from the room of the index case. A disease scattered at random throughout the hospital is compatible with an endogenous source, widespread distribution of a contaminated common source, or an extensive breakdown in patient-care practices.

Not only should the place of primary residence of patients be considered, but their exposures to other hospital areas should also be evaluated. Surgical wound infections, for example, may be specifically associated with particular operating rooms.

Time and place descriptions can be combined to reconstruct the dynamic spread of infection through the hospital. Here again, graphic or pictorial representation may be useful. Geographic exposures may be added to a standard epidemic curve, or sequential spot maps may be constructed to trace the spread of disease.

PERSON. A thorough description of the case population is the most important part of this phase of the investigation. The goals of this description are to define the specific underlying host characteristics that predispose to infection and to evaluate all exposures that may alter susceptibility or provide an opportunity for contact with the infecting agent. Here, a deliberate, exhaustive search for common features shared by the cases of infection is crucial. Patient characteristics that may influence susceptibility to disease should be recorded; these characteristics include factors such as age, sex, race, religion, the types of underlying diseases, any history of active or passive immunization, and the receipt of antimicrobial or immunosuppressive medications. For some diseases, specific host factors are important. Patients with gastric achlorhydria are especially susceptible to shigellosis and other enteric diseases. The animate and inanimate exposures of infected patients

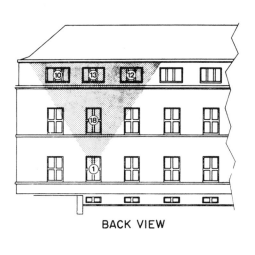

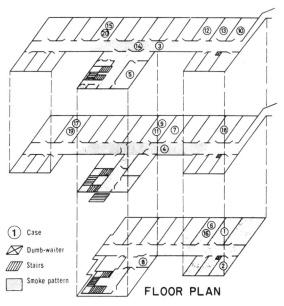

① Case
⊠ Dumb-waiter
▨ Stairs
▨ Smoke pattern

BACK VIEW

FLOOR PLAN

Figure 5-3. Spot map showing location of patients with nosocomial smallpox and relationship to air-flow patterns in hospital in Meschede, Germany [2]. Patient 1 was the index case. Shaded areas show flow of air from the room of patient 1 to other areas of the hospital.

should also be evaluated. The possibility of contact with people cannot be ignored, even in cases of diseases usually believed to be acquired from endogenous sources. The source for gram-negative microorganisms such as *Escherichia coli,* for example, is usually thought to be endogenous carriage or exogenous acquisition from the inanimate environment. These infections may, however, be transmitted from person to person; frequently, such spread occurs by way of patient-care personnel.

Therapeutic measures may alter intrinsic host susceptibility or provide the opportunity for contact with the infecting pathogen. Antimicrobial therapy should be invariably considered. It may predispose to colonization or disease if the infecting strain is resistant, or it may prevent disease if the strain is susceptible. Specific treatments may provide a portal of entry for the infecting microorganism: urinary catheterization, for example, provides a direct route by which bacteria may enter the bladder, and intravenous cannulas provide direct access to the vascular system. Knowledge of such expo-

sure may point to the source of the infecting strain.

METHODS FOR OBTAINING AND PROCESSING DATA. When possible, the clinical record of every case should be reviewed. When large numbers of patients are involved, however, this may be impractical. Although there are no rules to follow in deciding how many records need to be evaluated, broad guidelines can be offered. Generally, if fewer than 50 cases of disease are known, records for each should be reviewed. If substantially more patients are involved, a sample of records can be selected for review. Care must be taken so a representative sample is selected and obtained. The clinical records of seriously ill or unusual cases are often difficult to retrieve from the Medical Records Department because they have been signed out to staff physicians. If these records are not obtained, important information may be lost.

The case review may be aided by careful design of the data-collection forms. It should be remembered that the goal of the investigation is to characterize selected aspects of the entire affected population, not all the details about each individual case. Thus, simple descriptive characteristics (e.g., age, sex, nature of underlying diseases, and so on) and notations as to the presence or absence of selected exposures (e.g., geographic areas, personnel, medications,

CASE NO.	PATIENT I.D. NO.	DATES			AGE	SEX	SERVICE	WARD	SITE INFCT	DATE ONSET	ANTIMICROBIAL RESISTANCE (X)													IV	URINE CATH
		Adm	Disch	Death							1	2	3	4	5	6	7	8	9	10	11	12		
1	42266	4/27	6/1		46	M	Surg	4B	Blood	5/16	X	X		X	X	X		X	X	I	X	X	5/15-5/28	4/27-6/1
2	05819	5/17		5/24	32	F	OB	6A	Blood	5/18	X	X		X	X	X		X	X	I	X	X	5/18-5/19	5/18-9/19
3	38776	5/13		5/18	76	M	Med	2B	Blood	5/18	X	X		X	X	X		X	X	X	X	X	5/8-5/18	5/12-5/18

Figure 5-4. A portion of a typical line-listing form used to tabulate data during an epidemiologic investigation. The items to be tabulated are determined by the nature of the problem under investigation.

procedures, and the like) are all that are generally required. A simple line-listing form is usually the most efficient way to record these data (Fig. 5-4). On the form, each patient is listed and the appropriate characteristics checked off or otherwise simply summarized.

If many patients must be evaluated or if numerous host and exposure factors must be analyzed, data-processing techniques may aid the analysis of data. Marginal punch cards (Fig. 5-5) can be coded, punched, and sorted rapidly to make tabulations. Epidemiologic data may also be coded on computer cards and mechanically sorted or analyzed by computer. However, unless extensive data are collected and the investigators have ready access to adequate data-processing support, computerization of the investigation is likely to require more work than if the data were tabulated manually.

Formulating Tentative Hypotheses

After completing the review of the clinical and exposure data available for affected patients, the epidemiologist prepares a profile of cases. The profile is a summary of host factors and exposures of patient cases and is developed by tabulating the presence or absence of the time, place, and person characteristics just described. In this profile, the epidemiologist seeks to identify common features among the cases, the assumption being that at least one of these common features will account for the susceptibility to infection.

The list of common features may be short or long. On rare occasions, one feature is so prominent among cases that only a single explanation for the infection problem need reasonably be considered. More often, a large list is developed, and there are numerous reasonable hypotheses that may be advanced to explain the problem. The following hypothetical example illustrates the process of hypothesis formulation:

An investigation of epidemic *Proteus rettgeri* urinary tract infection (UTI) shows that all patients infected with the epidemic strain were hospitalized on a single ward, and each had indwelling urinary catheterization before the onset of infection. The epidemic strain neither had been isolated elsewhere in the hospital nor had it caused disease other than UTI.

From the case review, the problem appears uniquely to affect patients on a single ward who have been catheterized. These two associations suggest a number of hypotheses, some of which follow. The geographic clustering may have several explanations: it may result from practices in obtaining culture specimens that are unique to the affected ward, a common source such as a medication or an infected staff member may be present on the ward, or ward patients themselves who are already infected may provide a source for the epidemic strain. The association with urinary catheterization also suggests several hypotheses. The catheter may be related because it leads to a breach in bladder defenses. Alternatively, the catheter, or some agent associated with catheter insertion, may be contaminated with an epidemic strain. The catheter may be a proxy for the true risk factor, urinary irrigation, which is not routinely recorded in the patient record. Finally, if every patient on the ward is catheterized, catheterization may be quite unrelated to the risk of disease.

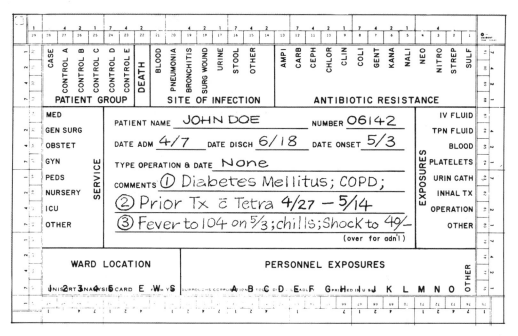

Figure 5-5. A sample marginal punch card used to tabulate data during an epidemiologic investigation. This card allows rapid sorting of large numbers of patient reports and convenient tabulation of susceptibility and exposure factors.

It should again be stressed that no factor can be excluded as unimportant simply because it is not present in each patient defined as a case. As noted earlier, rarely are all host and exposure factors identified with certainty, and, furthermore, sporadic cases of disease—those that are, in fact, unrelated to the problem being investigated—may occur during an outbreak; these cases may be difficult to identify.

Refining the Hypotheses
A valid hypothesis should not only explain why some patients acquire disease, but it should also explain why other patients do not. Most of the explanations in the example provided above are reasonable to explain UTI due to *Proteus* organisms, but if information is obtained only about the infected patients, the absence of disease in other patients remains an enigma. The crucial next step of the investigation allows refinement of the hypotheses so fortuitous associations can be discarded and causal factors can be more clearly delineated.

Three basic techniques are commonly used to refine hypotheses: case-control, cohort, and prospective intervention studies.

CASE-CONTROL STUDY. Retrospectively conducted case-control evaluation is the most effective technique for investigating most hospital epidemics, and it is also often useful for investigating hyperendemic problems. In such a study, a group of uninfected patients (the *control group*) is compared with infected patients (the *case group*), and differences in susceptibility and exposure factors are examined. If a proper control group is selected, statistically significant differences between groups are likely to identify the cause of the problem. The value of the case-control study is illustrated in the following example, which, although simplified, is based on an actual investigation:

Over a four-month period, 50 patients on a urology service had UTI due to *Pseudomonas cepacia*. A review of the charts of the patient cases showed that 48 (96 percent) had urinary tract irrigation prior to infection. No other factor was seen so often: prior cystoscopy was performed in 45 (90 percent), no single physician treated more than 20 percent of infected patients, and only 62 percent could be documented to have had contact with another known case.

From the case data, urinary tract irrigation appeared to be strongly implicated. To test this hypothesis, a control population comprising 84 uninfected urology patients hospitalized in the

Table 5-1. Pseudomonas cepacia *Urinary Tract Infection Outbreak: Exposures of Cases and Controls*

Patient category	Cases (%)	Controls (%)
Total patients	50	84
Exposed to urinary irrigation	48 (96)	80 (95)
Exposed to cystoscopy	45 (90)	24 (29)

same period was evaluated. In this control population, it was found that irrigation was indeed common; uninfected control patients had irrigation almost as often as did cases (Table 5-1). Only 24 of the 84 control patients, however, had prior cystoscopy. This suggested that the cystoscopy procedure may have been more important. Even this association, however, did not prove that cystoscopy was responsible for the outbreak. Why did some cystoscopy patients acquire [develop] infection, while others did not?

Uninfected cystoscopy patients were used as a second control group, and comparison of the data pointed up yet another significant association: there was a marked difference between the groups of physicians who treated the cases and controls (Table 5-2). In this analysis, treatment by one group of urologists (group A) was associated with only two cases of infection, but these physicians treated 12 of the uninfected control patients (attack rate: $2/14 = 14$ percent). In contrast, infection occurred in 43 of 55 cystoscopy patients treated by the other group (group B) of urologists (attack rate: $43/55 = 78$ percent). Further investigation revealed that the group having fewer cases disinfected cystoscopy instruments with glutaraldehyde, whereas the group with the

Table 5-2. Pseudomonas cepacia *Urinary Tract Infection Outbreak: Exposures to Two Physician Groups, Cystoscopy Cases Versus Cystocopy Controls*

Patient category	Cystoscopy cases	Cystoscopy controls	Total exposed	Attack rates
Total patients	45	24	69	—
Exposed to group A	2	12	14	14%
Exposed to group B	43	12	55	78%

higher attack rate preferred the use of an aqueous quaternary ammonium disinfectant. Upon culture the quaternary ammonium disinfectant yielded the epidemic strain of *P. cepacia.*

This hypothetical example based on an actual outbreak illustrates that several control groups are often required to identify the susceptibility and exposure factors responsible for an outbreak of disease. It is also apparent that the epidemiologist selects each control group to test one or more specific hypotheses. A basic strategy for selecting control groups in a stepwise manner can now be described.

First, the epidemiologist should identify important host factors that influence susceptibility to infection. How, for example, do cases differ from other hospitalized patients in terms of age, sex, underlying disease, immune status, antimicrobial therapy, and so forth? Often, it is not necessary to select a formal control group to evaluate some of these factors. If disease occurs only in neonates, it is not necessary to use a formal control group of the general hospital population to show that age is an important factor. It may be necessary, however, to compare gestational age, birth weight, or Apgar score of infected and uninfected infants.

Since susceptibility alone is not sufficient to explain infection (appropriate exposure to a pathogen is also required), one must next evaluate exposure factors. As with the case review, time, place, and person characteristics should be studied. In this phase of the investigation, susceptibility factors should be controlled for by using patients in the control group with similar susceptibility factors; for example, if patients with disease are significantly older than control patients, subsequent control populations should be selected to contain an age distribution comparable to that found for cases. As another example, if patients with gastroenteritis due to *Salmonella* have a significantly higher occurrence of peptic ulcer disease, subsequent control groups should be selected to include a comparable proportion of patients with ulcer.

If all cases have a single susceptibility factor, all controls should have that factor. More commonly, several susceptibility factors occur in varying proportions and with varying degrees

Table 5-3. Percentage Distribution of Patient Ages: Cases of Disease Compared with Random Control Population

Age range (years)	Cases (%)	Controls (%)
Birth–9	0	7
10–19	0	4
20–29	0	12
30–39	2	9
40–49	22	18
50–59	26	21
60–69	28	18
70–79	18	8
80 and over	4	3

of statistical significance when case populations are compared with controls. To deal with this problem, the control populations should be stratified to assure comparability. Age is one such susceptibility variable that is amenable to stratification. Table 5-3 shows the distribution of ages for hypothetical case and control populations. Although the patients with cases of disease are significantly older than the patients in the control population, young patients also have disease. To control for age adequately, subsequent control populations should be stratified to assure that they have a similar age distribution as the case group.

If an outbreak occurs during a discrete period, two control populations are possible. First, uninfected patients hospitalized before or after the outbreak may be compared with those with disease to identify significantly different exposures to people, procedures, or other factors. Next, uninfected patients hospitalized during the epidemic period may be studied to test whether these differences are important; that is, if the differences remain, such exposures may be important.

Exposure to various hospital locations can be similarly examined. If hemodialysis patients with hepatitis B had a significantly higher exposure to a single dialysis station than dialysis patients without hepatitis who were treated during the same period, the dialysis station is implicated as potentially important.

Finally, exposures to personnel, other patients, procedures, and medications should be

evaluated. Using a control population that is similar to the case group in terms of disease susceptibility and time and place characteristics, the exposure to the infecting pathogen should be found to occur significantly more frequently among cases than controls.

This progressive use of multiple control populations, controlling at each step for previously identified significant factors, may seem tedious and arduous. It is, but in fact, this description of the process overemphasizes the number of separate steps required. The steps listed separately above can often be combined, for it is usually possible to evaluate several time, place, and person exposures at the same time by using the same carefully selected control group. It must be recognized, however, that the process described above should not be ignored lest the chance of bias, with the resulting risk of deriving a faulty conclusion, be introduced.

On rare occasions, no difference in host susceptibility can be established upon comparison of cases and controls. This occurs most frequently when the infecting agent is quite virulent or when the portal of infection is such that, upon exposure, every patient develops disease. Similarly, the case-control evaluation may fail to demonstrate significant differences in exposures between infected and uninfected patients. Most commonly this occurs when there is widespread or unrecognized infection in the control population, when the disease results from endogenous colonization present at the time of admission, or when case records do not document the truly significant exposure. Each of these possibilities must be evaluated with the prospective techniques described below.

Hospitalization itself can have a profound effect upon host susceptibility, and this can complicate the interpretation of case-control studies. As an illustration, patients with lymphoma may have similar susceptibilities to infection at time of admission to the hospital. After treatment is initiated, however, their susceptibilities are altered. If infected and uninfected lymphoma patients are compared for host factors apparent at the time of their admission, no major differences in susceptibility may be apparent. To obtain a clearer definition of susceptibility factors, it may be necessary to compare these factors after a period of hospitalization. In this example, the epidemiologist might calculate the average interval between the time of admission and that of the onset of disease in case patients and then compare the host characteristics of cases and controls at that point.

METHODS FOR SELECTION OF CONTROL GROUPS. Before actually selecting the members of a control group, the epidemiologist must decide the number of control patients required and the specific technique for determining which uninfected patients will be selected.

The number of control patients required to show differences between case and control patients depends upon a number of factors, including the relative frequencies with which the factor to be compared occurs in each population and the statistical certainty required by the investigator in showing differences or no differences. Statistical techniques are available for estimating the size of control groups, but it is often unnecessary to calculate the control-group size precisely. If the factor to be compared occurs either very frequently or very infrequently in patients with cases of disease, one control patient for each case patient is usually sufficient; on the other hand, if the factor occurs in approximately half of the case patients, several control patients for each case are usually necessary. Almost always, at least one control patient for each case patient should be chosen.

Next, the epidemiologist must select a method to choose control patients. Individual control patients may be selected by including all in the pool of appropriate uninfected patients (a universal sample) or by taking a portion of that pool according to a sampling scheme.

When small populations are studied, all available controls may be required. If the potential pool of control patients is large, this universal sampling method is inefficient, since more control patients than are necessary will be evaluated. In such circumstances, matched, random, or stratified random-sampling schemes may be used.

A *matched sample* may be used when there are only a few general factors that must be controlled, such as age or date of hospitalization. With the matching procedure, each case patient is matched with one or more uninfected control patients according to specified matching characteristics. It is relatively easy to find an appropriate match when a single factor needs to be controlled. As the number of factors increases or as the matching factors become quite specific (e.g., the type and duration of surgical procedure), matching becomes more difficult. Even if successful, large numbers of records of potential control patients must be reviewed and discarded in order to obtain each successful match.

A *random sample* does not require the tedious selection process used in developing a matched sample. Instead, the epidemiologist relies on the powerful effect of random chance to assure that a representative, nonbiased population is selected. Various randomization schemes are available, but the use of a random number table is probably simplest for the hospital epidemiologist. To use a random number table for selecting 20 patients from a pool of 200 potential controls, for example, each potential control is given a number between 001 and 200. The first 20 three-digit numbers found in the table that fall within the range 001 to 200 identify the patients to be selected. Other techniques have been used, such as using patient record numbers, selecting control patients admitted just before or after case patients, or selecting every *n*th patient (e.g., every fifth bacteremia case or every seventh admission). These methods may lead to nonrandom selection, however; for example, patients are neither admitted nor operated on randomly, few elective surgical patients are admitted on Saturdays, and more difficult surgical procedures are usually scheduled early in the day.

The random selection of control patients is most useful when one does not need to control for specific factors within the pool of patients available as controls. If there are no age, sex, or other susceptibility factors identified as important in an outbreak of wound infection following cardiac surgery, for example, one can quickly obtain an appropriate control group by randomly selecting uninfected patients who had cardiac surgery in the appropriate period.

How could a control population be selected if it were necessary to control for numerous factors such as age, sex, and types of operation? As noted, matching on these factors would be quite tedious, and, furthermore, one might have difficulty finding control patients who match appropriately each case patient with regard to each factor. For this problem, a *stratified random sample* can be used. It is almost as convenient to select as a true random sample, and it allows almost the same degree of control over important variables as does the matching strategy. To draw a stratified random sample, the potential pool of control patients is divided into groups that correspond to the factors that must be controlled. Then, from each group, a separate random sample is chosen. To illustrate, consider the need to control for the type of operation when 50 percent of case patients had cholecystectomy, 30 percent had herniorrhaphy, and 20 percent had chest surgery. Potential control patients would be divided into groups according to the type of surgery. The epidemiologist would then select, with a separate random pick, half of the controls from the cholecystectomy group, 30 percent from the herniorrhaphy group, and the remainder from the chest-surgery group.

ANALYSIS OF CASE-CONTROL DATA. The frequencies of various susceptibility and exposure factors among cases and controls are tabulated. All differences between the two groups are considered potentially important. When possible, statistical techniques should be used to calculate the probabilities that the observed differences could have occurred by chance. Statistically significant differences are highly suggestive, but, of course, the presence or absence of statistical significance does not prove or disprove causation.

The case-control study may not provide the solution for a problem. Under such circumstances, other epidemiologic techniques—such as a cohort study or a prospective intervention study—may be employed.

COHORT STUDY. A cohort study (see also Part I, Chapter 2) may be conducted prospectively or retrospectively. For the investigation of nosocomial infection problems, a retrospective cohort study is seldom useful, since case-control techniques are generally more powerful. If, however, a case-control review fails to solve a problem because the data available retrospectively are inadequate or, as noted in the next section, it is necessary to confirm the results of the case-control study, then a defined high-risk population (the cohort) may be identified and followed prospectively. Necessary clinical and laboratory observations can then be made. After a period of time, differences in susceptibility or host factors among ill and well patients may become apparent that will identify the source of the infection problem.

Rarely is a cohort study conducted independently of a retrospective case-control study. Usually, the case-control study is used to narrow the list of hypotheses and to identify the high-risk populations that are studied prospectively.

PROSPECTIVE INTERVENTION STUDY. The prospective trial (an experimental epidemiologic study; see also Part I, Chapter 2), like the cohort study, is rarely used primarily in studying nosocomial infection problems. It also usually grows out of the findings of a retrospective case-control study. Here, a hypothesis is tested experimentally by intervening with specific measures to correct a presumed infection problem and measuring the impact of that intervention on infection rates. When feasible, such trials should be controlled; that is, the intervention should be applied to one segment of the population at risk but not to a comparable group of control patients. Only by comparing disease risk in the treated group versus the control group can one reliably interpret the results of such a trial.

Illustrations of the ways that uncontrolled trials have been misleading are legion and fall into several broad groups. First, disease occurrence may decline independently of the intervention; without a control group, the drop in infection rate may inappropriately be attributed to a beneficial effect of the intervention. Of course, it is also possible that the treatment regimen may be harmful; again, the use of an untreated control group allows documentation of this effect. It is also possible that an intervention may be beneficial but fail to alter the observed disease risk in the treated population.

This might occur if the benefit were offset by some new event that independently increased the disease risk. When a control group is used for comparison, disease risk would presumably increase more in the untreated population, thereby indicating benefit in the treated group. Of course, there are situations in which a controlled trial is difficult to justify; this occurs, for example, when the disease under study is very serious and when the intervention measures are highly likely to be useful. Even in these circumstances, however, a controlled trial should be strongly considered for the reasons outlined above.

MICROBIOLOGIC STUDY. It is a common mistake, when an infection problem is first investigated, to obtain large numbers of microbiologic cultures. As noted earlier, some carefully selected culture specimens may be obtained from persons or the inanimate environment if they will not be available later because of the institution of control measures. It must be stressed, however, that such surveys should supplement the epidemiologic investigation, not direct it. Furthermore, the cultures should be obtained only from sites that are likely to be epidemiologically relevant.

Beginning epidemiologists at CDC are cautioned, only partly in jest, that if the epidemiologic and laboratory data disagree, they should disregard the laboratory data. This advice may seem radical, especially to those who consider laboratory data to be "hard" and real and who view statistical and epidemiologic data as "soft" and speculative. The above advice, however, is valuable for several reasons.

First, the isolation of a microorganism by itself rarely explains the occurrence of a disease. The hospital is not a sterile environment, and viable, pathogenic microorganisms may be isolated from most hospital locations. As one example, large numbers of personnel are often colonized by the epidemic strain during a staphylococcal outbreak; however, most of these personnel are, like the affected patients, victims of the outbreak rather than its causes. Similar arguments can be made about isolation of microorganisms from sink drains, floors, air, or whatever. Unless there is an epidemiologic link between the source of the isolate and the occurrence of patient disease, the mere isolation of a microorganism, even of an epidemic strain, may mean little.

Second, the failure to isolate a microorganism from a presumed source or reservoir does not vindicate that site. The culture determinations may be negative because they were improperly collected or processed, because adequate technologic procedures were not available for primary isolation, or because too few specimen samples were obtained. This last possibility is dramatically illustrated by the outbreaks of disease caused by contaminated, commercially supplied intravenous medications. In several of these outbreaks, contamination had occurred in a very small proportion of individual units (approximately one in 5000 to 10,000 units in some outbreaks), and many negative culture specimens were processed before the first positive result was obtained. If the epidemiologic data had not strongly implicated intrinsic contamination of such fluids, extensive culturing could not have been justified and would not have been undertaken. With direction provided by the epidemiologic findings, however, examinations continued until positive results were obtained. As another example, several outbreaks of group-A streptococcal surgical wound infections have been traced to medical personnel who had negative pharyngeal culture specimens for group-A streptococci. Because of the epidemiologic association of the disease with these persons, extensive examinations were conducted, and asymptomatic anal carriage of the epidemic strain was documented. The initial failure to isolate a strain does not discredit the epidemiologic findings; instead, it requires that both the epidemiologic and microbiologic techniques be reevaluated.

Instituting and Evaluating Control Measures

As soon as the explanation for a nosocomial infection problem is found, control measures should be vigorously applied. These control measures may be used to confirm the validity of that explanation. The effectiveness of such control measures should be evaluated by continued surveillance for disease and, if necessary, by prospective study.

Evaluating Other Hospital Practices

A thorough epidemiologic investigation of a nosomomial infection problem often leads to improved infection control practices not only in the areas where the problem occurred but also throughout the hospital. An outbreak of disease might be considered an experiment of nature; that is, the factors that permit epidemic infections to occur are often responsible for endemic infections as well. Investigations of UTIs caused by multiple-drug-resistant Enterobacteriaceae, for example, have documented that many of these infections are transmitted by way of personnel from infected, catheterized patients to neighboring patients who are also catheterized. It is obvious that infections with other microorganisms are also transmitted by this mechanism, but the mode is more difficult to recognize if common pathogens are involved. Thus, measures to control the spread of an epidemic strain may also be expected to control the spread of other strains. The epidemiologist should therefore review practices and procedures throughout the hospital when an epidemiologic study is completed and should institute reasonable control or preventive measures throughout the institution. Hospital personnel should be informed about the investigation and its results.

Responsibilities for Dissemination of Information

Hospitals are an integral part of other and larger communities. They interact with their own geographic community in that personnel and patients come from and return to that community. Infection problems in the community influence the hospital, and, conversely, infection problems within the hospital may be spread to the community by patients or personnel. Because of this intimate association between the community and the hospital, the institution's infection control program must cooperate with local public health authorities by reporting and assisting in the investigation of problems.

Each hospital is also a part of the larger community of other hospitals. Patients may be transferred from one institution to another and carry their infections with them. Accordingly, frank and frequent exchanges of information between hospitals are important. Although each hospital has its unique practices and policies, a problem in one institution may also be a problem in other hospitals that have the same practices. Thus, the results of epidemiologic investigations should be disseminated widely. Finally, hospitals may be affected by outbreaks caused by a contaminated common vehicle that is commercially available to other institutions. When problems with such products are discovered, the hospital epidemiologist has the responsibility to notify promptly not only the manufacturer or distributor of the product, but also the appropriate public health authorities. Local and state health authorities, FDA, and CDC cooperate closely in monitoring and attempting to control the contamination of such products, and if such a problem is suspected, these agencies should be notified immediately.

Administrative Aspects

It should be obvious that an epidemiologic investigation requires vigorous action by hospital personnel. Because of this, each hospital should have an administrative structure that will allow uninhibited investigation of infection problems. The requirements are several.

First, the hospital must have access to someone trained and interested in hospital epidemiology. Often, responsibilities for infection control are delegated to an infection control team composed of one or more infection control nurses and a physician hospital epidemiologist (see Part I, Chapter 3). This team should be given adequate resources to conduct investigations. Their continuing education should be supported. Sufficient time should be set aside in advance and adequate financial backing must be available to support investigations. The infection control team should have the administrative authority to conduct efficient and wide-range investigations, and they should specifically have the authority to evaluate patients, take appropriate culture specimens from patients and personnel, and consult with outside experts. That administrative authority must also provide a mechanism that allows the team to make emergency decisions when an infection problem threatens the health and safety of patients and personnel.

Most importantly, the infection control effort must have adequate support from other divisions in the hospital. The microbiology laboratory must maintain the ability to process the specimens required for an epidemiologic investigation, and laboratory personnel should be able to serve as expert consultants in selecting the appropriate microbiologic and serologic techniques required in these investigations. The hospital's engineering and housekeeping departments must be ready to provide consultation regarding environmental control. Nursing services must work with the infection control program in conducting epidemiologic studies as well as in applying control measures. Finally, the infection control program must have the wholehearted support and assistance of the medical staff. If the infection control effort takes place without the interest or support of other personnel in the hospital, little can be accomplished.

References

1. Committee on Control of Surgical Infections of the Committee on Pre- and Postoperative Care, American College of Surgeons. *Manual on Control of Infections in Surgical Patients.* Philadelphia: Lippincott, 1976, pp. 29–30.
2. Center for Disease Control. Follow-up smallpox—Federal Republic of Germany. *Morbid. Mortal. Weekly Rep.* 19:234, 1970. (Adopted from World Health Organization. Smallpox Surveillance. *Weekly Epidemiological Record* 45:249, 1970.)

6

The Inanimate Environment

George F. Mallison

Epidemiology: General Principles

The inanimate environment present throughout the hospital is closely related to nosocomial infections, and it may contribute to sporadic cases of disease or outbreaks in institutions by providing sources for contact, common-vehicle, airborne, or vectorborne transmission (see Part I, Chapter 2).

Examples of contact transmission from environmental sources are enteric disease transmitted to a susceptible host by an endoscope contaminated with *Salmonella* or pneumonia transmitted by respiratory therapy equipment contaminated with *Pseudomonas aeruginosa*. Contaminated medicines, blood, intravenous fluids, food, and water cause sporadic cases and provide common sources for outbreaks of nosocomial disease.

In airborne transmission of disease, the air as part of the inanimate environment serves as the means through which infectious microorganisms from animate or inanimate sources are transmitted by droplet nuclei or dust; an example is the transmission of *Mycobacterium tuberculosis* on droplet nuclei. In vectorborne disease, the inanimate environment supports the presence of the vector that either carries or is itself the causative agent.

The inanimate environment is an area of concern in infection control because of the prominent role it plays as a source and a means for transmission of nosocomial infections. The inanimate environment is in constant contact with the animate environment, patients, and staff. Prevention of nosocomial infections is partly directed at controlling this contact in order to achieve the desired relationships and prevent the transmission of microorganisms.

Assigning the inanimate environment its proper role as a source and a means for the transmission of infections—that is, without over- or underestimating the contribution of the inanimate environment—should allow an assessment of the most effective means to prevent and control environmentally spread disease. Excessive attention to the inanimate environment occurs when the presence of microorganisms is assumed to represent evidence per se of a hazardous source of nosocomial infection. Such an assumption is often inappropriate; it may lead to inefficiency by allowing overemphasis to be placed on environmental control that does not meet the need. In such a case, the need may in fact be for much greater emphasis on the prevention and control of direct-contact spread, which is the major route of transmission of nosocomial disease.

There have been unrealistic and unnecessary attempts to "sterilize" the inanimate institutional environment when its real epidemiologic relevance has been overestimated. The historical overemphasis on the inanimate environment, particularly in the 1960s, is now being counteracted as a result of more information being obtained on the specific role of the inanimate environment in nosocomial disease. This chapter attempts to place the inanimate environment in its proper perspective in relation to the prevention and control of nosocomial infections.

Transmission

Epidemiologic Aspects

It is important to keep in mind some general epidemiologic aspects of the environmental transmission of nosocomial infections. Most species of microorganisms in the air or on the inanimate surfaces of institutions rarely cause disease. No matter how highly contaminated with pathogens they may be, objects that never contact an individual are rarely involved in transmitting disease. However, if either a pathogen-contaminated object is placed onto or into the body, or if microbial contamination in the air or on an object is directly introduced into a wound, the bloodstream, bladder, or lungs (thus avoiding some of the body's natural defense mechanisms), then the chance that disease will result may be great. Thus, environmental microbial contamination most frequently serves as a source for transmission of nosocomial disease when contaminated patient-care equipment, instruments, or medicines introduce pathogenic microorganisms through any bodily orifice or directly into a wound.

Gram-positive nosocomial pathogens may persist in the inanimate hospital environment, but they do not usually multiply there. On the contrary, gram-negative organisms and funguses may persist as well as multiply in a moist or wet environment, and these are more frequently associated with environmentally transmitted infections than gram-positive organisms or other microorganisms.

Contact Transmission in General

Contact with contaminated inanimate objects can transfer pathogenic agents that may cause disease in a susceptible person. Hands of either personnel or patients, when contaminated by contact with the inanimate environment and unwashed or inadequately washed, may transfer contamination that results in infections. Microbial contamination on various types of patient-care supplies and equipment obviously may be more hazardous to patients whose resistance to infection is compromised in some manner to make them highly susceptible to infection, for example, immunosuppressed patients, patients with underlying disease (including other infections), and patients receiving antibiotics to which the organisms are resistant. Fewer numbers of microorganisms will be more likely to cause infections in such patients than in normal, healthy persons, and organisms that are not generally considered pathogenic may infect such patients and cause significant disease.

The importance of contaminated syringes and needles in the transmission of viral hepatitis and the reduction of such transmission by the widespread use of sterile, disposable equipment for injection are well known. Nosocomial pulmonary infection acquired by contact with contaminated respiratory therapy and anesthesia equipment also is well known, and this topic is discussed in Part II, Chapter 15.

In addition to these sources, contact with a variety of other contaminated inanimate objects has sometimes served as a source for transmission of nosocomial infections. Such objects include the following: urinary catheters or cystoscopes; rectal thermometers and barium enema equipment; bedpans and urinals; infant bottle nipples and heating baths for bottles; aspiration and suction equipment; oxygenators; renal dialyzers; indwelling or other therapeutic or diagnostic venous or arterial catheters; pressure transducers; shaving brushes; fabrics; faucet hoses and aerators; hydrotherapy equipment; unsterile supplies that contact patients' wounds during surgical procedures, including implants, surgical gloves, sutures, sponges, surgical instruments, and the like; tonometers; wadding under casts; antiseptics and disinfectants; thermometers; and endoscopic apparatus [2,8,15]. Medicines, blood, food, and water are additional examples of contamination sources and are discussed later in this chapter.

Hospital laboratory personnel are at high risk of acquiring viral hepatitis or certain bacterial or parasitic infections from pathogenic agents that have low infectious doses and are present in diagnostic specimens. Prevention of skin contamination, hand-washing, and avoidance of smoking, eating, and drinking in clinical laboratories reduce the risk of such indirect transmission (see Part I, Chapter 7, The Clinical Laboratory).

There have been spurious reports of outbreaks of disease resulting from the laboratory identification of pathogens from clinical specimens that were subsequently shown to represent contamination of the specimen-collecting equipment, blood-collection tubes, skin antiseptics, and blood-culture media (see Part I, Chapter 8; Part II, Chapter 29).

Common-Vehicle Transmission

MEDICINES AND BLOOD. Perhaps the most dramatic incident of contamination associated with nosocomial disease in recent years was the national epidemic in the United States of septicemia caused by contaminated intravenous fluids manufactured by one company (see Part II, Chapter 26). Between mid-1970 and April 1971, 378 cases of *Enterobacter* septicemia resulting in 40 deaths were documented in patients receiving the contaminated fluids [6]. Septicemia was epidemiologically and microbiologically traced to intrinsic contamination of a screw-cap closure for infusion bottles that was sealed with a newly introduced elastomer liner [5].

Notwithstanding such dramatic common-source outbreaks, I believe that much more sporadic than outbreak transmission occurs in hospitals due to contaminated medicines and blood. Contaminated eye drops, cosmetics, and irrigants; antibiotics and ointments; diagnostic dyes; bronchodilators; parenteral fluids; and multiple-use medications also have been responsible for sporadic cases and outbreaks of nosocomial disease. In addition, contaminated blood and blood products (see Part II, Chapter 28) have transmitted not only viral hepatitis but also other viral infections as well as malaria and syphilis.

FOOD AND WATER. Food and water may serve as sources for direct or indirect contact transmission of enteric or other pathogens within the hospital (see Part I, Chapter 7, Food Services); such spread often is recognized as common-vehicle transmission (see Part I, Chapter 2). Contamination may occur before the vehicle is brought to the hospital or in the hospital itself during processing or handling. Some cases of nosocomial disease due to contaminated food and water occur sporadically, but the true number of cases from sporadic sources, in contrast to common-vehicle sources, is unknown.

Shigella or *Salmonella* organisms are the most frequent enteric pathogens encountered. Viral hepatitis also may be caused by the ingestion of contaminated food. Disease caused by other common enteric microorganisms is not generally spread by food or water in hospitals. Enteric colonization followed by subsequent nosocomial disease, however, may clearly occur following contact with food or water contaminated with gram-negative organisms such as *Escherichia coli, Klebsiella* species, and *Pseudomonas aeruginosa.* Nosocomial disease may be preceded by colonization due to *Pseudomonas,* for instance, on raw vegetables, in drinking water, or both. The administration of antibiotics, the lowering of stomach acidity, or both readily increase the likelihood of intestinal colonization by ingested microorganisms from environmental sources.

Contaminated ice has been associated directly and indirectly with outbreaks of nosocomial disease, but apparently this rarely occurs.

Because of the extremely low infective dose of *Giardia lamblia* and *Entamoeba histolytica,* sporadic cases or common-vehicle nosocomial outbreaks due to contaminated food or water could occur; however, we know of no such instances that have been documented.

Airborne Transmission

The air can serve as the vehicle through which microorganisms can travel from source to host. Airborne nosocomial disease may be exemplified by pulmonary tuberculosis, herpes zoster, influenza, measles, rubella, diphtheria, mumps, smallpox, chickenpox, *Staphylococcus aureus* pneumonia, and some wound and burn infections. Among the above listed diseases, probably only tuberculosis, herpes zoster, smallpox, chickenpox, and possibly influenza and rubella infections carry a high risk of airborne nosocomial transmission.

One group of investigators has theorized that the increase in nosocomial gram-negative infections in their institution was associated with airborne (not droplet) microbial contamination by gram-negative organisms from a large, wet solid-waste pulping device; discontinuing the use of the device was associated with the disappearance of airborne enteric and *Pseudomonas* organisms and a reduced frequency of gram-negative septicemias. Dustborne *Salmonella* infection has been reported. The vast bulk of data, however, indicate little overall importance for the airborne spread of gram-negative infections.

Although the great majority of postoperative infections are the result of either endogenous organisms or spread by person-to-person contact, there is evidence that airborne transmission may account for a relatively small percentage of such infections (see Part II, Chapter 16). Little evidence exists to show that the use of unidirectional, or so-called laminar flow, air systems significantly reduces the incidence of postoperative infections. Additionally, some research has been done on the use of unidirectional air flow in the protective isolation of burned or immunosuppressed, highly susceptible patients, but this research also indicates that large quantities of extremely clean ventilating air have relatively little value in actually reducing the number of infections.

The classic studies done by Gonzaga and colleagues [4] designed to define the route of spread of staphylococcal colonization in nurseries clearly showed that colonization of infants was primarily due to spread via unwashed hands, although some spread was demonstrated to result from airborne transmission. Walter and co-workers [16] have reported on two cases of apparently true airborne spread of staphylococcal postoperative infections. Such gram-positive infections, however, are mainly spread by contact.

British investigators have long considered that the maintenance of staphylococcal colonization in staff and patients, which is largely supported through the airborne route (see Part II, Chapter 20), is responsible for postoperative staphylococcal infection in hospitals.

The precise source of many laboratory-acquired infections in hospitals is not known, but a substantial proportion of such infections is probably associated with airborne spread.

Vectorborne Transmission

The great majority of insect problems in hospitals are infestations with cockroaches or adult flies. Rarely do either create disease problems; however, nosocomial myiasis is reported sporadically to the Center for Disease Control, and flies in critical hospital areas may contaminate sterile items, such as unwrapped instruments in operating rooms. Patients with scabies are occasionally admitted to hospitals; outbreaks of nosocomial transmission, generally from infested patients to staff members, do occur as a result of close personal contact.

Disinfection

Disinfection is a process in which only certain infectious agents, usually the vegetative forms of pathogenic bacteria or funguses, are destroyed. Objects that contact mucous membranes should receive *at least* a high level of disinfection; these objects include various endoscopic instruments, oral and rectal thermometers, medication and humidification apparatus, masks and tubing for respiratory therapy, and anesthesia equipment. Effective disinfection should destroy viruses and all common vegetative nosocomial pathogens.

Table 6-1 summarizes the recommendations for disinfection and sterilization of various items, depending on the type of use after processing. All items and surfaces *must be thoroughly cleaned* before disinfection or sterilization. It should be noted that certain agents tend to cause some materials to corrode: alcohol, formalin, formaldehyde alcohol, quaternary ammonium, and iodophor solutions should contain 0.2% sodium nitrite (or some other inhibitor) to prevent corrosion; phenolic solutions should contain 0.5% sodium bicarbonate to prevent corrosion.

The chemical used most frequently for high-level disinfection is glutaraldehyde (Table 6-1). If reusable endoscopy equipment or tubing, valves, nebulizers, and so on, for respiratory therapy or anesthesia are chemically disinfected because sterilization (or pasteurization) is impractical, then at least 30 minutes of treatment with 2% aqueous glutaraldehyde is recommended. Such treatment should be followed by rinsing three times with sterile or chlorinated water (10 mg. free chlorine per liter), drying with filtered hot air, and packaging for storage prior to reuse. Microbiologic monitoring to confirm the effectiveness of disinfection of such items should be carried out periodically, preferably using a swab or rinse procedure to collect specimens followed by culturing of the samples in brain-heart infusion broth with added beef extract (see Part I, Chapter 8).

When using liquid chemical disinfectants, gloves generally are recommended to protect against the skin toxicity of many products, particularly disinfectant concentrates. Care should be taken, however, to prevent disinfectant from spilling into the gloves or onto the hands when gloves are worn, because occlusion will accelerate toxic reactions. Skin contact with glutaraldehyde preparations over a period of months or years may cause serious allergic reactions. Inhalation toxicity may possibly occur when gaseous or vaporized disinfectants are used. Dermal or other types of toxicity have been as-

sociated with chemical residues in or on disinfected objects that are subsequently used in or on the body, so thorough rinsing of the items is essential.

In addition to disinfection with chemicals, good results in disinfecting previously washed anesthesia or respiratory-therapy equipment also have been obtained with 30 minutes of wet pasteurization at 71°C to 74°C (160°F to 165°F). Items should be dried with filtered hot air and packaged after wet pasteurization. Periodic microbiologic monitoring is recommended, using the same method recommended above for monitoring disinfection with glutaraldehyde.

Dry thermometer-care systems—that is, in which an oral thermometer for each patient is kept at the bedside, is washed before and after each use under the faucet with soap and friction, and is then wiped dry (or is washed and then wiped with 70% to 90% alcohol)—provide a reasonable and safe alternative to disinfection with liquids.

Sterilization

Sterilization is a process that has as its objective the removal, destruction, or both of *all* living organisms that may exist on or in an article. Instruments, catheters, or fluids that enter tissues or the vascular system as well as extracorporeal equipment through which blood circulates *must* be subjected to sterilizing procedures. Endoscopic instruments, though often disinfected in hospitals, should preferably be sterilized.

Because some sterilization processes (particularly those using steam) may be less expensive and are more effective than disinfecting processes, sterilization should be used whenever possible, even when it is not essential to prevent disease transmission. Reusable tubing and other supplies that may be steam sterilized are available for use in anesthesia and respiratory therapy; in fact, even steam-sterilizable conductive tubing is now available. Clean or sterile disposable tubing is available for respiratory therapy. The use of individually wrapped sterile goods is a desirable alternative to the

Table 6-1. Recommendations for Disinfection and Sterilization

Object	Disinfection — Will not come in contact with skin or tissue		Disinfection — Will come in contact with skin or mucous membrane		Sterilization (Will enter tissue or vascular system)	
	Procedure	Minutes	Procedure	Minutes	Procedure	Hours
Smooth, hard-surfaced objects	A	$\geqq 10$	A	$\geqq 30$	C	18
	D	$\geqq 10$	C	$\geqq 30$	K	mfr. rec.
	E	$\geqq 10$	F	$\geqq 30$	L	12
	G	$\geqq 10$	H	$\geqq 30$	M	10
	I	$\geqq 10$	J[a]	$\geqq 30$	P	mfr. rec.
			L	$\geqq 30$		
			M	$\geqq 30$		
			N	$\geqq 30$		
Rubber tubing and catheters			F	$\geqq 30$	K	mfr. rec.
			H	$\geqq 30$	P	mfr. rec.
			M	$\geqq 30$		
			N	$\geqq 30$		
Polyethylene tubing and catheters[b, c, d]			A	$\geqq 30$	C	18
			F	$\geqq 30$	K	mfr. rec.
			H	$\geqq 30$	L	12
			M	$\geqq 30$	M	10
			N	$\geqq 30$	P	mfr. rec.
Lensed instruments			L	$\geqq 30$	K	mfr. rec.
			M	$\geqq 30$	L	12
					M	12
Thermometers (oral & rectal)[e]			B	$\geqq 30$	C	18
			M	$\geqq 30$	K	mfr. rec.
					L	12
					M	10
Hinged instruments					K	mfr. rec.
					L	12
					M	10
					P	mfr. rec.

Key:
A   Ethyl or isopropyl alcohol (70%–90%)
B   Ethyl alcohol (70%–90%)
C   Formaldehyde (8%)-alcohol (70%) solution
D   Quaternary ammonium germicidal detergent solution (2% aqueous solution of concentrate)
E   Iodophor germicidal detergent (100 p.p.m. available iodine)
F   Iodophor (500 p.p.m. available iodine)
G   Phenolic germicidal detergent solution (1% aqueous solution of concentrate)
H   Phenolic solutions (3% aqueous solution of concentrate)
I   Sodium hypochlorite (100 p.p.m. available chlorine)
J   Sodium hypochlorite (1000 p.p.m. available chlorine)
K   Ethylene oxide gas (for time, see manufacturer's recommendations)
L   Aqueous formaline (40% formaldehyde)
M   Glutaraldehyde (2% aqueous solution)
N   Wet pasteurization at 75°C after detergent cleaning
P   Heat sterilization (see manufacturer's recommendations)

Notes:
[a] Not recommended for metal instruments.
[b] Tubing must be completely filled for disinfection.
[c] Instruments or catheters that enter tissue or the vascular system should be sterilized.
[d] Thermostability should be investigated when indicated.
[e] Thermometers must be thoroughly wiped, preferably with soap and water, before disinfection or sterilization. Alcohol-iodine solutions will remove markings on poor-grade thermometers. Do not mix rectal and oral thermometers at any stage of handling or processing.

Modified from U.S. Department of Health, Education, and Welfare. *Isolation Techniques for Use in Hospitals* (2d ed.). DHEW Publication No. (CDC) 76–8314. Atlanta: Center for Disease Control, 1975.

handling of batch-sterilized items with transfer forceps. Sterilization generally is accomplished in hospitals by exposing articles to moist or dry heat or to gaseous ethylene oxide (EtO).

Moist Heat

Moist heat, applied as steam under pressure in autoclaves, is used for the great majority of sterilizations by hospitals. Both the heat and the moisture that are supplied by steam are essential for sterilization; therefore, each bundle or pack placed in a steam autoclave must be free from air pockets, seals, or wrappers that can block ready penetration of steam. Pressure has no influence per se on sterilization; pressure is used in autoclaves only to obtain the high temperatures necessary for killing microorganisms quickly, to keep fluids from boiling, or both. Exposure to saturated steam at 250°F to 253°F (121°C to 123°C) for 15 to 45 minutes (depending on pack size) accomplishes sterilization dependably without extensive damage to most materials. Conventional gravity-displacement sterilizers operate by removing air from the chamber by displacement with steam until the sterilizing temperature is achieved. High-vacuum, short-cycle sterilizers, including washer sterilizers (see Part I, Chapter 7, Central Service), are also used in hospitals; they permit a total sterilization cycle time that is considerably shorter than that obtained with a gravity sterilizer, because of nearly instantaneous penetration of steam as well as higher sterilization temperatures (270°F to 275°F or 132°C to 135°C). Both types of autoclaves require routine maintenance and careful operation. In larger hospitals with heavy demands for sterile goods, the high-vacuum sterilizers are recommended for the terminal processing of sterile goods for patient-care uses because of their speed of operation, but they are relatively more expensive than conventional sterilizers, and they require more skill in operation and maintenance.

At least weekly testing of all steam sterilizers is recommended using a commercial preparation of spores of *Bacillus stearothermophilus.*

Dry Heat

Dry heat can be used for sterilization when direct contact between saturated steam and all surfaces of the articles is unattainable. Materials that should be sterilized by dry heat include anhydrous oils, petroleum products, powders, certain instruments that cannot be disassembled, sharp instruments that might be damaged by moist heat, and glassware. Specially designed, electrically heated, hot-air sterilizers are required, and units with forced-air circulation are most efficient. Muslin or foil are satisfactory wrappers for items sterilized by dry heat.

Operation of sterilizers using steam or dry heat should be carefully monitored by recording the times and temperatures of all cycles. A chemical color-change indicator should be used on the outside of each wrapped pack that is sterilized to indicate that the pack was indeed cycled through a sterilizer. Such indicators do not prove that a pack is sterile, however. To monitor the efficiency of dry-heat sterilizers, at least weekly testing of each unit is recommended with spores of *B. stearothermophilus.*

Ethylene Oxide

Sterilization with gaseous ethylene oxide (EtO) is recommended for reusable items that must be sterile but that might be damaged by sterilization processes using heat, moisture, or both. Commercial gas sterilizers are available that permit hospital sterilization in periods of about 3 to 8 hours. Items to be sterilized by gaseous EtO should be held at a relative humidity above 30 percent or should be rehydrated by washing (followed by the removal of all visible moisture) just prior to sterilization. Porous materials—such as rubber, various types of plastic, or leather—accumulate residues of EtO during sterilization, and thus they must be well aerated before they are allowed to come in contact with any body tissues, including blood and skin. Aeration cabinets operating at approximately 131°F (55°C) reduce aeration times to 8 to 12 hours; at room temperature, aeration for as long as a week may be necessary.

Items sterilized with gas should be wrapped with materials that are highly permeable to EtO, such as muslin, paper, and films no greater than 3-mil in thickness of cellophane, polypropylene, polyvinylchloride, or low-density polyethylene.

Each package of any kind that is sterilized by gaseous EtO should be monitored by a color-change indicator. At least weekly testing of gas sterilizers is recommended using spores of *Bacillus subtilis* (*globigii*) that have been prepared commercially. If items that *must* be sterilized are processed by EtO sterilization (e.g., intravascular catheters, surgical gloves, or heart valves), then each load from the gas sterilizer should be monitored using spores of *B. subtilis.*

Liquid Chemicals

A few liquid disinfecting chemicals (see Table 6-1) will produce results comparable to those attained by the above sterilizing processes, but very long contact times are required. After such processing, three rinses with *sterile* water are necessary, followed by manual drying and packaging of the items in a sterile field by masked individuals wearing sterile gloves. Such expensive processing is seldom recommended over one of the alternatives of steam, hot-air, or gas sterilization.

Summary of Sterilization Procedures

The data listed under "sterilization" in Table 6-1 summarize the recommendations for sterilizing various items used within the hospital. These recommendations for sterilization will dependably kill hepatitis viruses. In addition, high concentrations of hepatitis viruses in protective media, such as might occur in laboratory spills of blood or serum, may be readily destroyed by liberal application of 5% sodium hypochlorite (laundry bleach); damage to surfaces from such an application is probable.

In-hospital sterilization of some items is not recommended. The manufacture and sterilization of parenteral or irrigation fluids should not be undertaken by a hospital, because of the expense of adequate quality control, including sterility and pyrogen testing of each autoclave lot. Nor is in-hospital resterilization recommended for gloves, surgical or isolation masks, sponges of any kind, or any but the most sophisticated syringes; dependable, high-quality disposable equipment is now available that is less expensive and safer than reusing these items.

Other Control Measures

Design of Hospital

Aseptic practice to prevent infection is much easier in a well-designed hospital. Design features that promote infection control include the ready availability of sinks for hand-washing, sufficient and properly designed isolation rooms, separation of clean and dirty areas, and sufficient and convenient space to facilitate adequate patient-care practices that are essential to the prevention of infections [14]. Unfortunately, many hospitals built in recent years have been overdesigned, often in misguided attempts to prevent nosocomial infections by the provision of expensive architectural barriers and unnecessary material-handling or disinfection and sterilization systems. Such attempts have resulted in greater costs in operation as well as in construction, but there has been no evidence of reduction in the frequency of infections.

Engineering and Maintenance

Most hospitals do not have adequately trained and supervised maintenance personnel. An important aid for proper operation, as well as for infection prevention, is a schedule for the regular checking and maintenance of water and sewerage systems, solid-waste disposal systems and equipment, ventilation that facilitates isolation and operating-room asepsis, sterilization and disinfection, laundry operations, food-handling and storage, and emergency operations. There should be a written manual of procedures for all major hospital equipment. Every hospital should have a hospital-experienced, registered, professional engineer on its staff or as a consultant. This person should assist in the direction of all engineering and maintenance activities and should also be consulted on nonmedical aspects of occupational safety and employee health.

Hand-washing

Hand-washing is all-important to prevent nosocomial disease transmission by direct or indirect contact [10]. Hand-washing facilities with hot and cold water, preferably with wrist-blade faucet operation, should be readily available throughout a hospital, particularly in patient-care areas. Briefly, hospital personnel should wash their hands after handling any object that might be contaminated with pathogens and before and after any significant patient contact. Patients at greatest risk from contaminated hands are surgical patients, those with catheters, and newborn infants. The hands should be vigorously lathered and rubbed together for at least 15 seconds in a stream of warm water; if a sink has hand-blade or wrist-blade operated faucet handles, the water should be turned off by touching the handles only with a paper towel, after the hands are dried. Faucet aerators may become contaminated, and, as a preventive measure, it is recommended that they not be used on faucets.

Antiseptic soaps—that is, those containing antimicrobial agents—are recommended for use before surgery and other invasive procedures, in isolation units, and in the care of newborn infants; soaps without antimicrobials are recommended for all other hand-washing. Bar, liquid, granule, or leaflet soaps or soap-impregnated tissues are acceptable. If liquid soap dispensers are used, they should be emptied, thoroughly cleaned, and refilled with new solution on a regular basis. Only a wedding ring that a person prefers to wear permanently should be worn at work by patient-care personnel, and nail polish should not be worn. Rings and nail polish make hands difficult to decontaminate.

Housekeeping

Housekeeping operations in hospitals are directed toward esthetics, safety, and the reduction of direct and indirect contact-transmission of infections from environmental sources. There is very little documentation of the relationship between general surface contamination in hospitals (e.g., of floors) and the spread of infection; however, improper housekeeping operations can spread pathogenic organisms to areas where they may be touched or actually increase the contamination of surfaces. Detailed recommendations for operating-suite and isolation-area housekeeping have been published [7,12]. Double-bucket floor-cleaning systems are recommended, as are daily laundering and thorough drying of the mops. Use of EPA-

registered disinfectant-detergent products is recommended for surface cleaning. A spray-on, wipe-off system should be used for other surfaces in patient-care areas, using large quantities of clean wipes. Disinfectant fogging is *not* recommended. A continuous and effective program of training, as well as adequate supervision, are essential for housekeeping personnel.

Proper disposal of hospital solid wastes is a housekeeping responsibility that is not complex and should result in no risk of disease to employees, patients, or the community. Special procedures have been recommended for the safe, in-hospital handling of high-risk materials, including laboratory and isolation-ward wastes and wastes capable of causing physical injury [13].

Kitchen and Food-handling Operations

Numerous outbreaks of infection in hospitals due to contaminated food or drink attest to the need for the careful maintenance of appropriate standards for food-service operations that will help to prevent disease transmission [11] (see also Part I, Chapter 7, Food Services). Adequate training is essential for all food handlers. Perishable food must be stored at temperatures below 45°F (7°C) to prevent the growth of microorganisms that could cause foodborne disease; hot food must be kept above 140°F (60°C) for the same reason. Hot food to be reused *must* be cooled quickly; frozen food should be thawed in a refrigerator. Meat slicers and grinders should be cleaned three times daily when in use. Raw eggs should not be used in any hospital diet.

Laundry

Laundry operations to provide dependable, acceptable, and safe linens for patient-care purposes are described in the next chapter (Part I, Chapter 7, Linens and Laundry). Soiled linens should be placed into bags or carts at the location where they are used. They should never be thrown on the floor, where they may present a fire or accident hazard as well as spread microbial contamination. Soiled isolation and nursery linens should be placed in impervious bags. Sorting of soiled linen should be minimized.

Washing at temperatures above 160°F (71°C) for 25 minutes makes all linens safe for reuse; sterilization prior to washing is not recommended. Surgical linens are normally the only type sterilized (after laundering) prior to use.

Sanitation

A hospital should have available the services of a professional sanitarian for consultation and assistance in such areas as the sanitation of potable water systems and hydrotherapy equipment, kitchen and food sanitation, ice handling, and liquid and solid-waste handling and disposal. Such services are commonly available free on request from local or state health departments, or both. Written sanitation programs and good training and supervision are essential for persons who maintain a safe and sanitary hospital environment.

Unless sewage from a hospital is discharged directly into a body of water that is used without treatment as a potable water supply, all fecal material may and should be disposed of without treatment directly to the hospital sewerage system.

Vector Control

Control of insects and rodents is principally an esthetic problem, rather than a disease problem, in hospitals. During the warmest months, continuing measures to prevent flies from entering are indicated, principally through the use of window screening and by using doors at either end of short halls or foyers at major hospital entrances. Only pyrethrum aerosols may be used for fly control in patient-care areas of hospitals. Cockroach and rodent control requires not only efforts to prevent their entry in bulk supplies or hospital food, but also prompt control by competent pest control operators whenever infestations are found.

Early diagnosis and prompt treatment of scabietic patients with 1% lindane will quickly reduce the risk of transfer to hospital staff members with close patient contact. Clothing and bedding used by infested patients should be machine washed and dried at hot temperatures (see Part I, Chapter 7, Linens and Laundry). Mattresses without plastic covers should

be left unused for at least ten days, but special environmental cleaning of the patient's room is not necessary after discharge.

Ventilation

Most "standards" or recommendations [3] for ventilation of health-care facilities have little or no known relationship to the reduction of airborne (or droplet-spread) infections; rather, comfort and ready achievability have been the primary criteria used for design. Hospitals that are constructed and operated to meet current minimum construction requirements with respect to air changes and filtration [14] are probably more than sufficiently safe from any significant risk of airborne infection.

Hospital air is conventionally furnished at a rate of two air changes per hour to most patient rooms. Air is preferably exhausted through a vent in the patient bathroom. Patient rooms should normally be at the same air pressure as the corridor. Isolation-room doors must be kept closed except for necessary entrances and exits; six air changes per hour are recommended. Ultraviolet disinfection of the air is rarely useful for infection control. Recirculation of most air from critical hospital areas (e.g., to conserve energy) is possible and safe after high-efficiency filtration. "Laminar flow" or unidirectional air systems are not recommended for general hospital use in operating or patient rooms.

Environmental Surveillance

It is now widely accepted that good patient-care practices—not environmental-control programs—constitute the most important single factor for minimizing nosocomial disease [9]. The large-scale, nonepidemiologically directed or related, environmental sampling programs that existed widely in the 1960s in hospitals in the United States have been actively decried and discouraged in recent years [1].

Routine sampling of the general inanimate environment in hospitals for culture studies does not contribute to the prevention of nosocomial infections, nor does it permit one to predict when or where nosocomial infections may be most likely to occur. Since rates of nosocomial disease have not been correlated with levels of general environmental contamination, standards for "acceptable" levels of environmental contamination are arbitrary at best. Programs of routine environmental surveillance not only are expensive and time-consuming, but they may also generate large quantities of data that are difficult to interpret and may be falsely relied upon.

The preferable alternative is to maintain surveillance of nosocomial infections in patients and employees (see Part I, Chapter 4). When the results of patient-oriented and employee-oriented disease surveillance suggest that contaminated environmental reservoirs or sources of disease exist, investigations should be promptly initiated—with environmental samples being taken for culture studies if appropriate—to identify and eliminate any such environmental sources of infection.

The only routine environmental microbiologic monitoring that is recommended for infection control includes culture determinations on critical patient-care equipment after disinfection and the use of spores for microbiologic monitoring of sterilization processes. Steam and hot-air sterilizers should be checked with live spores at least once a week; those utilizing ethylene oxide for critical patient-care equipment or implantable items that must be sterile should be checked with live spores at each use. Hospital-prepared infant formulas should be tested by culture study once a week (see Part I, Chapter 8).

Microbiologic sampling of items sold to hospitals as "sterile" is not recommended, not only because of the low frequency of microbial contamination of such items in the United States, but also because of the great difficulty and expense of adequate sterility testing. Rather, surveillance data regarding disease in patients should be monitored carefully to insure that a common source of infection is noted promptly. If a commercial "sterile" product is suspected of causing disease, all items with the same lot number should immediately be quarantined and held by the hospital, and the local or state health department and the district office of the U.S. Food and Drug Administration should be informed promptly so they may investigate the potential problem with guaranteed access to any or all of the suspect items.

Any environmental microbial sampling program should be supervised by the Infection Control Committee, follow a carefully prepared protocol, and be done by competent individuals. A decision should be made *before* the sampling regarding what action will (or will not) be taken, depending on results of sampling. All sampling data should be reviewed immediately and appropriate action taken.

References

1. American Hospital Association. *Infection Control in the Hospital* (3d ed.). Chicago: American Hospital Association, 1974.
2. Bassett, D. J. C. Causes and prevention of sepsis due to Gram-negative bacteria: Common-source outbreaks. *Proc. R. Soc. Med.* 64:980, 1971.
3. Committee on Environment of Hospitals and Other Medical Care Facilities, Engineering and Sanitation Section, American Public Health Association. Guidelines for hospital operating and delivery room air conditioning systems. *Am. J. Public Health* 57:1053, 1967.
4. Gonzaga, A. J., Mortimer, E. A., Jr., Wolinsky, E., and Rammelkamp, C. H., Jr. Transmission of staphylococci by fomites. *J.A.M.A.* 189:711, 1964.
5. Mackel, D. C., Maki, D. G., Anderson, R. L., Rhame, F. S., and Bennett, J. V. Nationwide epidemic of septicemia caused by contaminated intravenous products: Mechanisms of intrinsic contamination. *J. Clin. Microbiol.* 2:486, 1975.
6. Maki, D. G., Rhame, F. S., Mackel, D. C., and Bennett, J. V. Nationwide epidemic of septicemia caused by contaminated intravenous products. I. Epidemiologic and clinical features. *Am. J. Med.* 60:471, 1976.
7. Mallison, G. F. Housekeeping in operating suites. *A.O.R.N. J.* 21:213, 1975.
8. Mallison, G. F. Introduction to Microbiology of the Institutional Environment. In *Proceedings of the Fourth Annual Technical Meeting of the American Association for Contamination Control.* Miami Beach, 1975.
9. Stamm, W. E. Elements of an active, effective infection control program. *Hospitals* 50:60, 1976.
10. Steere, A. C., and Mallison, G. F. Hand-

washing practices for the prevention of nosocomial infections. *Ann. Intern. Med.* 83:683, 1975.

11. U.S. Department of Health, Education, and Welfare. *Food Service Sanitation Manual Including a Model Food Service Sanitation Ordinance.* Washington, D.C.: Food and Drug Administration, Division of Food Service, 1976.

12. U.S. Department of Health, Education, and Welfare. *Isolation Techniques for Use in Hospitals* (2d ed.). DHEW Publication No. (CDC) 76–8314. Atlanta: Center for Disease Control, 1975.

13. U.S. Department of Health, Education, and Welfare. *Disposal of Solid Wastes from Hos-*

pitals. National Nosocomial Infections Study. DHEW Publication No. (CDC) 74–8257. Atlanta: Center for Disease Control, 1974.

14. U.S. Department of Health, Education, and Welfare. *Minimum Requirements of Construction and Equipment for Hospital and Medical Facilities.* DHEW Publication No. (HRA) 74–4000. Rockville, Md.: Health Resources Administration, 1973.

15. von Graevenitz, A., and Pantelick, E. Should Potential Sources of Hospital-Acquired Infections be Monitored– *Jahrgang* 3:1, 1975.

16. Walter, C. W., Kundsin, R. B., and Brubaker, M. M. The incidence of airborne wound infection during operation. *J.A.M.A.* 186:908, 1963.

7

Areas of Special Concern

Section A. The Hemodialysis Unit

John A. Bryan

Most hemodialysis units in the United States have been plagued with problems related to infections [1,3,4]. Bacterial infections, both local and generalized, and viral infections comprise those most commonly encountered. Bacterial infections are usually localized and most often affect arteriovenous shunts and fistulas, but bacteremia, septicemia, and other such generalized infections can also occur and cause death in a substantial number of patients. The "endemic" or background rate of bacterial infections was found to be between six and eight infections per 100 patient-months in one study of five chronic dialysis units, and it rose to levels twice as high during "epidemic" periods [5]. On occasion, epidemics of pyrogenic reactions (probably due to endotoxin in the dialysate) have developed in some dialysis units [10]. Viral infections—especially viral hepatitis—have also been common in hemodialysis units [16]. The viral hepatitis seems to be predominantly type B (hepatitis B); however, infections with non-B hepatitis viruses and agents such as cytomegalovirus and Epstein-Barr virus have been recognized. One recent report of a serologic epidemiologic survey of patients and staff in 15 United States centers for cases of hepatitis A virus infection documented that hepatitis A was no more frequent in hemodialysis units than in the general population not exposed to hemodialysis [14].

Infection problems in hemodialysis units undoubtedly are accentuated by the increased susceptibility to infection present in many patients with chronic renal failure, some of whom may have undergone renal transplantation and immunosuppression, as well as by the necessity for the regular use of indwelling catheters and cannulas. In addition, faulty dialysis technique has resulted in epidemics of disease in some units and probably contributes to a low level of endemic infection problems as well. A wide variety of bacteria have been identified as the causative agents of infection in hemodialysis patients; however, coagulase-positive staphylococci and *Pseudomonas* species have been most commonly incriminated in shunt infections and bacteremias.

Viral hepatitis infections—predominantly positive for hepatitis B surface antigen (HB$_s$Ag) and therefore caused by hepatitis B virus (HBV)—occur in the majority of hemodialysis units. Of the units surveyed by the Center for Disease Control (CDC) in 1970, 80 percent had experienced hepatitis in patients, staff, or both [3]. A survey for 1972 revealed that 3 percent of the more than 8000 patients dialyzed acquired HB$_s$Ag, and 75 percent were persistently positive after three months. Furthermore, almost 3 percent of staff developed clinical hepatitis, two-thirds of which was due to HBV. In 1974, a similar survey of 312 units with a total of 15,382 patients revealed an HBV attack rate of 6.2 percent for patients and 5.8 percent for staff. Almost 90 percent of patients who acquired HBV infection remained persistently HB$_s$Ag-positive [12].

Epidemics of hepatitis have occurred in some units, while in others, hepatitis has been endemic, with cases occurring regularly over a period of several years. Some units have reported high mortality rates among staff. Outbreaks of hepatitis have been reported from units in England, the Scandinavian countries, and the United States. The chronic nature of the problem is underscored not only by American data but also by data from the European Dialysis and Transplant Association that indicate annual rates for hepatitis during "endemic" periods of between 5 and 10 percent; case rates go much higher during "epidemic" periods, and recent estimates indicate that from 25 to 50 percent of patients and staff in renal hemodialysis units can develop hepatitis B on such occasions [11].

HBV infections have a significant disruptive impact on the operation of the hemodialysis unit, because frequently *both* patients and staff are affected. Staff are more likely to have an associated clinical illness than are patients; however, a majority of the infections in either group may go undetected unless frequent screening for HB$_s$Ag and antibody to HB$_s$Ag

(anti-HB$_s$) is conducted. Cytomegalovirus and Epstein-Barr virus infections have also been reported in chronic dialysis patients, but these and other viral diseases are not believed to occur frequently in the hemodialysis setting.

Epidemiologic Aspects of Hemodialysis
Bacterial infections in hemodialysis units usually occur because of lapses in aseptic technique, such as contamination of the surgical wound during placement of an arteriovenous shunt or creation of the fistula, improper technique in shunt care and maintenance, and unsterile cannulation of fistulized veins. Most infections occur as a result of direct contact with a contaminated surface or object, and frequently the infecting organism is derived from the patient's own skin flora. Use of unsterile equipment could also account for such infections, but the rapid decrease in shunt infections that was observed in several units following the institution of rigidly practiced and enforced aseptic techniques suggests that faulty handling of shunts or fistulas is often responsible.

Because of the virtual predominance of HBV among viral infections affecting hemodialysis-unit patients and staff, and because of the likelihood that other infections may be spread within units via the same mechanisms, the remainder of this section will be devoted to a discussion of the epidemiology, control, and prevention of HBV in the hemodialysis unit [2, 7,13].

Introduction and Modes of Transmission
of Hepatitis B Virus
Hepatitis B virus can be introduced into the hemodialysis unit environment by the following means:

1. by the admission of patients, staff personnel, or both, who are infected with HBV,
2. by patient(s) or staff currently enrolled in the unit acquiring infection, either in the community or in other areas of the hospital (i.e., while being treated on surgical or medical services), or
3. occasionally by transfusion of infected

blood, plasma, or blood products to patients.

Once it is introduced into the dialysis-unit environment, HBV can be acquired by patients during personal contact with other patients or staff, through the use of contaminated equipment, dialyzers, or dialysis-monitoring devices, or possibly through other environmental contact, for example, with surfaces (floors, walls, tabletops, and the like) that are contaminated. Infection can be transmitted parenterally by contaminated dialysis equipment or during the process of giving injections and obtaining blood samples; direct entry of infectious inocula through cuts, scratches, or other breaks in the skin may also occur. Other possible means of exposure include the inapparent ingestion of virus-containing material, the accidental inoculation of mucous membranes during splattering, and possibly (but less likely), the inhalation of aerosols containing the virus.

Once one or more patients in the hemodialysis unit are infected, spread to staff is a likely possibility because of such occurrences as inadvertent self-inoculation (e.g., through breaks in the skin or accidental needle puncture) and because of the nature of the hemodialysis environment, which necessitates frequent contact with blood. Inapparent ingestion of virus-contaminated materials and accidental inoculation of mucous membranes provide means of exposure, and these routes present an even greater risk for staff than for patients. Hemodialysis technicians have frequent contact with both dialysis equipment and patients, and they are at risk when obtaining specimens from patients, handling blood-stained equipment, and dismantling and rebuilding dialyzers.

Methods of Infection Control
Surveillance
Surveillance of hemodialysis patients and staff for HBV infection should be undertaken on a regular basis. Patients and staff should be closely observed for symptoms and signs indicative of the presence of infection. Periodic questioning of patients about symptoms suggestive of infection, physical examination, and review of clinical and laboratory data should be routine parts of the hemodialysis operation. Staff members should immediately report the presence of any signs or symptoms of infection. In addition to observation to identify hepatitis infections, patients and staff should be periodically monitored with blood tests for HB_sAg, anti-HB_s, and serum glutamate-oxaloacetate transaminase (SGOT), glutamate-pyruvate transaminase (SGPT), or both. Transaminase determinations are of value in identifying cases of HB_sAg-negative hepatitis and in confirming the presence of active hepatocellular inflammation in persons with persistent HB_sAg. Anti-HB_s screening is necessary to detect HBV infections that are transient and asymptomatic. The frequency of screening should depend on whether or not infection is occurring in a unit. If no seroconversions have occurred in six to twelve months, then sampling intervals of two to four months might be reasonable; however, if seroconversions are regularly observed, then monthly sampling should be considered.

Candidates for hemodialysis programs and those being considered for employment should be screened for HB_sAg and anti-HB_s *before* admission or employment in order to establish their HBV susceptibility or immunity as well as to recognize a need to institute precautions for the management of patients or employees with HB_sAg. Identification of the potential sources of infection in the unit is the first step in the control of infection.

Safety Officer
Many hemodialysis units have found it helpful to have a member of the staff who acts as a safety officer. Working closely with the Infection Control Committee, this person serves as the source of information for the unit about the control of infections and performs periodic evaluations of the hemodialysis staff. This individual insures that a log is kept of accidents, unusual events, or exposures (skin penetrations, heavy blood contamination, and so on). Such a log enables the evaluation of the progress of the staff in improving technique and the correlation of cases of infection with the history of accidents and exposures.

Disinfection and Sterilization

Heat sterilization is the treatment of choice for instruments and other objects that can be conveniently handled this way [8,17]. The importance of thoroughly cleansing instruments, containers, or surfaces to remove adherent material before treatment cannot be overemphasized. HBV can be inactivated by (1) boiling in water (100°C or 212°F) for 10 to 20 minutes, (2) steam under pressure (autoclaving) at 121°C (253°F) and 15 pounds per square inch pressure for 15 minutes, or (3) dry heat (170°C or 338°F) for two hours. In addition to heat, certain chemical disinfectants are presumed to be effective in inactivating HBV: (1) solutions of sodium hypochlorite, 0.5% to 1.0% (5000 to 10,000 p.p.m. available chlorine) for 30 minutes, (2) 40% aqueous formalin (16% aqueous formaldehyde) for 12 hours; 20% formalin in 70% alcohol for 18 hours, (3) 2% aqueous alkalinized glutaraldehyde for 10 hours, and (4) gas sterilization with ethylene oxide (check manufacturer's recommendations). Compatibility of the item being treated with the disinfectant must be considered (e.g., hypochlorite will corrode metal).

Protection of Patients

Patients need to be educated in the principles and practice of aseptic technique and shunt care, and they should be carefully observed periodically to assure that their technique is acceptable.

Transfusions should be kept to a minimum, but if required, HB_sAg-negative blood should be given. The use of blood from commercial sources and of blood products such as fibrinogen, antihemophilic factor concentrate, and factor-IX complex is associated with a high risk of hepatitis. The utilization of frozen packed red cells, which minimize exposure to leukocyte antigens, may be associated with less risk of viral hepatitis; however, the cost may be prohibitive. Detailed records of blood and blood products transfused (i.e., recipient, lot number, date, and so on) should be maintained to assist in monitoring and evaluating reactions, especially if hepatitis occurs.

Using individual supplies and equipment can help reduce the opportunity for the spread of hepatitis, as well as of other infections, that may occur through the use of shared items. In addition, sharing food, cigarettes, or other items among patients presents a risk of ingesting contaminated material and should not be permitted during the dialysis operation.

Protection of Staff

Techniques of scrupulous personal hygiene and asepsis must be emphasized to the staff to minimize the risk of infection. Thorough handwashing after contact with each patient minimizes the risk of infection. Accidental punctures and inoculations—a frequent source of exposure to HBV—can be minimized if:

1. needles for discard are not recapped but rather are deposited into disposable plastic containers (e.g., plastic milk cartons) placed at each bedside (when full, the containers can be capped and incinerated or discarded),
2. microhematocrit tubes are flame-sealed (instead of using clay) in order to reduce the danger of breakage and accidental puncture, and
3. minor abrasions, lacerations, or other breaks in the skin are routinely cleaned, disinfected, and covered with a watertight dressing to reduce the risk of contact with infectious material.

If patients with arteriovenous fistulas were trained to cannulate themselves, this would reduce or eliminate the substantial contact with blood that staff must have when they perform such cannulations themselves.

Protective clothing can reduce the hepatitis risk. It is advised that disposable gloves be available at each patient's bedside for use in attending the patient and that a fresh pair of gloves should be used with each patient. Gloves also should be worn during any procedure (e.g., handling shunts, drawing blood, dismantling dialysis machinery, or changing bedpans) in which hands might be contaminated with blood or other body fluids. However, gloves are not a substitute for good technique and proper personal hygiene. Gowns or scrub clothes can protect skin and clothing from blood and fluids, and an outer garment (i.e., a laboratory coat or apron) worn over the uniform when temporarily leaving the dialysis unit can restrict the spread of infection to other areas of the hospital. Surgical-type masks and protective shielding for the eyes might be considered when personnel are engaged in procedures where splattering of blood would likely occur.

The Environment

The dialysis working area should be as spacious as possible in order to avoid overcrowding and cramped conditions. Separate cubicles for individual dialysis patients would provide the best arrangement to minimize cross-infection. Surfaces in the dialysis area (i.e., floors, walls, tabletops, and the like) that are frequently blood-splattered should be cleaned and disinfected regularly to reduce environmental contamination. Bed linens should be changed (especially if soiled), individual dialysis areas cleaned after each dialysis, and prompt attention given to the cleanup of any spilled blood.

Hand-washing areas should be conveniently located, and sinks should be equipped, if possible, with knee-operated faucets and pedal-operated soap dispensers to reduce the possibility of contamination. A separate area of the hemodialysis unit should be specifically designated for the decontamination and maintenance of the dialysis equipment. To protect those handling them, contaminated disposable items should be placed in tightly sealed containers (e.g., plastic bags) for incineration or disposal. Alternatively, such items could be soaked overnight in hypochlorite solution or autoclaved prior to disposal. Linens and other contaminated items should also be bagged, and if they are from infected patients, they should be so labeled.

The Equipment

Each patient should have an individual dialysis machine that is not shared with others; dialysis-monitoring and other equipment that must be shared should be assigned to a constant, limited number of patients to minimize the number of persons exposed. Records of the dates when monitors and dialyzers were used should be maintained to correlate any infections that de-velop with specific pieces of equipment. An outbreak of Epstein-Barr virus hepatitis, for example, has been traced to a contaminated venous pressure gauge. Assigning patients to specific shifts and bed positions on a permanent basis is helpful in minimizing the effect of variables related to the transmision of disease. For safety's sake, all equipment that is exposed to blood should be either disposable or capable of being sterilized after thorough cleaning. Nondisposable components that cannot be subjected to standard methods of sterilization can be chemically treated with one of the disinfectants mentioned previously (see Disinfection and Sterilization, above).

Many units disinfect dialyzers as follows: first, the blood compartment of the dialyzer is filled with one of the appropriate disinfectants and allowed to stand for one hour. The machine is then disassembled, and the disposable portion is bagged and incinerated or autoclaved. Nondisposable parts are rinsed with tap water and reassembled. A disinfectant is again instilled into the blood compartment and then flushed out with sterile saline. Finally, the dialysis compartment is rinsed with tap water. The dialysis-monitoring equipment will also periodically require sterilization or disinfection. Special attention in cleaning should be given to equipment that is shared (e.g., venous pressure gauges), because contamination of these devices (e.g., by reflux of blood into nondisposable portions of the equipment) can result in cross-infection. Impermeable disposable diaphragms should be considered to prevent reflux or other means of contamination of such equipment.

Precautions for Patients with Hepatitis Infection

Patients infected with HBV should be handled with caution and dialyzed in an area of the hemodialysis unit that, if not physically separate from the HB$_s$Ag-negative dialysis area, is at least removed from the mainstream of activity. In the most recent CDC survey, patients in units with a separate room for HB$_s$Ag-positive patients had a significantly lower attack rate than patients in units that did not (p < .01). Also, the rate for patients in the units with separate rooms was slightly lower than the attack rate in units that separated HB$_s$Ag-positive from HB$_s$Ag-negative patients without using a separate room (7.2 percent versus 9.4 percent). Some units with HB$_s$Ag-positive patients have found it helpful to assign staff with the most dialysis experience and best technique to care for these infected patients. Staff members with anti-HB$_s$ antibody have at least partial (if not complete) immunity to repeat HBV infection, and they therefore are less likely to become ill as a result of exposure to such patients. Because of the risk of cross-infection, staff should be assigned to HB$_s$Ag-positive or HB$_s$Ag-negative patients only during a given shift, and they should not attend both simultaneously. Blood and other specimens from a patient with HBV that are sent to the clinical laboratories from the dialysis unit should be clearly marked for hepatitis precautions. If possible, patients with persistent HB$_s$Ag should be strongly considered for home training programs, because their removal from the dialysis unit environment would reduce the total reservoir of antigen.

Passive and Active Immunization against Hepatitis B Virus

Since dialysis-associated hepatitis occurs in the setting where contact with HB$_s$Ag-positive patients and their blood and other body fluids is frequent and where HB$_s$Ag can often be demonstrated on environmental surfaces and equipment, most cases are thought to be due to HBV infection. In view of this and the data from studies of immunoglobulin prophylaxis [6,9] (see also Part II, Chapter 24), the following recommendations are made for prophylaxis of hepatitis B in hemodialysis settings using currently available immunoglobulin preparations.

Postexposure Prophylaxis

When single exposures occur involving HB$_s$Ag-positive inocula (e.g., resulting from accidental needle punctures, ingestion, or contact with mucosal surfaces), hepatitis B immune globulin (HB-Ig) in a dose of 0.03 ml. per pound (0.06 ml. per kilogram) of body weight should be administered *intramuscularly* as soon as possible within a seven-day period after exposure. The usual adult dose is 3 to 5 ml., and a second identical dose should be given four weeks (25 to 30 days) after the first. If HB-Ig is not available, standard immune serum globulin (ISG) should be given according to the same recommended dosage and schedule.

Preexposure Prophylaxis

Routine preexposure immunoglobulin prophylaxis is not recommended for patients and staff of most hemodialysis units, because conventional control and prevention methods should be sufficient. In certain units where HBV infection is endemic and chronic virus transmission continues to occur, however, immunoprophylaxis may be considered for HB$_s$Ag-negative and anti-HB$_s$-negative patients and staff. Standard ISG in a dose of 0.03 ml. per pound (0.06 ml. per kilogram) of body weight given *intramuscularly* every four months is recommended for this purpose; there is no convincing evidence for the superior efficacy of HB-Ig in such situations, and acquisition of passive-active immunity is more likely to occur with standard ISG. Individuals to be immunized should be periodically tested for anti-HB$_s$, and if such tests are positive, these persons should not receive further immunoprophylaxis.

On occasion, hepatitis A infections may occur in the hemodialysis unit. When hepatitis A is strongly suspected on the basis of epidemiologic or laboratory studies, ISG should be given to those exposed in a dose of 0.01 ml. per pound (0.02 ml. per kilogram) of body weight [15]. If the exact diagnosis is not known, the dose of ISG should be that given for HBV prophylaxis (see above).

Vaccines for active immunization against hepatitis B are being developed and tested for safety and efficacy. These preparations are inactivated HBV vaccines that, when licensed by the Bureau of Biologics, Food and Drug Administration, may be used to prevent or attenuate infection in individuals at high risk of hepatitis B by virtue of continuous exposure to HB$_s$Ag-positive individuals and blood. Since dialysis-unit personnel fall into this category and have about the highest risk of hepatitis B infection of any group of persons in the United States, they will undoubtedly be a target population for the use of such vaccines when they become available.

References

1. Bailey, G. L. (Ed.). *Hemodialysis: Principles and Practice.* New York: Academic Press, 1972.
2. Center for Disease Control. Perspectives on the control of viral hepatitis, type B. *Morbid. Mortal. Weekly Rep.* Suppl. 25(17):3, 1976.
3. Garibaldi, R. A., Bryan, J. A., Forrest, J. F., Hanson, B. F., and Dismukes, W. E. Hemodialysis-associated hepatitis. *J.A.M.A.* 225:384, 1973.
4. Gutch, C. F., and Stoner, M. H. *Review of Hemodialysis for Nurses and Dialysis Personnel.* St. Louis: C. V. Mosby, 1971.
5. Kaslow, R. A., and Zellner, S. R. Infection in patients on maintenance hemodialysis. *Lancet* 2:117, 1972.
6. Krugman, S., and Giles, J. P. Viral hepatitis, type B (MS-2 strain): Natural history and prevention. *N. Engl. J. Med.* 288:755, 1972.
7. Marmion, B. P., and Tonkin, R. W. Control of hepatitis in dialysis units. *Br. Med. Bull.* 28(2):169, 1972.
8. Perkins, S. S. *Principles and Methods of Sterilization in Health Sciences.* Springfield, Ill.: Charles C Thomas, 1970.
9. Prince, A. M., Szmuness, W., Mann, M. K., et al. Hepatitis B "immune" globulin: Effectiveness in prevention of dialysis-associated hepatitis. *N. Engl. J. Med.* 293:1063, 1975.
10. Raij, L., Shapiro, F. L., and Michael, A. F. Endotoxemia in febrile reactions during hemodialysis. *Kidney Int.* 4:57, 1973.
11. Rosenheim, L. (Chairman). *Report of the Advisory Group 1970–1972: Hepatitis and the Treatment of Chronic Renal Failure.* Department of Health and Social Security, Scottish Home and Health Department, Welsh Office, 1973.
12. Snydman, D. R., Bregman, D. J., and Bryan, J. A. Hemodialysis-associated hepatitis in the United States—1974. *J. Infect. Dis.* 135:687, 1977.
13. Snydman, D. R., Bryan, J. A., and Dixon, R. E. Prevention of nosocomial viral hepatitis, type B (hepatitis B). *Ann. Intern. Med.* 83:838, 1975.
14. Szmuness, W., Dienstag, J. L., Purcell, R. H., Prince, A. M., Stevens, C. E., and Levine, R. W. Hepatitis A and hemodialysis. A seroepidemiological study in 15 U.S. centers. *Ann. Intern. Med.* 87:8, 1977.
15. U.S. Public Health Service Advisory Committee. Immune serum globulin for protection against viral hepatitis. *Ann. Intern. Med.* 77:427, 1972.
16. W.H.O. Expert Committee Report. Advances in viral hepatitis. *W.H.O. Tech. Rep. Ser.* 602:1, 1977.
17. Working Party of the Central Pathology Committee. *Safety in Pathology Laboratories, 1972.* London: Department of Health and Social Security, Alexander Fleming House. Elephant & Castle, 1972.

Section B. The Intensive-Care Unit

Alfred E. Buxton

As the technology of medicine has progressed over the past 15 years, there has been a proliferation of specialized units designed to render intensive therapy to seriously ill patients. The original medical-surgical intensive-care unit (ICU) has now been subdivided into coronary-care units, respiratory ICUs, oncology units, burn units, neurosurgery units, and pediatric and neonatal ICUs. Along with the benefits to patient care that have accrued from the development of these specialized facilities are certain hazards, notably that of producing a concentration of highly susceptible patients at great risk of acquiring nosocomial infections.

Several factors are responsible for the high-risk status of ICU patients. Many ICU patients have specific underlying illnesses that compromise host resistance. Changes in patients' flora that accompany serious illness undoubtedly play some role [2,3]. Some antibiotics used to treat life-threatening diseases change the host's flora, predisposing to colonization with multiple-drug-resistant bacteria, while others impair host defense mechanisms. In addition, when a patient enters an ICU, he or she is subjected to a variety of invasive procedures, both for therapeutic and monitoring purposes, that are potential vehicles of infection. Frequently, life-saving procedures must be performed on an emergency basis, compromising the usual infection control measures. Finally, the concentration of patients in close proximity to others predisposed to similar infections creates a situation in which an infectious illness acquired by one patient may be easily transmitted to others in the same unit.

Since the purpose of the ICU is to give the special care needed by critically ill patients, effective provision of these services should be the primary consideration in formulating policies for admitting patients to and performing procedures in the unit. However, whenever possible without jeopardizing patient care, infection control procedures should be stressed as much as those that are more directly related to the medical care of patients. It should be recognized, of course, that the former may have to be compromised occasionally because of practical considerations.

The question often arises whether patients with recognized or suspected infections should be admitted to the ICU. Although their admission should be avoided if possible, the medical needs of the individual patient are the primary consideration, and if the care of a patient will suffer outside an ICU, he or she must be admitted and placed under the appropriate isolation precautions. Rarely, instances will arise in which a patient in need of intensive care has an infection which, if it spread to medical staff or other patients, could be disastrous (e.g., pneumonic plague, smallpox, or certain exotic viral infections such as Lassa fever or Marburg disease). It would be preferable to have a private medical staff attend such patients in a remote area of the hospital or out of the hospital; however, judgment must be made by the physicians caring for the patient, and the potential risk to other patients and staff must be balanced against the needs of the individual patient. Ideally, all hospitals should have an ICU available solely for infected patients, but this is not economically feasible unless an institution houses large numbers of infected patients and has constant need for such a unit.

Operationally, the problems of infection control in the ICU are threefold. The first type of problems are those related to handling patients with known infections. In these cases, isolation measures appropriate for the disease concerned should be applied. The second kind are those arising from patients with subclinical or incubating infections or with active infections recognized late; for example, when a patient is admitted to the ICU with apparently typical pulmonary edema and is later found to have active, disseminated, pulmonary tuberculosis. Third are problems resulting from gross breakdowns in isolation techniques that occur despite ongoing isolation procedures or routine infection control measures. This type of case is exemplified by a cardiac arrest that necessitates cardiopulmonary resuscitation in a patient with meningococcic meningitis or, more likely, in a patient with hepatitis B antigenemia. In these last two situations, individual judgments have to be made about actions to be taken, such as possibly providing prophylaxis for medical personnel and other patients or maintaining a period of intensive surveillance for specific illnesses. Such situations emphasize the importance of keeping ICU personnel constantly aware of the potential for spread of infections in this unique setting. In addition, these eventualities must be considered when ICUs are being designed and constructed.

In addition to the prevention of transmission of recognized infections, transfer of endogenous flora among patients and personnel must be avoided, because an organism that is a harmless commensal on the skin of a nurse or in the intestinal flora of one patient may become a virulent pathogen in the patient whose host defenses are impaired [1].

This section reviews general principles for design and operation of ICUs that may be applied to all such facilities. Specific procedures are discussed elsewhere in this book.

Structural Aspects of the ICU

When an ICU is designed, the relative importance of the various modes of disease transmission (airborne, contact, common-vehicle, and vectorborne) should be taken into account, in addition to aspects relating more directly to the medical care of patients. This may entail making compromises in the design of facilities to best accommodate the medical needs of patients and, at the same time, to permit the use of appropriate techniques to prevent transmission of disease by people and inanimate objects.

Airborne Transmission

The control of airborne contamination is being approached in several ways: the use of ultraviolet irradiation of the air, laminar-flow ventilation with or without additional physical barriers, positive-negative air-pressure relationships between rooms and corridors, filtered ventilation with and without physical barriers, and private rooms. Ultraviolet irradiation of the air can be effective, but it is somewhat impractical because the light source must be kept free of dust and the airflow in the room must be controlled so that the air passes close enough to the light source for the radiation to be effective. Laminar airflow, too, is effective, but it has the disadvantage of being expensive. Most important, these devices do not seem to be necessary for most ICUs, because the airborne route is not a common route for disease transmission in ICUs.

The importance of the airborne mode of spread varies according to the patient population being considered: it may play a role in patients with extensive burns and in immunosuppressed patients. In contrast, for most patients receiving intensive respiratory care, contact spread of endogenous flora and other patients' flora is far more important. Therefore, although many air-control systems have been shown to control levels of airborne bacteria effectively, few valid studies have shown any positive effect of such measures on actual infection rates. If established standards of ventilation are maintained (six exchanges per hour minimum), it appears adequate to maintain the ICU air under positive pressure relative to the corridors to minimize air exchange with the rest of the hospital and to exhaust air directly to the outside or filter it before recirculation [10]. In addition, there should be one or more private rooms that can be placed under negative air pressure if the need arises to provide strict or respiratory isolation.

Contact Transmission: Direct

Although it is clear that certain diseases are transmitted by the airborne route, at the present time it would appear that by far the most important mechanism for the transmission of infections in ICUs is contact spread from patient to patient on the hands of hospital personnel. Thus, the most effective means of controlling the spread of nosocomial infections is diligent hand-washing by personnel between patient contacts. To encourage hand-washing by personnel, sinks must be placed near all beds, and the ratio of sinks to beds in a multiple-bed unit should be about 1 to 6. A sink should be provided in each isolation room [10].

The most important design factor in preventing the transmission of microorganisms is the separation of patients, both spatially and by physical barriers. Surrounding each patient with a cubicle is probably the most efficient and economical way of doing this. However, no matter how patients are separated, each bed should have adequate space around it to contain all anticipated patient-care equipment—such as respirators, dialysis machines, and the like—and still provide adequate access for physicians and nurses. Standards for construction of intensive-therapy areas specify the minimum clearance between beds in multiple-bed rooms (7 feet) and the minimum clear area around beds in cubicles or single rooms (120 square feet) [10]. The principal reasons for providing a physical barrier between patients are to decrease the likelihood that materials and medications being used on one patient will be used for a patient in an adjacent bed and to lessen the chances of hospital personnel going from one patient to the next without washing their hands.

The concept of physical barriers can be carried one step farther by providing single rooms for each patient. Unfortunately, with such an arrangement, the ability of personnel to observe patients closely may suffer, even if remote monitoring systems are available. While there is no doubt that single rooms may be more effective in preventing cross-infection, the instances in which they are really needed are relatively few; they are needed, for example, for immunosuppressed patients and patients with tuberculosis, certain viral diseases (e.g., measles, mumps, rubella, smallpox, and varicella), and a few other highly communicable diseases (e.g., Lassa fever, congenital rubella syndrome, and *Staphylococcus aureus* pneumonia). Therefore, although private rooms in which the air pressure can be controlled should be available, such facilities are not needed for most patients with infection.

Contact Transmission: Indirect
Contact spread of microorganisms from the inanimate environment is also a potential problem in ICUs, and an important inanimate source of microorganisms has been room nebulizers and humidifiers. Large-volume reservoirs for such apparatus rapidly become contaminated with gram-negative bacteria and can act as reservoirs of infection if not cleaned and changed at appropriate intervals. Since there is little indication for such therapy, its use should be condemned as a hazard to ICU patients.

It is essential to have enough equipment to provide for the needs of individual patients adequately. Because certain items such as pressure transducers are expensive, they may be in short supply. This may lead to sharing of these devices by patients or to their reuse after an inadequate sterilization process. Similarly, because of expense or inadequate supplies, tubing on respiratory therapy equipment is sometimes used on several patients. Although this could happen on any hospital ward, it is more likely to occur in the ICU because of frequent emergencies and because the beds are often so close to each other. These practices create the potential for cross-infection between patients, and they have been documented as causing and perpetuating outbreaks of infection in ICUs [11]. The most effective plans for isolation are useless if contaminated equipment is transferred among patients. Therefore, care should be taken to provide an adequate amount of equipment to supply the greatest anticipated demands of the unit, and the frequent occurrence of emergencies should be taken into account.

Functional Aspects of ICU Infection Control
Prevention of cross-infection among ICU patients is dependent on the medical personnel's maintaining a high level of awareness of the susceptibility of such patients to nosocomial in-

fections. Employee attitudes toward this problem are crucial in controlling infections in this setting, and constant in-service education must be carried out. Hospital personnel are responsible for most instances of cross-contamination, and hand-washing between patient contacts remains the principal mode of prevention [4].

Gloves
Wearing gloves would undoubtedly be more effective than just hand-washing, and personnel should be encouraged to do this, especially when manipulating apparatus such as intravenous and intraarterial catheters, open wounds, and indwelling urinary catheters [5]. Cross-contamination via hands probably occurs less often during routine, noninvasive tasks performed by physicians, such as physical examination of patients without skin lesions [8,9]. Gloving of *both* hands should be mandatory for persons handling endotracheal tubes and performing endotracheal suction, not only to decrease contamination of this highly vulnerable orifice, but also for protection of personnel against herpetic whitlow and hepatitis B infection [7]. Unfortunately, gloving consumes time, is seen as interfering with the performance of many patient-care tasks, and is therefore difficult to enforce. In addition, gloving may be impractical at times when it is needed most, such as during cardiopulmonary resuscitation. Under these circumstances, emergency procedures must come first; later, defects in infection control should be corrected when possible.

Gowns
Another approach to preventing cross-infection is to require all personnel to gown upon entering the ICU, as is done in some pediatric units. Gowns themselves, however, are probably of little importance other than to remind personnel of the need for good patient-care procedures, including hand-washing precautions.

Invasive Procedures
Because of limitations in ancillary services, space, and environmental control, invasive procedures such as tracheostomies and venous cutdowns should not be performed in the ICU

routinely if more appropriate facilities are available. To lessen the chances of perioperative infections, these operations should be performed in standard operating rooms equipped for this purpose, where lighting and space are better controlled. It must be anticipated, however, that such procedures will often need to be done in emergencies in the ICU. Contingency plans for preventing infections in these circumstances should be prepared, appropriate equipment must be available, and personnel should be educated in the techniques of these procedures and made aware of potential problems.

Visitors

The time allowed for visitors must be limited so as not to interfere with medical care of ICU patients, but more importantly, the number of visitors to the unit should be restricted to decrease the traffic in the unit, to make it easier for the staff to monitor visitors, and to decrease the chances of introducing community infections into the unit.

Patient Spacing

Spatial separation of patients may be effected not only by the permanent arrangement of beds and barriers in the unit, but also by placement of patients in the unit. Medical personnel often tend to place patients requiring similar care near each other, hoping to facilitate medical and nursing care. This practice may be beneficial in some situations, but in others—such as with groups of patients having tracheostomies, endotracheal tubes, or indwelling urinary catheters—hazards arise. It is likely that any potential benefits gained from this arrangement, such as saved nursing time, are far outweighed by the potential hazards of cross-infection from one patient to the next. Because patients having similar illnesses and similar procedures may be susceptible to colonization and subsequent infection by similar organisms, close grouping of these patients increases the potential for cross-contamination. Almost invariably, if one patient with an endotracheal tube becomes colonized with *Acinetobacter,* a patient in an adjacent bed with an endotracheal tube will eventually become colonized. The likelihood of spread decreases the farther away in

the ICU one gets from the infected or colonized patient. Another example of this is the observation that grouping patients with Foley catheters facilitates spread of *Serratia* urinary tract infections among them and that transmission is interrupted by dispersing such patients [6].

One also increases the chances of transmission between patients of organisms on the hands of personnel by placing patients with similar tubes or catheters in adjacent beds. In addition, this increases the chances that common irrigating or other solutions from multidose vials may be used on more than one patient. Therefore, rather than grouping such patients together, they should be spread out through the ICU as much as possible.

Surveillance

In spite of diligent application of these principles, nosocomial infections in ICU patients will continue to occur. By monitoring the occurrence of such infections through an ongoing surveillance program (see Part I, Chapter 4), one may assess the effects of changes in procedures, therapy, and infection control measures on rates of infection. Because infection rates in many ICUs are noticeably higher than in other hospital areas, the magnitude of changes in infection rates may be accentuated by procedural changes, thereby providing a relatively sensitive indication of the revised procedure's effects on nosocomial infections. In addition, increases in rates of various infections might be noted early enough that corrective steps may be taken to avert actual epidemics.

References

1. Holzman, R. S., Florman, A. L., Podrid, P. J., Simberkoff, M. S., and Toharsky, B. Drug-associated diarrhea as a potential reservoir for hospital infections. *Lancet* 1:1195, 1974.
2. Johanson, W. G., Pierce, A. K., and Sanford, J. P. Changing pharyngeal bacterial flora of hospitalized patients. *N. Engl. J. Med.* 281: 1137, 1969.
3. Johanson, W. G., Pierce, A. K., Sanford, J. P., and Thomas, G. D. Nosocomial respiratory infections with gram-negative bacilli. *Ann. Intern. Med.* 77:701, 1972.
4. Knittle, M. A., Eitzman, D. V., and Baer, H.

Role of hand contamination of personnel in the epidemiology of gram-negative nosocomial infections. *J. Pediatr.* 86:433, 1975.

5. Lowbury, E. J. L., Thom, B. T., Lilly, H. A., Babb, J. R., and Whittall, K. Sources of infection with *Pseudomonas aeruginosa* in patients with tracheostomy. *J. Med. Microbiol.* 3:39, 1970.

6. Maki, D. G., Hennekens, C. H., and Bennett, J. V. Prevention of catheter-associated urinary tract infection—An additional measure. *J.A.M.A.* 221:1270, 1972.

7. Rosato, F. E., Rosato, E. F., and Plotkin, S. A. Herpetic paronychia—An occupational hazard of medical personnel. *N. Engl. J. Med.* 283:804, 1970.

8. Salzman, T. C., Clark, J. J., and Klemm, L. Hand contamination of personnel as a mechanism of cross-infection in nosocomial infections with antibiotic-resistant *Escherichia coli* and *Klebsiella aerobacter. Antimicrob. Agents Chemother.* 7:97, 1967.

9. Steere, A. C., and Mallison, G. F. Handwashing practices for the prevention of nosocomial infections. *Ann. Intern. Med.* 83:683, 1975.

10. U.S. Department of Health, Education, and Welfare. *Minimum Requirements of Construction and Equipment for Hospital and Medical Facilities.* Washington, D.C.: U.S. Government Printing Office, DHEW Publ. No. (HRA) 74-4000, 1974.

11. Weinstein, R. A., Stamm, W. E., Kramer, L., and Corey, L. Pressure monitoring devices: Overlooked source of nosocomial infection. *J.A.M.A.* 236:936, 1976.

Section C. The Newborn Nursery

James R. Allen and Thomas K. Oliver, Jr.

Nosocomial Nursery Infections

Striking changes have occurred in the medical and surgical care provided for neonates during the last decade and a half. While standards have continued to improve for infants cared for in term newborn nurseries, the quality and sophistication of care provided for the premature infant and the sick newborn in neonatal intensive-care units (NICU) have improved manyfold. These advances, however, have been accompanied by significant risks of nosocomial infection.

Predisposing Factors

Neonates are particularly susceptible to infection for several reasons. Up to the time of birth, most fetuses have been living in sterile environments. During the first hours and days following birth, infants are exposed to numerous organisms that readily colonize the open umbilical wound, circumcision site, skin, nares, throat, and gastrointestinal tract. Without the inhibition provided by a balanced normal flora, very heavy colonization with various bacteria may occur. The immune system of infants, particularly of pre-term (premature) or sick infants, is not fully developed. All neonates have physiologic dysgammaglobulinemia. Maternal immunoglobulin G (IgG) crosses the placenta readily, but IgM and IgE pass in miniscule amounts and IgA not at all. In addition, the polymorphonuclear leukocytes of a neonate, particularly those of a stressed infant, are less functional at phagocytizing and killing organisms than are those of an older person. Other factors, including opsonins and chemotactic factors, may also be depressed in the neonate. Many infants cared for in an NICU are extremely ill with other complicated medical and surgical problems, including prematurity, respiratory disease, cardiovascular diseases, and poor nutritional status. Because of this, many high-risk infants require invasive diagnostic, monitoring, and therapeutic procedures, all of which are associated with increased risk of infection.

Classification

Infections occurring in neonates are acquired from one of four sources:

1. A small percentage of infections are acquired transplacentally, such as congenital syphilis or rubella.

2. Some infections are transmitted from the mother during labor and delivery.

3. Most infections are produced by organisms acquired in the hospital, although it is often difficult to determine whether the organism was originally acquired from maternal or hospital sources.

4. A small proportion of infections are ac-

quired prior to admission to the nursery in infants born outside the hospital or in those who are readmitted to the nursery from home.

Because the majority of infants are born in a hospital, and because it frequently is highly impractical (if not impossible) to determine whether an organism causing infection in an infant is acquired from maternal or hospital sources, the Center for Disease Control National Nosocomial Infections Study (NNIS) has chosen to define all neonatal infections—acquired either intrapartum or during hospitalization—as nosocomial.

Incidence

Using the above definition, the five categories of NNIS hospitals have reported a combined nosocomial infection rate of 1.7 percent for all infants discharged from the newborn nursery service (term plus NICU). Approximately 70 percent of the infants are discharged from community or community-teaching hospitals, with a reported neonatal nosocomial infection rate of 0.9 to 1.1 percent. In contrast, the NICUs of two university medical centers have recently reported nosocomial infection rates of about 24 percent [19,42], with over 15 percent of the infants in one NICU developing one or more infections [19].

Pathogens

About 35 percent of the infections reported by the NNIS hospitals (Table 7-1) were caused by *Staphylococcus aureus,* most of which were superficial cutaneous or eye infections (conjunctivitis). *Escherichia coli* caused over 12 percent of the reported infections, including most of the urinary tract infections and gastrointestinal infections where a pathogen was identified. *E. coli* or group-B *Streptococcus* was isolated from almost 32 percent of neonatal meningitis cases. *Pseudomonas* species, *Klebsiella* species, and *S. aureus* caused most of the pneumonia and other lower respiratory tract infections in this series, while various pathogens were frequently isolated as the cause of primary bacteremia. Although group-B

Streptococcus (see also Part II, Chapters 22 and 23) caused only 2.5 percent of the nursery-associated infections in the NNIS hospitals, it presents one of the most significant threats of serious infections to infants in this country [20]. Nosocomial viral and fungal infections as well as those with delayed clinical expression are incompletely reported through NNIS hospital surveillance.

Although staphylococcal infections are still common in neonates, most infections during the 1970s were less serious than those occurring during the pandemic years of the mid-1950s through the early 1960s, when phage group-I *S. aureus,* particularly phage type 80/81, was prevalent. Many staphylococcal infections currently seen in neonates are caused by phage group-II staphylococci; these occasionally result in exfoliative infections.

Infants during the first few days of life frequently become colonized at one or more skin sites with one of the strains of *S. aureus* prevalent in the nursery; the umbilicus, groin, or circumcision site is usually the first site to become colonized. The most common means of transmission of staphylococcus in the nursery is from infant to infant on the inadequately washed hands of personnel; only rarely is an outbreak of disease in the nursery traced to an asymptomatic carrier (see Part II, Chapter 20).

The epidemiologic characteristics of colonization and infection of infants with group-B streptococci have not been completely defined. Estimates of the neonatal colonization rate with this organism range around 25 percent and the disease rate around 0.3 percent. Most disease with onset during the first several days of life probably results directly from in utero or intrapartum acquisition of the organism. The source of organisms that cause disease with later onset is less certain; colonization and subsequent clinical infection in at least some infants occur as the result of infant-to-infant transmission of the organism on the hands of nursery personnel. The role that the colonization of personnel plays in the transmission of infection to infants has not been determined.

Screening programs to identify infants who are colonized with group-B streptococci do not

Table 7-1. Rate of Nursery-Associated Nosocomial Infections[a] Reported by Hospitals in the National Nosocomial Infections Study, by Site and Pathogen, July 1974 to December 1976[b]

Pathogen	Site of Infection[c]										Percentage for this pathogen
	Skin	Eye	Primary blood	LRT	GU	GI	CNS	URT	Misc.	Total	
Staphylococcus aureus	434.0	89.3	21.7	18.7	9.0	8.7	3.0	14.4	15.7	614.5	35.2
Escherichia coli	73.2	23.1	28.4	9.7	35.4	27.8	7.0	3.0	9.0	216.7	12.4
Staphylococcus epidermidis	53.2	39.1	21.1	4.3	5.0	0.7	2.3	1.7	2.0	129.4	7.4
Klebsiella spp.	44.1	15.7	12.4	14.4	11.7	2.3	3.3	1.7	7.4	113.0	6.5
Streptococcus, group D	56.5	10.7	13.7	3.0	7.4	1.3	2.0	0.3	3.0	98.0	5.6
Candida spp.	28.8	0.3	2.3	1.0	2.0	1.3	1.0	1.0	48.5	86.3	4.9
Pseudomonas spp.	15.7	22.4	3.0	19.7	2.7	2.3	1.0	1.0	3.0	70.9	4.1
Streptococcus, not group B or D	22.4	17.1	15.0	3.3	3.3	0.3	3.0	2.3	1.3	68.2	3.9
Streptococcus, group B	12.7	0.7	12.7	4.3	3.7	0.7	6.4	1.0	1.7	43.8	2.5
Miscellaneous gram-negative bacteria	14.0	8.7	7.4	2.3	1.3	1.0	3.0	0.0	1.3	39.1	2.2
Proteus spp.	27.1	3.3	3.7	0.0	2.0	0.7	1.7	0.0	0.7	39.1	2.2
Enterobacter spp.	18.1	5.0	3.0	3.7	1.7	1.0	0.7	0.0	2.3	35.4	2.0
Serratia spp.	4.3	3.0	1.7	1.0	0.3	0.0	1.3	0.0	3.3	15.0	0.9
Miscellaneous gram-positive bacteria	3.0	2.3	0.7	0.0	0.0	0.0	1.3	0.0	0.3	7.7	0.4
Unreported and other pathogens	92.9	29.8	2.0	15.4	1.7	14.0	5.3	1.7	3.7	166.5	9.5
Total	900.0	270.5	148.8	101.0	87.3	62.2	42.5	28.1	103.3	1743.6	100
Percentage for this site	51.6%	15.5%	8.5%	5.8%	5.0%	3.6%	2.4%	1.6%	5.9%	100%	—

[a] Per 100,000 discharges

[b] 5212 infections; 299,099 discharges

[c] "Skin" includes umbilicus, external genitalia and circumcision site, superficial surgical wounds, and breast; "Eye" includes conjunctiva; LRT = lower respiratory tract; GU = genitourinary tract; GI = gastrointestinal tract; CNS = central nervous system; URT = upper respiratory tract

need to be conducted except during an epidemic. Routine care of infants in the nursery with all personnel washing their hands carefully between handling infants is usually sufficient to prevent transmission of this organism. The relative efficacy of various agents (e.g., triple dye) that are applied to the umbilical stump to prevent or eliminate colonization of infants with group-B streptococci is unknown.

Attempts to use systemic or topical antibiotics to eradicate colonization with this organism have not been successful.

Much information remains to be learned about the biology and epidemiology of gram-negative bacillus infections in infants. *E. coli* is the most common organism causing serious neonatal infections; most strains of this organism are acquired from the infants' mothers.

The majority of other gram-negative bacilli that cause neonatal infection are probably acquired within the nursery [28]. Although contaminated fomites can play an important role in some common-source epidemics, the most important source of gram-negative organisms is the inadequately washed hands of nursery personnel [9]. Although nursery personnel occasionally are colonized with the same strains of enteric bacteria as those that are causing infections within a nursery, personnel carrying these organisms at intestinal or other sites only rarely are the source of a problem within the nursery [8]. The usual pattern of infection is for an infant to become heavily colonized in the intestinal tract, upper respiratory tract, umbilical stump, or skin site with a gram-negative organism that is prevalent in the nursery [18]; subsequent procedures or manipulation of the infant allow invasion of the organism to occur and disease to develop. This sequence of events is well described in the report by Stamm and co-workers, in which infants colonized with *Serratia marcescens* developed cutaneous abscesses and bacteremia following the insertion of scalp-vein needles [38].

Patterns of Infection
Most clinical infections in nurseries develop as sporadic or endemic disease rather than as an epidemic problem. In part, this occurs because the majority of infants who become colonized with a particular organism do not develop disease with that organism. This is the case not only with colonization of the umbilicus or nares with *S. aureus,* but also with colonization of the gastrointestinal tract with *Klebsiella* species or *Pseudomonas* species. Because of the potential presence of a large reservoir of asymptomatic infants who are colonized with pathogenic organisms, it is important to evaluate carefully even the small clusters of infectious disease within a nursery that appear to be nosocomial.

In addition, infections acquired within the hospital may not become clinically manifest until after discharge. The median age of infants developing staphylococcal skin disease, for example, is usually seven to ten days. A small cluster of infants with disease in the hospital may therefore portend that a large number of infants recently discharged from the nursery will have nosocomial infection.

Many infections in infants can be diagnosed more rapidly and precautionary steps can be taken to prevent further transmission of the organism within the nursery if there is close cooperation between the obstetric and the neonatal or pediatric medical personnel. It is important for the nursery to be informed of a suspected or diagnosed infection in a mother, such as gonorrhea, salmonellosis, or shigellosis. Similarly, if an obstetric procedure is causing morbidity in infants, such as infections following the use of scalp electrodes for fetal monitoring, it is important that the obstetric personnel be informed of the problem and steps be taken jointly to solve it.

General Prevention and Control Measures
Nursery Design
Until relatively recently, most nurseries were designed with special rooms, separate from the regular nursery, called "suspect nurseries." These were used to house infants with suspected infection or an increased potential for developing infection, such as the infant of a mother with prolonged rupture of the membranes. Because of the inconvenience of caring for them, the infants at increased risk of illness often received poorer care and less frequent observation than the nonsuspect babies. Infants with proved infection were immediately removed from the nursery and frequently placed in isolation on the pediatric ward, where they did not receive the special medical and nursing care they needed. The advent of the NICU has changed this in many hospitals by providing graded care facilities, including an observation unit, an intensive-care unit, and an intermediate-care or long-term growth unit. In general, infants with many types of infections can be managed successfully in these relatively open units if techniques to prevent transmission of organisms from one infant to the next are meticulously followed. Adequate space must be provided for each infant, including those requiring special procedures such as ventilatory assistance; recommendations for

minimum floor space and facilities per infant have been published [2]. The intensive-care unit especially should be designed to be flexible in use to allow optimal care to be provided for varying numbers of infants and to meet the special needs of each [33,41].

Isolation Procedures

The general principles of isolation technique (see Part I, Chapter 9) apply to the nursery, although unique problems and circumstances in this area require amplification of the established procedures. Infants with most types of infection can be managed within the nursery area or NICU, as can infants who are born under nonsterile conditions or who are considered to be at increased risk of developing an infection. Factors that must be considered in each individual case include the type of infectious agent, the site of infection, the source of the infection, and the mode of transmission of the infection. In practice, infants with deep bacterial infections usually can be managed safely within the nursery area. Infants with gastroenteritis or draining skin lesions probably can also be managed safely in these areas, if necessary, provided that enteric or wound precautions (see Part I, Chapter 9), including meticulous hand-washing, are strictly followed. Infants with infections that can be spread by the airborne route, however, must be separated from the other infants, preferably by moving them out of the nursery area.

In the past, it has been felt that enclosed incubators with access to the infant through portholes provided adequate isolation, both for the protection of the infant from disease as well as for the prevention of spread of infection. No clinical studies have confirmed either hypothesis. Although many enclosed incubators manufactured today use high-efficiency intake air filters, opening and closing of the units to provide care for the infant effectively nullify the value of this filtration. Air leaving the incubators is not filtered. Manipulation of the units can allow cross-contamination, and at least one epidemic has been traced to contamination of the porthole covers of the incubators [4]. Recently, open incubators using radiant heat as the warming source have become increasingly popular, because they allow easy access to infants requiring intensive care. These units do not provide any isolation from the airborne spread of organisms. Although an experimental open incubator has been constructed that provides forced air isolation (air curtain) through high-efficiency particulate air (HEPA) filters [27], this system has not been extensively evaluated for isolation purposes and is not in commercial production.

Prophylactic Antibiotics

Signs of serious infection in newborns are nonspecific and extremely subtle, and the mortality rate from infections is high [19]. Because infants in an NICU are frequently seriously ill, have had invasive procedures performed, and are at high risk of developing an infection, a large proportion of them (frequently 50 percent or greater) are given broad-spectrum "prophylactic" antibiotics. Very few controlled, double-blind studies have been conducted to demonstrate the efficacy of this approach to prevention. Antibiotics, for example, are not useful in preventing infections from venous catheters for total parenteral nutrition or from umbilical vessel catheters for monitoring and fluid therapy [3,7], although they may be useful in preventing colonization and clinical infection in a selected group of high-risk infants with endotracheal intubation and respiratory support [18].

The frequent use of antibiotics in an NICU enhances the emergence of organisms resistant to the antibiotics and increases the likelihood that the infants will be colonized with the resistant strains. Infants heavily colonized with resistant bacteria are probably at greater risk of developing clinical infections caused by their own flora, particularly if they have had a complicated course and have been subjected to invasive procedures [18]. Similarly, with the exception of group-A streptococcal outbreaks and some enteric bacterial gastroenteritis outbreaks, the use of prophylactic systemic antibiotic therapy for all neonates in a unit has not been an effective way of dealing with nursery epidemics. Prophylactic systemic antibiotics should not, therefore, be given as a routine procedure following prolonged rupture of the maternal membranes, insertion of an umbilical vessel catheter, or following exchange transfusion.

Employee Health

Employee health services should function to protect the infant from being exposed to infectious diseases carried by nursery personnel as well as to protect personnel from infections carried by infants (see Part I, Chapter 3). In addition to the well-described problems of staphylococcal and streptococcal disseminators among personnel, recent reports have described the transmission of pertussis [24], tuberculosis [40], and influenza [5] from nursery personnel to the infants. An individual with an acute respiratory tract infection (including pharyngitis), a nonspecific febrile illness, gastroenteritis, open or draining skin lesions, or active herpesvirus hominis infection should not work in the nursery for the duration of the illness. Individuals with chronic dermatitis should be carefully evaluated to determine whether they can safely work in the nursery. Female personnel of child-bearing age should have a rubella antibody titer obtained and be vaccinated against rubella if antibodies are not detectable (rubella vaccination is contraindicated for any woman who is pregnant or might become pregnant within three months of vaccine administration). Female personnel should also be warned about the potential transmission of cytomegalovirus from infected infants and the potential danger of contact during the first trimester of pregnancy with any virus-infected infant.

Surveillance for Infections

A surveillance program using multiple techniques to detect infections and problems within a nursery is essential to detect as rapidly as possible any pattern of infections that could indicate a break in patient-care practices or herald an epidemic (see Part I, Chapter 4). The potential usefulness of obtaining routine or periodic nasal cultures for staphylococci from infants in the nursery to detect lapses in pa-

tient-care techniques [44] must be balanced against the time and expense of such surveillance. Routine culture testing of nursery personnel is not useful and is to be discouraged.

An active and continuing in-service educational program is essential to remind personnel of the potential problems that can arise in the nursery and to review the correct techniques for using all equipment and performing all procedures. The hospital epidemiologist as well as the physicians responsible for the nursery must be constantly sensitive to changes in frequency and patterns of infections and to changes in antimicrobial sensitivity of bacteria causing infections. Since infections may first become apparent after the patients are discharged from the nursery, it is imperative to establish good contact with pediatricians in the community in order to learn rapidly about infections that may be nosocomial in origin. Postdischarge surveillance by hospital personnel to obtain this information from mothers is effective but time-consuming.

Evaluation of New Procedures

As new procedures and techniques are introduced into the nursery, each needs to be critically evaluated for its efficacy and safety, including its risk of introducing nosocomial infection. Examples of infectious hazards associated with minor procedures include staphylococcal enterocolitis developing in infants who had an indwelling nasoduodenal feeding catheter passed through nares colonized with *S. aureus* [17], cutaneous abscesses developing at the site where needle leads were inserted for electrocardiographic monitoring [19], and scalp abscesses or skull osteomyelitis developing at the site where the intrauterine fetal-monitoring lead was attached to the scalp [29,31,46].

Specific Nursery Routines to Prevent Infections

Many nursery routines have been developed over the years and frequently have been incorporated into state codes for nursery operation. A number of these nursery routines are little more than ceremonial, as has been clearly shown by Williams and Oliver [44]. These investigators demonstrated that nasal colonization with *S. aureus* in neonates was unaffected by discontinuing the use of caps and masks, delaying the initial bath after birth until thermal homeostasis was achieved, discontinuing the use of hairnets, allowing medical students into the nursery, permitting parents to enter the nurseries and handle their infants provided they used good hand-washing techniques, discontinuing the use of brushes in initial hand-washing, and discontinuing the use of gowns except when handling an infant outside a closed incubator. Others have confirmed these results [10,14]. Procedures or routines found through controlled studies to be unnecessary or ineffective should be eliminated, not only because they may be expensive and time-consuming, but also because they may discourage personnel from giving optimal care to ill infants and may dilute the emphasis given to effective procedures [36].

Gowns, Caps, and Masks

Caps, beard-bags, and masks are not necessary for routine nursery activities, but they are recommended for special procedures such as catheterization of an umbilical vessel. Gowns should be used for handling infants outside of incubators and bassinets. The clothing and unscrubbed skin areas of nursery personnel should not come into contact with the infants.

Hand-Washing

The major mode of transmission of organisms to an infant is on the hands of personnel [26]. Hand-washing is therefore the most crucial element in infection control in the nursery [39]. Although transient surface bacteria can be largely eliminated simply by washing one's hands in tap water for 15 seconds with vigorous rubbing [37], even careful hand-washing with antiseptic compounds is not always adequate to eliminate organisms on the hands that can be transmitted to infants [9].

Antiseptic agents should be used by nursery personnel for all hand-washing. Preferably, these should contain either 3% hexachlorophene, an iodophor, or 4% chlorhexidine.

Persons sensitive to these agents should use plain soap or detergent compounds. Personnel coming on duty should use an initial three-minute scrub to the elbows. Immediately *before* and *after* handling each infant or after handling contaminated objects, the hands should be washed for 15 seconds.

Gloves

Any infant with diarrhea or with a draining skin infection should be considered potentially infective regardless of whether a pathogenic organism has been identified. Such an infant should receive the appropriate enteric or wound and skin precautions, both of which require gloves for direct handling of the patient (see Part I, Chapter 9).

Cohort Programs

For the purposes of hospital epidemiology, a *cohort* is a group of individuals kept together to minimize contact between members of the cohort and other patients (cohorts) or personnel to decrease opportunities for the transmission of infectious agents. The success of a cohort program at limiting the spread of infectious disease depends significantly on the willingness of hospital personnel to cooperate fully with its objectives.

Many hospitals, particularly those with large nurseries, use routine cohorting of neonates to minimize the risk of transmission of *S. aureus* or other infectious agents to noninfected infants. The common characteristic of the infants in any given cohort is that they have been born within the same 24- or 48-hour period. The group of infants is admitted to one room of the nursery, and following the end of the admitting period for that cohort, no additional infants are admitted to that nursery room until all the infants have been discharged and the room has undergone thorough cleaning. The most successful cohort programs are those in which personnel during any one shift work only with one group of infants and do not work even temporarily with any infants other than those in their assigned cohort. Separate facilities should be provided for handling any infant who needs special observation or care or who will be remaining in the hospital longer than other members of his cohort.

During a nursery epidemic, cohorting of infants and personnel frequently can provide effective isolation of infected infants from noninfected infants. The success of the separation depends heavily on the rapidity and thoroughness with which different aspects of the program are conducted. All infants who have overt clinical disease or who are colonized with the epidemic organism must be identified and placed in the cohort of infected infants. If rapid identification of infected infants is not possible, then all exposed and potentially infected infants should be placed in a cohort separate from new admissions to the nursery. Regular nursery personnel should be assigned to work with only one cohort and should not be permitted to work even temporarily with other groups. Physicians, laboratory technicians, and other transient personnel in the nursery either must work only with one cohort or else must take meticulous precautions to prevent transmission of infection between groups; if they are to handle more than one infant on a single visit, they should move from the noninfected cohort to the infected cohort. If the infection can be transmitted from asymptomatic colonized personnel to infants, personnel should be screened, and those who are found to be infected should be assigned to care only for the group of infants already infected.

Term nurseries that have sufficient admissions to justify the program should be arranged so that infants can be cohorted routinely; nurseries that are being constructed or remodeled should be designed to facilitate this. Routine cohorting of infants in an NICU is not usually practical. The technique may be used during epidemics, however, by forming groups in different rooms of the NICU or simply by establishing groups of infected and noninfected infants and providing physical separation within a common room with strict assignment of personnel and equipment to each group. NICUs that have sufficient floor space for each infant and that are flexible in arrangement facilitate the implementation of this system. Diseases that are spread by the airborne route cannot be managed in this manner.

Care of Equipment

Bassinets, incubators, nebulization and humidification equipment, resuscitation equipment, oxygen hoods, and any other equipment used directly with infants must be dismantled, thoroughly cleaned to remove all organic material, and then sterilized or disinfected (see Part I, Chapter 6). Diagnostic instruments such as stethoscopes and otoscopes should be disinfected with alcohol or an iodophor compound prior to use on each infant. Preferably, each infant in the NICU will be assigned specific equipment, such as a stethoscope, so these instruments will not be carried from infant to infant.

One of the most serious problems affecting nurseries is what Wheeler has described as "water bugs in the bassinet" [43]. Any container or device filled with water or a solution may potentially be contaminated with organisms that thrive in water. Such devices include nebulization and humidification equipment, plastic squeeze bottles used for eyewashes or eye rinsing, and bowls used for bath or rinse water. All such devices should be cleaned and sterilized or disinfected at frequent intervals. Unit-dose medications and drugs should be used if possible. Water or other solutions used should be sterile (distilled water is not synonymous with sterile water). Once opened, bottles of sterile water should no longer be considered sterile. No container such as that used for an infant bath or for moistening sponges for wiping an infant's buttocks should be allowed to remain standing; the water must be discarded and the container cleaned, disinfected, and dried prior to its next use.

Infant Bathing and Cord Care

Numerous studies have demonstrated the effectiveness of routine bathing of infants with a 3% hexachlorophene (HCP) preparation in reducing the rate of colonization of infants with *S. aureus* [15]. Bathing infants with this agent has also been useful as an adjunctive control measure in stopping epidemics of staphylococcal disease, although a few published reports suggest that it has not been effective for this task [23]. Within the last several years, the neuropathologic toxicity of HCP when absorbed percutaneously has become apparent [25]. The retrospective autopsy studies on human infants reported to date suggest that as few as three baths with HCP can produce neuropathologic changes in small premature infants similar to those seen in experimental animals with HCP toxicity [34]. Despite this, no clinical signs have been correlated with the use of HCP for bathing of infants, and no deaths or residual neurologic dysfunctions have been attributed to the topical use of this agent for bathing. The current recommendation is that HCP not be used for routine bathing of infants. Its usefulness as an adjunctive measure in controlling an epidemic of staphylococcal disease must be weighed against its potential toxic effects (see Part II, Chapter 20).

No other topical preparations for bathing infants have unequivocally been proved to be both safe and effective in reducing colonization and disease with *S. aureus* or other organisms. In view of this, the American Academy of Pediatrics has recommended that it is best to handle the infant's skin as little as possible and has suggested a return to "dry skin care" [1].

Numerous methods of caring for the umbilical stump have been recommended, but no one method has proved to be clearly superior at preventing colonization or disease with *S. aureus*. Initial trials with bacitracin ointment [15, 22] and with triple dye [30] applied to the umbilical cord stump suggest that these agents are effective in preventing colonization. The potential toxicity of the latter compound has not been adequately studied, however. Alcohol has also been widely applied to the umbilical stump, both for its antiseptic effect as well as to hasten drying of the cord; its effectiveness in limiting colonization and disease is in doubt, however [22].

Special Considerations Involving Neonatal Intensive-Care Units (NICU)

Equipment and Procedures

The equipment used to care for infants in the NICU is extremely sophisticated and expensive. The diagnostic, monitoring, or therapeutic procedures associated with the use of such equipment are frequently invasive and associated with a high risk of infection. It is imperative that these procedures be conducted using aseptic technique and that the devices, when in use, be regularly inspected and cared for. Examples of such equipment include ventilators, humidifiers, and other equipment used in respiratory therapy or ventilatory support; pressure transducers and lines for monitoring intraarterial pressures; umbilical vessel catheters for fluid therapy, blood-gas monitoring, or other reasons; or central venous catheters for total parenteral nutrition. Procedures employing any of these devices can be safely conducted if the correct techniques are carefully followed; such techniques are discussed in several chapters of this text as well as elsewhere [45].

The demand within a nursery for much of the equipment, particularly for expensive items, will occasionally exceed the supply, but it is extremely important that the equipment be carefully cleaned and sterilized between use on each patient. Many of the sophisticated devices available for use have not been adequately tested for their ease of cleaning and sterilization or for their safety from a microbiologic viewpoint. These factors must be considered when equipment is being evaluated before purchase. New equipment that is being developed will hopefully decrease the risk of nosocomial infection by reducing the frequency of invasive procedures. Transcutaneous oxygen electrodes, for example, should reduce the need for indwelling arterial cannulas and blood sampling for monitoring blood gases.

Human Milk

Accompanying the recent increased interest in breast feeding for infants has come a demand to provide human milk for premature infants in hospital nurseries. The primary reasons cited are for psychologic, nutritional, and immunologic benefits. The psychologic benefits, are quite clear, and families should be encouraged to interact with and support the premature infant in many different ways. The second reason—nutritional benefits—has not been as clearly defined, and authorities in the field are not in agreement on the value of breast milk compared with commercially prepared formulas for feeding premature infants. The third reason—the immunologic benefits—is also not clearly defined. Although a number of studies have strongly suggested that the incidence of serious infections and gastroenteritis is less frequent in breast-fed infants compared to formula-fed infants, this correlation was not demonstrated with premature infants in a nursery who were fed with fresh human milk and compared to those fed with formula [16]. Similarly, although several investigators have suggested that fresh human milk may help prevent necrotizing enterocolitis from developing in infants, this has not been demonstrated in controlled clinical trials.

Fresh human milk contains several components that enhance the resistance of neonates to infection, although the precise role of each component has not been defined [6,16]. Such factors include active leukocytes, over 80 percent of which are monocytic phagocytes with the remainder being lymphocytes; immunoglobulins, primarily secretory IgA; enzymes such as lysozyme and lactoperoxidase; the iron-binding protein lactoferrin; and other factors such as an antistaphylococcal factor. In addition, because of intrinsic factors, breast milk promotes heavy intestinal colonization with *Lactobacillus* rather than with a mixed bacterial flora, predominantly *E. coli*.

Several potential risks of feeding human milk to premature infants also exist, however. Breast milk frequently is contaminated with skin bacteria at the time of collection; although this is not a significant problem for an infant who is nursing or if the milk is used promptly, prolonged or inadequate storage of the milk can result in proliferation of the bacteria to levels that might cause adverse effects. Two outbreaks of *Salmonella kottbus* have been traced to contamination of human milk collected to feed premature infants [32]. Although it is unclear whether the breast milk was primarily or secondarily contaminated, inadequate storage and handling of the milk after collection allowed proliferation of the organisms to significant levels. Because of the immaturity of the premature infant, normal intestinal mucosal barriers may not be competent, and several investigators have raised questions about the immunologic hazards of feeding fresh

human milk containing active leukocytes from unrelated donors to premature infants [6].

Both of these potential risks can be prevented by freezing or pasteurizing the milk prior to feeding it to an infant. Such treatment methods will destroy living cells, and additionally, heat treatment may denature protective proteins in the milk [13]. By processing the milk to make it safer for the infants, therefore, the protective factors in the milk may be destroyed. Studies have not been conducted that demonstrate any protective benefit of frozen or heat-processed milk in preventing septicemia or gastroenteritis in neonates or premature infants.

Studies are being conducted to assess the benefits and hazards of providing fresh or processed human milk for premature infants in a nursery [11,12]. These studies include methods for collection, transportation, storage, processing, and feeding milk to infants. Collection of fresh breast milk from a mother for feeding to her own premature infant appears to be safe and probably beneficial. The mother must be instructed in the careful collection and storage of the milk; even with refrigeration, it should be fed to the infant within 24 hours of collection. Until standards have been established for operating a nonrelated donor milk bank and until it is known whether or not processed human milk enhances the resistance of premature infants to infection, hospitals are to be discouraged from establishing this complex service without giving extremely careful consideration to all aspects of operating a human milk bank and to the benefits that are expected to accrue to the infants.

References

1. American Academy of Pediatrics, Committee on Fetus and Newborn. Skin care of newborns. *Pediatrics* 54:682, 1974.
2. American Academy of Pediatrics, Committee on Fetus and Newborn. *Standards and Recommendations for Hospital Care of Newborn Infants* (6th ed). Evanston, Ill: American Academy of Pediatrics, 1977.
3. Anagnostakis, D., Kamba, A., Petrochilou, V., Arseni, A., and Matsaniotis, N. Risk of infection associated with umbilical vein catheterization. *J. Pediatr.* 86:759, 1975.

4. Barrie, D. Incubator-borne *Pseudomonas pyocyanea* infection in a newborn nursery. *Arch. Dis. Child.* 40:555, 1965.

5. Bauer, C. R., Elie, K., Spence, L., and Stern, L. Hong Kong influenza in a neonatal unit. *J.A.M.A.* 223:1233, 1973.

6. Beer, A. F., and Billingham, R. E. Immunologic benefits and hazards of milk in maternal-perinatal relationship. *Ann. Intern. Med.* 83:865, 1975.

7. Bhatt, D. R., Hodgman, J. E., and Tatter, D. Evaluation of prophylactic antibiotics during umbilical catheterization in newborns (Abstract). *Clin. Res.* 18:217, 1970.

8. Burke, J. P., Ingall, D., Klein, J. O., Gezon, H. M., and Finland, M. *Proteus mirabilis* infections in a hospital nursery traced to a human carrier. *N. Engl. J. Med.* 284:115, 1971.

9. Eisenoch, K. D., Reber, R. M., Eitzman, D. V., and Baer, H. Nosocomial infections due to kanamycin-resistant, (R)-factor carrying enteric organisms in an intensive care nursery. *Pediatrics* 50:395, 1972.

10. Evans, H. E., Akpata, S. O., and Baki, A. Bacteriologic and clinical evaluation of gowning in a premature nursery. *J. Pediatr.* 78:883, 1971.

11. Fomon, S. J., et al. Human milk in premature infant feeding: Summary of a workshop. *Pediatrics* 57:741, 1976.

12. Fomon, S. J. Human milk in premature infant feeding: Report of a second workshop. *Am. J. Public Health* 67:361, 1977.

13. Ford, J. E., Law, B. A., Marshall, V. M. E., and Reiter, B. Influence of the heat treatment of human milk on some of its protective constituents. *J. Pediatr.* 90:29, 1977.

14. Forfar, J. O., and MacCabe, A. F. Masking and gowning in nurseries for the newborn infant: Effect on staphylococcal carriage and infection. *Br. Med. J.* 1:76, 1958.

15. Gezon, H. M., Thompson, D. J., Rogers, K. D., Hatch, T. F., Rycheck, R. R., and Yee, R. B. Control of staphylococcal infections and disease in the newborn through the use of hexachlorophene bathing. *Pediatrics* 51 (Suppl):331, 1973.

16. Goldman, A. S., and Smith, C. W. Host resistance factors in human milk. *J. Pediatr.* 82:1082, 1973.

17. Gutman, L. T., Idriss, Z. H., Gehlbach, S., and Blackmon, L. Neonatal staphylococcal enterocolitis: Association with indwelling feeding catheters and *S. aureus* colonization. *J. Pediatr.* 88:836, 1976.

18. Harris, H., Wirtschafter, D., and Cassady, G. Endotracheal intubation and its relationship to bacterial colonization and systemic infection of newborn infants. *Pediatrics* 58:816, 1976.

19. Hemming, V. G., Overall, J. C., and Britt, M. R. Nosocomial infections in a newborn intensive-care unit: Results of forty-one months of surveillance. *N. Engl. J. Med.* 294:1310, 1976.

20. Howard, J. B., and McCracken, G. H. The spectrum of group B streptococcal infections in infancy. *Am. J. Dis. Child.* 128:815, 1974.

21. Hurst, V. Colonization in the Newborn. In Maibach, H. I., and Hildick-Smith, G. (Eds.), *Skin Bacteria and Their Role in Infection.* New York: McGraw-Hill, 1965, pp. 127–141.

22. Johnson, J. D., Malachowski, N. C., Vosti, K. L., and Sunshine, P. A sequential study of various modes of skin and umbilical care and the incidence of staphylococcal colonization and infection in the neonate. *Pediatrics* 58:354, 1976.

23. Light, I. J., and Sutherland, J. M. What is the evidence that hexachlorophene is not effective? *Pediatrics* 51 (Suppl.):345, 1973.

24. Linnemann, C. C., Ramundo, N., Perlstein, P. H., Minton, S. D., Englender, G. S., McCormick, J. B., and Hayes, P. S. Use of pertussis vaccine in an epidemic involving hospital staff. *Lancet* 2:540, 1975.

25. Lockhart, J. D. How toxic is hexachlorophene? *Pediatrics* 50:229, 1972.

26. Mortimer, E. A., Lipsitz, P. J., Wolinski, E., Gonzaga, A. J., and Rammelkamp, C. H. Transmission of staphylococci between newborns: Importance of hands of personnel. *Am. J. Dis. Child.* 104:289, 1962.

27. Musch, B., Adams, J. L., and Sunshine, P. An air curtain incubator for use in an intensive-care nursery. *J. Pediatr.* 79:1024, 1971.

28. Noy, J. H., Ayliffe, G. A. J., and Linton, K. B. Antibiotic-resistant gram-negative bacilli in the faeces of neonates. *J. Med. Microbiol.* 7:509, 1974.

29. Overturf, G. D., and Balfour, G. Osteomyelitis and sepsis: Severe complications of fetal monitoring. *Pediatrics* 55:244, 1975.

30. Pildes, R. S., Ramamurthy, R. S., and Vidyasagar, D. Effect of triple dye on staphylococcal colonization in the newborn infant. *J. Pediatr.* 82:987, 1973.

31. Plavidal, F. J., and Werch, A. Fetal scalp abscess secondary to intrauterine monitoring. *Am. J. Obstet. Gynecol.* 125:65, 1976.

32. Ryder, R. W., Crosby-Ritchie, A., McDonough, B., and Hall, W. J. Human milk contaminated with *Salmonella kottbus*—A cause of nosocomial illness in infants. *J.A.M.A.* 283:1533, 1977.

33. Segal, S. Neonatal intensive care: A prediction of continuing development. *Pediatr. Clin. North Am.* 13:1149, 1966.

34. Shuman, R. M., Leech, R. W., and Alvord, E. D. Neurotoxicity of hexachlorophene in humans: II. A clinicopathological study of 46 premature infants. *Arch. Neurol.* 32:320, 1975.

35. Siber, G. R., Alpert, S., Smith, A. L., Lin, J. S. L., and McCormick, W. M. Neonatal central nervous system infection due to *Mycoplasma hominis. J. Pediatr.* 90:625, 1977.

36. Silverman, W. A., and Sinclair, J. C. Evaluation of precautions before entering a neonatal unit. *Pediatrics* 40:900, 1967.

37. Sprunt, K., Redman, W., and Leidy, G. Antibacterial effectiveness of routine handwashing. *Pediatrics* 52:264, 1973.

38. Stamm, W. E., Kolff, C. A., Dones, E. M., Javariz, R., Anderson, R. L., Farmer, J. J., and de Quinones, H. R. A nursery outbreak caused by *Serratia marcescens:* Scalp-vein needles as a portal of entry. *J. Pediatr.* 89:96, 1976.

39. Steere, A. C., and Mallison, G. F. Handwashing practices for the prevention of nosocomial infections. *Ann. Intern. Med.* 83:683, 1975.

40. Steiner, P., Rao, M., Victoria, M. S., Rudolph, N., and Buynoski, G. Miliary tuberculosis in two infants after nursery exposure: Epidemiologic, clinical, and laboratory findings. *Am. Rev. Respir. Dis.* 113:267, 1976.

41. Tyne, M. D. Concepts for improved nursery design. *Hospitals* 48:66, 1974.

42. Wenzel, R. P., Osterman, C. A., and Hunting, K. J. Hospital-acquired infections. II. Infection rates by site, service and common procedures in a university hospital. *Am. J. Epidemiol.* 104:645, 1976.

43. Wheeler, W. E. Water bugs in the bassinet (Editorial). *Am. J. Dis. Child.* 101:273, 1961.

44. Williams, C. P. S., and Oliver, T. K., Jr. Nursery routines and staphylococcal colonization of the newborn. *Pediatrics* 44:640, 1969.

45. Wilmore, D. W., and Dudrick, S. J. Safe long-term venous catheterization. *Arch. Surg.* 98:256, 1969.

46. Winkel, C. A., Snyder, D. L., and Schaerth, J. B. Scalp abscess: A complication of the spiral fetal electrode. *Am. J. Obstet. Gynecol.* 126:720, 1976.

Section D. The Pharmacy

Stephen R. Zellner and Leighton E. Cluff

The hospital pharmacist is responsible for dispensing drugs and often adds drugs to solutions for intravenous administration. The pharmacist, the hospital pharmacy, and the therapeutics committee frequently monitor drug utilization in the hospital and are an important source of drug information. Hospital pharmacies may thus be involved both in the occurrence and in the control of nosocomial infections.

Dispensing and Compounding of Drugs

Pharmacists compound drugs less frequently than previously, insofar as the manufacture of drugs has become progressively more industrialized. Drug manufacturers are required by the Food and Drug Administration (FDA) to adhere to standards assuring the sterility of their products. These standards, however, have not always prevented microbial contamination of drugs [2,3,9]. In addition, sterile items may become contaminated after distribution to hospital pharmacies [5]. Even though intravenous fluids and medications may be sterile, devices used for their administration have been found to be contaminated with microorganisms and responsible for causing infection [6].

Medications purchased from commercial sources have been found to be contaminated with strains of *Salmonella, Proteus, Pseudomonas, Escherichia coli,* and other potential pathogens [4,12]. These drugs have included digitalis alkaloids, barbiturates, and tranquilizers for oral use [10]. Carmine dye, used in gastrointestinal physiologic studies, has been contaminated with *Salmonella cubana,* which produced acute gastroenteritis in hospitalized patients [11]. Fluorescein ophthalmic solutions contaminated with *Pseudomonas aeruginosa* have been responsible for epidemic nosocomial eye infections [1]. Multidose drug vials contaminated during repeated use have been responsible for cross-infections in patients [9].

Although the hospital pharmacist may not be directly responsible for the surveillance of nosocomial infection, it must be appreciated that there is the potential for infecting patients if they are given contaminated medications as well as the possibility that drugs may not be sterile when received from distributors or manufacturers. Packaging or bottling of drugs in the pharmacy must be done in such a way as to eliminate the possibility of contamination.

When surveillance data suggest that materials provided by the pharmacy may be the source of nosocomial infection, the pharmacist must cooperate and participate in investigating and controlling the problem. Pharmacies actively involved in compounding drugs and in adding drugs to intravenous solutions must provide facilities that avoid microbial contamination. Laminar-flow hoods and personnel trained in sterile technique are necessary. Bacteremia due to *Enterobacter cloacae, Enterobacter agglomerans,* and *Candida albicans* has resulted from contaminated fluids and drugs given intravenously that were prepared or administered improperly [8].

Antiseptics and Disinfectants

Hospital pharmacies may stock large quantities of antiseptics and disinfectants, dispensing small quantities for use in patient care. Some of these compounds support bacterial growth and may even selectively foster the growth of microorganisms; for example, aqueous benzalkonium chloride, a quaternary ammonium compound, has been the vehicle responsible for the spread of *Pseudomonas* infections [13]. Often, contamination of these antiseptics occurs after they are stocked in the pharmacy, and the methods used for dispensing them in small quantities may be responsible. Antiseptics for patient care should be dispensed aseptically into sterile containers.

Antibiotic Surveillance and Control

The hospital pharmacy and the Committee on Pharmacy and Therapeutics should monitor the utilization of antimicrobial drugs and their associated adverse effects. These bodies should also establish an effective hospital formulary system that insures the availability of antimicrobial drugs needed for patient care, but which eliminates or controls the use of those determined to be duplicative, unnecessary, or excessively hazardous. Surveillance of antibiotic utilization is one mechanism by which the pharmacy may aid the prescribing physician, the hospital Infection Control Committee, and the patient. Widespread, often inappropriate use of antimicrobials within the hospital may result in the emergence of resistant bacterial strains. This phenomenon has been repeatedly observed in the United States and England. Correlation of the frequency with which each antibiotic is used and the sensitivity patterns of organisms isolated from patient material over a period of time may prove helpful to the hospital as an early warning sign of emerging microbial resistance. In a recent epidemic of *Klebsiella* infections occurring in a newborn nursery, 80 percent of the isolated strains were resistant to kanamycin [7]. Investigation revealed that this agent had been frequently used, often without justification. Two months after kanamycin usage was discontinued, 20 percent of the organisms isolated were resistant to kanamycin, and the incidence of *Klebsiella* infections had declined significantly.

Continuing education of physicians in the correct use of antibiotics is necessary in order to avoid inappropriate use. A program for surveillance of antibiotic usage may best be accomplished through the joint efforts of the pharmacist, hospital epidemiologist, and physicians. The charts of patients treated with antibiotics can be reviewed, and data regarding the diagnosis of infection, the appropriateness of drug selection, and the proper course of therapy as determined by designated physicians are useful in identifying misuse of these drugs. Such information and recommendations to the prescribing physician on the proper use of antibiotics in particular clinical situations serve as an effective means of continuing education and improving drug utilization. The pharmacy, through its program of antibiotic utilization review, may also provide the physician with research data on new agents, the cost of these agents, and the efficacy of such agents as they become available. Establishment of a drug-monitoring program may soon be a requirement for hospital accreditation. Guidelines have recently been formulated by the American Medical Association and the American Hospital Association to aid hospitals in reviewing their patterns of antibiotic utilization, and there may be further guidelines and requirements developed by the Professional Standards Review Organization activities.

Conclusions

The hospital pharmacist, the hospital Committee on Pharmacy and Therapeutics, and the hospital Infection Control Committee should collaborate and cooperate in controlling nosocomial infections. The pharmacist can discharge this responsibility by (1) controlling the techniques in the pharmacy that may contribute to microbial contamination of oral and parental medications, antiseptic agents, and disinfectants; (2) monitoring the use of antimicrobial drugs in the hospital and providing this information to the Infection Control Committee or hospital epidemiologist; (3) serving as a source of drug information that is pertinent to the hospital staff; and (4) establishing an effective formulary system in the hospital. The Infection Control Committee should also be made aware of the importance of the pharmacy and of the drugs dispensed as potential sources of nosocomial infection, and it should assist in establishing and assuring aseptic and sterile procedures in drug compounding and in the formulation of intravenous fluids, as well as assist in the control of multidose vials used for parenterally administered drugs.

References

1. Ayliffe, G. A. J., Barry, D. R., Lowbury, E. J. L., Roper-Hall, M. J., and Walker, W. M. Post-operative infection with *Pseudomonas aeruginosa* in an eye hospital. *Lancet* 1:1113, 1966.
2. Bruch, C. W. Sterility or Microbial Control of Commercially Supplied Items. In Brachman, P. S., and Eickhoff, T. C. (Eds.), *Proceedings of the International Conference on Nosocomial Infections,* August 3–6, 1970. Chicago: American Hospital Association, 1971, p. 236.
3. Bruch, C. W. Possible modification of USP microbial limits and tests. *Drug and Cosmetic Industry* 110:6, 1972.
4. Bruch, C. W. Objectionable microorganisms in non-sterile drugs and cosmetics. *Drug and Cosmetic Industry* 111:11, 1972.
5. Center for Disease Control. Nosocomial bacteremias associated with intravenous fluid therapy. 20(Suppl.):91, 1971.
6. Center for Disease Control. Recall of contaminated intravenous cannulae. *Morbid. Mortal. Weekly Rep.* 23:57, 1974.
7. Franco, J. A., Eitzman, D. V., and Baer, H. Antibiotic usage and microbial resistance in an intensive care nursery. *Am. J. Dis. Child.* 126:318, 1974.
8. Goldmann, D. A., Martin, W. T., and Worthington, J. W. Growth of bacteria and fungi in total parenteral nutrition solutions. *Am. J. Surg.* 126:314, 1973.
9. Herman, L. G. A critical evaluation of microbiological hazards associated with the pharmacy and the hospital. *Am. J. Hosp. Pharm.* 27:56, 1970.
10. Kallings, L. O. Contamination of therapeutic agents. In Brachman, P. S., and Eickhoff, T. C. (Eds.), *Proceedings of the International Conference on Nosocomial Infections,* August 3–6, 1970. Chicago: American Hospital Association, 1971, p. 241.
11. Lang, D. J., Kunz, L. J., Martin, A. R., Schroeder, S. A., and Thomson, L. A. Carmine as a source of nosocomial salmonellosis. *N. Engl. J. Med.* 276:829, 1967.
12. Morse, L. J., and Scholeck, L. E. Hand lotions—A potential nosocomial hazard. *N. Engl. J. Med.* 278:376, 1968.
13. Ogden, A. E., and Rathnell, T. K. Infections and benzalkonium solutions. *J.A.M.A.* 193:978, 1965.

Section E. Food Services

Eugene J. Gangarosa

The food service has the job of providing food for patients and hospital staff that is wholesome, appetizing, economical, and safe to eat. The safety of food is always important, but it is particularly so for hospitalized patients. Patients are unusually susceptible to diseases transmitted by food because of constitutional factors (e.g., malignancy, immunopathy, achlorhydria, and old age) or iatrogenic factors (e.g., antibiotic, immunosuppressive, or antacid therapy and gastric surgery). Persons ill enough to be hospitalized are more likely not only to acquire disease when exposed to foodborne agents, but also to develop the various sequelae associated with such diseases. Small inocula of enteric pathogens that might be innocuous to most healthy people can cause disease and even death in certain highly susceptible hospitalized patients.

Secondary transmission may also occur when hospital staff become infected and they in turn unknowingly expose patients as a consequence of poor personal hygiene and faulty patient-care technique. This was vividly illustrated in a serious outbreak of nosocomial *Salmonella derby* infections in 1963 that were initially transmitted by raw and undercooked eggs and were secondarily transmitted by hospital staff [17]. The chain of transmission may be even further extended by hospital staff, patients, or both, who may transmit disease to visitors or others removed from the hospital setting.

The problems of the hospital food services generally parallel those of a large restaurant or catering firm. Food services frequently operate with restricted budgets, which sometimes necessitates purchasing foods of questionable purity, such as checked (cracked) eggs, or employing some permanent and temporary kitchen helpers who, because of limited education or training, may have poor sanitary habits. The problem is further magnified by the need to purchase and rapidly process quantities of food that require large working surfaces, numerous utensils, and many working hands and by pressure to adhere to tight schedules to ensure rapid preparation and safe storage of a variety of foods. Besides these common issues, hospital food services have additional unique problems created by the need for a wide variety of special diets that are often nutritionally exacting. Meals and supplemental feedings must be provided not only from a central kitchen but often from decentralized kitchens on wards. These problems challenge the food manager to plan effectively and to purchase, process, store, and serve foods that are nutritious, tasty, and safe.

Epidemiologic Aspects of Foodborne Disease
Statistics are not available to delineate the types and frequency of foodborne diseases that specifically occur in hospitals. It seems reasonable to postulate that most of the types of foodborne illness seen in the community also occur in hospitals. According to reports of foodborne illness received at the Center for Disease Control (CDC) during the period 1969 to 1975, the agents most often responsible for foodborne outbreaks were staphylococcal enterotoxins, *Clostridium perfringens*, salmonellae, shigellae,

and hepatitis A [3,10]. Parasitic infections are only rarely transmitted by food (e.g., trichinosis [16]). For details of infection problems caused by these foodborne agents and others that may be transmitted by food, the reader is advised to consult the comprehensive reviews of foodborne diseases written by Merson and co-authors [15] and Bryan [4–9].

The best documented disease transmitted by food in the hospital setting is salmonellosis. In a review of the problem of nosocomial salmonellosis covering the period 1963 to 1972, Baine and co-workers [1] found that 112 (28 percent) of 395 outbreaks of salmonellosis in the United States reported to CDC occurred in institutions (hospitals, mental institutions, and nursing homes); 3496 cases in patients and staff were associated with these 112 outbreaks. Institutions ranked second to the home in frequency of place of occurrence of reported salmonellosis outbreaks. The potential severity of foodborne salmonellosis was underscored by an outbreak due to *Salmonella enteritidis* that occurred in a nursing home in which 25 of 104 affected patients died, an unusually high case–fatality ratio of 24 percent [11].

Inferences can be made from reported data regarding the importance of various factors related to the occurrence of foodborne disease outbreaks. In the period 1961 to 1972, there were 725 community outbreaks in which the factors responsible for the outbreaks were known (Table 7-2). Inadequate refrigeration, which was reported in 46 percent of the outbreaks, was the leading contributing factor. Others were inadequate cooking or heat processing, preparing foods far in advance of planned service, food-handling by infected persons who practiced poor personal hygiene, holding food in warming devices at bacteria-incubating temperatures, using contaminated raw ingredients in uncooked foods, inadequate reheating, cross-contamination, and improper cleaning of equipment. Clearly, training and planning can eliminate these contributing factors and thereby prevent outbreaks.

In a hospital setting, there is also at least the theoretical risk that food can serve as a vehicle of transmission of organisms that rarely cause disease in healthy persons but which can cause

Table 7-2. Factors that Contributed to 725 Reported Foodborne Disease Outbreaks, 1961–1972

Factor	Frequency (%)[a]
Inadequate refrigeration	336 (46)
Preparing food far in advance of planned service	156 (22)
Infected persons practicing poor personal hygiene	151 (21)
Inadequate cooking or heat processing	140 (19)
Holding food in warming devices at bacteria-incubating temperatures	114 (16)
Contaminated raw ingredient in uncooked foods	84 (12)
Inadequate reheating	66 (9)
Cross-contamination	58 (8)
Inadequate cleaning of equipment	52 (7)
Obtaining foods from unsafe sources	44 (6)
Using leftovers	23 (3)
Storing acid foods in toxic containers	19 (3)
Intentional additives	17 (2)
Incidental additives	8 (1)

[a] More than one factor was identified in many of the outbreaks.
Modified from Bryan, F. L. Status of foodborne diseases in the United States. *J. Environ. Health* 38: 74, 1975.

disease in a compromised host. Kominos and colleagues [12] found *Pseudomonas aeruginosa* of the same pyocine type in clinical specimens and on raw vegetables served patients from a kitchen in a general hospital, for example. Intestinal organisms (e.g., *Escherichia coli*) or other organisms (e.g., *Klebsiella*) that are commonly found as contaminants of a variety of foods may subsequently colonize patients—particularly those receiving antimicrobial agents to which the ingested strain is resistant—and thus serve as the causative agent in diseases of the urinary, respiratory, and other systems. In recognition of this possibility, certain patients who may be extremely susceptible to infection (e.g., leukemia patients receiving immunosuppressive therapy) may require as a complement to protective isolation procedures food free of all such contaminants [2,18].

Food served from a hospital kitchen can be contaminated before, during, or after preparation. Raw poultry and red meat are often already contaminated with organisms such as *Salmonella* and *Clostridium perfringens* when purchased. In several surveys of dressed poultry collected from poultry processing plants or from retail markets, levels of *Salmonella* contamination were as high as 50 percent [4,5]. Raw fish may be contaminated with such pathogens as *Vibrio parahaemolyticus* and *C. perfringens*. Fecal matter on the external surface of unprocessed eggs is often contaminated with *Salmonella*. Food may also become contaminated while being processed; organisms come from soiled hands, coughing, and sneezing as well as from contaminated equipment or working surfaces. Finally, bacterial growth may occur while food is in storage, for example, when cooked foods are stored with raw foods or when foods are held at inadequate temperatures.

The hazard of cross-contamination of food is illustrated by an outbreak of salmonellosis in a Missouri hospital in August and September 1976. Fifteen cases of diarrhea occurred intermittently in patients and staff in a seven-week period. This suggested person-to-person transmission, but epidemiologic and microbiologic evidence incriminated tuna fish salad and macaroni salad as the vehicles of infection. Further studies demonstrated that raw meat served as the source of contamination. The salad was prepared in an area of the kitchen where frozen raw meat was thawed [21].

Prevention of Foodborne Transmission
Prevention may be considered from two aspects: food hygiene (i.e., in the preparation, storage, and distribution of food) and personal health and hygiene of food handlers. Prevention—limiting contamination and destroying or inhibiting the growth of potential pathogens—is simple in principle but may be difficult in practice. A dietician with special training in food-service sanitation, a sanitarian, or both should be consulted in the formulation and monitoring of all food-handling operations and procedures. Consultants should be available from local or state health departments.

Food Hygiene

Food must be purchased from reliable sources. Microbial contaminants already on some raw foods must be kept from multiplying during processing; proper storage practices and adequate heat treatment must be used. Work surfaces, knives, slicers, pots, pans, and other kitchen equipment can serve as a means of conveying bacteria by cross-contamination from contaminated food to other foods. All product-contact surfaces of equipment and utensils must be cleaned and decontaminated after use. All workers must thoroughly wash their hands when they enter the food-processing area after handling raw poultry, meat, and fish and always after going to the toilet. Food spillage should be cleaned up immediately. Equipment and kitchen layout should be designed to promote rapid processing in order to minimize chances for cross-contamination; to avoid producing aerosols, sprays, or splashing during processing; and to facilitate cleaning and sanitizing operations [20]. Contamination by insects, birds, rodents, sewage backflow, and drips must be prevented by screening and proper storage, including the segregation of raw meats from processed foods. Garbage from hospital kitchens and the wards should be enclosed and protected from insects and rodents and transported or disposed of in a sanitary manner [13].

The chances of cross-contamination can be minimized by the adoption of standard operating techniques for all cleaning procedures to ensure that working surfaces and kitchen utensils will be sanitized after use and that raw foods will be processed in areas of the kitchen and on working surfaces that are not subsequently used for cooked foods. These procedures should be reviewed periodically, especially when there is a change of personnel, when physical changes are made in the kitchen, or when new equipment is put into use.

Some common mistakes that have caused foodborne diseases have been the result of poor planning or simply a lack of understanding. A typical example is not allowing enough time for poultry to thaw, or assuming that thawing is complete, and thus undercooking it. This problem is sometimes compounded by keeping undercooked food in the oven after the heat has been shut off, thus providing bacteria that survived the initial cooking with ideal incubation conditions. Potentially harmful bacteria in foods must be destroyed by thorough cooking or reheating to internal temperatures that reach 74°C (165°F); meat temperature should be measured by bayonet-type thermometers. Cooked foods should be served hot (60°C or 140°F) or cold (below 7°C or 45°F). Periodically, the internal temperature of foods in serving lines should be checked.

In some outbreaks, even when refrigerator temperatures were adequate, the center temperature of perishable foods was high enough to permit bacteria to grow or toxin to develop. When cooked foods are kept at room temperature (or are refrigerated in large quantities) for a period of four or more hours, certain pathogens remaining in the food may be able to multiply to a high enough level or produce enough toxin to cause disease. The usual reasons for keeping cooked foods at room temperature long enough for potential pathogens to replicate are inadequate refrigerator space, poor utilization of kitchen facilities, or failure to perceive the importance of refrigeration. In general, food that requires refrigeration should be stored at 7°C (45°F) or below in shallow containers so the food is no more than 3 inches deep.

Problems also arise because of certain real or imagined preferences for raw or undercooked foods, such as eggnog. Eggnog prepared from undercooked or raw eggs was an important cause of foodborne salmonellosis prior to the regulation requiring the pasteurization of eggs that are to be dried or frozen. An outbreak of diarrhea, however, was caused by *Salmonella typhimurium* in 1973 in a hospital that prepared eggnog from fresh eggs purchased directly from a farm [19]. Such direct farm purchases of eggs may be economically expedient but can be dangerous, as demonstrated by this outbreak. Nonpasteurized milk, ungraded eggs, and nonpasteurized bulk egg products should not be used in hospitals.

Storage is a particular problem when food must be delivered from a central kitchen to peripheral areas of the hospital or other buildings either by truck or by food carts. Procedures for transporting food must include facilities for keeping hot food hot and cold food cold. Thermometers to measure food temperatures should be standard equipment in such conveyances. Standby equipment should be on hand or alternative plans formulated to handle emergency conditions arising from equipment failure. Food delivered to a kitchen or a ward should be stored so as to prevent growth of bacteria, and it should be distributed with minimum handling by ward personnel. Ward personnel who must handle food should be carefully supervised to ensure that the same high standards required of kitchen personnel are maintained.

Personal Health and Hygiene of Food Service Personnel

Supervision of employees requires attention not only to culinary matters but also to work habits, personal hygiene, and health. Hands of food service personnel may become contaminated not only by raw foods (*Salmonella* and *C. perfringens*) but also by human excreta (*Salmonella, Shigella, C. perfringens,* and hepatitis A virus) as well as by secretions from the respiratory tract or from infected wounds (*Streptococcus* and *Staphylococcus*).

There has been a tendency for management to rely on laboratory tests to ensure that food service personnel do not transmit diseases to others. Various health-monitoring means have been employed, which have traditionally included periodic chest roentgenograms for tuberculosis, serologic tests for syphilis, and stool examinations for ova and parasites, certain enteric bacterial pathogens, or both. These measures may be important to the health of individual workers and perhaps may be justified in preemployment physical examinations, but they usually are not relevant to the issue of whether workers can transmit foodborne diseases. It is particularly important to recognize that a single stool culture will often not detect the small number of organisms present in an individual who does not have diarrhea but is infected with enteric

pathogens. McCall and co-workers [14] found, for example, that the probability of obtaining a positive culture from any chronic *S. derby* carrier by taking one rectal swab was 0.47 and that seven consecutive daily swabs were needed to detect 95 percent of known carriers. Obviously, such extensive culturing is impractical and costly. Furthermore, a person may not be infected on the day when the culture specimen is taken, but the same person may later acquire infection. Also, a carrier may excrete organisms intermittently, so sporadic sampling for culture tests may never reveal the true carriage status. Finally, cultures of nose and throat secretions and the feces of many persons may reveal potential foodborne pathogens such as *S. aureus,* but this carriage may be of no danger to others; that is, the carrier may not be disseminating the organisms. Thus, there is no scientific justification for conducting or requiring routine laboratory testing.

Laboratory monitoring of food handlers may actually be counterproductive by giving the food handler and hospital administrators a false sense of security. Negative reports are likely to be interpreted by the employee to mean that he or she is not capable of transmitting foodborne pathogens to food. From the standpoint of management, laboratory monitoring of food handlers may convey the false assurance that something meaningful is being accomplished to ensure continuing food safety.

The proper approach is to establish and pursue a policy of training food service managers and workers. The hospital Infection Control Committee should plan a program that includes an initial comprehensive training course for all new employees as well as refresher courses for all food service personnel to be given at regular intervals. These courses should include the basic principles of personal and food hygiene. For such training, lectures and seminars are best, but self-instructional material may be useful. It may be necessary to give courses in a foreign language or to translate the course materials into a foreign language. CDC will provide on request training aids, including reprints and kits, for food service managers. The kit entitled *Control of Foodborne Diseases in the Food Service Industry** is particularly recommended. Other study programs are also available, and some states have training and certification programs for food service supervisors and managers. Incentives should be provided for food service personnel to participate in such training.

The courses should emphasize the reasons why food handlers should wash their hands after using the toilet and after handling such foods as raw poultry, fish, and meats. They should emphasize the importance of reporting to supervisors acute intestinal diseases, boils, and any skin infection, particularly on the fingers and hands. In addition to these personal aspects of hygiene, the principles of food sanitation should be stressed. Food service personnel should be taught the hazards associated with their work and how to prevent them. Emphasis must be on rapid and effective cooling, adequate holding of hot foods, and efficient reheating of foods. An environment should be created in which the important, contributory role of food service personnel toward taking care of patients is stressed.

Surveillance

Responsibility for the prevention, detection, and investigation of foodborne disease outbreaks should be an integral part of the activity of the hospital Infection Control Committee. The causes of acute illness and absenteeism among food service workers should be promptly determined. It is important that an atmosphere be created that does not penalize food handlers for reporting illness. Whenever possible, workers who report acute intestinal or respiratory illness should be given sick leave or assigned alternative jobs that have no risk for the transmission of foodborne diseases. There should be no loss of pay or vacation leave for reporting illness (see Part I, Chapter 3).

* Available from Applied Food Service Sanitation, National Institution for the Food Service Industry, 120 S. Riverside Plaza, Chicago, Ill. 60606, and Sanitation in the Retail Food Service Operation, Educational Institute of the American Hotel and Motel Association, Kellog Center, Michigan State University, East Lansing, Mich. 48823.

Appropriate culture specimens should be taken and processed during such illnesses. Rectal swab or fecal specimens promptly inoculated into appropriate laboratory media are recommended in cases of acute diarrhea. In cases in which enteric pathogens have been identified, workers should be permitted to return to their assigned jobs only after their symptoms have disappeared and they have had at least one negative stool culture after completing drug treatment if drugs are used. The same procedure is recommended with streptococcal infections of the throat or tonsils. Boils, open sores, and cellulitis of the fingers, hands, and face are particularly dangerous. Food handlers with any of these infections should be under a physician's care. That physician's judgment should prevail in the decision as to when the worker can return to work. Medical and laboratory services should be provided by the hospital without cost to the employee, at least for acute respiratory, intestinal, and dermatologic illnesses.

Routine surveillance of patients and employees should detect any cases of gastrointestinal disease related to the hospital's food service. Clusters of such cases according to time and place should alert the infection control officer to the possibility of an outbreak; any cluster should be investigated promptly.

References

1. Baine, W. B., Gangarosa, E. J., Bennett, J. V., Barker, W. H.   Institutional salmonellosis. *J. Infect. Dis.* 128:357, 1973.
2. Bodey, G. P.   Isolation for the compromised host. *J.A.M.A.* 233:543, 1975.
3. Brachman, P. S., Taylor, A., Gangarosa, E. J., Merson, M. H., Barker, W. H.   Food Poisoning in the U.S.A. In Hobbs, B. C., and Christian, J. H. G. (Eds.), *Microbiological Safety of Food*. New York: Academic Press, 1973, p. 143.
4. Bryan, F. L.   What the sanitarian should know about staphylococci and salmonellae in non-dairy products. I. Staphylococci. *J. Milk Food Technol.* 31:110, 1968.
5. Bryan, F. L.   What the sanitarian should know about staphylococci and salmonellae in non-dairy products. II. Salmonellae. *J. Milk Food Technol.* 31:131, 1968.
6. Bryan, F. L.   What the sanitarian should know about *Clostridium perfringens* food-

borne illness. *J. Milk Food Technol.* 32:383, 1969.

7. Bryan, F. L. Emerging foodborne diseases. I. Their surveillance and epidemiology. *J. Milk Food Technol.* 35:618, 1972.

8. Bryan, F. L. Emerging foodborne diseases. II. Factors that contribute to outbreaks and their control. *J. Milk Food Technol.* 35:632, 1972.

9. Bryan, F. L. Microbiological food hazards today—Based on epidemiological information. *Food Technol.* 28:52, 1974.

10. Bryan, F. L. Status of foodborne diseases in the United States. *J. Environ. Health* 38:74, 1975.

11. Center for Disease Control. Salmonellosis—Baltimore, Maryland. *Morbid. Mortal. Weekly Rep.* 19:314, 1970.

12. Kominos, S. D., Copeland, C. E., Grosiak, B., Postic, B. Introduction of *Pseudomonas aeruginosa* into a hospital via vegetables. *Appl. Microbiol.* 24:567, 1972.

13. Kotschevar, L. H. *Food Service Planning: Layout and Equipment.* New York: John Wiley & Sons, 1961.

14. McCall, C. E., Sanders, W. E., Boring, J. R., Brachman, P. S., Wikingsson, M. Delineation of chronic carriers of *Salmonella derby* within an institution for incurables. *Antimicrob. Agents Chemother.*, 1964, p. 717.

15. Merson, M. H., Hughes, J. M., and Gangarosa, E. J. Miscellaneous Food Poisoning. In Eickhoff, T. C. (Ed.), *Tice's Practice of Medicine.* Hagerstown, Md.: Harper & Row, 1976, pp. 1–24.

16. Pocock, D. G., Schnurrenberger, P. R., Ziegler, A. D., Wentworth, F. H., Winslow, J. B. Trichinosis—A point source outbreak. *Ann. Intern. Med.* 59:323, 1963.

17. Sanders, E., Sweeney, F. J., Friedman, E. A., Boring, J. R., Randall, E. L., Polk, L. D. An outbreak of hospital-associated infections due to *Salmonella derby.* *J.A.M.A.* 186:984, 1963.

18. Schimpff, S. C., Greene, W. H., Young, V. M., Fortner, C. L., Jepsen, L., Cusack, N., Block, J. B., Wiernik, P. H. Infection prevention in acute nonlymphocytic leukemia: Laminar air flow room reverse isolation with oral, nonabsorbable antibiotic prophylaxis. *Ann. Intern. Med.* 82:351, 1975.

19. Steere, A., Hall, W., Gangarosa, E. J., Craven, P. J., Leotsakis, N., Farmer, J. J., Wells, J. G. Person-to-person spread of *Salmonella typhimurium* after a hospital common-source outbreak. *Lancet* 1:319, 1975.

20. U.S. Public Health Service. *Food Service Sanitation Manual.* Washington, D.C.: Food and Drug Administration, 1962.

21. West, C. M., Gunn, R. A., and Klass, J. Nosocomial salmonellosis acquired from an

intermittent common source masquerading as person-to-person transmission. (In preparation.)

Section F. Central Service

George F. Mallison

Functions of Central Service

A Central Service Department (CSD) in hospitals should process, store, and dispense the supplies and equipment required for all aspects of care, diagnosis, and treatment of patients [5]. In carrying out these functions, a CSD removes or destroys infectious contamination on reusable items and redistributes them; it also distributes safe, single-use items. The role of the CSD in the prevention of nosocomial disease is clear, because improperly sterilized or disinfected reusable items—including endoscopic equipment, thermometers, bedpans and urinals, respiratory therapy and anesthesia supplies, equipment for aspiration and suction, pressure transducers, and surgical instruments—have been directly responsible for the transmission of infection.

Hospitals have found for economic reasons, as well as for efficiency and maintenance of high standards, that it is preferable for all reusable supplies and equipment requiring special cleaning, disinfection, or sterilization, to be handled centrally whenever possible; it is also preferable, for the same reasons, that prepackaged supplies purchased for patient care be handled centrally [2].

Precleaning reusable supplies and equipment in patient-care areas is seldom recommended now, because such cleaning is inefficient, expensive, unsafe, and obviously unnecessary with central processing. Rather, items for reprocessing should simply be packaged, clearly marked as to their contents (if not obvious), and returned to the CSD. If they are potentially contaminated with infectious material, items should be placed in impervious plastic bags labeled "contaminated." Items for reprocessing should be placed in designated areas for pickup and subsequent transfer to the CSD. To prevent the risk of viral hepatitis or other infections to personnel, used surgical instruments should not be cleaned by hand; rather, they should be processed through a washer-sterilizer in the operating room before being sent to the CSD. Reusable linens should be returned to the laundry, not to the CSD.

Details of the requirements and recommendations for the disinfection and sterilization processes to be carried out in a CSD are given in Part I, Chapter 6.

Designated Areas of the CSD

A CSD should have separate receiving areas for new single-use items and for soiled reusable items that have been returned for reprocessing. Separate decontamination, disinfection, sterilization, and packaging areas and facilities also are required. A storage area should be provided for clean or disinfected nonsterile items that are ready for reuse, such as carts, stands, lamps, heaters, wheelchairs, ice mattresses, and the like. Additionally, a storage area is necessary for sterile items, both hospital-processed and new. Finally, an area for dispensing items and an administrative area are necessary in a well-organized CSD [5].

In the design of a new hospital or in major renovation of an old one, the CSD should be planned to provide efficiency and safety of operation. In planning, consideration should be given to the location of the CSD in relationship to the major hospital locations from which goods are received or distributed, such as the loading dock, laundry, operating and obstetric suites, emergency rooms, respiratory therapy and intensive-care units, and major patient-care areas. The best location for the CSD with respect to these other areas is one that minimizes the costs of construction and operation of the entire hospital. Highly sophisticated, "automated" handling systems for supplies proposed for and installed in some hospitals in recent years have not been proved to be economical to the hospital in terms of total costs (i.e., space requirements; costs of installation, operation, maintenance; and cost of replacement services during downtime).

Initial Processing of Supplies
Sorting and Decontamination

Sorting and decontamination (i.e., the preliminary processing required to make items safe for subsequent handling with reasonable care) should be carried out in a room that is under negative pressure and is ventilated by at least six air changes per hour. Decontamination by vigorous physical scrubbing—using either a detergent or a disinfectant-detergent solution in hot water and preferably machine washing—greatly reduces microbial contamination on the surfaces of items. Sometimes such decontamination processing may be sufficient, and no further processing is necessary. Some items (e.g., heating lamps, carts, wheelchairs, crutches, and headboards) need only to be scrubbed with detergent before being stored for reuse. However, patient-care items that are contaminated with excretions or secretions, that become wet in use (e.g., ice mattresses and flotation pads), that have been used by or for isolated patients, or that may have had significant, direct, skin contact with patients while in use (e.g., perineal lamps, toys, and portable commodes) should be scrubbed with a fresh disinfectant-detergent solution before being stored for reuse.

Washer-Sterilizers and Ultrasonic Cleaners

Washer-sterilizers, which are recommended for the initial decontamination of surgical instruments, provide an agitated, high-temperature, detergent bath followed by steam sterilization. The washing and the sterilization of a load of unwrapped used instruments are possible in about 20 minutes. After processing in a washer-sterilizer, surgical instruments should be further processed through an ultrasonic cleaner in the CSD; dried, inspected, and cleaned further by hand if necessary; assembled into appropriate packs; and then terminally sterilized.

Linen Packs

Linen packs should be assembled in the hospital laundry and transferred to the CSD for sterilization. These packs should weigh no more than 5.5 kg. (12 pounds) and be no larger than 30 by 30 by 50 cm. (12 by 12 by 20 inches). Cotton cloth, paper, and cellophane wrappers have been used for linen and other packs that have been sterilized by steam; only tape should be used to seal packs.

Storage of Sterile Goods

Storage Areas

Storage areas for hospital-processed or other sterile items should be ventilated with at least two air changes per hour, and the temperature should be maintained at between 18°C and 25°C (64°F and 77°F). Prevention of excessive humidity in storage areas is also necessary to preclude any possibility of condensation of water on cold surfaces that could wet packages of sterile goods, as well as to prevent mold or mildew growth; at no time should a relative humidity above 75 percent be permitted in areas where sterile goods are stored. Low humidity is also undesirable, because excessive drying may result in fabric damage due to superheating of outdated linen packs during resterilization; if a relative humidity above 30 percent is maintained, it should not be necessary to disassemble, relaunder, and repack outdated linen packs for resterilization. The relative humidity should be measured continuously, and the measuring device should be checked at least monthly with a sling psychrometer. All storage of sterile goods should be at least 30 cm. (12 inches) above floor level; no sterile items should ever be placed on the floor. A thorough, continuous program for insect and rodent exclusion and control is necessary in an area for sterile storage. No hanging steam, potable-water, or waste-water pipes should be permitted in a room used for sterile storage. Light levels of at least 110 lumens per square meter (10 foot-candles) should be present in all locations in a sterile storage area.

Safe Storage Times

Many types of wrappers used for packs sterilized in hospitals have not been tested under carefully controlled, comparable conditions. It is recommended that most types of packs sterilized in hospitals—whether by gas or steam—be double-wrapped with cotton muslin, with each wrapper consisting of two fabric layers (a total of four layers). Such a wrapper will maintain sterility of the pack contents for three weeks when stored on open shelves (Table 7-3). The use of single-wrapped muslin packs (one or two layers) is not recommended [4]. All sterile packs wrapped in pervious wrappers should be handled as little as possible to reduce the opportunity for microbial contamination of the contents.

Closed-cabinet storage clearly is preferable to storage on open shelves, but the extra labor required to move supplies in and out of closed cabinets and the extra costs for the cabinets should be considered when weighing the advantages against those of open-shelf storage for shorter times. Long-term (at least nine months) sterile storage is possible if packs are sealed in sterile, 3-mil polyethylene bags [4]. However, long storage times may be uneconomical, even if safe, because they reflect an unused inventory of sterile items. Nonetheless, a hospital may wish to maintain in storage a

Table 7-3. Storage Times During Which Packs Remained Sterile

	Duration of Sterility[a]	
Wrapping	In closed cabinet	On open shelves
Single-wrapped muslin (two layers)	1 week	2 days
Double-wrapped muslin (each two layers)	7 weeks	3 weeks
Single-wrapped two-way crepe paper (single layer)	At least 8 weeks	3 weeks
Tightly woven pima cotton (single layer) over single-wrapped muslin (two layers)	—	8 weeks
Two-way crepe paper (single layer) over single-wrapped muslin (two layers)	—	10 weeks
Single-wrapped muslin (two layers) sealed in 3-mil polyethylene	—	At least 9 months

[a] Sterility was checked daily for the first week of storage and weekly thereafter.
From Mallison, G. F., and Standard, P. G. Safe storage times for sterile packs. *Hospitals* 48:77, Oct. 16, 1974.

supply of sterile, disposable, nonwoven fabric packs for emergency use in the event of laundry or sterilizer problems or disasters. Routine use of such packs is not recommended, however, because of excessive costs [1].

A pack should not be considered sterile if it becomes wet, it has been dropped onto the floor, or the tape seal has been broken. An expiration date should be marked clearly on each pack immediately *after* sterilization. A procedure is needed for the regular review of all hospital-sterilized and commercially sterilized packs and items in storage to insure that no outdated materials are ever present [3].

References

1. Bodner, B., Zelner, L., Merchant, R., and Laufman, H.   Costs of linen versus disposable O.R. packs. *Hospitals* 47:76, Dec. 1, 1973.
2. Committee on Infection Control. *Infection Control in the Hospital* (3d ed.). Chicago: American Hospital Association, 1974.
3. Joint Commission on Accreditation of Hospitals. *Accreditation Manual for Hospitals.* Chicago: Joint Commission on Accreditation of Hospitals, 1976.
4. Mallison, G. F., and Standard, P. G.   Safe storage times for sterile packs. *Hospitals* 48:77, Oct. 16, 1974.
5. U.S. Department of Health, Education, and Welfare. *A Manual for Hospital Central Services.* Washington, D.C.: U.S. Government Printing Office, DHEW Publication No. (ARA) 74-4012, 1975.

Section G. Linens and Laundry

George F. Mallison

Hospitals in the United States produce an estimated 6 billion pounds of linens annually, much of which is potentially contaminated with microbial pathogens. These pathogens could be the source of infections for patients or the hospital staff, especially those who handle the soiled linens. Linens are handled throughout the hospital by many people; once in the laundry, complex linen-handling and processing operations are usually necessary in preparing the linen for reuse. The purpose of the laundry is to process soiled and contaminated linen into clean linen that aids patient comfort and care and is not a vehicle of infection. The processing of linens should not cause infections among employees.

A review of scientific literature reveals at least five documented instances where hospital employees handling soiled linens have acquired infectious disease from these linens: Q fever [10], salmonellosis [6,7,11], and smallpox [5]. Fungal infections can be spread from contaminated fabrics in the hospital; for example, wool socks washed at low temperatures without a disinfectant added to the wash water have spread "ringworm" of the feet in an extended-care hospital. Urinary catheters contaminated by direct contact with patient linens have caused patient infections. In the classic studies by Gonzaga, Mortimer, Wolinsky, and Rammelkamp [8] on transmission of *Staphylococcus aureus* to infants in hospital nurseries, heavily contaminated linens as well as hands caused transfer of staphylococcal colonization to exposed infants. Streptococcal infections, however, were not transmitted to well military recruits exposed to streptococci on blankets. Undoubtedly, more episodes of infections due to contamination of linens with pathogens have occurred in hospitals, but, because of the lack of recognition of an association or of failure to report them, such episodes have not been investigated or have not been published in the scientific literature.

Linens may cause noninfectious problems in hospitals, including dermal irritation of employees or patients who handle glass-fiber fabrics or who use linens that have been washed with glass-fiber fabrics. Residues of aniline dyes and phenols on diapers have caused illness and death in newborns.

Notwithstanding the potential for transmission of pathogens, the actual occurrence of disease related to contaminated fabrics in hospitals apparently is rare, even among hospital staff who have direct and frequent contact with soiled linens as a part of their work. Nonetheless, adequate procedures for the collection, transportation, processing, and storage of hospital linens are essential, not only to limit the possibility of disease in patients who may be unusually susceptible or in hospital employees who may handle soiled linens, but also for esthetic reasons.

Handling of Soiled Linens
Bagging and Pickup
All soiled linens should be bagged or placed into covered carts *at the location where used.* Soiled linens should be handled with a minimum of agitation during bed making or while being changed in order to prevent contamination of the air with microorganisms, particularly from patients on strict and respiratory isolation [12]. One's hands should be washed after handling soiled linens. Soiled linens should not be sorted or pre-rinsed in patient-care units. Soiled linens should be removed at least daily from patient-care units and at least thrice daily from nurseries [1]; soiled nursery linen should be stored and transported in impervious bags [1]. If soiled linens must be temporarily stored prior to laundering, well-lighted and ventilated rooms should be used for this purpose.

Transportation
Soiled linens should be transported in well-covered and identified carts that should be used exclusively for this purpose. The linings of these carts should be cleaned or laundered frequently. If laundry chutes are used, all soiled linens so transported should be bagged. Chutes should be cleaned on a regular basis. Charging doors for chutes should preferably be located in well-ventilated, fireproof rooms, not on corridors [13]. Laundry chutes can readily be exhaust-ventilated to reduce airborne microbial contamination when the chute doors are opened.

Linens known to be contaminated with infectious microorganisms—particularly linens from strict and respiratory isolation facilities and from enteric and wound and skin precaution areas [12]—should be clearly labeled and handled with special care. Impervious bags are recommended, and hot-water-soluble bags are particularly useful, because they can be placed into the washing machine without sorting the contents [12]; however, they are expensive.

Sorting
Soiled linens should be handled and sorted as little as practical. If sorting is done, it should be in a room separate from the main laundering area. Consideration should be given to the wearing of protective clothing and gloves by laundry personnel who sort soiled linens prior to washing. There is no evidence that masks are necessary, and few individuals who sort linens are willing to wear even comfortable surgical masks. Frequent hand-washing by individuals who sort soiled linens is essential; thus, hand-washing facilities must be convenient to laundry personnel. Cloth bags for soiled linens require the same laundering as their contents each time the bags are used.

Laundry
Washing
A hospital laundry should be designed to wash seven days of soiled linens within any work week. There is no evidence that "continuous-flow" washers or "pass-through" washer-extractors [14] reduce contamination of linens or reduce the risk of disease to laundry workers. The floor and all equipment in a hospital laundry should be cleaned at the end of each work day, and a regular schedule should be established to clean the overhead and hard-to-reach areas of the laundry. The flow of ventilating air in the laundry should be from the cleanest to the dirtiest area.

Thorough washing action using hot water and effective detergents is essential to highly efficient removal of soil and microbial contamination in the actual laundering process. An accurate thermometer should be used to measure water temperatures. Water temperatures above 71°C (160°F) for 25 minutes kill nearly all microorganisms other than spores, and such temperatures are recommended for use except with delicate fabrics [2,3]. The use of cotton thermal blankets is preferable to that of wool blankets because of ease of laundering. Laundering at lower temperatures may result in much lower effectiveness in the removal of microbial contamination [3]. The use of bleach (or other chemicals) in the laundering process may provide further reduction in microbial contamination beyond the effects of hot water. Although some recontamination of washed linens may occur during extraction, drying and ironing ultimately reduce microbial contamination of well-processed hospital linens to insignificant levels for routine patient use [3].

It is recommended that all heavily soiled launderable items (e.g., web-footed mops or the "step-off mats" used just inside the outdoor entrances to hospitals) be washed separately from other hospital linens. Mops must be thoroughly dried after laundering, or they will likely become heavily contaminated with microorganisms before reuse [9].

Additives

There are a number of advantages to treating linens with safe and effective combination textile softeners and bacteriostatic agents that are incorporated in the laundry process. Softeners make the linen easier to wash and handle, softer for the patient, and reduce linting. Effective bacteriostatic agents will help to prevent putrefaction in soiled and wet linen, thus increasing its useful life. These agents will help to prevent the growth of potentially pathogenic microorganisms in soiled, wet linen, and the use of such bacteriostatic agents may reduce the incidence of ammonia dermatitis.

Storage

To minimize microbial contamination after washing and ironing, clean linen should be handled as little as possible and stored wrapped or covered. The clean linen storage room(s) should be separate from the main laundering area, and personnel who work with clean linens should have this as their exclusive activity. Storage in enclosed linen carts that are wheeled to patient areas helps to minimize handling (and thus lowers costs) and also helps to protect from contamination by dust. Shelves of carts or of closets where clean linens are stored should be cleaned on a regular basis; at least weekly cleaning is suggested.

Sterilization of Linens

It is recommended that surgical gowns and linens used in or on patients in the operating

and delivery rooms be sterilized after laundering and sterilized again before use by autoclaving. Neither the American Academy of Pediatrics (AAP) nor the Center for Disease Control, however, require the use of sterile nursery linens [1]; also, the AAP has stated that the use of clean disposable diapers should be satisfactory for normal, well infants [1]. In some hospitals, all linens in direct contact with patients in protective isolation are sterilized.

Disposable Linens

Disposable sheets, mattress covers, drapes, gowns, curtains, and the like are improving in quality, and the use of such items in hospitals to promote sanitation and improve patient care has been increasing. As with soiled linens, however, sanitary techniques are necessary for the handling (and disposal) of soiled disposable linens. Recent evaluations have also shown that such disposables (except for small items such as sponges, masks, diapers, caps, and so on) generally are considerably more expensive than reusable linens [4].

References

1. American Academy of Pediatrics. *Hospital Care of Newborn Infants* (5th ed.). Evanston, Ill., 1971.
2. American Hospital Association. *Hospital Laundry Manual of Operation.* Chicago: American Hospital Association, 1949.
3. Arnold, L.   A sanitary study of commercial laundry practices. *Am. J. Public Health* 28: 839, 1938.
4. Badner, B., Zelner, L., Merchant, R., and Laufman, H.   Costs of linen *vs.* disposable OR packs. *Hospitals* 47:76, Dec. 1, 1973.
5. British Medical Journal.   Smallpox. *Br. Med. J.* 1:288, 1951.
6. Canadian Epidemiology Bulletin. *Salmonella typhi. Can. Epidemiol. Bull.* 16:128, 1972.
7. Datta, N., Pridie, R. B., and Anderson, E. S. An outbreak of infection with *Salmonella typhimurium* in a general hospital. *J. Hyg. (Camb.)* 58:229, 1960.
8. Gonzaga, A. J., Mortimer, E. A., Jr., Wolinsky, E., and Rammelkamp, C. H., Jr.   Transmission of staphylococci by fomites. *J.A.M.A.* 189:711, 1964.
9. Mallison, G. F.   Housekeeping in operating

suites. *A.O.R.N. J.* 21:213, 1975.

10. Oliphant, J. W., Gordon, D. A., Meis, A., and Parker, R. R. Q fever in laundry workers, presumably transmitted from contaminated clothing. *Am. J. Hyg.* 49:76, 1949.

11. Steere, A. C., Craven, P. J., Hall, W. J., III, Leotsakis, N., Wells, J. G., Farmer, J. J., III, and Gangarosa, E. J. Person-to-person spread of *Salmonella typhimurium* after a hospital common-source outbreak. *Lancet* 1: 319, 1975.

12. U.S. Department of Health, Education, and Welfare. *Isolation Techniques for Use in Hospitals* (2d ed.). Washington, D.C.: U.S. Government Printing Office, DHEW Publ. No. (CDC) 76-8314, 1975.

13. U.S. Department of Health, Education, and Welfare. *Minimum Requirements of Construction and Equipment for Hospital and Medical Facilities.* Washington, D.C.: U.S. Government Printing Office, DHEW Publ. No. (HRA) 74-4000, 1974.

14. U.S. Department of Health, Education, and Welfare. *The Hospital Laundry.* Washington, D.C.: U.S. Government Printing Office, DHEW Publ. No. 930-D-24, 1966.

Section H. The Operating Room
Harold Laufman

Critical analysis of the operating-room environment in recent years has given rise to certain basic principles of architecture and engineering, on one hand, and exposed misdirected but expensive developments on the other. Despite a host of existing codes and guidelines directed at minimizing hazards, these hazards until recently have been ill-defined and, in some cases, exaggerated. Identifiable operating-room hazards include infection, power failure, electrical and mechanical malfunctions, flame, and explosion. Inherent in all these hazards in the physical environment is the pervading effect of human failure. The danger associated with unskilled, poorly trained, or untrustworthy personnel who may abuse an otherwise satisfactory environment constitutes an insidious, but perhaps the most important, aspect of hazard control in the operating room. Human failure is especially related to the problem of infection control.

Environmental Design of the Surgical Suite

Design and equipment of a surgical suite can affect utilization patterns, material handling, and traffic and commerce in and around the suite. To a certain extent, design and equipment have an influence on the effectiveness of people, of machines, and of the various systems in which there is interaction between people and things. Insofar as there is an interrelationship between design, efficiency, methods, economy, and the human element, the architectural configuration and the equipment of a surgical suite indirectly affect the incidence of surgical infection [8].

From an architectural point of view, a number of design concepts have arisen that are directed at the control of surgical infection. Most planners of surgical suites acknowledge that people rather than things are the chief problem in the control of wound infection. Although both surgeons and planners agree that the environmental approach cannot be ignored, proof of the effects of architecture on infection is almost impossible to obtain. It is widely agreed that the surgical suite should be located to provide isolation from the mainstreams of common corridor traffic.

An effort at developing traffic patterns that would separate "clean" from "dirty" traffic in a surgical suite has resulted in the architectural concepts known as the clean central core and the peripheral corridor. Although these concepts were experimented with by American architects since the late 1920s, British architects developed them in the post-World War II years. In principle, these concepts were developed on the proposition that the site of the operation in the center of each operating room is considered the cleanest spot, the periphery of the room less clean, the corridors of the surgical suite less clean, and so on, toward the periphery of the suite. The central core of the suite serves as the supply center and therefore is supposedly cleanest of all. The clean core and inner corridors are designated for use by clean traffic (patients before elective, clean operations, as well as surgeons and nurses before operating), whereas the peripheral corridors are designated for so-called dirty traffic (patients after operation, as well as surgeons and nurses after operating). If the patient is considered infected before operation, he is brought in and taken out of the operating room through the dirty corridors.

A number of suites now in use have been the subject of criticism. Observations made in them reveal that, unfortunately, almost none is being used as planned [6]. The existing traffic pattern does not conform with the one conceived by the architect. People tend to take the shortest distance between two points, rather than a roundabout way. Moreover, in those suites being used almost as planned, no notable reduction in infection rates has been observed over previous rates or over those found with other architectural designs. The peripheral corridors, occupying thousands of square feet of otherwise valuable space, have become long storage halls for expensive floor-standing equipment that should have been accorded legitimate storage space inside the suite. While no one is willing to argue against the theory of the clean-core concept, the actual use of such layouts, as with the peripheral corridor suites, does not usually fulfill the intent of their designers. The clean core in its pure form is intended to be an area of the surgical suite that is virtually as clean as any operating room, where only such clean activities as clean storage, instrument packing, and autoclaving are done, or that serves as a supply port for adjacent operating rooms. All traffic from this area is intended to be in the direction of the operating rooms, and all traffic out of the operating rooms is intended to be in the direction of the peripheral corridor. In practice, however, we have observed that personnel working in the clean-core area do not usually wear masks and are not confined to the clean core. Clean storage in this area may contain cartons that often come directly off the truck that delivered them to the hospital. In this area, short sleeves on personnel is the rule. The shedding of bacteria-carrying squamae from exposed skin is well documented. Of necessity, people go into and come out of the operating rooms into the clean core in the course of their work. This unavoidable activity, plus the other abuses mentioned, give one pause to ponder the validity of the clean-core concept, as well as to wonder about the absence of studies concerned with it.

The architectural configurations of surgical suites fall into four categories, each with variations: (1) the central corridor or hotel plan with "L" or "T" variations; (2) the double central corridor, multiple corridors, or clean-core plan; (3) the grouping or cluster plan, and (4) the peripheral corridor, ring, or racetrack plan. A partial or complete peripheral corridor may be designed for any of these plans.

The fact that equally good surgery can be done in any of these suites at equally low risk and with equally good results, provided the surgery is done well and is supported by efficient support personnel who do not abuse their environment, may mean one of three things: (1) traffic patterns within the surgical suite are not important; (2) traffic patterns are important, but architects are not planning them realistically, or (3) current ideas on designing surgical suites and traffic patterns are in need of revision in concept. One is inclined to see a bit of truth in all three possibilities.

Recovery Areas
Recovery areas have emerged from their original designation as a place for a patient to recover from anesthesia to a place where intensive nursing care can be given to a critically ill patient postoperatively. Especially since the advent of open-heart surgery, organ transplantation, and other types of major surgery, the recovery "room" has become an intensive-care suite of windowed cubicles. Patients with severe infections can be given care as good as that given to patients whose defense mechanisms may be suppressed, and all patients are under close surveillance. Thus, the open, Florence Nightingale-type of recovery room, although still in wide use, is giving way to a recovery area of isolation cubicles, located immediately adjacent to, or as part of, the surgical suite.

Transfer Areas
A transfer area is ordinarily considered desirable. In this area, the patient is transferred from the "outside" cart to an "inside" cart,

ostensibly to prevent the tracking of hospital dirt into the surgical suite. Although this practice is acknowledged to have theoretical validity, no hard evidence is available that traces surgical infections to the wheels of carts. Some costly devices are available for patient transfer, including mechanical transfer-board arrangements. The same procedure, however, can be simply, effectively, and economically carried out at any counter-height barrier. Many hospitals continue to bring the hospital cart into the operating room and to transfer the patient directly to the operating table. No reported infections thus far have been traced to this practice.

Other Areas

A conference room, nurses' offices, a scheduling area, holding and preparation areas, an adequate vestibular area, and appropriately sized and located locker rooms and lounges are all considered essential to an up-to-date surgical suite. All require significant space in terms of square footage, but a good case can be made for them on the basis of hazard control alone. At the entrance to a surgical suite, for example, the frequent opening and closing of the doors to the common corridor or to a bank of elevators causes an inevitable influx of unfiltered air, regardless of the pressurizing of the air in the operating rooms. For this reason, a well-ventilated, generously proportioned, vestibular space, preferably demarcated by a second set of doors, will permit appropriate dilution of airborne contamination and thus serve as a sort of airlock. Opening on this vestibular space are the offices mentioned above, the transfer area, surgeons' lockers, the scheduling desk, and other spaces requiring an outside and inside interface. Through such an arrangement, these spaces need not open directly to a common corridor.

Number of Operating Rooms

The number of operating rooms is relevant to hazard control only as it relates to the economy of scheduling, housekeeping practices, and staffing. For most hospitals, the "five-percent formula" works quite well: the number of operating rooms should be 5 percent of the total number of surgical beds. Thus, for a hospital with 100 surgical beds utilized by all surgical specialties combined, there should be five or six operating rooms. Cystoscopy and endoscopy rooms are additional. Overuse of operating rooms gives rise to the risk of personnel fatigue and incomplete cleansing practices. If a room is used for many lengthy operations so that only one operation per room per day can be performed, more rooms will be required.

Size of Operating Rooms

The size of operating rooms that is considered optimal for most operations is 20 by 20 feet and 10 feet high. Although some procedures—such as those in ophthalmology, otolaryngology, and cystoscopy—can be done comfortably in smaller rooms, the primary requisite regarding size is that all maneuvers, including gowning and draping, the circulation of personnel, and the use of equipment, should be executable without the risk of contact contamination. Because of the space requirements of the extracorporeal pump, the pump team, and other additional people, a somewhat larger room, such as 24 by 26 feet, is recommended for open-heart surgery. When one dimension of a room exceeds 30 feet, however, something is lost in personnel efficiency.

Methods of Infection Control
Operating-Room Surfaces

In general, the harder and less porous the floor, walls, ceilings, and other surfaces, the more dirt-resistant the surface will be and the easier it will be to clean. Ceramic tile has been criticized because the rough surfaces of grouting may attract bacteria. A new grouting material is now available, however, that has a surface as smooth as ceramic tile itself. Other wall materials suitable for operating-room use include laminated polyester with an epoxy finish, hard vinyl coverings that can be heat-sealed at the seams, and other hard building materials such as formica.

Tacky mats with replaceable sheets have been widely promoted and used in front of the doors leading to the surgical suite on the pretext that they prevent the tracking in of dirt from common corridors. Our test results have shown that these mats do not remove bacteria but in fact transfer tagged bacteria to new contacts [8]. Wet-mopping of hard-surfaced floors with a phenolic solution between each patient in the operating room as well as every several hours during the working day in the corridors of the suite with wet-vacuuming at night is an unsurpassed method of keeping the floors clean.

Air-Handling Systems

Most conventional operating rooms are, or should be, ventilated by efficient, well-maintained, bag-filtered or high-efficiency particulate air-filtered (HEPA) systems. The environment of such operating rooms suffers only by abuse, but otherwise it has been shown to be virtually as effectively clean as that of costly special chambers. Defective air-handling systems, on the other hand, may be considered hazardous under special circumstances.

The significance of airborne contamination as a cause of wound infection has gone through several cycles of argument. Today's consensus holds that airborne organisms assume a significant role in causing wound infections only when (1) an air-handling system is grossly contaminated [5], (2) an otherwise effective air-handling system is abused, or possibly (3) in occasional instances of highly specialized procedures in which a large foreign body is implanted (the last point is still controversial). Additionally, an occasional infection in clean surgical wounds occurs in which the route of infection appears to have been the air, but which is unassociated with any of the above three factors. The infrequency of this occurrence probably is the result of the low numbers of airborne bacteria and the attention paid to the air in operating rooms.

It must be emphasized that no matter how clean the air may be in an operating room and no matter in what direction it is blown, the air system will not have any effect upon contact contamination from the patient himself or from the surgical team.

Abuse of the operating-room environment by personnel includes such practices as leaving a door open to the corridor during operative procedures; permitting unrestricted opening and closing of the operating-room doors as people come and go; not covering long hair, sideburns, or beards; and allowing technical, nursing, and anesthesia-administering personnel to circulate in and out of operating rooms while wearing short-sleeve shirts. No matter how particulate-free the air may be that is blown into a room, the particulate biologic matter that inevitably is circulated around the room is quantitatively in direct proportion to the number and movement of people in the room and the amount of exposed hair and skin. Shed particles tend to mount exponentially when excessive numbers of improperly covered visitors are present and when unnecessary activity of people occurs, including the flapping of drapes, towels, and gowns as well as any other maneuver that may unsettle previously shed particles from horizontal surfaces.

Current U.S. Public Health Service and National Fire Protection Association (NFPA) minimum requirements for operating-room air call for a minimum of 25 changes per hour, positive pressure compared with corridors, temperatures between 18°C and 24°C (65°F to 75°F), humidity of 50 to 55 percent, and, depending upon the locality, up to 80 percent recirculation with the use of effective filtering. In some states, 100 percent outside air with no recirculation is still required. Recently, engineers are suggesting an upgrading of these requirements for new hospitals in which high-risk surgery is to be performed. They are specifying that air be supplied into the operating room through ceiling panels (approximately 10 by 10 feet) directly over the operating table at 60 feet per minute face velocity. This high-flow system delivers 6000 cubic feet of air per minute and would result in one and a half air changes per minute (or 90 per hour) in a room 20 by 20 by 10 feet. When the air flow is this great, an important feature is adequate exhaust; this should be located on the walls above the baseboard in order to maintain some directionality and prevent great turbulence. If the inflow is reduced to 30 feet per minute face velocity, it will result in 45 air changes per hour, a figure considered highly satisfactory by many authorities.

Our own investigations, which were carried

out in collaboration with engineers and micro-biologists, have convinced us that corridor air in a surgical suite should be as clean as the air in the operating room. Indeed, we believe that the air in the entire surgical suite—including closets, storage areas, personnel areas, and re-covery-room areas—should be equally well-filtered and ventilated as the air in the operat-ing room.

Several questions remain unanswered with respect to laminar flow in the operating room. These questions relate largely to whether this method of diffusing air has any effect on infec-tion control, and, indeed, whether it is relevant at all to hospital use. The term "laminar" is being applied or misapplied to many types of unidirectional air-blowing systems, ranging from virtually any type of ceiling or wall dif-fuser to a variety of "curtain effect" air sys-tems. The use of the term, erroneous though it may be, appears to be here to stay. So-called laminar flow can be delivered in a horizontal or vertical direction. Although there are pro-ponents of each, neither method has been shown to be superior to the other; indeed, it has not been shown whether either is superior to nonlaminar flow. The British surgeon, Charn-ley, gave impetus to the promotion of laminar-flow chambers by claiming that his reduction of wound infections following hip replacement operations from 9 percent to 1 percent was due to the use of the chamber [3]. Charnley's crit-ics point out that this improvement in results over the six-year study period could well have been the result of several other changes in technique that he employed, including the use of a coverall surgical gown as well as changes in a number of technical maneuvers [9].

Most bacteria are in the 0.5 to 5.0 μ diame-ter range. Thus, if HEPA filtering is used, the first air downstream from the filter is virtually bacteria-free. HEPA-filtered air, however, is often confused with laminar air flow. One is a filtering capability; the other, a method of dif-fusion or distribution of air into a space in a more or less unidirectional manner. Thus, lam-inar flow may be imparted to air that is either filtered or unfiltered, and HEPA-filtered air can be delivered by any type or size of dif-fusing method, laminar or nonlaminar, high

speed or low speed. It must be remembered that HEPA filtering does nothing to filter par-ticles produced in the room; it merely produces almost particle-free first air as it leaves the diffuser.

Although ambient bacterial counts can be reduced by large-volume unidirectional air flow, no evidence has been presented to show that this alone has any effect on the incidence of surgical wound infections or whether uni-directional flow is or is not superior to a well-functioning, properly installed, conventional, nonlaminar system in this respect.

A number of American orthopedic surgeons who have performed thousands of hip replace-ment operations in conventional operating rooms without laminar-flow chambers report a combined two-year infection rate of 0.45 percent, a figure as low as or lower than that reported by surgeons with comparable num-bers of operations performed in laminar-flow chambers [9]. Moreover, the bacteria cultured from wound infections following hip replace-ment surgery have been shown to correlate poorly with those found in the air of the room or chamber. Air is only one of several possible sources of microorganisms; others include en-dogenous sources, person-to-person transmis-sion, and the inanimate environment (equip-ment and the like).

Use of Ultraviolet Light
The bactericidal effect of ultraviolet (UV) light is undeniable. Many European hospitals use UV in the empty operating room, either overnight or during protracted periods of non-use of the room. The use of UV is limited by the possibility of burns as well as by the fact that, because it is a ray, it can only strike ex-posed surfaces. In a large, rather well-con-trolled study, the use of UV was not shown to influence the overall incidence of wound infec-tion [1], although it did appear to have an ef-fect on the incidence of infection in clean pro-cedures.

Cleaning Methods
Every major surgical operation is now consid-ered to be "dirty," because evidence is avail-able to show that saprophytic organisms pre-

viously considered harmless may occasionally be responsible for severe sepsis. Also, viral hepatitis type B may be unsuspectedly carried in the blood of any surgical patient. Therefore, the current recommendation is for terminal sterilization of all instruments upon completion of an operation. If the instruments must leave the operating room in order to be terminally sterilized, they must be placed in containers as should all other used materials. Only after terminal sterilization are instruments to be handled and examined by personnel. These points speak in favor of an on-site instrument-processing operation in the surgical suite, instead of having it carried out in a distant central supply area.

There remains some difference of opinion on the virtues of ultrasonic cleaning over other methods, but many hospitals use commercially available ultrasonic devices, either as a separate operation or in combination with automatic washing of instruments.

The contaminated or "dirty" case is commonly considered as one in which frank pus was encountered during the operation. In a few hospitals, it is still the practice to clean the room thoroughly where such an operation was performed and keep it sealed for up to 48 hours before another operation is permitted in it. This practice is no longer considered necessary, provided the appropriate clean-up techniques are used and the air-handling system is adequate. Even with a minimum of 12 air changes per hour, the air in an operating room is exchanged every five minutes. Therefore, the usual clean-up period of 20 or 30 minutes should allow four to six complete air changes, provided the doors are kept closed. This should be adequate to dispose of any airborne bacteria that may have resulted from the contaminated case. The air systems of many modern operating rooms provide 25, 30, or more changes of air per hour, thus insuring faster clean-out of any residual airborne contamination.

The technique of cleaning a "contaminated" room consists of wet mopping or flooding with a good phenolic detergent, wiping down all metal furniture and plastic surfaces with a germicidal detergent or with 70% alcohol, and

changing all rubber or plastic tubing that may be in the room [10]. It is not considered necessary any longer to clean the walls any more than what is provided by the usual routine at the end of each day, unless, of course, direct contamination such as splashing has occurred. One of the common defects in cleaning methods is to scrub walls unnecessarily while neglecting to clean the anesthesia equipment. The instruments, linen, and waste should be placed separately and carefully in containers before they are taken from the room. All gowns, masks, and shoe covers used during the procedure and in the clean-up must be left in the room to be put in containers [7].

Scheduling of Operations

Scheduling practices also may have a bearing on infection hazard, especially in terms of the type of case scheduled to follow another. In some hospitals, it is the policy to schedule all "dirty" operations at the end of the day. In others, a septic room is set aside for such cases. Some surgeons believe the risk of wound infection in an otherwise "clean" case is greater if the operation is performed late in the day.

It is no longer deemed advisable to set aside a room for septic surgery. Current thinking considers every case to be potentially, if not actually, infected. Clean-up techniques have made such separate, low-usage facilities unnecessary. Nonetheless, on doctrinaire grounds, an open-heart operation would not be scheduled to follow the drainage of an abscess in the same room if it could be avoided. Many times, however, a "clean" emergency operation must of necessity be performed late in the day or following a septic case. Yet, with appropriate clean-up techniques, there is no evidence of increased risk of infection in such instances.

Operating-Room Personnel

Routine culture testing of specimens from the nasopharynx or other sites of personnel who work in operating rooms is no longer considered mandatory or necessary. In tracking down possible sources of infection, however, it is necessary to review not only the microbiologic contribution of such sources as the nasopharynx, hair [4], skin, and even occasionally the respiratory and gastrointestinal tracts of all concerned personnel, but also all applicable cleaning methods and routines as well. An additional factor is the personal integrity and work ethics of the personnel. All duties may be well performed while under surveillance but may be poorly done or even omitted when the employee is on his own. Clean-up methods should be checked for efficacy at regular intervals [7].

Personnel may be the source of organisms that cause disease when transmitted to patients. These personnel may be classified as carriers or disseminators (or shedders). A *carrier* is an infected person who harbors a specific infectious agent but shows no evidence of clinical disease. If this individual sheds these organisms, he or she is referred to as a *shedder* or *disseminator,* and if disease results in another individual, then the shedder may be referred to as a *dangerous disseminator* (see Part I, Chapter 2). Organisms can be disseminated on skin squamae, from the oral or nasal pharynx, in the blood, and in secretions or excretions.

Nasopharyngeal droplets expelled by talking, coughing, or yawning are usually entrapped in the mask, but a certain portion will manage to escape around the mask or through a damp or defective mask. Face masks should therefore cover the nose and mouth snugly. Permeation of moisture and bacteria through the mask will depend on the barrier qualities of the material of the mask. Moreover, face masks should not be allowed to hang under the chin when not in place, since they may be a disseminating source. A mask should also not be reused after being used once and then carried under the chin.

There are many different types of surgical masks that have been developed for use in the operating room. The literature on their evaluations is voluminous and difficult to summarize. The best universal recommendation is to use a high-efficiency, filter mask that is properly worn at all times while in the operating room.

Operating-Room Garb

The purpose of operating-room clothing is primarily to provide a barrier to contamination that may pass from personnel to the patient as well as from the patient to personnel. Traditional garb consists of gowns, caps, masks, and shoe covers, made either of woven launderable materials or of nonwoven disposable materials. Impermeability to moisture is an important property of any barrier material, because the wicking effect tends to transmit bacteria. Surgical gowns reinforced on the front and sleeves with a tightly woven material (Barbac) and treated with waterproofing have been shown to be impermeable at the areas of reinforcement through up to 100 launderings [2]. Drapes of this material are equally impermeable. Among the nonwoven materials, however, very few stand up to the stresses of stretch, pressure, and friction common to operating-room usage without becoming permeable to a moist contaminant. Equally disturbing is the fact that manufacturing standards for surgical gloves permit at least two holes per hundred gloves. Gloves are only spot-checked for holes, and therefore many more defective gloves are used than are realized by surgeons.

In an effort to prevent shedding at its source —that is, the skin of personnel—a variety of coverall hoods and gowns are available that are used in conjunction with a plastic mask or helmet and are designed to cover the entire head and body of the surgeon and his team members. These outfits are highly effective in virtually eliminating shedding. Because of the discomfort due to retained heat under such outfits, however, it is necessary to use vacuum to exhaust the space between wearer and uniform in order to keep the wearer comfortable. Such precautions may be more than what is required for everyday surgery, except for types of surgery in which the risk of contamination may be exceptionally great, as in the implantation of large devices (e.g., joint replacements).

Hoods rather than caps are now being recommended for all operating-room personnel. Since it is known that hair may acquire and might shed bacterial particles, it is recommended that all hair on the face and head be covered in the operating room.

The usual practice of wearing white shoes with dried secretions on the leather is condemned as unsanitary for a number of reasons, one of which is the tendency for flakes to come off with motion and enter the general ambience. Thus, shoe covers are recommended for use in the surgical suite. Disposable, easy to put on, and equipped with a conductive strip, nonwoven shoe covers should be put on fresh every time a person enters the surgical suite from the outside.

The search goes on for the ideal material for operating-room garb, both disposable and reusable. Materials sought are those that are impervious to bacteria and moisture; resistant to the stresses of stretch, pressure, and friction; relatively nonretentive of heat; flame retardant; low in static; and economical. None of the disposable materials now in use fulfills all these requirements.

The Scrub and Skin Preparation

The surgeon's hands and forearms, as well as those of his assistants and scrub nurse, must be washed prior to operation. Experience has shown that this "scrub" should take at least 10 minutes and should consist of constant friction, soaping, and repeated rinsings. Scrubbing much longer will often result in raising bacteria from deep dermal layers to the surface and lead to higher bacterial counts on the surface. Although scrubbings for shorter periods than 10 minutes have been shown to be virtually as effective, the full period is still advocated for scrubbing. The lubricating material may be soap or a detergent that contains either iodophor or hexachlorophene. In recent years, hexachlorophene has been shown to be absorbed under certain circumstances into the blood, fat cells, and brain cells. The Food and Drug Administration has therefore banned its routine use for newborn infants (see Part I, Chapter 7, The Newborn Nursery); however, it can still be used by surgeons and other hospital personnel for washing their hands. Soap and detergent dispensers have been shown to support the growth of gram-negative bacteria sometimes. Hence, the most expedient and safest scrub technique today consists of using a disposable brush or sponge impregnated with detergent that contains iodophor solution. For iodine-sensitive surgical personnel, 3% hexachlorophene or chlorhexidine may be used.

Scrub sinks are traditionally fitted with foot, knee, or elbow pedals to allow operation of the sink without using one's hands. New sinks are activated either with an electric eye or electrical field of flux for no-touch operation. They have additional features such as no-splash streams, controlled water temperature, and filtered water. If sprinklers or aerators are used, they should be periodically washed in a high-temperature washer or autoclaved.

The skin of the patient is prepared by shaving the operative site, if necessary, as short a time as possible before surgery. Just prior to surgery, the operative site should be scrubbed with soap and water or a detergent solution, dried with a sterile towel, and then painted with an iodophor or with tincture of chlorhexidine.

The skin preparation ritual is followed by appropriate draping to protect the clean field from the unprepared parts of the patient.

Record Keeping

Guidelines of the Joint Commission on Accreditation of Hospitals contain standards requiring the existence of an Infection Control Committee in all hospitals. In large hospitals, there may be a separate committee or subcommittee on surgical infections. The purpose of such committees is not only to define, monitor, and investigate all infections within its purview, but also to keep a careful record or log of such infections. Unfortunately, the methods used by hospitals in complying with these standards vary greatly. Surgeons do not always agree on the definition of a wound infection, for example. Some anesthetists are unwilling to ascribe postoperative fever accompanying pulmonary "congestion" to a respiratory tract infection acquired during anesthesia administration and therefore do not gather follow-up statistics. In many cases, the infection of a wound does not become evident until after the patient leaves the hospital and so is lost to the record. If the patient is readmitted with an established infection, the infection is rarely recorded as a complication, especially if the original operation was performed at another hospital. For these reasons and others, a standard method should be formulated and adopted by all hospitals. Amazingly, no such standard exists.

References

1. Ad Hoc Committee on Trauma, NAS-NRC. Post operative wound infections. *Ann. Surg.* 160(Suppl.):August, 1964.
2. Badner, B., Zelner, L., Merchant, R., and Laufman, H. Costs of linen *vs.* disposable OR packs. *Hospitals* 47:78, 1973.
3. Charnley, J., and Eftekhar, N. Postoperative infection in total prosthetic replacement arthroplasty of the hip joint. *Br. J. Surg.* 56:641, 1969.
4. Dineen, P., and Drusin, L. Epidemics of postoperative wound infections associated with hair carriers. *Lancet* 2:1157, 1973.
5. Gage, A. A., Dean, D. C., Schimert, G., and Minsky, N. *Aspergillus* infection after cardiac surgery. *Arch. Surg.* 101:384, 1970.
6. Laufman, H. What's wrong with our operating rooms? *Am. J. Surg.* 122:332, 1971.
7. Laufman, H. Cleanup techniques in the operating room. *Med. Surg. Rev.* pp. 1–4, October–November, 1971.
8. Laufman, H. Surgical hazard control: Effect of architecture and engineering. *Arch. Surg.* 107:552, 1973.
9. Laufman, H. Current status of special air handling systems in operating rooms. *Med. Instrum.* 7:7, 1973.
10. Mallison, G. F. Housekeeping in operating suites. *A.O.R.N. J.* 21:213, 1975.

Section I. The Admitting and Outpatient Departments
Kathryn S. Wenzel Owens

The admitting and outpatient facilities should be considered as part of the inpatient facilities of the hospital insofar as infection control activities are concerned. It may be necessary, however, to give some special consideration to certain aspects of an efficient and sensitive surveillance program and to establishing effective cleaning procedures in some areas of these two departments because of the rapidity and frequency of patient movement through such areas. A specific plan needs to be developed and implemented with the infection control nurse (ICN) and with other infection control personnel, because infection control is as important in these areas as it is within the inpatient facilities.

Admitting Department
The Facility

The admitting department should not be overlooked in the overall infection control program within the hospital. Although patients with infectious diseases may be properly managed on the nursing unit, planning for the patient's management should begin prior to the time of admission and be carried out in consultation with the admitting department. Because of lack of space and personnel, few hospitals are able to care for patients adequately for long periods of time in the admitting area. This then presents a potential problem as concerns patients with infectious diseases if beds are not immediately available for admission. Ideally, the admitting area should include facilities for these patients in case there is a delay in admitting procedures or if a bed is not available.

Admitting Procedures

Anxiety on the part of the patient and personnel can be averted with a definitive plan providing for the direct admission, bypassing the Admitting Department if necessary, of infected patients. The plan should be initiated by the physician at the time the request for admission is made. The physician should keep in mind the hospital policy for isolation or other special precautions and may want to speak to the ICN, the hospital epidemiologist, or both, as well as with the admitting personnel. The admitting department or physician should notify the ICN, who in turn can alert the nursing unit regarding the special needs for these patients. A good example of the confusion that can arise within the admitting department and on the nursing units is provided by a community outbreak of disease such as influenza. Without a priority or plan developed by the Infection Control Committee to cover such a situation, the patients, families, and personnel may be unduly upset by additional bed transfers and inconsistent practices.

Patients

Patient transfers, being usually arranged through the admitting department, represent another area of attention for infection control. The ICN, the head nurse, or clinical coordinator must communicate the special needs of patients with an infectious disease to admitting personnel as well as to personnel on the transfer unit.

Patients who return to the hospital with a nosocomial infection that requires their having a private room should not necessarily be financially penalized for the entire cost of the private room. There should be a mechanism by which an adjustment to this cost can be considered if it is indicated according to hospital policy or recommended by the Infection Control Committee or its designate.

Personnel

Admitting-department personnel should be included in orientation sessions for new personnel regarding infection control. These introductory classes should include a discussion of the primary goal of the infection control program (i.e., that of preventing nosocomial infection) as well as a review of departmental infection control policies regarding patients and personnel. In-service classes should be conducted periodically on pertinent topics or changes in infection control policies.

The admitting department should be represented on the Infection Control Committee or a subcommittee thereof to keep abreast of changes in infection control policies and to provide necessary input from the admitting department.

The continuity of patient care is enhanced by efficient and informed patient management, which begins within the admitting department.

Outpatient Departments

The outpatient departments (including all clinics, the emergency room, and outpatient surgery) are not often considered within the framework of acute care, but they represent essential patient services and should be within the purview of the Infection Control Committee. Because patients with infections are seen in clinics, outpatient operating rooms, and emergency rooms, many of the inpatient infection control policies should also be applied in these departments.

The Facility

Outpatient departments should be designed to accommodate patients with infections. Appropriate facilities should be available for such procedures as the incision and drainage of abscesses or the examination of patients with infectious disease. Isolation procedures should be in accord with the hospital policy. Busy, overcrowded clinics may occasionally overlook the potential for spread of infectious disease in waiting areas. Clinics should have designated rooms available for these patients prior to their arrival to prevent exposure of susceptible patients. Adequate ventilation should be provided in waiting areas as well as in examining and treatment rooms and operating rooms.

Surveillance

The ICN should appropriate his or her time to include patient surveillance in these areas. The ICN, who is responsible for identifying nosocomial infections, should have frequent contact with the head nurses of these departments as well as with the microbiology laboratories to insure accurate reporting of the infections that occur after discharge from the hospital. The laboratory reports of outpatient culture determinations may provide a starting point for the follow-up of nosocomial infections. Personnel records as well as medical records may provide additional information needed to determine the presence or absence of nosocomial infection. Attenting physicians may need to be contacted as well. These infections should be included in the regularly prepared summary reports of nosocomial infections for the hospital and should be available to personnel in each area.

Community Outbreaks

The ICN may detect, if communication is encouraged, community outbreaks through the outpatient departments. In this setting, if a reportable disease is involved, reports should be made to the local health officer by use of the morbidity form or by telephone. Physicians, who should be consulted prior to reporting, are usually grateful for this assistance.

Personnel

Personnel practices may influence infection rates in the outpatient departments as well as inpatient services. Personnel in these areas should be included in the initial orientation to the infection control program as well as in frequent in-service programs in matters related to the prevention, surveillance, and control of infection in this patient population.

Personnel health practices should be in accord with the hospital policies, including those regarding employment physicals; tuberculin tests, chest roentgenograms, or both; and various immunizations. Consideration should be given to policies involving inadvertent exposure of pregnant personnel to cytomegalovirus infection or rubella, and personnel should be included in tuberculin follow-up studies after exposure to open pulmonary tuberculosis (see Part I, Chapter 3).

The Environment

A review of the sanitation of the environment should be regularly scheduled, as throughout the rest of the hospital, in order to identify actual or potential problem areas. Environmental cleaning procedures should be similar to those established for the inpatient services, except a special routine may be necessary for some outpatient areas because of the frequency of use by patients. Aseptic procedures and methods of cleaning, disinfection, and sterilization should be periodically reviewed to insure optimum practices. Particular attention should be devoted in busy clinic areas to processing of cystoscopes, sigmoidoscopes, and tonometers, and sterilization procedures, rather than disinfection, should be used (see Part I, Chapter 6). Sterilizers should be monitored on a weekly basis by utilizing spore test strips. The nursing procedure committee should include a representative from the outpatient departments, because aseptic practices are as vital in the outpatient setting as they are for the inpatient population. The ICN can provide assistance to the outpatient departments through teaching, consultation, and patient and environmental surveillance.

A successful nosocomial infection control program must include the outpatient departments for comprehensive surveillance, control, and prevention of infection.

Section J. The Clinical Laboratory

Marie B. Coyle and John C. Sherris

The clinical laboratory is an area of special concern, both because it is a focus for the handling and processing of potentially hazardous materials from infectious patients and because it generates a considerable volume of pathogenic organisms in its microbiologic work. The risks are greatest for the laboratory personnel, but visitors to the laboratory area may also be exposed to infectious organisms. Poor design and operation can allow accidentally generated aerosols to extend beyond the confines of the laboratory and, at least potentially, be a hazard to other areas of the institution.

This section will consider the nature and extent of these problems and practical means of controlling them. In particular, we will discuss infection control in the clinical microbiology laboratory and the more general problem of the control of hepatitis B infections in all areas of clinical laboratory work. We will not deal with the special problems associated with diagnostic virology laboratories or the large-scale handling of pathogenic microorganisms in research or manufacturing facilities.

Extent of the Laboratory-Acquired Infection Problem

The incidence of clinical laboratory-acquired infections is unknown, because many are unrecognized and most are probably never recorded. The literature contains numerous reports of individual infections and occasionally small groups of infections, and certain organisms can be recognized as being especially liable to produce severe or fatal disease in laboratory workers or as having unusual infectivity. Sulkin and Pike [12,15] tabulated valuable information on laboratory-acquired infections. Their early data [15] were based on a questionnaire covering the period 1930 to 1950, while more recent information was gained either from reports in the literature or from personal communications. They compiled data on about 3900 cases of overt laboratory infections with an overall case fatality rate of 4.1 percent. Many of these infections, however,

Table 7-4. Sources of 3921 Laboratory Infections

Known accident	Number of infections	Percentage of total[a]
Cut, bite, or scratch	207	6.6
Spill or spatter	188	6.0
Syringe and needle	177	5.6
Pipetting	92	2.9
All other	39	1.2
Subtotal	703	22.3
No known accident, most likely source		
Working with agent	827	26.2
Animal, egg, or arthropod	659	20.9
Aerosol	522	16.6
Clinical specimen	287	9.1
Human autopsy	75	2.4
Discarded glassware	46	1.5
Other	35	1.1
Subtotal	2451	77.8
Total[a]	3154	100.1

[a] Excluding 767 infections with unknown accident status and source.

From Pike, R. M. [12].

occurred in research departments, not in clinical laboratories.

The overall pattern that emerges from these reports and other published literature is that infections sufficiently severe to be recognized or reported usually involve a small group of infectious organisms. These include *Mycobacterium tuberculosis*, *Brucella* species, *Francisella tularensis*, *Coxiella burnetii*, various other *Rickettsia*, *Coccidioides immitis*, *Salmonella* species causing enteric fever, *Shigella*, and hepatitis B virus. These have the common characteristic of being able to initiate infections in the susceptible subject with a relatively small challenge dose. The potential for infection exists, however, with all pathogenic species, and it may be realized following a laboratory accident involving the introduction of an unusually large number of organisms.

Sources and Routes of Spread

Pike's review showed that only about 20 percent of laboratory-acquired infections were preceded by a known accident (Table 7-4). Self-inoculation with a needle and syringe and aspiration while pipetting by mouth accounted for over one-third of the known accidents but only about 9 percent of all laboratory-associated infections.

The identities of the agents most commonly involved in these laboratory infections suggest that the inhalation of aerosols produced during routine laboratory manipulations and the ingestion of pathogenic microorganisms were the commonest means by which they were acquired. Only 17 percent of all the respondents, however, associated their infections with a specific, aerosol-generating procedure (Table 7-4). The manipulation of liquids always results in some aerosol production, but the amount is highly dependent on the particular procedure used as well as on the adequacy of the technique of the individual worker. Table 7-5 contains some data of Reitman and Wedum [13,17] comparing aerosol production during some commonly used bacteriologic procedures. Considerable dissemination may occur, and most of the droplets produced are between 2 and 5 μ in diameter [10]. Particles of

Table 7-5. Bacteria Recovered by Air-Sampling Within Two Feet of the Site of Common Bacteriologic Procedures

Procedure	Colonies obtained per operation
Removing tight cover of standard blender immediately after mixing cultures	Too numerous to count
Opening lyophilized culture tube	86
Decanting centrifuged fluid into flask	17
Inserting hot loop in culture flask	9
Removing dry cotton plug from shaken culture flask	5
Pipetting 1 ml. of inoculum to poured agar in Petri plate	3
Pipetting 1 ml. of culture into 50 ml. of broth	1

Adapted from Wedum, A. G., Laboratory safety in research with infectious aerosols. *Public Health Rep.* 76:619, 1964; and Reitman, M., and Wedum, A. G., Microbiologic safety, *Public Health Rep.* 71:659, 1956.

this size are capable of bypassing the defenses of the upper respiratory tract, and they can be drawn into the alveoli [2] where fewer organisms may be required to establish an infection [6].

These data emphasize the need for special safety procedures when dealing with agents known to be highly infective. Whenever it becomes apparent from a suspected clinical diagnosis or from the laboratory workup of a specimen that such an agent may be present, additional safety precautions appropriate for the suspected agent should be employed. Operational requirements for safe handling of specific microbiologic agents have been published by the Center for Disease Control (CDC) [4,5].

General Control Measures

Education and Training

There is little doubt that the most important factors in preventing laboratory-acquired infections are the knowledge, training, and techniques of the individual laboratory worker. The other methods and procedures discussed in this section are adjunctive and may be rendered ineffective by carelessness and lack of understanding of the hazards and routes of infection.

It is critical, as in hospital infection control generally, that examples of good technique and safe practices be provided by those in supervisory positions and that the operating regulations be rigidly enforced. A laboratory director who smokes, eats, or drinks in the laboratory or who fails to wash and change coats before leaving the laboratory area encourages an environment in which accidents are more prone to occur. Training must be supplemented with a written manual that details the routine and emergency procedures to be employed as well as with continuing programs of safety education and monitoring of the effectiveness of equipment designed to contain infection.

Laboratory Design

From the point of view of microbiologic safety, the microbiology laboratory would ideally be a self-contained unit isolated from the rest of the hospital environment. This is essentially impractical if important consultative interactions between the laboratory and the clinical staff are to be maintained. Within the laboratory, however, work areas can be set up to minimize the risk of spread of infectious particles. Some form of partitioning of such work spaces has two advantages: it prevents traffic patterns passing behind the technologist and creating unnecessary air currents, and it also helps to contain any aerosols that may be produced by accidents. Certain spaces should be set aside for particularly hazardous operations, such as handling *Mycobacterium tuberculosis* and funguses. These should be self-contained, provided with sterilizing equipment and hand-washing facilities, and equipped with the appropriate safety hoods to prevent dispersion of organisms into the general laboratory environment.

The general plan for the laboratory should include provisions for an adequate number and placement of autoclaves, adequate disposal containers, and an adequate number and placement of sinks. Surfaces should be nonporous, without cracks, and easy to clean.

The overall ventilation system of the laboratory should be capable of diluting aerosols and insuring a flow of air from "clean" to "dirty" zones. [5]. The ventilation system for laboratories should be completely separate from that of the rest of the hospital, and air should be vented at least 25 feet from any windows, doors, or air intakes.

Laboratories should be designed to prevent overcrowding and to avoid needless personnel movement, which may in itself contribute to accidents.

Specific regulations and recommendations governing procedures for particular classes of pathogenic agents [4] have been and are being developed at both national and state levels. It is essential that laboratory directors become acquainted through their state health departments with the current requirements.

Specialized Equipment

Safety working hoods should be available for handling especially hazardous specimens and cultures, such as those involved in the diagnosis of tuberculosis or cultures of certain systemic fungi. Various safety cabinets are available, and the best are those that depend on high-efficiency particulate aerosol (HEPA) filters. The entrances for one's hands into the working space should be kept at a minimum and yet be sufficiently large to permit easy manipulation, and there should be an air flow rate of 50 to 75 linear feet per minute through this area [3]. The exhaust from the hood should be vented through the HEPA filter to the outside.

The efficiency of safety hoods depends on proper construction to eliminate all leakage around seams, gaskets, fans, filters, and other component parts. Hoods should be monitored after installation as well as after each filter change and at yearly intervals to insure that they are operating effectively and that there is no discharge of potentially contaminated material into the laboratory environment. Routine quality control procedures are also needed for ultraviolet lamps in safety cabinets. These cannot be considered germicidal just because they are emitting blue light; they must be routinely cleansed to avoid any grease that may be deposited and checked for germicidal efficiency. The CDC has published a brochure on maintaining both biologic safety cabinets and ultraviolet lamps [3].

Other laboratory equipment also needs regular inspection and monitoring to avoid accidents. Routine records should be maintained of discharge valve temperatures, pressures, and times of sterilization of autoclaves. They may be tested on a weekly basis for the capacity to kill spores during a routine cycle by using commercially available products. Autoclave tape serves to insure that items have gone through an autoclave cycle, but it is not designed to indicate sterility. Deep freezes should be organized into well-labeled compartments that permit easy identification of the vials of infected materials or cultures that are being sought. This permits shorter search periods and less chance of breakage. Gloves and a surgical mask should be worn while cleaning freezers that may contain vials of infectious material and also when changing filters of safety cabinets that may have taken up infected material.

Routine Prophylaxis
Specific immunization of laboratory personnel will reduce the risk of infection with some of the pathogenic organisms that may be encountered (see Part I, Chapter 3). All personnel working in clinical microbiology laboratories should have up-to-date tetanus and diphtheria immunization, and immunization for any other infectious disease for which adult immunization in the community is recommended. All individuals who handle specimens should receive a skin test with purified protein derivative (PPD) of tuberculin every six months if their initial test is negative. If the previous skin test was positive, a yearly chest roentgenogram is recommended. If reactivity is primarily to PPD-S, skin test converters should be medically evaluated for currently recommended prophylaxis (see Part II, Chapter 15).

Immunization against typhoid should be required if the disease is endemic in the area, although careful attention to simple laboratory techniques should avoid the risk of contracting this infection.

Specific Technical Routines
Standard Precautions
Certain routines and procedures are mandatory to reduce the risk of laboratory-acquired infection. These are stated below as a number of specfic guidelines. Other lists have been prepared by other authors [6,15,17]. Laboratories engaged in mycobacteriology should follow the guidelines specified by CDC [16].

1. Personnel hygiene in the laboratory:
   A. No eating, drinking, or smoking should be allowed.
   B. Hands should be washed before one leaves the laboratory.
   C. Laboratory coats should be removed before leaving the laboratory area.
   D. No food may be stored in refrigerators that contain specimens or serum products.
2. Routine culture procedures:
   A. Pipetting by mouth—this includes *all* solutions—is to be prohibited.
   B. While pipetting, bubble production is to be avoided.
   C. A cool inoculating loop should be used.
   D. Cylindrical burners should be used when culturing tuberculosis specimens.

E. Petri dishes should be inoculated without striking their walls.

F. Before flaming loops with excess material, they should be precleaned in a container of alcohol and sand.

G. When removing rubber stoppers from vacutainers, the tops should be covered with an alcohol-moistened towel.

3. Hazardous procedures that should be carried out in a biologic safety cabinet:

A. Opening lyophilized cultures (a safe and simple procedure has recently been reported that greatly reduces the risk of dispersal [8]),

B. Homogenizing with a mortar and pestle or a high-speed blender, and

C. Decanting supernatants.

4. Centrifugation: Operate centrifuge in a well-ventilated room that can be closed off in case of an accident (see 7.B below). Careful balancing is critical. Sturdy plastic screw-top tubes are recommended.

5. Syringes and needles:

A. Only needle-locking syringes may be used.

B. An alcohol swab should be placed around the stopper and needle when withdrawing the needle from a rubber-stoppered vial.

C. Excess air and bubbles should be expelled into an alcohol swab.

D. Animals are to be swabbed with antiseptic both before and after inoculation.

E. Used needles should be immediately placed in a narrow-mouthed metal or glass container for disposal.

6. Discarding contaminated materials:

A. All contaminated slides and pipettes are to be placed in a jar of disinfectant until they are autoclaved.

B. All specimens—including urine and those for immunoserology—are to be autoclaved before they are discarded.

C. All contaminated materials are autoclaved (heat-resistant plastic bags eliminate the mess from melted plastic laboratory ware).

D. Stools should be collected in a separate, lined container and incinerated.

7. Spills and accidents:

A. A wash bottle of disinfectant should be kept at hand to carry out emergency decontamination in the event of a spill. Phenolics are most useful in clinical laboratories that do not culture for viruses, while hypochlorites are recommended for discard jars where contamination by viruses is expected. (Some recent references on disinfectants have been listed [9,14].)

B. Accidents involving the potential of major aerosol generation, such as breakage in a centrifuge, should receive special handling. The room should be evacuated and closed off for at least an hour or until eight to ten air changes have occurred and the larger droplets have settled out. Decontamination should be done by senior personnel, and they should be protected by mask and gloves.

8. Shipping specimens to reference laboratories: Postal regulations should be observed. (They have been included in Bodily's recommendations [1]).

Hepatitis B Precautions

Hepatitis has long been recognized as a special hazard for laboratory workers, particularly those working with blood or serum samples (see Part I, Chapter 3 and Part II, Chapter 24). Thus, the risk has been greatest for those working in hematology, biochemistry, and serology laboratories. Several recent episodes of hepatitis B infection involving a number of laboratory workers have been recorded. One outbreak in a university hospital involved 74 cases of viral hepatitis, including one fatality within a four-year period [18]. Almost half the cases were associated with the clinical laboratories, but no cases occurred among laboratory personnel who did not routinely handle blood specimens.

Hepatitis B virus (HBV) can be acquired by the alimentary or conjunctival routes as well as by the respiratory route and transdermal inoculation through cuts and needle punctures. The infectivity of specimens can be very high. There should be special identification and flagging of all blood and urine samples from patients with hepatitis, patients who are known to be hepatitis B antigen-positive, or patients from high-risk groups such as drug addicts, recipients of multiple transfusions, and those who have recently received transplants and are on immunosuppressive therapy. Specimens from such patients should be double-bagged on collection and handled with special care within the laboratory. The risk, however, is not restricted to these specimens, because any serum sample may be infected and pose a hazard. Thus, laboratory personnel should not develop a false sense of security in handling unflagged specimens. Even control sera employed in clinical chemistry laboratories frequently contain hepatitis B antigen [18]. Some measures that may reduce the risk of infection are listed below:

1. Personnel working with blood or serum should wear specially colored gowns that may not be worn outside the laboratory area.
2. The contamination of hands with blood should be avoided, as should all mouth pipetting. When contamination is unavoidable or when specimens of known hazard are being processed, plastic gloves should be worn.
3. Rubber stoppers should be removed by gentle twisting to avoid aerosol production.
4. All sera should be transferred by bulb suctioning.
5. All spills should be immediately cleaned up with a 1% solution of hypochlorite (1 : 5 solution of Chlorox).
6. All discarded blood samples, clots, and sera and the glassware or other equipment used in processing them should be autoclaved. Disposable glass or plastic pipettes and tubes should be used whenever possible. These may be incinerated rather than autoclaved if preferred.
7. Stringent regulations should be enforced to insure that hands are washed and that outer clothing is changed before one leaves the laboratory area. Eating, drinking, or smoking in the laboratory should be totally prohibited.

8. Accident documentation:
   A. Any employee who sustains a cut or needle-puncture wound or who swallows any blood or blood product should report it to the supervisor immediately.
   B. A baseline blood sample for hepatitis B antigen testing should be drawn.
   C. Information should be obtained concerning the person from whom the blood products were obtained.
   D. At this writing, hepatitis B immune globulin is recommended for post-exposure prophylaxis of individuals sustaining an accidental needle stick or mucosal exposure to blood known to contain HB_sAg. If this product is not readily available, local public health authorities should be consulted for the current recommendation regarding standard immunoglobulin prophylaxis [11].

Accident and Illness Reporting

Medical records of infectious diseases—including hepatitis—should be maintained for all personnel. It is a wise precaution to file a sample of serum from each laboratory worker annually. In the event of subsequent illness, a rising titer may be rapidly detected, which will facilitate diagnosis and recognition of the source of the infection.

It is the responsibility of the hospital to provide sufficient funds and to appoint competent supervisory staff in order to insure the safe operation of clinical microbiology laboratories. Laboratory supervisors should maintain a high index of suspicion of possible job-related infections when employees become ill and, when indicated, assure that appropriate steps are taken to evaluate this possibility. Infections that are job-related should not result in financial penalty to the employee.

There should be a policy of reporting all accidents to the employee health clinic regardless of how minor they might seem to be. This is beneficial because (1) it permits appropriate prophylaxis, (2) a review of reports can lead to the recognition of special hazards and the introduction of safer techniques and equipment, and (3) reports provide the data for an accurate assessment of the hazards of various pathogens and attack rates. Also, forms are being developed by the CDC that will be available through state laboratories for the reporting of infections resulting from laboratory work.

Summary and Conclusions

Laboratory infections pose a particular risk to the staff of the clinical microbiology laboratories and to those handling discarded materials, whereas hepatitis B antigen poses a serious hazard to all laboratories handling blood specimens. The frequency of laboratory infections in clinical laboratories is unknown, and prospective studies to compare sickness rates with matched groups in less potentially hazardous occupations would be desirable.

Good training, ongoing educational programs, and scrupulous technique are the main factors protecting against laboratory infection. Special attention to laboratory design can reduce the risk, as can the use of adequate safety hoods. Routine immunization and tuberculin testing is mandatory, and health and accident records must be maintained. Significant accidental exposure to pathogens should be considered a medical emergency and a basis for consideration of prophylactic chemotherapy or immunotherapy.

Stringent procedures, little used up until this time, are needed in biochemistry and hematology laboratories to lessen the risk of hepatitis B infections, which have increased substantially with the expansion of renal dialysis, immunosuppressive therapy, and drug abuse.

References

1. Bodily, H. L. General Administration of the Laboratory. In Bodily, H. L. (Ed.), *Diagnostic Procedures for Bacterial, Mycotic and Parasitic Infections* (5th ed.). New York: American Public Health Association, 1970.
2. Brown, J. H., Cook, K. M., Ney, F. G., and Hatch, T. Influence of particle size upon retention of particulate matter in the human lung. *Am. J. Public Health* 40:450, 1950.
3. Center for Disease Control. *Biological Safety Cabinet.* Atlanta: Center for Disease Control, 1971.
4. Center for Disease Control. *Classification of Etiologic Agents on the Basis of Hazard.* Atlanta: Center for Disease Control, 1972.
5. Center for Disease Control. *Laboratory Safety at the Center for Disease Control.* Washington, D.C.: U.S. Government Printing Office, DHEW Publ. No. (HSM) 72-8118, 1972.
6. Darlow, H. M. Safety in the Microbiological Laboratory. In Norris, J. R., and Ribbons, D. W. (Eds.), *Methods in Microbiology,* Vol. 1. New York: Academic Press, 1969.
7. Darlow, H. M. Safety in the Microbiological Laboratory: An Introduction. In Shapton, D. A., and Board, R. G. (Eds.), *Safety in Microbiology: The Society for Applied Bacteriology, Technical Series No. 6.* New York: Academic Press, 1972.
8. Grief, D. Safe procedure for opening evacuated glass ampoules containing dried pathogens. *Appl. Microbiol.* 18:130, 1969.
9. Hugo, W. B. *Inhibition and Destruction of the Microbial Cell.* New York: Academic Press, 1971.
10. Kenny, M. T., and Sabel, F. L. Particle size distribution of *Serratia marcescens* aerosols created during common laboratory procedures and simulated laboratory accidents. *Appl. Microbiol.* 16:1146, 1968.
11. Maynard, J. E. Passive immunization against hepatitis B: A review of recent studies and comment on current aspects of control. *Am. J. Epidem.* 107:77, 1978.
12. Pike, R. M. Laboratory-associated infections: Summary and analysis of 3921 cases. *Health Lab. Sci.* 13:105, 1976.
13. Reitman, M., and Wedum, A. G. Microbiological safety. *Public Health Rep.* 71:659, 1956.
14. Spaulding, E. H. Chemical disinfection and antisepsis in the hospital. *J. Hosp. Res.* 9:7, 1972.
15. Sulkin, S. E., Long, E. R., Pike, R. M., Sigel, M. M., Smith, C. E., and Wedum, A. G. Laboratory Infections and Accidents. In Harris, A. H., and Coleman, M. B. (Eds.), *Diagnostic Procedures and Reagents* (4th ed.). New York: American Public Health Association, 1963.
16. Vestal, A. L. *Procedures for the Isolation and Identification of Mycobacteria.* Atlanta: Center for Disease Control, 1969.
17. Wedum, A. G. Laboratory safety in research with infectious aerosols. *Public Health Rep.* 76:619, 1964.
18. Wetli, C. V., Heal, A. V., and Miale, J. B. A previously unrecognized laboratory hazard: Hepatitis B antigen-positive control and diagnostic sera. *Am. J. Clin. Pathol.* 59:684, 1973.
19. Williams, S. V., Huff, J. C., Feinglass, E. J., Gregg, M. B., Hatch, M. H., and Matsen, J. M. Epidemic viral hepatitis type B in hospital personnel. *Am. J. Med.* 57:904, 1974.

8

The Microbiology Laboratory: Its Role in Surveillance, Investigation, and Control

Raymond C. Bartlett, John V. Bennett, Robert A. Weinstein, and George F. Mallison

Although hospital laboratory capacities are often strained by the large number of routine specimens to be processed, each hospital laboratory is also responsible for the special support activities related to the prevention, surveillance, and control of nosocomial infections. Each hospital microbiology laboratory can and should make major contributions toward infection control.

Surveillance and Control

Endemic Infections

Laboratory records are an important tool for the surveillance of infections. More than 80 percent of infections subsequently judged to be nosocomial may be discovered by culture determinations in those hospitals with active infection surveillance and control programs [57]. Thus, the data gathered by infection control personnel during laboratory rounds together with the data gathered from clinical rounds form an important base for the calculation of infection rates for various pathogens according to the site of infection and the hospital service (see Part I, Chapter 4).

Detection of Outbreaks

Laboratory records may provide early warning of the emergence within a hospital of highly infectious pathogens, multiple-drug-resistant organisms, and clusters of unusual infections. In hospitals where formal programs of surveillance have not yet been established, laboratory workers may therefore be the only personnel in a position to detect trends of infection.

Routine Environmental Sampling

The microbiology laboratory is often called upon to provide expertise in the microbiologic sampling of the hospital environment: this includes knowing not only which sampling and isolation techniques are best for each specific situation, but also which circumstances are appropriate for conducting sampling. In general, the surveillance of patient disease and the improvement of patient-care policies should be the primary focuses of infection control programs, and microbiology and infection control personnel should be firm in not conducting indiscriminate, routine, microbiologic sampling and testing (see Part I, Chapter 6). Routine checks on the adequacy of sterilizer function and the microbiologic quality of infant formula prepared in the hospital as well as periodic checks on the effectiveness of disinfection of the equipment that directly contacts tissues other than skin may, however, help prevent infections from these sources.

Surveys During Outbreaks

During nosocomial epidemics, laboratory personnel may conduct culture surveys of patients, hospital personnel, and the environment. Large numbers of cultures may have to be obtained, processed, and evaluated over a short period of time. Special typing procedures may need to be performed in the laboratory, or arrangements may be made for submitting samples to reference laboratories for this purpose. Data gathered by microbiology personnel in such surveys may be crucial in identifying the reservoir and mode of spread of the epidemic organisms.

Administrative Aspects

Relationship to Infection Control Committee

The adequacy of the basic techniques for primary isolation, speciation, and antimicrobial susceptibility testing should be discussed and agreed upon jointly by the microbiologist and the Infection Control Committee. The diagnostic microbiology laboratory is primarily engaged in the evaluation of isolates that are directly related to infection. The use of its resources to assess colonization states or to sample personnel and the environment for bacteria should never be permitted when the epidemiologic indications are unclear. Such activities should be closely coordinated with the Infection Control Committee.

A clinically oriented member of the laboratory staff can contribute significantly by serving on the Infection Control Committee. This member of the committee is essential in contributing to a harmonious relationship among clinical, infection control, and microbiology personnel.

Budgetary Considerations

Salaries for nurse epidemiologists or other personnel assigned to infection control as well as the costs of the bacteriologic sampling of personnel and the environment should be borne by a budget separate from that of the laboratory. To facilitate all the microbiologic activities that are necessitated by an outbreak, the laboratory (or Infection Control Committee) should have a contingency fund to enable personnel, materials, and space to be temporarily assigned to epidemic aid support. An investigation of an outbreak should not be financed by charging the patients cultured during the study.

Reporting of Results

Although time may allow progressive academic refinement of the microbiologic report, increased reporting time bears an inverse relation to the value of the report for patient care. This problem could be minimized if observations were reported at each progressive step of development. Unfortunately, most laboratories are limited to one preliminary report.

Limited space on laboratory report forms often results in handwritten phrasing that may be illegible and misinterpreted. Development of automatic or semiautomatic data systems is contributing to the solution of such problems, but most laboratories will be dependent upon handwritten forms and manual sorting and filing for several years. A comprehensive discussion of the problems associated with the reporting of information from clinical microbiology laboratories appears elsewhere and will not be repeated; here, attention will be drawn specifically to those aspects that relate to infection control [6].

To facilitate the surveillance of nosocomial infections and of all infections requiring isolation or notification of public health authorities, a copy of positive culture results should be sent to the infection control nurse. Physicians and nurses are typically lax about notifying public health authorities of reportable diseases. Isolation of such organisms will be reported to health authorities more efficiently if these responsibilities are delegated to the infection control nurse or some other individual designated by the Infection Control Committee.

Prompt reporting by telephone to both clinicians and infection control personnel of presumptively identified isolates that are of nosocomial significance is essential to insure proper treatment of the patient and the application of proper control measures. Such reporting should be used when presumptive identification is made of the causative agents of meningitis as well as of salmonellae or shigellae from stool specimens. Positive smears and cultures of tuberculosis bacilli from any patient or employee as well as the isolation of *Staphylococcus aureus* from any culture taken of an employee or of lesions of a newborn should also be reported promptly to the epidemiologist.

Laboratory Records
Laboratory records should be retained at least three years to facilitate retrospective epidemiologic investigations and quality-control activities. Culture data on inpatients and outpatients should be maintained separately. The source of each specimen; the date of collection; the patient's full name, hospital number, hospital service, and ward; and the organism(s) identified in the final isolate should be recorded. Records should also be kept of the results of antimicrobial sensitivity tests and of any special biochemical or typing reactions.

All cultures should be recorded so that results are readily available by date, by type of specimen, and by pathogen(s) isolated. Simple, inexpensive, and epidemiologically useful records that include these results are provided best by bound log books, which are kept chronologically for each major type of specimen (i.e., blood, wound and skin, cerebrospinal fluid, urine, stool, sputum and respiratory, and others). Sole reliance on a filing system of loose lab slips is not desirable because specific data are difficult to retrieve and are easily lost. If available, computer storage of all results is advantageous; noncomputerized rapid retrieval and sorting systems may also be useful [56].

The permanent records of the microbiologic laboratory should include dates and other details of any major changes in culturing techniques or laboratory procedures. Dates of changes in the criteria and for identification and taxonomic designations applied to isolates should be recorded so that the memory of the staff is not the only method for interpreting past data on the isolation and identification of microorganisms.

Identification and Typing of Clinical Isolates
Selection of Specimens for Processing
COLLECTION AND TRANSPORT PROBLEMS. Specimens that are not collected or transported properly may give inaccurate results, even in the best clinical laboratories. In turn, inaccurate results may lead to improper clinical decisions by physicians, unnecessary labor by laboratory personnel, excessive patient charges, and misleading epidemiologic data. Certain laboratory findings suggest specific handling errors; for example, a frequent failure to isolate organisms from the deep abscesses of patients who are not on antibiotics or pathogens that are seen on Gram stain in cases of presumed anaerobic infections suggests the use of aerobic transport vials, delay or inappropriate refrigeration of specimens in transit, or use of inadequate isolation techniques for isolating anaerobes. The frequent recovery of two or more different organisms or of 10^3 to 10^4 organisms per milliliter in clean-voided urine specimens strongly suggests unsatisfactory technique in collecting specimens, a delay in transporting specimens to the laboratory, or a delay in culturing the specimens. The finding of negative acid-fast cultures from a high percentage of specimens with positive acid-fast smears suggests unsatisfactory sputum collection and handling, errors in staining, or errors in culture techniques [74].

Specimen collection and handling should be regularly assessed to detect and correct such problems. An ongoing analysis of the frequency with which probable contaminants are isolated from clinical specimens provides an indirect measure of the quality of specimen collection on the ward. Wards with high frequencies of polymicrobial urine specimens can be singled out for evaluation and, if necessary, have intensive in-service education instituted by laboratory or infection control personnel. In addition, personnel who draw blood cultures that frequently contain diphtheroids, coagulase-negative staphylococci, or other probable skin contaminants should be reinstructed in aseptic technique. Periodic review of the relative incidence of false-positive, acid-fast smears may highlight problems in sputum collection and processing.

Some hospitals use laboratory slips with space to record both the time the specimen was collected and the time the laboratory received it, so transport time can be continuously monitored and the culturing of old specimens avoided.

MICROSCOPIC EVALUATION OF SPECIMENS. Microscopic review of certain types of specimens may help to avoid the culturing of inadequately collected material. Criteria used at Hartford Hospital for several years [6] have classified sputum specimens containing more than 25 squamous cells and less than 10 neutrophils per low-power (×100) field as primarily oropharyngeal material. Such specimens are not cultured and requests for recollection are issued. Also, a prospective study at the Mayo Clinic, showed that sputum specimens with more than ten squamous epithelial cells per low-power (×100) Gram-stained field were usually contaminated with oropharyngeal secretions; therefore, all such specimens at that institution are rejected for bacteriologic culture, and the staff member who submitted the specimen is notified [49]. This system has been analyzed and modified slightly [69]. Scoring systems for use in determining acceptable sputum, wound, vaginal, cervical, and other specimens have also been described [2,4]. Application of these discriminating criteria will not only reduce unnecessary costs but will also produce information on isolates for which the probability of association with infection is high. A repeated collection should be requested or limited speciation and antimicrobial susceptibility testing performed on bacteria isolated from specimens that show evidence of superficial contamination. A qualifying statement should be inserted on the report to alert the clinician to the questionable value of the specimen for guidance in diagnosis and treatment. These efforts will substantially reduce errors in diagnosis and the unnecessary antimicrobial therapy that might otherwise occur. Such an approach will also improve the specificity of infection surveillance data, which might otherwise include a substantial number of isolates of questionable infectious significance.

The unqualified reporting of the morphologic characteristics of bacteria seen in Gram stains of sputum and exudate from wounds without a statement regarding the presence or absence of white blood cells may be more misleading than enlightening. Both sites may be extensively contaminated with cutaneous, oropharyngeal, or intestinal bacterial flora. The presence of abundant squamous cells in the absence of leukocytes should not be overlooked or go unmentioned, or the clinician may gain the erroneous impression that a mixed infection is present from a Gram stain report of a superficial and contaminated specimen. Even the finding of predominating numbers of gram-positive cocci, perhaps lancet-shaped in the case of sputum, is in no way suggestive of staphylococcal or pneumococcal infection if there is an abundance of squamous cells in the absence of leukocytes. Substantial effort will be conserved and superior information will ultimately be provided if repeated collection is requested for such specimens.

Anaerobic culture of specimens should be limited either to those that show leukocytes on Gram stain, no evidence of contaminating squamous cells, and organisms suggestive of anaerobic species or to those specimens that are received with a specific request for anaerobic culture. This limitation results in the reporting of isolates that have a much higher probability of association with infection. Although sensitive new techniques for culturing and identification of anaerobes are available [17], their application to specimens that contain indigenous facultative and strictly anaerobic flora is costly and productive of misleading information. It has been estimated that the cost for processing wound and cervical cultures would increase 107 percent if direct anaerobic culturing was done for all specimens [5]. Large numbers of anaerobic organisms are present in the normal flora of the skin, oral cavity, and the genital and gastrointestinal tracts. Thus, swabs from superficial portions of skin or mucous membrane lesions, specimens of expectorated sputum, and any materials contaminated with feces should be considered inappropriate for anaerobic culture. The frequent submission for anaerobic culture of such specimens or of specimens from sites that are rarely infected by anaerobes (e.g., urine) [57] suggests the need for in-service education of hospital personnel.

Isolation of *Candida* from a series of specimens together with the demonstration of abundant pseudohyphae is required before serious consideration is to be given to their pathogenicity. Yeasts are frequently isolated from respiratory tract secretions and other clinical specimens, but most represent colonization and are not causing infection. Microbiologists should store cultures of yeasts that are isolated in pure culture, or from several consecutive specimens, for two or three days and append a comment to the report requesting the physician to consult the laboratory if complete identification is indicated. Few requests will be received, thus substantially reducing unnecessary work. When specific requests for fungus culture of sputum are received, wet preparations and periodic acid Schiff stained–smears should be examined and the specimen should be inoculated onto Sabouraud's agar with and without bacterial inhibitors.

Identification of Isolates

NEED FOR ACCURACY AND CONSISTENCY. When the need for complete identification of isolates has been ascertained, it is important that standard criteria and nomenclature be consistently applied. Otherwise, attack rates for nosocomial infections with various species may identify false problems (e.g., because of the appearance of previously unreported species or strains) or fail to identify true problems. Furthermore, such surveillance data may not be usefully compared with data developed in other institutions or in cooperative surveillance programs.

Many spurious outbreaks have been traced to inaccurate or inconsistent microbiologic procedures. An "outbreak" of *Staphylococcus aureus* infection, for example, may have been caused by delayed reading of coagulase tests, resulting in the misidentification of coagulase-negative organisms as coagulase-positive. Improvements in laboratory technique that allowed the accurate identification of *Acinetobacter calcoaceticus* var. *anitratus* (*Herellea vaginicola*) organisms for the first time in an institution have also resulted in apparent "outbreaks."

Even more important, incomplete or incorrect identification of organisms may obscure real problems and make retrospective epidemiologic investigation impossible. A report of "*Klebsiella-Aerobacter* group," for example, not only uses obsolete terminology but also fails to distinguish between *Klebsiella* and *Enterobacter* organisms that are characterized by different antimicrobial sensitivities and that have different epidemiologic patterns within the hospital [65]. Similarly, identifying an isolate as *Pseudomonas cepacia,* an organism frequently associated with illness caused by contaminated dilute aqueous benzalkonium chloride or similar antiseptics [22], provides much more epidemiologic information than identifying it as "*Pseudomonas* species."

We believe that each hospital microbiology laboratory should maintain the capability of identifying gram-negative organisms to the genus level with at least 95 percent accuracy. Speciation depends upon application of appropriate criteria, including biochemical reactions, and cannot be based on colonial morphology alone. Isolates from normally sterile specimens such as blood or cerebrospinal fluid should be completely speciated. Isolates whose colonial morphology suggests indigenous flora may be reported generically or as "respiratory flora," etc. without performing specific tests for identification. The problems of the evaluation of clinical significance and need for speciation of all isolates in mixed cultures, especially when there is evidence of superficial contamination, have been the subject of several recent reports [4,5,72].

Many hospitals find it advantageous to employ commercial, multiple test-media kits for biochemical testing [20,36,40,42,52,53,62–64]. Information on various systems may be obtained from state public health laboratories or from the Bureau of Laboratories, Center for

Disease Control (CDC). In addition, public health and other reference laboratories can provide assistance in identifying unusual isolates. Acceptable methods for microbiologic procedures are described in detail elsewhere [11,13].

QUALITY CONTROL. Just as an effective clinical microbiology laboratory is essential to an effective infection control program, adequate quality control is essential to insure the practice of good clinical microbiology. A more complete presentation of this subject is found elsewhere [6]. Such a program begins with a comprehensive procedure manual that establishes standards of operations, including definitions of acceptable and unacceptable quality of specimens and containers, permissible delay between collection and processing, and times during which specimens are accepted for processing. It should define the action to be taken by workers when specimens are not submitted in accordance with these established standards. This portion of the procedure manual should be made known to clinicians and nurses verbally and in writing.

Other portions of the procedure manual should cover administrative aspects of laboratory operation, including infection control and microbiologic safety. Minimum standards for the identification of isolates are to be provided. The program includes a schedule of equipment and reagents to be monitored and measures to be conducted with all tests to insure reproducible and accurate performance. The periodic evaluation of the skills of part-time workers or those who cover nights and holidays will be useful in minimizing errors that might otherwise occur at those times.

Participating in proficiency testing programs helps the laboratory maintain competence, particularly if proficiency test specimens are submitted to the laboratory in a blind fashion and are handled routinely. The submission of blind, unknown specimens is somewhat difficult but extremely useful in insuring the correct performance of equipment and materials as well as the proper interpretation of results by personnel.

Hospital-supported, continuing education is very important for "personnel quality control," particularly if small laboratories are to remain abreast of technologic advances [33]. In addition to these and the other quality control activities that are discussed above, selected laboratory materials, media, and methods may be examined periodically. A manual on quality control procedures for microbiologic laboratories [28], which is available from the CDC Bureau of Laboratories, offers a comprehensive discussion of this subject.

Despite quality control within the laboratory, erroneous microbiology results related to the inadvertent use of faulty or contaminated materials may occur and be overlooked by both clinician and microbiologist. An example is an "outbreak" of false-positive Gram stains of cerebrospinal fluid caused by nonviable contaminants in the specimen tubes in a lot of commercial lumbar puncture trays [73]. In addition, contaminated skin antiseptics, vacutainer tubes, penicillinase, and blood-culturing media and equipment have all been implicated in spurious outbreaks of pseudobacteremia. Such sources of error should be considered when culture or stain results do not appear to reflect clinical or epidemiologic findings.

Typing of Isolates

GENERAL ASPECTS. Epidemiologically important isolates may need special typing, and if so, they should be forwarded to state or local reference laboratories. Potentially pathogenic materials should be packaged for air transport in conformance with federal regulations [38]. Although hospital laboratory personnel may not have the facilities to perform specialized typing procedures, they should know which organisms are typeable and which laboratories can perform the procedures. Furthermore, in cooperation with infection control personnel, the laboratory personnel should subculture and save epidemiologically important isolates, whether such isolates are from outbreaks or from single cases of unusual or potentially epidemic diseases. A system for reviewing and periodically discarding these isolates must also be established.

TYPING SYSTEMS. Selected typing systems of special value in investigating nosocomial infection problems are summarized in Table 8-1. When indicated by epidemiologic circum-

Table 8-1. Selected Typing Systems and Bibliographic References[a]

Organism	Bacteriocin typing	Bacteriophage typing	Serotyping	Other
Escherichia coli	[37]	[14,47]	[24]	Resistogram typing [26]
Klebsiella sp.	—	—	Quellung reaction [15,24]	—
Proteus mirabilis	[51]	[54]	[21]	Dienes' typing [21]
Pseudomonas aeruginosa	[12,31]	[60]	[12]	—
Salmonella sp.	—	[1,39]	Definitive Spicer-Edwards technique [23,24]	—
Serratia marcescens	[29,30]	[35]	[24]	—
Shigella spp.	(*S. sonnei*) [48]	(*S. sonnei*) [41]	(*S. dysenteriae, boydii, flexneri*) [24]	Resistotyping (*S. sonnei*) [25]
Staphylococcus aureus	—	[61]	[16]	—
Staphylococcus epidermidis	—	[69]	[16]	Biotyping [10]
Streptococcus pyogenes				
Group A	—	—	Precipitin; T-agglutination [34,66]	—
Group B	—	—	Precipitin [45,75]	—
Group D	—	—	Precipitin [27]	—

[a] Reference numbers (brackets) given when a test is available.
Source: Data was compiled with the assistance of Frederic J. Marsik, Ph.D., Microbiology Section, Department of Clinical Pathology, University of Virginia School of Medicine, Charlottesville, Virginia.

stances (see Part II, Chapter 21), the following examinations for enteropathogenic *E. coli* can be performed by clinical laboratories. At least six colonies should be picked from blood-agar plates (not bile-containing media) inoculated with feces. These colonies should be pooled and tested with polyvalent O and B antisera for enteropathogenic strains. False-positive reports commonly occur because of misinterpretation of agglutination, and some cross-reactions with the nonenteropathogenic strains sometimes occur. A lower frequency of false-positive results occurs with fluorescent antibody methods, which may be applied directly to fecal specimens. Although fluorescent antibody techniques are not recommended as routine diagnostic tools, laboratory workers may wish to familiarize themselves with this approach because the technique has merit when multiple specimens are being collected from infants and personnel if an outbreak is suspected. Cultures that are positive or suspect should be submitted to reference laboratories for complete serotyping of O, H, and K antigens. A viable stock should be maintained until the results are returned. Additional procedures for typing *E. coli* strains (colicin typing, resistogram, and phage typing) may be available from reference laboratories or those engaged in research with these techniques (see Table 8-1).

The cost of routinely serotyping *Klebsiella*

pneumoniae isolates is not justified by the benefit that accrues to diagnosis and treatment.

Methods for subtyping *Proteus mirabilis* are referred to in Table 8-1. Dienes' typing [21] can readily be performed by clinical laboratories on swarming strains. A line of demarcation develops at the swarming junction when unrelated strains are simultaneously inoculated on the same agar plate, but it does not appear when the same strains are simultaneously inoculated.

Pyocine typing of *Pseudomonas aeruginosa* is probably the single most useful typing procedure for these organisms. Serotyping and bacteriophage typing often permit further subdivisions of strains of the same pyocine type; for maximum usefulness, all three procedures should probably be performed.

Bacteriophage typing of *Staphylococcus aureus* is a useful epidemiologic tool. The test is usually available only through reference laboratories. The technique continues to be of value in relating isolates obtained from patients, personnel, and the environment under epidemic conditions. It is often desirable to have the bacteriophage types of numerous isolates obtained prior to an outbreak. Although the cost of bacteriophage typing of all *S. aureus* isolates is not justifiable, isolates may be inexpensively and conveniently stored by placing a small amount of growth on a blank paper disc that is then placed in a 2-ml., glass, screw-cap vial that contains a few granules of silica gel. If the vial is kept tightly closed, isolates may be retrieved by placing the disc in broth up to six months later if an outbreak should occur.

Biotyping has been proposed as a convenient means for clinical laboratories to subtype *Staphylococcus epidermidis*. This method can establish whether the cultures are being derived from an infection that is caused by a single strain, or whether they may represent spurious contaminants of heterogeneous biotypes.

M-typing of group-A *Streptococcus pyogenes* is epidemiologically useful and also of clinical value because of the association between certain M types of glomerulonephritis. T-typing can be of epidemiologic value because of the large number of identifiable antigens. The latter test is generally available only through reference laboratories.

Antibiotic Susceptibility Testing
General Aspects

METHODS. A standardized method of antimicrobial susceptibility testing that is subject to minimum quality control is essential in any clinical microbiology laboratory. The Kirby-Bauer single disc diffusion method [9] or an equivalent test system is recommended for routine antibiotic sensitivity testing of bacteria. Other sources may be consulted for a detailed discussion of the performance and quality control of this procedure [6,68]. Tube dilution or other methods of establishing minimal inhibitory concentrations of antibiotics must be used for organisms that have not been standardized for testing by this procedure, including many anaerobic bacteria, funguses, and yeast. Testing for the latter should be performed only by specialized mycology laboratories.

While disc tests are probably the most widely used and convenient method of routinely establishing resistance, other methods for determining susceptibility can be useful for both clinical and epidemiologic purposes, provided the methods are consistent and the results reproducible over time.

SELECTION OF STRAINS. Application of susceptibility tests to bacteria that are doubtfully related to infection must be avoided, and specific guidelines for the selection of isolates for susceptibility testing should be established in the laboratory. The practice of performing tests only because they have been requested is being progressively abandoned. Certainly, such a request should not be construed as a justifiable reason for testing indigenous bacteria from sites where they demonstrate little or no recognized pathogenicity. Similarly, the testing of mixed cultures should not be performed, because of the significant number of erroneous results that are known to occur [3]. Direct testing of urine and spinal fluid is not clinically essential. Direct testing of isolates from blood cultures is useful, however, but the results must be confirmed by the standard procedure. Potential pathogens with well-established susceptibility to antimicrobial agents should not be tested routinely; these presently include *Streptococcus pyogenes* and *S. pneumoniae,* although occasional strains of the latter that are resistant to penicillin are being reported.

Modified methods are required for the testing of *Neisseria* species and *Hemophilus influenzae. Neisseria* species do not need to be routinely tested; infections due to *N. gonorrhoeae* and *N. meningitidis* should be treated with ample doses of penicillin. Patients who fail to respond to adequate doses of penicillin for gonorrhea may be treated with other drugs instead of waiting for the laboratory to demonstrate penicillin resistance. Penicillin resistance caused by β-lactamase-producing strains is being reported primarily from the Far East and Europe, but routine testing for β-lactamase is not yet indicated in this country. Resistance of *H. influenzae* type b to ampicillin has now been reported from many different areas of the United States, and testing for ampicillin resistance and/or production of β-lactamase may now be advocated as a routine clinical laboratory procedure.

SELECTION OF DRUGS. Introduction of Food and Drug Administration (FDA) controls on the certification of discs for use in the Kirby-Bauer method has substantially reduced the unnecessary and wasteful testing of related antimicrobials. Generally, only one drug of a particular class of antibiotics needs to be tested, since the results will pertain to all members of that class. The selection of drugs for routine testing should be jointly determined by the Infection Control Committee and the clinical laboratory, and the drugs may consist of a mixture of agents providing useful clinical, taxonomic, and epidemiologic data. The Infection Control Committee may decide not to include in clinical reports the results of antimicrobial sensitivity tests performed for epidemiologic purposes only or those performed on antibiotics the hospital wishes to control. If this is done, clinicians should be told which antibiotics are being tested routinely but not reported.

The epidemiologic value of sensitivity patterns may be enhanced by including certain antibiotics that do not necessarily provide useful clinical information. Two disc sets of 12 antibiotics each, one for gram-negative and another for gram-positive organisms, have been recommended by the Hospital Infections Branch at CDC. Drugs used in each set should be decided on and periodically updated by the Infection Control Committee. Although alternative sets employing fewer discs have been advocated for routine clinical use [50] based on the site of infection or the identity of infecting organisms, the few extra discs selected primarily for epidemiologic purposes are inexpensive, and all 12 discs can be placed in the same dispenser and applied simultaneously to an agar plate. Moreover, while the results from a limited disc set allow treatment decisions for individual patients, the results obtained from using the additional discs have proved valuable to some institutions in identifying and evaluating episodes of cross-infection and common-source infection. Results from these discs have also been helpful in tracing infections that occur at low frequency in many different hospitals. During a recent nationwide outbreak of bacteremia, for example, susceptibility patterns of *Enterobacter agglomerans* blood isolates to nitrofurantoin and the cephalosporins assisted in identifying the epidemic strains in contaminated commercial intravenous products [46]. Furthermore, comparison of the expected and observed susceptibility patterns for organisms can provide valuable taxonomic and quality control information [59].

QUALITY CONTROL. Errors in the performance of susceptibility tests occur and may result in information that may be misleading not only for diagnosis and treatment but also for relating isolates epidemiologically. Antibiotic discs should be stored at 4°C to 8°C (39°F to 46°F) except for those containing synthetic penicillins and cephalosporins, which must be stored at −20°C (−4°F). Desiccant must be provided, and dispensers should be protected from intermittent exposure to refrigerator temperatures and warm humid air. Whether prepared in the laboratory or bought commercially prepared, every batch of Mueller-Hinton medium should have its pH tested. This is easily accomplished using a surface electrode, or the medium may be broken into a slurry and placed in a small cup and the pH measured with an ordinary immersion electrode. A pH range of 7.2 to 7.4 is acceptable. Before either a new batch of medium or any new lot numbers of discs are put into use, cultures of control strains of *Staphylococcus aureus* ATCC 25923, *Pseudomonas aeruginosa* ATCC 27853, and *Escherichia coli* ATCC 25922 should be tested to insure that zone diameters fall within the range of acceptability established by the FDA and listed on the disc package insert. In addition, these cultures should be tested several times a week to insure that turbidity standards and interpretive criteria are producing correct results. Susceptibility tests should be routinely performed at an incubator temperature of 35°C (95°F).

When results exceed acceptable limits, reports on clinical isolates can be withheld until acceptable control results are obtained. Alternatively, results on clinical isolates may be reported with a note indicating "accuracy of result questionable; control values unacceptable." The reader is referred elsewhere for a more detailed presentation of the performance of this test and the investigation of erratic control results [6].

The reproducibility of susceptibility tests can also be assessed, as an adjunct to an infection control program, by resubmitting a blind culture containing an organism that has been previously tested by the laboratory. Furthermore, selected important strains—such as a methicillin-resistant *S. aureus* strain—can be blindly submitted. If the strain is correctly identified, the committee will be assured that the laboratory applies proper techniques and skills. Such unknown specimens may be used to supplement the internal quality control of procedures provided by the ATCC strains.

Consistent and accurate identification of organisms over time is necessary in order for susceptibility data to be useful for clinical and epidemiologic purposes.

Typing of Organisms by Resistances

OVERALL RESISTANCE PATTERN. Epidemic strains of organisms of the same genus and species can sometimes be detected by distinctive overall susceptibility patterns, or antibiograms. The value of any particular antibiotic for typing purposes varies with the expected frequency of susceptibility in a population of strains of the same genus and species in the same locale at the same time. Knowledge of the susceptibility profiles of organisms in a particular hospital may therefore be very helpful in identifying an unusual susceptibility finding, which may be of great value for epidemiologic purposes.

The stability of a particular acquired resistance in an epidemic strain is also important. Chromosomal resistance tends to be more stable than episomal, and therefore such resistances may prove totally stable throughout an epidemic that extends over a long period of time.

A variety of antibiograms may be found within many common species of bacteria isolated from clinical material. This provides an inexpensive, rapid source of information for relating strains that may be linked to cross-infection. It may allow retrospective correlation of isolates that may no longer be available for study. Additional antimicrobial agents may be used to provide markers, even though the results are not reported for use in diagnosis and treatment. Subsequent serotyping or bacteriophage typing may be restricted to those isolates that show the same antibiogram.

EXACT ZONE SIZE. Even when the antibiograms are essentially the same, there are additional ways to subdivide and establish a unique epidemic strain by utilizing the susceptibility data. One of the simplest of these is to use the actual zone size or minimal inhibitory concentrations. The former method is preferable, however, because disc tests provide a more precise quantitation of the susceptibility of the strains that are being compared; a continuous gradient of antibiotic surrounds a disc, whereas abrupt, two-fold changes in concentration are used in dilution tests. Organisms that are sensitive or resistant to a particular drug may still have zone diameters sufficiently different to exclude variation in the testing method as the cause. This occurs because the interpretive schemata for susceptibilities in the Kirby-Bauer technique often have broad ranges of zone sizes that signify sensitivity or resistance. Quantitative differences in the susceptibility of strains to different drugs, despite identical qualitative antibiograms, may therefore be used when the differences in zone diameters exceed those expected from method variation alone, as determined on quality control strains.

R-PLASMID CHARACTERIZATION. Strains with similar antibiograms may be further characterized by their plasmids. Some of these procedures are too complex for general application, but others can be done by clinical laboratories. Strains with the same qualitative patterns of resistance may be used as the donors in conjugation experiments with a recipient strain that is sensitive to antibiotics to which the donor strains are resistant; the transconjugants are thus selectively cultured from mixtures of donor and recipient strains on the basis of unique properties. Donor strains are then compared with respect to their ability to transfer resistance, the frequency of transfer, and the resistance pattern of transconjugants. Additional, more complex tests have also been used to type R plasmids, such as qualitative and quantitative analysis of the enzymes involved in resistance, determination of the compatibility status with F factor or other R plasmids, and analysis of R plasmid DNA.

*Factors Influencing Usefulness
of Antibiotic Typing*

ORGANISM. Experiences in the investigation of *S. aureus* outbreaks have strongly corroborated the meaningfulness and utility of susceptibility data. The susceptibility patterns of isolates from lesions are often sufficient to demonstrate the presence of a common epidemic strain and to identify accurately personnel who are carriers of such strains. The accuracy of antibiograms in marking epidemic strains of Enterobacteriaceae has generally been less, but the accuracy of this method varies with the mode of spread and the clinical site involved (see below). Enterobacteria are often capable of conjugally transferring their resistances, especially in the intestinal tract. Such transfers may create strains with the same antibiograms as those of autogenous flora of the same or

other genera, or they may result in the epidemic strain's acquiring new resistances from existing flora. *Pseudomonas aeruginosa* typing by antibiograms is comparatively less valuable, because their patterns may also change through the acquisition of resistance determinants by resistance transfer, as in the case of the enterobacterial patterns, and pseudomonads are so uniformly resistant to many antibiotics that only a few drugs may be useful in differentiating strains.

MODE OF SPREAD. Antibiograms are very useful when the mode of spread involves a common source, such as an intermittent positive pressure breathing apparatus, intravenous fluid, food, and the like. In a common-source outbreak, each infected patient receives the same organisms from the source. Organisms that are spread from person to person, however, are more likely to acquire new resistances, most commonly by R-plasmid transfer, but also through mutation and transduction. The means by which resistances to specific antimicrobial agents are acquired vary with the organism and the antimicrobial agent. Antibiograms from strains involved in common-source outbreaks tend to be more uniform than those associated with other forms of transmission. The frequency and nature of newly acquired resistances also depend on the frequency of occurrence of specific R plasmids within the hospital and the frequency of exposure of patients to antimicrobial agents.

CLINICAL SITE. Because of exposure to a variety of other organisms potentially capable of transferring resistances, isolates of an epidemic strain from gastrointestinal sites are likely to show greater variation in antibiotic susceptibility patterns than do those organisms from other sites of infection. In contrast, the antibiograms of epidemic strains isolated from sites where contact with other organisms is unlikely (e.g., spinal fluid and blood) may be very uniform in their susceptibility patterns.

Other Uses of Susceptibility Data

TAXONOMIC USES. Gram-negative rods that are susceptible to all tested antimicrobials are very likely to be *E. coli;* such findings are uncommon or rare among other gram-negative rods. Cephalosporin susceptibility may sometimes be useful in separating *Klebsiella* from Enterobacteriaceae species; in some institutions, *Klebsiella* species have been found to be almost uniformly sensitive to these drugs, whereas high frequencies of resistance have been found in Enterobacteriaceae. Ampicillin sensitivity can be used to distinguish *Proteus mirabilis* from *P. vulgaris*. *Pseudomonas cepacia* usually appears resistant to gentamicin and polymyxins and thus can be presumptively differentiated from *P. aeruginosa* before speciation is confirmed biochemically. In laboratories that do not speciate *Pseudomonas,* such susceptibility patterns may be one of the few means by which an epidemic strain of *P. cepacia* can be retrospectively distinguished in laboratory records from unspeciated *Pseudomonas* isolates. Nontransferable resistance to the polymyxins is almost uniformly found in *Serratia marcescens*. Resistance of a staphylococcal strain to methicillin or other penicillinase-resistant semisynthetic penicillins should suggest *S. epidermidis* rather than *S. aureus,* because such resistances are commonly found at present among the former but only very rarely among the latter in the United States. Bacitracin susceptibility is sufficient to identify presumptively group-A *Streptococcus pyogenes,* although up to 10 percent of susceptible isolates may be other than group-A streptococci. Other taxonomic uses have also been described [59].

OUTBREAK DETECTION. Computer programs have been developed to identify clusters of infections with the same organism and susceptibilities that occur at the same time in the same patient-care area (service or ward). Such programs are still investigational, but they have permitted the identification of outbreaks with strains with one antibiogram to be identified; these outbreaks could otherwise have been masked by the large amount of data on commonly occurring organisms such as *S. aureus* and *E. coli.* The overall incidences of infections caused by common nosocomial pathogens may remain essentially constant, even though an outbreak with a particular substrain is occurring. Analyses of such incidences are generally too te-

dious and difficult to be performed without computer assistance.

SELECTIVE MEDIA FOR SURVEYS. Susceptibility data on epidemic strains may also be used to construct selective media for use in microbiologic surveys of the animate and inanimate environments. Once the pathogen is isolated and pretested on the appropriate media containing one or more antibiotics to which it is resistant, the media can then be used to exclude numerous bacteria unrelated to the outbreak, which may accelerate the detection of contaminated equipment or infected patients. Pretesting is essential because of possible synergism or antagonism between drugs or between the drugs and the media; these phenomena could cause inhibition of the growth of the epidemic strain or failure to inhibit the growth of "sensitive" organisms.

SUMMARY REPORTS FOR CLINICAL USE. Development of profiles of the susceptibility of common, rapidly growing pathogens to drugs commonly in use is of considerable assistance in guiding therapy and providing a rational method of selecting treatment for sepsis of unknown cause as well as for other infections. Testing of slow-growing bacteria, such as *Bacteroides* species, may be performed in batches to allow the development of a profile of susceptibility for this genus; such testing would be more helpful than testing individual isolates, which usually would not produce results until four or five days after the specimens are submitted to the laboratory.

In cooperation with the Infection Control Committee, the laboratory should distribute at least annually a summary of sensitivity patterns to all clinicians. The Infection Control Committee, a medical staff committee, or both may wish to review antibiotic utilization at this time [44,58,76]. Furthermore, if a list of the cost (e.g., per unit dose) of each antibiotic is included in the summary, clinicians may be motivated to reduce costs of patient care.

Two separate tabulations of data are suggested: (1) tabulation of the frequency of sensitivity to individual drugs by site of infection (this may provide guidance in selecting drugs for therapy of a newly diagnosed infection before organisms have been isolated from cultures) and (2) tabulation of the frequency of sensitivity to individual drugs by pathogen (this may prove useful in redirecting therapy after an organism is isolated from cultures of serious infections and before susceptibility tests on the isolate have been completed). For maximal value, separate compilations should be made for community-acquired and nosocomial infections and isolates, and multiple isolates of the same organism from an infection should be excluded.

Microbiologic Sampling and Surveys
General Aspects

ENVIRONMENTAL SAMPLING. In the absence of an epidemic, sampling should be minimal. All steam and ethylene oxide gas sterilizers should be checked at least once each week with a suitable live-spore preparation [7]; ethylene oxide gas sterilizers should also be checked with each load of items that will come into contact with blood or other tissues. Hospital-prepared infant formulas should be tested by culturing each week. Instruments that touch mucous membranes but are disinfected rather than sterilized before use, such as inhalation and anesthesia equipment and endoscopes, may be sampled on a spot-check basis as needed to insure adequacy of disinfection. Although commercial patient-care items that are labeled "sterile" (e.g., intravascular catheters and fluids) have occasionally been contaminated with viable organisms that can cause patient disease, routine sampling of these items is not recommended, because of the low frequency of contamination and because of the difficulty and expense of performing adequate sterility testing. If contamination of commercial products sold as sterile is suspected, the FDA should be telephoned immediately.

Depending on the size of the institution and the magnitude of the infection control program, it may be desirable to develop experience and confidence with other survey methods that may have specific usefulness in investigating outbreaks. These methods include surface-sampling techniques applicable to floors and other environmental surfaces, air sampling, and the testing of medicines, antiseptics, soap dispensers, lubricants, hand lotion, food, kitchen equipment, water, and ice. Standard techniques for many of these determinations do not exist, and consultation with a public health or other laboratory should take place before large surveys involving these items are undertaken.

Sampling techniques that are not directly related to epidemiologic surveys may prove useful in educational programs where visible evidence of contamination of hands, clothing, equipment, and surfaces may serve to drive home the need for effective aseptic technique and sanitation. Levels of environmental contamination in hospitals, however, have not been shown to correlate with the incidence of nosocomial disease, and routine environmental sampling of this type should not be construed to be an element of an infection control program. Furthermore, in-use testing of antiseptics and disinfectants should not be a routine procedure for hospital microbiology laboratories.

DIFFERENTIAL AND SELECTIVE SURVEY MEDIA. Routine culturing of patients or hospital personnel for microbial carriage is not generally recommended. Surveys may clearly be indicated during outbreak investigations and should be responsive to and directed by epidemiologic findings. Sampling sites relevant to infections caused by specific pathogens are described in Part II of this text.

To reduce the work load in the laboratory and to expedite the processing of specimens, selective survey media should be used whenever possible for culturing specimens from the patients, staff, and environment during outbreak investigations. Use of media that contain antibiotics to which an epidemic strain is resistant is often possible, but, as mentioned earlier, such media should be pretested on epidemic isolates before use. Other selective media may also be extremely useful. Cetrimide or a commercial medium such as Pseudosel (BBL), for example, may be extremely helpful in selectively isolating *Pseudomonas aeruginosa* from contaminated material or mixed cultures. Tetrathionate broth is an excellent medium for selective preenrichment of *Salmonella* cultures. Mueller-Hinton agar containing sorbitol, a pH indicator, and commercially prepared antibiotics for use in Thayer-Martin medium (vancomycin, colistin, and nystatin) provide selective differentiation of *Serratia* species. Many epidemic strains of *Staphylococcus aureus,* especially those lysed by phages of the 80/81 complex, are resistant to mercuric chloride, and the incorporation of small amounts in trypticase-soy agar (TSA) medium has been of great value in inhibiting nonepidemic strains of *S. aureus, S. epidermidis,* and most gram-negative organisms except *Pseudomonas.* The resistances of epidemic strains to other heavy metals, dyes, disinfectants, and other antimicrobial substances may also be used to construct selective media for surveys.

Routine Environmental Sampling

SPORE STRIP CULTURES TO MONITOR STERILIZATION. All sterilizers should be equipped with time-temperature recorders to provide evidence of adequate exposure for each load. Evidence that a sterilizing temperature has been held for an adequate time, however, does not insure sterilization, because the temperature is measured at the outlet valve and does not indicate whether adequate sterilization occurred within dense volumes of fluid or large, dense, fabric-wrapped packs. Residual air or superheating may also result in incomplete sterilization. The use of chemical monitors (e.g., test tapes or heat-sensitive color indicators) within the autoclave provides only an indication that a sterilizing temperature may have been reached, but such monitors do not show whether there was adequate exposure. The best means of insuring sterility is to contaminate the product to be sterilized intentionally and subsequently retrieve it for culture determinations. This is, unfortunately, an impractical approach. Thus, biologic monitoring with spore strips has generally been accepted as the most effective way to determine successful sterilization (see Part I, Chapter 6).

Microorganisms chosen for test spore strips are more resistant to sterilization than are most naturally occurring contaminants, and the test organisms are provided in relatively high con-

centrations to insure a margin of safety. The spores may be provided either in impregnated filter-paper strips or in solution in glass ampules. For steam and hot-air sterilization, the thermophile *Bacillus stearothermophilus* is used, and for ethylene oxide sterilization, *Bacillus subtilis* (strain *globigii,* variety niger) is used. Both species are frequently incorporated simultaneously in the test strips, and these can be used to test for adequate sterilization with either procedure.

Most spore strip preparations are provided in envelopes that contain one or two test strips and a control strip. The test strips are packaged in separate envelopes, which are removed and sterilized at the time other material is processed. Subsequently, the test strips and control strip are cultured by placing the strips in a tube of tryptic-digest casein-soy (TS) broth to be incubated at 37°C (99°F) for spores used to control gas sterilization and 56°C (133°F) for those used to monitor steam sterilization. It is not necessary to culture a positive control strip for each test; if strips are obtained from a single lot, only 10 percent of the positive control strips need to be tested.

Other types of spore preparations are commercially available and require, in some cases, unique handling. In each case, the manufacturer's directions should be closely followed. Spore solutions are prepared in sealed glass ampules for testing the adequacy of sterilization of fluids. These ampules should be incubated at 56°C (133°F) in a water bath. If there is no change in the indicator by seven days, the test is reported as negative. Alternatively, the fluid may be inoculated with a test culture, which may be subcultured after autoclaving.

Steam and hot-air sterilizers should be tested once a week. Every load of material sterilized with ethylene oxide that is to be placed in contact with deep tissues should be tested because of the frequency of sterilization failures that have been observed with this procedure. Goods should be impounded until test cultures are proved negative (see Part I, Chapter 7, Central Service).

Test strips or spore solutions should always be placed in the center of the specimen to be tested, never on an open shelf in the autoclave.

The center of a pack located near the bottom front exhaust valve will be exposed to the least adequate duration and temperature of sterilization. Testing of sterilization of fluids is accomplished by placing an ampule containing a spore solution in the largest vessel.

Ampules containing spore solutions should not be used to check the sterilization of bacteriologic culture media, because these do not require the duration of exposure that is required for sterilization of material known to contain large populations of bacteria. In fact, heating of bacteriologic culture media to a temperature sufficient to insure sterilization of a test strip or spore ampule will result in damage to the medium through overheating.

The handling of spore strips in the laboratory requires considerable care to prevent secondary contamination. A laminar-flow cabinet will be found extremely helpful. The transfer should be made with sterile forceps and scissors. Common sources of contamination include the forceps and scissors, which may be insufficiently sterilized by flaming or wiping with alcohol. Alcohol or flaming techniques should be avoided, because alcohol may contain viable spores that might not be killed by flaming, and flaming may be insufficient to heat instruments to a temperature that will destroy viable spores. Care should be taken not to cross-contaminate the sterilized spore strips with the control strips.

The likelihood of contamination can be reduced by minimizing the handling of the strip after sterilization. Test strips can be removed from their envelopes and placed in sterile glass tubes prior to sterilization. The tube is then sterilized with the screw-cap removed or with other closures permeable to steam in place. After sterilization, the tube is submitted to the laboratory, where the nutrient broth is added. Condensation on the cover of a 56°C (133°F) water bath may cause contamination of the caps and closures of tubes. A heating block may be used, or the bath may be left uncovered, although this will make it necessary to provide a reservoir to maintain the water level because of the high evaporation rate at this temperature. Uninoculated culture media should be incubated at 35°C (95°F) or 56°C

(133°F) to insure that contamination will not yield false-positive reports.

Gram staining and subculturing should be performed to prevent the false-positive reports that could result from secondary contamination of test cultures. If organisms other than gram-positive bacilli are observed, the test should be repeated and reported "equivocal results, potential laboratory contamination."

Whenever positive results are obtained, the sterilizers should be immediately retested, with careful examination of thermometer and pressure-gauge readings as well as review of recent time and temperature records. If any deficiency is observed or if the repeated sterility test still results in growth, engineering personnel and consultants expert in autoclave maintenance should be consulted promptly.

INFANT FORMULA. Several bottles of hospital-prepared infant formula selected at random from each lot produced should be tested once a week. Sampling of commercially prepared formula milk is less important, but it may be required by various state health codes.

Formula milk may be sampled by inoculating one milliliter into a pour plate of TS agar. After 48 hours, the plates are examined for surface and subsurface colonies. No more than 25 colonies of spore-forming organisms should be observed [18].

BLOOD COMPONENTS. The American Association of Blood Banks (AABB) had recommended [7]—but no longer recommends [67]—random culturing of units of blood to insure sterility. Culturing of components prepared in an open system, however, is advocated. Ten-milliliter samples of the component should be cultured both aerobically and anaerobically for ten days. Incubation at both 18°C to 20°C (64°F to 68°F) and 35°C to 37°C (95°F to 99°F) is probably advisable.

If a transfusion reaction occurs, the possibility of contamination should be considered. After immediate disconnection of the administration unit, sterile shields should be placed over the exposed ends of needles or tubing to prevent subsequent contamination. A 5-ml. sample should be removed aseptically from the administration tubing in the laboratory and processed according to the AABB-recommended method described above. It is desirable to collect several blood culture specimens simultaneously by venipuncture from the patient.

Periodic Sampling of Disinfected Equipment

INDICATIONS. Any article that makes direct contact with the vascular system or tissue other than unbroken skin should be sterile. Whenever possible, steam or gas sterilization should be applied. If chemical disinfection or pasteurization rather than sterilization is used on equipment such as cystoscopes and other endoscopic instruments, respiratory therapy apparatus, or anesthesia equipment, then periodic microbiologic sampling is desirable to insure the absence of pathogens after processing. (Disinfection of respiratory therapy and anesthesia equipment is discussed further in Part II, Chapter 15.)

The frequency of sampling of disinfected devices of the above types will depend on the results of intermittent sampling, any evidence that nosocomial infection is associated with their use, and an assessment by the Infection Control Committee of the adequacy of standards for control of contamination of such equipment.

Sampling of unused sterile disposable parts is not necessary, but they must not be reused. Samples should be taken of reusable equipment after it has been disinfected and made ready for use on patients.

METHODS OF CULTURE-SWAB-RINSE TECHNIQUE. Cultures of external surfaces or internal cavities (e.g., tubes and containers) may be conducted by a swab-rinse technique [8]. Brain-heart infusion broth (BHIB) supplemented with 0.5% beef extract is used. The broth should contain 0.07% lecithin and 0.5% polysorbate 80 as neutralizers whenever the cultured objects are likely to contain residual disinfectants.

A cotton applicator swab is immersed in this broth in a screw-cap tube, wrung out, and used to swab the surface to be sampled. The swab is returned to the tube after sampling; the portion of the stick handled by the operator should be broken off.

The same broth may be used to sample containers and the lumens of tubular structures by a rinse technique, which is a better and more convenient sampling method for such equipment than the application of swabs. The rinse technique involves introducing a suitable quantity of broth into the lumen of tubular structures (40 to 50 ml. for respiratory therapy tubing) and manually tilting the object to produce a rinsing action. Up to 50 agitations are desirable. A sample of the broth is then placed in a screw-cap tube. Bottles and containers such as nebulizer reservoirs may be sampled by adding 10 to 15 ml. of rinse broth, inserting a sterile stopper if required, and shaking vigorously for about 30 seconds. The broth is decanted or pipetted from the container into a sterile vessel.

Sample tubes should be thoroughly agitated to insure a homogeneous suspension, particularly when swabs are used. Plate counts are accomplished by preparing a series of tenfold solutions in tubes of TS broth using 1 ml. of the test sample for the first dilution. From each tube of the dilution series, 0.5 ml. is pipetted onto the surface of a TS agar plate, which is supplemented with 5% sheep or rabbit blood. The plate is rocked until the inoculum is thoroughly distributed, and it then is allowed to dry at 35°C (95°F). The plates are inverted and incubated for 24 hours, after which colony counts are made if colonies appear to be coalescing or spreading; otherwise, counts are made after 48 hours of incubation.

For specific identification of isolates, the original broth sample should be subcultured at 4 hours and at 24 hours after removal of the 1 ml. that was used for the dilution count. To perform each subculture, 0.5 ml. is pipetted onto the surfaces of TS blood agar, MacConkey agar, and cetrimide agar plates. They are rocked to distribute the inoculum and are allowed to dry prior to incubation at 35°C. At 24 hours, those same media are inoculated from the original BHIB rinse sample that was incubated at 35°C. If growth seems apparent on the basis of turbidity, only a loopful should be subcultured to provide isolated colonies. At least two colonies of each morphologic colony type should be picked for identification.

Other Environmental Cultures

As indicated earlier, a wide variety of items and substances can be responsible for cross-infection, and a detailed description of suitable culture techniques for each of these is beyond the practical scope of this chapter. Culture procedures for the following materials and objects should not be conducted unless surveillance of infections in patients specifically implicates these items as potential sources of infection. Because standard methods for the microbiologic evaluation of such procedures often do not exist or are of doubtful validity, considerable expense may be incurred in the production of information that is not only worthless but misleading.

WATER AND ICE TESTING. Water that meets U.S Public Health Service drinking water standards frequently contains 10^2 to 10^6 or more microorganisms per milliliter, some of which may be opportunistic pathogens. After melting, ice is sampled by the same procedures used for water.

Samples of water (or melted ice) can be cultured by passing large quantities through a $0.45-\mu$ (or $0.22-\mu$) Millipore filter and then culturing the filter in broth or directly on agar.

Maximum sensitivity is achieved when the previously described 24-hour BHIB dilution method is used. Substantial numbers of bacteria may be isolated by this technique, but there is no evidence that this is hazardous.

The finding of a most probable number of 2.2 or more colonies by the tube test or more than four colonies per 100 ml. by the millipore filtration test is considered abnormal for potable water [17].

PARENTERAL FLUID AND EQUIPMENT. The investigation of bacteremia associated with parenteral therapy may require investigation of the needle or catheter, portions of the administration set, the fluid being administered, and portions of the cap or closure provided with the fluid (see Part II, Chapters 25 and 26). Blood culture specimens should be collected simultaneously from the patient. It is especially important to keep careful track of lot numbers, which should be recorded on the pa-

tient's chart as well as on all subsequent laboratory records.

Because of the elaborate nature of the sampling of all potentially involved sites, the microbiologist should work closely with the Infection Control Committee, nurse epidemiologist, or clinicians to concentrate efforts on the most probable sites of contamination, so conducting comprehensive sampling on a routine basis each time some portion of the equipment is suspected may be avoided.

Needles and catheters must be submitted separately from the hubs and other portions of the administration set that may have been exposed to superficial contamination. If portions of the administration set are suspected, these must be received properly capped to exclude spurious contamination. The bottle and administration set should remain connected and be placed in a plastic bag to minimize contamination during delivery to the laboratory.

Catheters and needles may be cultured by a swab-rinse technique, but the semiquantitative culture methods described in Part II, Chapter 25 are preferable. Culture methods for intravenous fluid in containers or collected from administration lines are described in Part II, Chapter 26. Careful aseptic technique is critically important.

FLOORS AND OTHER SURFACES. Floors may be sampled by the swab technique previously described. In this case, a 2- by 2-inch square hole is cut from the center of a sheet of heavy paper, which is subsequently sterilized and wrapped. The culture is collected by placing the paper on the surface to be sampled. The swab is slowly rubbed in close, parallel streaks across the exposed area. This is repeated after moving the swab in a direction perpendicular to the first streaks.

Such surfaces may also be conveniently sampled using Rodac plates [32], which are designed to permit direct contact of agar with flat surfaces. Such plates should be filled with 16.5 ml. of TS agar containing 0.07% lecithin and 0.5% polysorbate 80 as neutralizers of disinfectant. The number of plates to use will depend on the size of the surface to be sampled and on the level of statistical significance that is required. Both the plates and the surface to be sampled should be dry at the time the sample is collected. Plates are pressed firmly against the surface without producing a rotary or sliding motion. Colonies are counted after incubation at 35°C to 37°C (95°F to 99°F) for 48 hours. The use of various types of automatic and semiautomatic colony counters will save time in counting large numbers of plates.

Standards for acceptable levels of contamination of floors and overbed tables sampled by the Rodac plate technique have been suggested by a committee of the American Public Health Association [19]. There is no evidence, however, that any particular level of contamination is directly correlated with an increased risk of infection, and such standards are probably only useful in assessing the adequacy of house-cleaning. Finding 25 or fewer colonies per plate is considered "good"; 26 to 50 colonies, "fair"; and more than 50 colonies, "poor." These values are based on samples taken about one-half hour after cleaning and do not reflect the levels of contamination that would progressively accumulate in the interval prior to the next cleaning of the surface. For this reason, random Rodac plate sampling conducted without reference to the time of cleaning will produce results that cannot be compared with these standards. Counts below five colonies per Rodac plate are achievable in some areas, such as in operating rooms.

AIR SAMPLING. Air sampling may be performed with either settling plates or sophisticated instruments. Airborne spread of nosocomial bacterial (or other) infections, however, is probably very uncommon, and, if suspected, it is best evaluated by someone with experience in this field.

Particles suspended in hospital air vary greatly in size and in the number of microorganisms they contain. The average diameter of airborne microbial particles in ward air is about 13 μ, but 7 percent are less than 4 μ in size and 30 percent are greater than 18μ. Particles with a mean size of 13μ settle at a rate of approximately one foot per minute. Since a standard 100-mm. Petri dish represents an area of about 1/15 square feet, and if the in-

stitutional air under study is assumed to contain particles of average size, then an open Petri dish in still air will sample microbial particles from about a cubic foot of air during 15 minutes of exposure. Brain-heart infusion (BHI) or trypticase-soy agar (TSA) are recommended media for such sampling. Although this is an inexpensive way to evaluate airborne microbial contamination, quantitative results may correlate poorly with those obtained with mechanical, volumetric, air samplers because of variation in particle size and unknown influences of air turbulence. Under low humidity conditions, droplet nuclei of about 3 μ can remain suspended indefinitely and can be collected only with high-velocity, volumetric, air samplers.

It must be recognized that the measurement of the number of airborne microbial "particles" as measured by their growth after impaction on an agar plate is not the same as the total number of airborne microorganisms; an airborne microbial particle may contain one too many viable bacterial or fungal cells (or viruses). Air-sampling techniques in which volumetric samples are taken by bubbling air through collection fluid will break up airborne particulate matter and provide higher counts per unit of air than will air samplers that impinge contaminated particles on agar.

A slit sampler from New Brunswick Scientific, Inc. (New Brunswick, N.J.) is suitable for most microbial air-sampling applications. BHI or TSA media should be used in sampling plates. The six-stage Andersen sampler (Andersen 2000, Inc., Atlanta, Ga.) should be used only when it is necessary to determine the size distribution of airborne microbial particles. Efficient vacuum sources must be used for both samplers, and the rate of flow of air must be properly calibrated to insure accurate results.

References

1. Anderson, E. S., and Williams, R. E. O. Bacteriophage typing of enteric pathogens and staphylococci and its use in epidemiology. *J. Clin. Pathol.* 9:94, 1956.
2. Balows, A., Dehaan, R. M., Dowell, V. R.,

and Guze, L. B. (Eds.). *Anaerobic Bacteria.* Springfield, Ill.: Charles C Thomas, 1974.

3. Barry, A. L., Joyce, L. J., Adams, A. P., and Benner, E. J. Rapid determination of antimicrobial susceptibility for urgent clinical situations. *Am. J. Clin. Pathol.* 59:693, 1973.

4. Bartlett, R. C. A plea for clinical relevance in medical microbiology. *Am. J. Clin. Pathol.* 61:867, 1974.

5. Bartlett, R. C. Control of cost and medical relevance in clinical microbiology. *Am. J. Clin. Pathol.* 64:518, 1975.

6. Bartlett, R. C. *Medical Microbiology, Quality, Cost and Clinical Relevance.* New York: Wiley Interscience, 1974.

7. Bartlett, R. C., Gröschell, D. H. M., Mackel, D. C., Mallison, G. F., and Spaulding, E. H. Control of Hospital-Associated Infections. In Lennette, E. H., Spaulding, E. H., and Truant, J. P. (Eds.), *Manual of Clinical Microbiology* (2d ed.). Washington, D.C.: American Society for Microbiology, 1974.

8. Bartlett, R. C., Gröschel, D. H. M., Mackel, D. C., Mallison, G. F., and Spaulding, E. H. Microbiologic Surveillance. In Lennette, E. H., Spaulding, E. H., and Truant, J. P. (Eds.), *Manual of Clinical Microbiology* (2d ed.). Washington, D.C.: American Society for Microbiology, 1974.

9. Bauer, A. W., Kirby, W. M., Sherris, J. C., and Turck, M. Antibiotic susceptibility testing by a standardized single disc method. *Am. J. Clin. Pathol.* 45:493, 1966.

10. Bentley, D. W., Hagne, R., Murphy, R. A., and Lepper, M. H. Biotyping, an epidemiological tool for coagulase-negative staphylococci. *Antimicrob. Agents Chemother.,* p. 54, 1967.

11. Blair, J. E., Lennette, E. H., and Truant, J. P. (Eds.). *Manual of Clinical Microbiology* (2d ed.). Washington, D.C.: American Society for Microbiology, 1974.

12. Bobo, R. A., Newton, E. J., Jones, L. F., Farmer, L. H., and Farmer, J. J., III. Nursery outbreak of *Pseudomonas aeruginosa:* Epidemiological conclusions from five different typing methods. *Appl. Microbiol.* 25:414, 1973.

13. Bodily, H. L., Updyke, E. L., and Mason, J. O. *Diagnostic Procedures for Bacterial, Mycotic and Parasitic Infections.* New York: American Public Health Association, 1970.

14. Brown, W. J., and Parisi, J. T. Bacteriophage typing of bacteriuric *Escherichia coli. Proc. Soc. Exp. Biol. Med.* 121:259, 1966.

15. Casewell, M. W. Experience in the use of commercial antisera for the capsular typing of *Klebsiella* species. *J. Clin. Pathol.* 25:734, 1972.

16. Cohen, J. O. Serotyping of Staphylococci. In Cohen, J. O. (Ed.), *The Staphylococci.* New York: Wiley Interscience, 1972.

17. Committee of American Public Health Association, American Water Works Association, and Water Prevention Commission. *Standard Methods for the Examination of Water and Waste Water* (13th ed.). New York: American Public Health Association, 1971.

18. Committee on Fetus and Newborn, American Academy of Pediatrics. *Standards and Recommendations for Hospital Care of Newborn Infants* (5th ed.). Evanston, Ill.: American Academy of Pediatrics, 1971.

19. Committee on Microbial Contamination of Surfaces, Laboratory Section, American Public Health Association. A comparative microbiological evaluation of floor-cleaning procedures in hospital patient rooms. *Health Lab. Sci.* 7:3, 1970.

20. Coppel, S. P., and Coppel, I. G. Comparison of the R-B System and the Enterotube for the identification of *Enterobacteriaceae. Am. J. Clin. Pathol.* 61:218, 1974.

21. deLouvois, J. Serotyping and the Dienes' reaction on *Proteus mirabilis* from hospital infection. *J. Clin. Pathol.* 22:263, 1969.

22. Ederer, G. M., and Matsen, J. M. Colonization and infection with *Pseudomonas cepacia. J. Infect. Dis.* 125:613, 1972.

23. Edwards, P. R. *Serological Examination of Salmonella Cultures for Epidemiological Purposes.* Atlanta: National Communicable Disease Center, 1962.

24. Edwards, P. R., and Ewing, W. H. *Identification of Enterobacteriaceae.* Minneapolis: Burgess Publishing, 1972.

25. Elek, S. D., Davies, J. R., and Miles, R. Resistotyping of *Shigella sonnei. J. Med. Microbiol.* 6:329, 1973.

26. Elek, S. D., and Higney, L. Resistogram typing—A new epidemiological tool: Application to *Escherichia coli. J. Med. Microbiol.* 3:103, 1970.

27. Elliot, S. D. Type and group polysaccharides of group D streptococci. *J. Exp. Med.* 3:621, 1960.

28. Ellis, R. J. *Quality Control Procedures for Microbiological Laboratories.* Atlanta: Center for Disease Control, 1974.

29. Farmer, J. J., III. Epidemiological differentiation of *Serratia marcescens:* Typing by bacteriocin production. *Appl. Microbiol.* 23:218, 1972.

30. Farmer, J. J., III. Epidemiological differentiation of *Serratia marcescens:* Typing by bacteriocin sensitivity. *Appl. Microbiol.* 23:226, 1972.

31. Farmer, J. J., III, and Herman, L. G. Epidemiological fingerprinting of *Pseudomonas aeruginosa* by the production of and sensitiv-

ity to pyocine and bacteriophage. *Appl. Microbiol.* 18:760, 1969.

32. Fincher, E. L. Surface sampling, application, methods, recommendations. In Berlin, B. S., and Hilbert, M. (Eds.), *Control of Infections in Hospitals.* Ann Arbor: University of Michigan, School of Public Health, 1966.
33. Fouty, R. A., Haggen, V. E., and Sattler, J. D. Problems, personnel, and proficiency of small hospital laboratories. *Public Health Rep.* 89:408, 1974.
34. Griffith, M. D. The serological classification of *Streptococcus pyogenes. J. Hyg.* (Camb.) 34:542, 1934.
35. Hamilton, R., and Brown, W. J. Bacteriophage typing of clinically isolated *Serratia marcescens. Appl. Microbiol.* 24:899, 1972.
36. Hansen, S. L., Hardesty, D. R., and Myers, B. M. Evaluation of the BBL Minitek System for the identification of *Enterobacteriaceae. Appl. Microbiol.* 28:798, 1974.
37. Hettiaratchy, I. G. T., Cooke, E. M., and Shooter, R. A. Colicine production as an epidemiological marker of *Escherichia coli. J. Med. Microbiol.* 6:1, 1973.
38. Huffaker, R. H. (Ed.). *Collection, Handling, and Shipment of Microbiological Specimens.* Atlanta: Center for Disease Control DHEW Publ. No. (CDC) 74-8263, 1973.
39. Ibrahim, A. E. Bacteriophage typing of salmonellae. II. New bacteriophage typing scheme. *Appl. Microbiol.* 18:748, 1969.
40. Isenberg, H. D., Scherber, J. S., and Cosgrove, J. O. Clinical laboratory evaluation of the further improved Enterotube and Encise II. *J. Clin. Microbiol.* 2:139, 1975.
41. Kallings, L. O., Lindberg, A. A., and Sjöberg, L. Phage typing of *Shigella sonnei. Arch. Immunol. Ther. Exp.* (Warsz.) 16:280, 1968.
42. Kiehn, T. E., Brennan, K., and Ellner, P. D. Evaluation of the Minitek System for identification of *Enterobacteriaceae. Appl. Microbiol.* 28:668, 1974.
43. Kunin, C. M. *Detection, Prevention, and Management of Urinary Tract Infections.* London: Kimpton, 1974.
44. Kunin, C. M., Tupasi, T., and Craig, W. A. Use of antibiotics. *Ann. Intern. Med.* 79:555, 1973.
45. Lancefield, R. C. Serological differentiation of specific types of bovine hemolytic streptococci (group B). *J. Exp. Med.* 59:441, 1934.
46. Maki, D. G., Rhame, F. S., Mackel, D. C., and Bennett, J. V. Nationwide epidemic of septicemia caused by contaminated intravenous products. *Am. J. Med.* 60:471, 1976.
47. Marsik, F. J., and Parisi, J. T. Bacteriophage types and O antigen groups of *Escherichia coli* from urine. *Appl. Microbiol.* 22:26, 1971.

48. Morris, G. K., and Wells, J. G. Colicin typing of *Shigella sonnei. Appl. Microbiol.* 27:312, 1974.
49. Murray, P. R., and Washington, J. A. Microscopic and bacteriologic analysis of expectorated sputum. *Mayo Clin. Proc.* 50:339, 1975.
50. National Committee for Clinical Laboratory Standards. *Performance Standards for Antimicrobial Disc Susceptibility Tests.* Villanova, Pa.: National Committee for Clinical Laboratory Standards, 1975.
51. Oonagh, T., and Thomson, E. J. An evaluation of three methods of typing organisms of the genus *Proteus. J. Clin. Pathol.* 25:69, 1972.
52. Rhoden, D. L., Tomfohrde, K. M., Smith, P. B., and Balows, A. Auxotab—A device for identifying enteric bacteria. *Appl. Microbiol.* 25:284, 1973.
53. Rhoden, D. L., Tomfohrde, K. M., Smith, P. B., and Balows, A. Evaluation of the improved Auxotab 1 System for identifying *Enterobacteriaceae. Appl. Microbiol.* 26:215, 1973.
54. Scheckler, W. E., Garner, J. S., Kaiser, A. B., and Bennett, J. V. Prevalence of infections and antibiotic usage in eight community hospitals. In Brachman, P. S., and Eickhoff, T. C. (Eds.), *Proceedings of the National Conference of Nosocomial Infections.* Chicago: American Hospital Association, 1971.
55. Schmidt, W. C., and Jefferies, C. D. Bacteriophage typing of *Proteus mirabilis, Proteus vulgaris,* and *Proteus morganii. Appl. Microbiol.* 27:47, 1974.
56. Schneierson, S. S., and Armsterdam, D. A manual punch card system for recording, filing, and analyzing antibiotic sensitivity test results. *Am. J. Clin. Pathol.* 47:818, 1967.
57. Segura, J. W., Kelalis, P. P., Martin, W. J., and Smith, L. H. Anaerobic bacteria in the urinary tract. *Mayo Clin. Proc.* 47:30, 1972.
58. Shoji, K. T., Axnick, K., and Rytel, M. W. Infections and antibiotic use in a large municipal hospital 1970–1972. *Health Lab. Sci.* 11:283, 1974.
59. Sielaff, B. H., Johnson, E. A., and Matsen, J. M. Computer-assisted bacterial identification utilizing antimicrobial susceptibility profiles generated by Autobac 1. *J. Clin. Microbiol.* 3:105, 1976.
60. Sjöberg, L., and Lindberg, A. A. Phage typing of *Pseudomonas aeruginosa. Acta Pathol. Microbiol. Scand.* 74:61, 1968.
61. Smith, P. B. Bacteriophage typing of *Staphylococcus aureus.* In Cohen, J. O. (Ed.), *The Staphylococci.* New York: Wiley Interscience, 1972.

62. Smith, P. B., Rhoden, D. L., and Tomfohrde, K. M. Evaluation of the Pathotec Rapid I-D System for identification of *Enterobacteriaceae*. *J. Clin. Microbiol.* 1:359, 1975.

63. Smith, P. B., Tomfohrde, K. M., Rhoden, D. L., and Balows, A. Evaluation of the modified R/B System for identification of *Enterobacteriaceae*. *Appl. Microbiol.* 22:928, 1971.

64. Smith, P. B., Tomfohrde, K. M., Rhoden, D. L., and Balows, A. API System: A multitube micro-method for identification of *Enterobacteriaceae*. *Appl. Microbiol.* 24:449, 1972.

65. Steinhauer, B. W., Eickhoff, T. C., Kislak, J. W., and Finland, M. The *Klebsiella-Enterobacter-Serratia* division. *Ann. Intern. Med.* 65:1163, 1966.

66. Swift, H. F., Wilson, A. T., and Lancefield, R. C. Typing hemolytic streptococci by M precipitin reactions in capillary pipettes. *J. Exp. Med.* 78:127, 1943.

67. *Technical Methods and Procedures* (6th ed.). Washington, D.C.: American Association of Blood Banks, 1974.

68. Thornsberry, C. The agar diffusion antimicrobial susceptibility test. In Balows, A. (Ed.), *Current Techniques for Antibiotic Suscepti-bility Testing*. Springfield, Ill.: Charles C Thomas, 1974.

69. Van Scoy, R. E. Bacterial sputum cultures: A clinician's reinterpretation. *Mayo Clin. Proc.* 52:39, 1977.

70. Verhoef, J., vanBoven, C. P. A., and Winkler, K. C. Phage-typing of coagulase-negative staphylococci. *J. Med. Microbiol.* 5:9, 1972.

71. Virginia Polytechnic Institute and State University Anaerobe Laboratory. *Outline of Clinical Methods in Anaerobic Bacteriology*. (2d ed.). Blacksburg, Va.: Virginia Polytechnic Institute, 1970.

72. Washington, J. A. Utilization of microbiologic data. *Hum. Pathol.* 6:267, 1975.

73. Weinstein, R. A., Bauer, F. W., Hoffman, R. D., Tyler, P. G., Anderson, R. L., and Stamm, W. E. Factitious meningitis. *J.A.M.A.* 233:878, 1975.

74. Weinstein, R. A., Stamm, W. E., and Anderson, R. L. Early detection of false-positive acid-fast smears. *Lancet* 2:174, 1975.

75. Wilkinson, H. W., and Eagon, R. G. Type specific antigens of group B type Ic streptococci. *Infect. Immun.* 4:596, 1971.

76. Zeman, B. T., Pike, M., and Samet, C. The antibiotic utilization committee. *Hospitals* 48:73, 1974.

9

Isolation Policies and Procedures

Julia S. Garner and Philip S. Brachman

Recommendations for isolation policy and procedures for patients with communicable diseases were included for the first time in hospital handbooks and nursing textbooks in the United States in 1877, when a hospital handbook recommended placing patients with communicable diseases in isolation huts [5]. Patients with communicable diseases were segregated into separate facilities, but problems with cross-infection soon resulted because the infected patients were not separated from each other according to their disease, and few, if any, aseptic procedures were practiced. To combat the problems of cross-infection, communicable disease hospitals as early as 1889 gradually began to isolate groups of patients by setting aside a floor or ward for housing patients with similar communicable diseases [2] and by putting into practice the aseptic procedures recommended in the nursing textbooks published from 1890 to 1900 [5].

In 1910 isolation practices in the United States were altered by the introduction of the cubicle system for isolating individual patients [2]. Under the cubicle system, patients in multiple-bed wards were managed for the first time as if they were in a room occupied solely by themselves; separate gowns were used by hospital personnel, who washed their hands with antiseptic solutions after contact with patients and disinfected objects contaminated by the patients. The nursing procedures used with the cubicle system to prevent transmission of pathogenic organisms to other patients or personnel became known as *barrier nursing*. The use of the cubicle system of isolation and barrier nursing spread rapidly not only to communicable disease hospitals, but also to pediatric and general hospital wards.

Within the past 20 years, further changes in isolation practices have occurred in the United States. The general contagious disease hospitals and wards gradually began to close in the 1950s, and patients with communicable diseases were provided care in the general hospital setting. Furthermore, in the mid-1960s, tuberculosis hospitals also began to close as general hospital or outpatient treatment became popular for patients with tuberculosis. Thus, in the 1970s, we find with few exceptions that patients needing isolation are housed in the general hospital on the ward to which they were admitted, either in a specially designed, single isolation room or in a regular, single or multiple-patient room. The Center for Disease Control's *Isolation Techniques for Use in Hospitals* [1], a detailed manual of isolation procedures that can be applied in small community hospitals with limited resources as well as in large metropolitan, university-associated medical centers, has facilitated the management of patients with any communicable disease. The recommendations presented here reflect the procedures outlined in that publication, which should be consulted for specific details not covered in this chapter.*

Strategies for Isolation

Isolation policies and procedures are established to prevent transmission of infectious agents from patients to other patients, hospital personnel, or visitors; protective isolation techniques are applied to protect highly susceptible patients from other patients, hospital personnel, or visitors. In speaking of "isolation," we are using the word in its broadest sense, that is, the prevention of the spread of an infectious agent from an infected person to another person. The spectrum of possible isolation techniques ranges from the most to the least demanding. The most stringent isolation strategy is that of strict isolation for all patients with any infectious disease. A second strategy would be to identify the specific needs for maintaining isolation for each specific disease and then group those diseases that demand identical actions; this would result in 20 to 30 different categories of isolation. Another strategy would be to develop a limited number of categories of isolation based upon mode of transmission and group the diseases with similar isolation requirements into these categories, making neces-

* For sale by Superintendent of Documents, U.S. Government Printing Office, Washington, D.C. 20402. Price $2.10; Supt. Docs. Stock #017-023-00094-2.

sary compromises in order to accommodate all the diseases into the limited number of categories. The least stringent isolation technique (or mechanism of preventing the spread of infectious agents) is to have no specific isolation precautions other than hand-washing between patient contacts.

The first method has the advantage of being a single system; thus, the staff would have little difficulty in remembering what actions and procedures are necessary in order to practice isolation. Theoretically, it presents less difficulty in maintaining isolation than the other methods outlined. Properly applied, it would prevent the transmission of all infectious diseases. Its disadvantages, however, are that most patients would be greatly over-isolated, it would increase the cost of isolation as well as the difficulties in patient care, and it would tend to dissuade attending and nursing staffs from ministering to the needs of the patient. It would also increase the number of patients that might have psychologic problems as a result of being isolated under the stringent procedures of strict isolation. The great disparity between the precautions being practiced and those necessary for the prevention of transmission would tend to erode staff compliance with implementing the recommended techniques.

The last strategy—that is, no specific isolation techniques except hand-washing—has the advantages of low cost, ease of application, and minimal psychological trauma to the patient. These advantages, however, would be overshadowed by not meeting the purpose of isolation, and thus the risk of nosocomial infections would be increased.

The two strategies that involve categories of isolation are the most practiced methods. The first of these—that is, instituting the isolation procedures necessary to control the spread of each infection according to its own specific epidemiologic characteristics—would result in an inordinately large number of categories of isolation. Although it incorporates specific methods of preventing the spread of each disease, it would be an awkward system to enforce because of the many different specific categories. It would increase the cost of practicing isolation, be difficult to enforce, and make it necessary for the staff to constantly review individual techniques.

The best strategy, therefore, is to develop a limited number of categories of isolation and group the diseases according to how they are transmitted. The advantages of this strategy are the limited number of different isolation categories, the ease of educating the staff in isolation techniques, and the ease of administration. Its only disadvantage is that in some instances, a preventive measure not related to the transmission of a particular disease would be recommended; however, this minor inconvenience is necessary in order to reduce the number of categories to a minimum. Any extraneous isolation procedure errs on the side of conservatism. This disadvantage is outweighed by the convenience resulting from the limited number of categories. Other advantages to using categories of isolation rather than a single, "strict isolation" system include the following:

1. *Release of private rooms.* By using a private room for patients with only certain communicable diseases, private rooms are released for patients who need them for other reasons. Moreover, some hospitals have a shortage of private rooms and often must use multiple-bed rooms to house a single isolation patient. Thus, more efficient room utilization can be accomplished by using categories of isolation.

2. *Saving of supplies.* By using gowns, masks, gloves, and other supplies only when these requirements closely correspond to needs based on the epidemiology of the disease, supplies and money are saved. Most hospitals have limited supplies, particularly of gowns; shortages may deprive staff of the use of these materials when they are really needed.

3. *Better care for isolation patients.* The excessive donning of gowns, masks, and gloves wastes time, is inconvenient, and may discourage the hospital staff from seeing the patient and giving the best care. Moreover, solitude deprives the patient of normal social relationships and may be psychologically injurious, especially for children. All activities that discourage proper patient contact should be held to the minimum.

4. *Greater acceptance of isolation procedures by hospital personnel, especially physicians.* It is not unreasonable to expect a physician to reject the details of a policy of stringent isolation for a patient when the physician knows that the epidemiologic nature of the disease and the mode of transmission do not warrant such extreme measures. When isolation is practical and the requirements closely correlate with needs dictated by factual epidemiologic and microbiologic data rather than by ritual, physicians as well as other hospital personnel show greater acceptance and conformity to the procedures.

Isolation Categories

We recommend the following categories of isolation for patients with infectious diseases: strict isolation, respiratory isolation, enteric precautions, wound and skin precautions, discharge precautions, and blood precautions; for noninfected patients who have seriously impaired resistance, we recommend protective isolation. The term "isolation" is used in general when a private room is indicated; the term "precaution" is used when a private room is optional or not indicated. The specifications for room, gown, mask, gloves, and hand-washing for each category of isolation are listed below:

1. Strict isolation:
   A. Private room necessary; door must be kept closed.
   B. Gowns must be worn by all persons entering room.
   C. Masks must be worn by all persons entering room.
   D. Hands must be washed on entering and leaving room.
   E. Gloves must be worn by all persons entering room.
   F. Articles must be discarded, or wrapped before being sent to Central Supply for disinfection or sterilization.
2. Respiratory isolation:
   A. Private room necessary; door must be kept closed.
   B. Gowns not necessary.
   C. Masks must be worn by any person en-

tering room unless that person is not susceptible to the disease.

D. Hands must be washed on entering and leaving room.

E. Gloves are not necessary.

F. Articles contaminated with secretions must be disinfected or discarded.

3. Enteric precautions:

A. Private room necessary for children only.

B. Gowns must be worn by all persons having direct contact with patient.

C. Masks are not necessary.

D. Hands must be washed on entering and leaving room.

E. Gloves must be worn by all persons having direct contact with the patient or with articles contaminated with fecal material.

F. Special precautions are necessary for articles contaminated with urine and feces; articles must be disinfected or discarded.

4. Wound and skin precautions:

A. Private room is desirable.

B. Gowns must be worn by all persons having direct contact with infected wound.

C. Masks are not necessary except during dressing changes.

D. Hands must be washed on entering and leaving room.

E. Gloves must be worn by all persons having direct contact with infected area.

F. Special precautions are necessary for articles such as instruments, dressings, and linen.

5. Discharge precautions:

A. Private room is not necessary.

B. Gowns are not necessary.

C. Masks are not necessary.

D. Hands must be washed before and after patient contact.

E. Gloves desirable but optional.

F. Articles contaminated with discharges must be disinfected or discarded.

6. Blood precautions:

A. Private room is not necessary.

B. Gowns are not necessary.

C. Masks are not necessary.

D. Hands must be washed before and after patient contact.

E. Gloves for contact with blood.

F. Used needles and syringes must be disinfected or discarded.

G. Blood specimens should be labeled.

7. Protective isolation:

A. Private room is necessary; door must be kept closed.

B. Gowns must be worn by all persons entering room.

C. Masks must be worn by all persons entering room.

D. Hands must be washed on entering and leaving room.

E. Gloves must be worn by all persons having direct contact with patient.

F. No special precautions are required for articles.

The compromises that have been made in developing a limited number of categories are toward being overly cautious. Diseases are listed by category of isolation in Table 9-1, and the compromises necessary to limit the number of individual categories may be noted in the table. The categories of isolation will be discussed individually.

Strict Isolation

This category is designed to prevent the transmission of highly communicable, often rapidly fatal, and usually rare diseases that are easily spread by direct contact with the patient, by the airborne route, or by indirect contact with inanimate articles that have become contaminated from contact with the patient. In addition to the specifications listed above, personnel who provide care for patients with diphtheria and smallpox should be immune by maintaining up-to-date vaccination status against these diseases. Those attending patients with congenital rubella syndrome should either have had rubella or have been immunized against rubella.

Respiratory Isolation

This category is designed to prevent the spread of organisms by the airborne route or by droplets. Additionally, some of the organisms responsible for illnesses listed in this category (specifically measles and rubella) are infrequently spread by indirect contact with freshly contaminated articles. In addition to the specifications listed above for this category, a room with suitable ventilation is required for patients with tuberculosis. Moreover, unless vaccination is contraindicated, personnel working on pediatric units who have not had mumps, measles, and rubella should be vaccinated if they have no evidence of having protective antibody levels. Furthermore, special attention should be given to preventing pregnant staff members who are susceptible to rubella from working in the newborn nursery, because of the possibility of fetal infections with the subsequent development of congenital rubella syndrome.

Enteric Precautions

These precautions are designed to prevent the spread of diseases that can be transmitted through the fecal-oral route, that is, by means of direct or indirect contact with infected feces and, in some instances, with heavily contaminated articles. Control is dependent on strict attention to careful hand-washing after any patient contact, and especially after direct or indirect contact with the patient's excretions. With constant attention to proper hand-washing, gloves could be omitted; however, practical experience suggests the need for the additional barrier of gloves to prevent transmission. The patient should be instructed to wash his or her hands carefully, especially after defecating. Viral hepatitis (including types A and B) is included in this category because of the difficulty in distinguishing between types A and B on clinical grounds and the lack of diagnostic laboratory support in many hospitals. As laboratory support becomes increasingly available, however, it should be possible to identify patients with either type and thus institute the precautions specific for hepatitis A or hepatitis B. Additionally, other types of hepatitis should be included in this category if their specific cause is in doubt.

Wound and Skin Precautions

These precautions are designed to prevent personnel and patients from acquiring infection from direct contact with wounds and articles contaminated with wound or skin secretions.

Wound infections caused by gram-positive microorganisms—such as *Staphylococcus aureus,* group-A *Streptococcus,* and *Clostridium perfringens*—have traditionally caused more concern than infections caused by gram-negative microorganisms. However, *Escherichia coli, Proteus, Pseudomonas,* and other gram-negative microorganisms can be transmitted by the contact route and cause wound infections. The extent of the wound, the amount and nature of drainage, and the causative agent determine whether wound and skin precautions or discharge precautions (see below) are to be followed. A moderate-size wound infected with *E. coli,* for example, may need to be handled by wound and skin precautions, whereas a stitch abscess infected with the same organism can be properly handled by discharge precautions.

Discharge Precautions

These precautions are designed to prevent the direct spread of infection by oral, lesion, or fecal discharges in those circumstances where the likelihood of cross-infection from such sites is slight. Patients with diseases requiring discharge precautions need not be managed differently from other patients in the hospital, except when handling their potentially infectious discharges. Separate precautions are recommended for lesion and oral secretions and for fecal excretions, and indications for the use of each type of precaution are primarily based on the cause of a patient's infection.

Discharge precautions for lesions are designed to prevent the spread of infection by direct contact with wounds that have a small infected area and from secretion-contaminated articles. Basically, a barrier to transmission is interposed by the use of the "no-touch" dressing technique (i.e., not touching the wound or dressings with one's hands) when changing dressings on these lesions and by use of proper hand-washing procedures.

Discharge precautions for oral secretions are designed to prevent the acquisition of infection through direct contact with oral secretions. The precautions include attention to the proper disposal of oral secretions and careful hand-washing to prevent spread of infection.

Discharge precautions for excretions are de-

Table 9.1. Infectious Diseases Grouped According to Degree of Recommended Isolation

Category of Isolation	Private Room	Mask	Gown	Gloves	Excreta and Excreta-Soiled Articles	Blood	Secreta and Secreta Soiled Articles
Strict isolation:							
Smallpox	X	X	X	X	X	X	X
Anthrax, inhalation; plague, pneumonic; vaccinia, generalized and progressive, and eczema vaccinatum	X	X	X	X	—	—	X
Burn, skin, or wound infection, major, with *Staphylococcus aureus* or group-A *Streptococcus* that is not covered by a dressing or that has copious purulent drainage	X	X	X	X	—	—	X
Lassa fever, Marburg virus disease	X	X	X	X	—	X	X
Pneumonia (*Staphylococcus aureus* or group-A *Streptococcus*)	X	X	X	X	—	—	X
Diphtheria (pharyngeal or cutaneous)	X	X	X	—	—	—	X
Varicella (chickenpox); herpes zoster, disseminated	X	X*	X	X	—	—	X
Congenital rubella syndrome; disseminated neonatal herpesvirus hominis (herpes simplex)	X	—	X	—	X	X	X
Rabies	X	—	—	X	—	—	X
Respiratory isolation:							
Tuberculosis, pulmonary (including tuberculosis of the respiratory tract), suspected or sputum-positive (smear)	X	X*	—	—	—	—	X
Meningococcal meningitis; meningococcemia	X	X	—	—	—	—	—
Measles (rubeola); mumps; rubella (German measles); pertussis (whooping cough)	X	X*	—	—	—	—	X
Enteric precautions:							
Cholera; enterocolitis, staphylococcal; gastroenteritis (enteropathogenic or enterotoxic *Escherichia coli, Salmonella* species, *Shigella* species, *Yersinia enterocolitica*); typhoid fever	D	—	X	X	X	—	—
Diarrhea, acute illness with suspected infectious cause	D	—	X	X	X	—	X
Hepatitis, viral, type A or unspecified	D	—	—	—	X	X	X
Hepatitis, viral, type B	D	—	—	—	—	X	X
Wound and skin precautions:							
Gas gangrene (due to *Clostridium perfringens*)	D	—	—	X	—	—	X
Herpes zoster, localized	D	X*	X	X	—	—	X
Burn, skin, or wound infections, limited (including infections with *Staphylo-*	D	X	X	X	—	—	X

Table 9-1 (Continued)

Category of Isolation	Private Room	Mask	Gown	Gloves	Excreta and Excreta-Soiled Articles	Blood	Secreta and Secreta Soiled Articles
coccus aureus or group-A *Streptococcus* that are covered by, and the discharge adequately contained by, a dressing); plague, bubonic							
Burn, skin, or wound infections, major (except *S. aureus* and group-A *Streptococcus; see* Strict isolation), that are not covered by a dressing or that have copious purulent drainage; melioidosis, extrapulmonary with draining sinuses	D	—	X	X	—	—	X

Discharge precautions—Oral and lesion secretions:

Actinomycosis, draining lesions; anthrax (cutaneous); brucellosis, draining lesions; burn infection, minor; candidiasis, mucocutaneous; coccidioidomycosis, draining lesions; conjunctivitis, acute bacterial (including gonococcal); conjunctivitis, viral; gonococcal ophthalmia neonatorum; gonorrhea; granuloma inguinale; herpangina; herpes oralis; herpesvirus hominis (herpes simplex), except disseminated neonatal disease; infectious mononucleosis; keratoconjunctivitis, infectious; listeriosis; lymphogranuloma venereum; melioidosis, pulmonary; *Mycoplasma pneumoniae* pneumonia; nocardiasis, draining lesions; orf; pneumonia, bacterial, if not covered elsewhere; psittacosis; Q fever; respiratory infectious disease, acute (if not covered elsewhere); scarlet fever; skin lesion, minor; streptococcal pharyngitis; syphilis, mucocutaneous; trachoma, acute; tuberculosis, extrapulmonary, draining lesions; tularemia, draining lesion; wound infections, minor	—	—	—	D	—	—	X

Discharge precautions—Excretions:

Amebiasis (amebic dysentery); *Clostridium perfringens* (*C. welchii*) food poisoning; enterobiasis; giardiasis; hand, foot, and mouth disease; herpangina; infectious lymphocytosis; leptospirosis (urine only); meningitis, aseptic; pleurodynia; poliomyelitis; staphylococcal food poisoning; tapeworm disease (only with *Hymenolepis nana* and *Taenia solium* [pork]); viral diseases, other (ECHO or Coxsackie gastro-	—	—	—	D	X	—	—

Table 9-1 (Continued)

Category of Isolation	Private Room	Mask	Gown	Gloves	Excreta and Excreta-Soiled Articles	Blood	Secreta and Secreta Soiled Articles
enteritis, pericarditis, myocarditis, meningitis)							
Blood precautions:							
Arthropodborne viral fevers (dengue, yellow fever, Colorado tick fever); hepatitis (viral; type A, B, or unspecified); malaria	—	—	—	D	—	X	—

Note: Legionnaires' disease—insufficient evidence to categorize (see Part II, Chapter 15).
Key:
 X = recommended at all times
X = with direct contact
X* = for susceptible persons
 D = desirable but optional
X = with direct wound contact

Adapted from Center for Disease Control. *Isolation Techniques for Use in Hospitals* (2d ed.). Washington, D.C.: U.S. Government Printing Office, DHEW Publ. No. (CDC) 76-8314, 1975.

signed to prevent the acquisition of infection by direct contact with contaminated fecal or urinary excretions from patients with diseases considered to be less contagious than those listed under specific isolation categories. Control is dependent on attention to careful handwashing following any patient contact and especially following contact with the patient's excretions. The patient should also be instructed in the need for careful hand-washing, especially after defecating. In the case of acute poliomyelitis, only hospital personnel who have been vaccinated with poliomyelitis vaccine should have direct contact with the patient.

Blood Precautions
These precautions are designed to prevent the acquisition of infection from contact with contaminated blood or items soiled with contaminated blood. The specific precautions primarily involve handling needles and syringes soiled with contaminated blood with extreme care, especially while disposing of them.

Protective Isolation
Unlike the other categories of isolation that are designed to prevent transmission of disease from infected patients to other patients, personnel, and visitors, protective isolation—also known as *reverse isolation*—is designed to protect noninfected patients who have seriously impaired resistance to infection from exposure to potentially pathogenic microorganisms (including commensal microorganisms) as well as to other patients, personnel, visitors, or objects. Because these patients are significantly more susceptible to infections than other patients, they may benefit from an attempt to reduce contact with microorganisms if they are placed in private rooms and personnel and visitors are required to wear gowns, masks, and gloves. More vigorous efforts to exclude all microorganisms—such as using patient-isolator units, eradicating endogenous flora, and sterilizing food, water, and fomites—may be warranted for certain patients.

Card System of Isolation
A card system that is designed to give concise information about the isolation procedures essential for each category of isolation is a practical method of informing people about isolation policies and procedures. This can be

accomplished by printing in a standardized manner the essential information for each category of isolation on the front of a card; the diseases included in the specific category can be listed on the back of the card. In addition, the use of color-coded cards facilitates rapid identification of the different categories of isolation. The colored cards should be attached to each isolated patient's door, bed, medical chart, or all three. The use of cards that provide readily available and easy-to-understand instructions is particularly important, not only because of the rapid turnover of hospital personnel, but also because of the rapid turnover of various students, who may not have been oriented to the hospital's isolation policies and procedures. In addition to providing specific instructions, the cards should instruct visitors to report to the nurses' station for further instructions before entering the isolation room or its environs. The card system should not be used as a substitute for formal instruction. Formal instruction about isolation policies and procedures should be included in employee and student orientation to the hospital, provided on an in-service basis when the policies and procedures are changed, or given on an individual basis when poor performance is observed.

Implementing Isolation Policies and Procedures

Infection Control Committee Responsibilities
That certain patients need isolation is usually well recognized. What isolation policies and procedures to adopt and how to implement them in an individual hospital are often controversial subjects. For this reason, the Infection Control Committee should be responsible for determining the isolation policies and procedures for the hospital, promoting their proper use, and enforcing their implementation. The policies and procedures for isolation and the responsibilities and methods of implementing them should be established, if possible, by a consensus of all departments; they should then be written and widely distributed throughout the hospital. Moreover, if the policies and procedures are designed in accordance with

what can be realistically accomplished in the hospital, they can be implemented with more willingness and ease.

Many hospitals have reviewed the Center for Disease Control's *Isolation Techniques for Use in Hospitals* [1] and have determined that the policies and procedures outlined in the CDC manual are applicable and thus have adopted them. In other hospitals, the Infection Control Committee has used the CDC recommendations, other published materials, or both as guidelines and have developed isolation policies and procedures tailored to their individual hospital situation.

In addition to deciding on isolation policies and procedures to use in the general areas of the hospital, the Infection Control Committee should determine whether isolation of patients should be permitted in critical-care areas of the hospital (e.g., intensive-care units, recovery rooms, newborn nursery, and so on), and if permitted, what special precautions should be used. The Infection Control Committee should also regularly review the policies and procedures for isolation within these areas and keep them up to date with new research findings and changes in the hospital facilities.

Orders for Isolation
Ideally, each physician should be responsible for ordering isolation for his or her patient. If the physician neglects to order isolation, then a simple reminder on the part of the head nurse or infection control nurse may be all that is necessary. It is also the responsibility of the physician who has a patient admitted to the hospital to alert the admission office to the infectiousness of the patient, in order that necessary isolation facilities can be arranged at the time of admission.

In some hospitals, the nurse in charge of a ward is given the responsibility for isolating a patient suspected of having a communicable disease if the physician neglects to do so or is not available; however, this responsibility necessitates that the charge nurse be extremely knowledgeable about diseases and conditions requiring isolation. Since this may not be the case and may place the charge nurse in a difficult position regarding his or her future contacts with physicians, an individual with delegated power to order isolation (e.g., the infection control nurse, hospital epidemiologist, or physician representative on the Infection Control Committee) should be available to the charge nurse to act as arbiter empowered to place a patient in isolation. Anytime a patient is placed in isolation by someone other than the patient's own physician, the latter should be notified as soon as possible of this action.

The charge nurse also must see that the appropriate card is conspicuously displayed in the immediate vicinity of the isolated patient and that the necessary equipment for the appropriate isolation procedure is obtained in sufficient quantities so as not to discourage proper patient contact. It is also the charge nurse's responsibility to make certain that the nursing staff under his or her supervision understand the procedures and techniques involved.

General Responsibilities of Staff
In addition to the specific responsibilities outlined for the Infection Control Committee, physician, and charge nurse, all hospital staff, including students, should know the policies and procedures for isolation, comply with them, promote their use, and tactfully call observed infractions to the attention of the offender, either directly or through the offender's supervisor. The physician plays an important role in the successful implementation of isolation and accordingly must observe the proper isolation procedures; the physician's actions must teach by example. Carelessness on the part of the physician in adhering to isolation policies and procedures or an attitude of negativism concerning them will inevitably undermine the morale of the other staff, who feel that their own efforts are thus rendered futile. In addition, patients and their visitors have a responsibility for preventing the spread of infection. These responsibilities must be brought to the attention of each patient and his or her visitors by the patient's physician, the nursing staff, or both. Intelligent rules and regulations should apply to everyone, and there should be

no exceptions: "the chain is no stronger than its weakest link."

Facilities Needed for Isolation
Isolation Beds
The facilities needed for isolation on general hospital units will vary according to the type of hospital and the specific service. In a prevalence study of 6000 patients conducted by CDC in eight hospitals that collaborated in the Comprehensive Hospital Infections Project (CHIP), the four major categories of isolation —strict, respiratory, enteric, and wound and skin—were required for 2 percent of the patients [3]. The prevalence rates for isolation needs, however, varied from 1.6 isolation beds per 100 patients for community hospitals to 4.9 isolation beds per 100 patients for city-county hospitals. The study also revealed that the overall rate of 2 percent for isolation needs was not equally applicable to all hospital services. The prevalence of patients needing isolation by service on which they received care ranged from a high of 10.8 percent on pediatric to a low of less than 1 percent on obstetric and psychiatric services. Most medical and surgical patients required isolation at rates of 1 to 2 percent.

We would anticipate from these data that there is a need for one isolation bed for every 62 patient beds for the community hospital and one isolation bed for every 20 patient beds for the city-county hospital; however, less than half of these beds need to be in single isolation rooms. Similar recommendations for isolation facilities have been promulgated by the Division of Facilities Utilization of the U.S. Public Health Service (formerly the Hill-Burton Program); they recommend that single rooms for patients who need to be isolated because of infection should be provided at a rate of one such room for each 30 hospital beds in general hospitals [4]. For specialty health-care facilities (e.g., those for psychiatric patients), these recommended ratios may not be applicable. Thus, each hospital should determine the number of rooms needed for isolation in accordance with the policies and procedures for isolation, the patient population served, and the incidence of infection requiring isolation in the patient population.

Physical Facilities

If the hospital allows patients who require isolation to be admitted to critical-care areas of the hospital (e.g., intensive-care units, the newborn nursery, recovery rooms, and the like), then separate isolation rooms that include hand-washing facilities should be provided in each area. Large viewing panels in the walls and doors of the isolation rooms will facilitate care. Separate isolation rooms may be indicated in critical-care areas, particularly in epidemic situations, even though the specific category of isolation that a patient needs may not normally require a separate room. Experience has shown that in these crowded units (where numerous patient-care activities, some emergency in nature, are foremost in mind), routine hand-washing between patient contacts is not always practiced; thus, the prevention of cross-infection is extremely difficult. Accordingly, infected patients should be physically separated, if possible, from the noninfected high-risk patients if disease transmission is to be prevented.

When the hospital's facilities for isolation—either in general or in special-care units—are less than ideal or are limited due to epidemic situations, compromises may have to be made. If the personnel involved understand the basic principles of isolation, then adjustments to conditions, personnel, equipment, and physical arrangements can be accomplished in such a way as to minimize the risk of spread of infection. Under these circumstances, it is usually wiser and more rational to insist on the rigid enforcement of a relatively few important procedures, such as hand-washing, than to make ineffective efforts to carry out every detail of an elaborate technique.

References

1. Center for Disease Control. *Isolation Techniques for Use in Hospitals* (2d ed.). Washington, D.C.: U.S. Government Printing Office, DHEW Publ. No. (CDC) 76-8314, 1975.
2. Gage, N. D., Landon, J. F., and Sider, M. T. *Communicable Disease*. Philadelphia: F. A. Davis, 1959.
3. Garner, J. S., and Kaiser, A. B. How often is isolation needed? *Am. J. Nurs.* 72:733, 1972.
4. Health Resources Administration. *Minimum Requirements of Construction and Equipment for Hospital and Medical Facilities*. Washington, D.C.: U.S. Government Printing Office, 1974.
5. Lynch, T. I. *Communicable Disease Nursing*. St. Louis: C. V. Mosby, 1949.

10

Legal Aspects of Nosocomial Infections

R. Crawford Morris

In the past, legal cases based on nosocomial infections have primarily fallen into two main categories: cases regarding patients who acquired infection through blood transfusion (e.g., hepatitis B) and those regarding patients with all other infections, mainly staphylococcal. During more recent years, the number of legal cases has increased significantly and has involved almost all categories of nosocomial infections; some cases have come to trial but many have been settled before coming to trial. Space does not allow an analysis of cases involving all these types of infections. Accordingly, I will primarily discuss cases regarding hepatitis associated with blood transfusion and those regarding staphylococcal infections; these will serve as examples of the field of the legal aspects of nosocomial infections.

Blood-Transfusion Cases

Blood from donors who have hepatitis B may give patients who receive transfusions hepatitis. During the past several years, laboratory tests have been developed that make it possible to identify at least half the blood donors with hepatitis B infection. There still is a risk, however, that the blood recipient will develop hepatitis. Why, then, should a doctor give blood transfusions? The answer is provided by the doctor's rule of thumb that I use for the jury, that is, the benefit-to-risk ratio. The benefit of saving lives by giving blood transfusions to people so far outweighs the low risk of getting hepatitis B that one must take the risk. Commercial suppliers of blood still put a warning on the label of the bottle, "Despite the utmost care in the selection of donors, human blood may contain the virus of homologous serum hepatitis." When the only cases regarding transfusion-associated hepatitis B were decided in court, there was no known way to detect the virus in blood.

The legal facts in blood-transfusion cases are not so simple. For every sale of every product, the law implies a warranty that it is reasonably fit for the purpose intended. If there is a sale, there is a product; if there is a defect in the product, "strict liability" applies. If so, the patient does not have to prove negligence. He merely says, "I took your blood and I got serum hepatitis, which shows the blood was defective. You breached your warranty; pay me."

To avoid this harsh doctrine of strict liability, when there is no totally reliable test available to insure the purity of blood, many courts have resorted to the legal fiction that blood transfusions do not involve a sale of a product, but only the sale of a service to which warranties and strict liability do not attach. Some legislatures have passed statutes so holding. Accordingly, in such jurisdictions, the patient's only route to obtaining a settlement is to attempt to prove negligence, which is by no means an easy task.

The Supreme Court of New Jersey, for example, heard a case [9] in 1969 involving an operation and the transfusion of five units of blood. The patient contracted serum hepatitis. The hospital obtained four of the five units from Blood Bank A and one unit from Blood Bank B. Blood Bank A got two of its four units from individual donors and two from Blood Bank C. The patient sued Blood Banks A and B and the hospital, but not Blood Bank C. The trial court threw the case out, but the Supreme Court wanted it tried because Blood Bank A was engaged in business for profit. It paid $8 per pint to blood donors and charged hospitals $18. The hospital charged its patients $25. The hospital's charge was purposely made high in order to provide an incentive for blood recipients to have a friend or relative donate blood, which it then applied to offset the charge. The hospital said that this was to avoid having to purchase blood from commercial blood banks, which usually use indigent donors, frequently including unhealthy derelicts. It was not known if the hospital told the patient the reason for the higher charge, but the hospital never notified the patient of the inherent danger nor even told him of the warning of the disclaimer on the label placed on the bottle by the blood bank. "The issue is very important therefore," said the Supreme Court, which sent the case back to the trial court for

trial with instructions that a complete new record be made, including detailed testimony as to the availability of any "test" to ascertain the presence of hepatitis virus in the blood, and that the incidence of viral hepatitis associated with blood received from commercial blood banks and from other sources must be brought into evidence.

Drug addicts sell their blood because they need money. In addition to hepatitis—which is one of the most prevalent blood transfusion-transmitted diseases—addicts may transmit malaria parasites or bacteria such as *Salmonella*. Screening blood in the laboratory for the presence of hepatitis B virus has reduced the risk of hepatitis, but a risk remains. This risk could be further reduced by an upgrading of where commercial blood banks get the blood.

It is also not easy to establish proximate cause. One of my cases [14] involved a young lady who had had a hemorrhage and had gone into shock. She was given fibrinogen and four units of blood from a blood bank. She contracted serum hepatitis, and she sued my client, the laboratory that made the fibrinogen. She also sued the hospital and the blood bank. Under Ohio law, she had to prove negligence and proximate cause. She could not prove whether her infection with serum hepatitis was due to contamination of my client's fibrinogen or of the blood supplied by the codefendant blood bank, and the jury cannot speculate. Because of the difficulty of proving the exact source of the patient's infection, the patient settled the case for a nominal amount.

To win a lawsuit involving staphylococcal or any other infection, the plaintiff must prove that he or she got that infection *in the hospital,* that the hospital was negligent in allowing the plaintiff to contract any infection, and that this negligence directly caused not only the infection but any injury that stemmed from it. The patient's attorney may claim that the hospital violated its own rules on housekeeping, he may try to show there was cross-infection from other patients, he may try to prove there was an epidemic and the hospital did not isolate the infected patients, and he may say that some of its personnel were carriers. This is the sort of attack seen in the legal suits, and the defense against such suits is, of course, good house-keeping and good infection control. One of the problems in such cases is that not all nosocomial infections are preventable; certain ones will occur in spite of the performance of all the proper techniques, including all the appropriate housekeeping procedures.

Of concern is the fact that to run a hospital correctly, there must be rules, and hospitals set high standards for themselves. The patient's lawyer, however, can turn these rules against the hospital for the benefit of the patient, because there is nothing more devastating than being caught violating one's own rules; it is *prima facie* negligence.

Many monographs on infection control in the hospital have been published [2,3,6]. These are valuable works from the point of view of hospital management. The plaintiff's attorney, however, may ask, "Did you have positive-pressure ventilation in this operating room, and did you have negative-pressure ventilation in that?" He will go through the lists published in such books until he finds something the hospital failed to do. Ever since the *Darling* decision [7], defense attorneys have had to fight the set of rules of the Joint Commission on Accreditation of Hospitals [10]. Most hospitals are accredited today, which has its merits until the defense attorneys get in court. The plaintiff's attorney may then produce a copy of the Joint Commission's rules and go down the list to find one the hospital violated in order to make the jury think that the hospital did not do something that it should have done. This is a game of the courtroom. Defense attorneys know that hospitals have to have rules, but when the hospital drafts them or redrafts them, it should be practical, not idealistic. The hospital should not set impossible standards or unreachable goals for its personnel.

Staphylococcal Infection Cases

Concrete examples from the trials of actual lawsuits perhaps best illustrate such cases. In one nosocomial infection case [8], the medical facts were these: Patient A was in an auto accident and had multiple fractures of the left hip and pelvis. Patient A was then taken to a hospital, admitted, and put in a two-bed room with Patient B. Patient B was paralyzed from the waist down. On August 1, extensive surgery was done on Patient A's hip, and he was returned to the room in good condition. On August 9, Patient B complained of a boil under his right arm; the boil was treated with hot compresses. On August 10, purulent discharge came from Patient B's boil. On August 13, the discharge was found to contain coagulase-positive *Staphylococcus aureus,* so Patient B was removed to an isolation ward. That same day, Patient A's surgical wound erupted and discharged pus. A culture was rushed to the laboratory. The laboratory reported the same *S. aureus* organism. For 12 days, the nurses had gone from one patient to the other, ministering to their needs. Patient A sued the hospital.

Testimony at the trial was that the nurses had gone from one patient to the other. Until they knew that Patient B had a staphylococcal infection, no phage typing was done, only antibiograms. The verdict of the jury was $69,-839.97 for Patient A against the hospital. The Supreme Court of the state affirmed the verdict in these words:

> Crucial . . . question . . . did [Patient A] show by substantial believable evidence, that he acquired his infection from his roommate [Patient B]? Essential to this finding is proof that these two patients were infected with the same strain of *Staphylococcus aureus,* coagulase-positive. It is undisputed that cross infection between patients would be a medical impossibility unless it was of the same strain.
>
> Two tests identify . . . these bacteria . . . . [One is] the antibiogram sensitivity test . . . [and the other, the really sophisticated test, is] the phage [type] test. . . .
>
> The phage-type test is not [used in hospitals in this area], but is used principally by governmental and centralized agencies for epidemiological investigation, that is, to locate the sources of staphylococcal infections which threaten to reach epidemic proportions. . . .
>
> [The plaintiff's experts,] a bacteriologist from Sacred Heart Hospital, and a professor of microbiology from the University of Washington Medical School, attributed definitive qualities to the antibiogram sensitivity test, which [the hospital's expert] witness, head of the bacteriological labora-

tory for the Idaho State Department of Health, found lacking.

Experts whose opinions shaded strongly toward the antibiogram test agreed that, although it was employed as a therapeutic tool to aid the physician in deciding which particular antibiotic medicine to prescribe, . . . the test then became a strong one to indicate which strains of staphylococci were present. [The hospital's expert,] on rebuttal, testified to the contrary, however; he testified that . . . he did not believe that the sensitivity test gave a reliable basis for determining strains of *Staphylococcus.* [He] held to the opinion that the only purpose of the antibiotic sensitivity test was to aid the physician in determining the best antibiotic to use on a particular patient. His laboratories never use this test to ascertain a strain of *Staphylococcus.* In his opinion, the sensitivity test is unreliable in determining strains because it is subject to too many variables . . . [8].

The court held there was no evidence of cross-infection from Patient B to Patient A. Then the court said:

We do not have an inference founded upon another inference or conjecture, but rather strong circumstances pointing one way or the other from which the jury could and did find the ultimate facts [8].

In another case [11], K. G., a high-school graduate, entered the navy as a WAVE and was sent to a Naval Hospital Corps school for four months of nurses' training, including service in the pediatric ward handling sick children during her last two weeks of training. After graduation, she was given a physical examination—which did not include a throat culture—and was assigned to the defendant Veterans Administration hospital. On reporting for duty, she had no physical examination and no throat culture. She was assigned to the nursery for premature babies.

One month later, a staff sergeant's wife gave premature birth to a baby girl, A, who weighed 2 pounds 15 ounces. The baby was placed in an isolette in the premature nursery. Shortly after birth, baby girl A appeared jaundiced. The jaundice was progressive, and the baby became increasingly lethargic. At the age of four days, she was put on the critical list. Three femoral taps over a five-day period were made for bilirubin determinations. These taps

were discontinued because the jaundice gradually cleared and the baby appeared to be recovering. When the umbilical cord fell off, there was some redness around the navel. This area contained *Proteus vulgaris,* and an antibiotic, bacitracin ointment, was applied.

The physician in charge of the nursery testified that:

The nurses called my attention to the fact that the child had not been wiggling her legs as much as usual on the 25th [age 11 days]. . . . [On] Sunday morning the 26th . . . there was obvious swelling and warmth in the child's hips. She had fever. She had not had fever before, and it was apparently an infectious process [11].

The child was transferred on the 26th from the premature nursery to the pediatric department. There, both hips were incised, drained, and irrigated with an irrigation drain. The child was started on antibiotic therapy. Roentgenography confirmed the initial diagnosis of osteomyelitis involving both the right and left femur, the pelvic girdle, and the right humerus.

Culture and antibiotic sensitivity studies showed the material from the left hip contained coagulase-positive *Staphylococcus aureus* organisms that were sensitive to chloramphenicol and nitrofurantoin. The material from the right hip contained *Pseudomonas.* It was suspected that this was an overgrowth and that this material actually also contained coagulase-positive *S. aureus.*

As a result of these laboratory findings, nose and throat cultures were done on all personnel in the nursery, and all were negative except that of WAVE K. G., whose nose culture showed coagulase-positive *S. aureus.* These microorganisms were sensitive to chlortetracycline hydrochloride, chloramphenicol, oxytetracycline, tetracycline, and nitrofurantoin.

The disease was finally arrested, but baby girl A was left permanently and severely handicapped.

The U.S. District Court, acting as jury, held for the plantiff and stated:

The degree of care exacted of private institutions toward their patients is such reasonable care and attention for their safety as their mental and physical condition, if known, may require, and should be in proportion to the physical and mental ailments of the patient, rendering him unable to look after his own safety.

Of course, a higher degree of care is required of a hospital in caring for a child than an adult. . . . A premature infant is entitled to the highest possible degree of care, consistent with good medical practice, because of its precarious toe-hold on life and its helplessness [11].

The hospital had broken its own rule forbidding Corps WAVES to handle or minister to premature infants of the plaintiff's age and development; WAVE K. G. was asked to and did pick up the baby, change her diapers, transfer her to the cart to take her for feedings, and feed her.

The staphylococci from the child and WAVE K. G. were not phage typed, because of the alleged unavailability of that kind of testing in the area in 1961. Instead, sensitivity tests (antibiograms) were done. They showed that organisms from the baby were sensitive to chloramphenicol and nitrofurantoin, whereas organisms from WAVE K. G. were sensitive to these as well as to chlortetracycline hydrochloride, oxytetracycline, and tetracycline. The court observed:

[D]oes this mean that the two strains were different?

The Court concludes that they were not different. . . .

It is clear that there is no direct evidence, as opposed to circumstantial evidence, upon which to make a determination of the identity of the strain, or the method of actual transmittal to the child. Nevertheless, circumstantial evidence is competent to show both. . . .

The mere fact of infection is not enough to open the door to the awarding of damages, but when the admitted direct evidence is considered in light of the different means of transmittal about which all the doctors testified, then it can be seen that plaintiff has met the burden of proof [11].

Concerning accepted practice of the community not being equal to the proper standard of care, the court observed:

[T]he testimony of Dr. John R. . . . , Chief of the Department of Pediatrics at the Medical College . . . , has given the Court great concern.

Q. Now with regard to the testing at the Medical College Hospital, did I understand that at one time there was testing [culturing], routine testing of the personnel in that nursery?

A. This was put into practice before I took over charge of the service. . . .

Q. And then, as you said, you forbade this particular practice?

A. Yes. . . .

Q. And you would prefer not to know whether you had such a carrier on the staff in the nursery?

A. Right.

Q. Because if you knew about it, it might upset whether you were able to assign these people or not?

A. It would make it impossible for us to run the nursery.

Q. Do you feel that it is better simply to be in ignorance as to whether you have carriers working in your nursery?

A. Yes.

Q. You don't think it would be better to have this knowledge and then make a determination based upon the other qualifications of the person and whether they had any other signs of disease?

A. We prefer not to know it. That is absolutely correct [11].

The court would not accept this. Quoting from another case, the court said:

To relieve a member of the medical profession from liability for injury to a patient on the ground that he followed a degree or standard of care practiced by others in the same locality is, in our opinion, unthinkable when the degree or standard of care in question is shown to constitute negligence because it fails to meet the test of reasonable care and diligence required by the medical profession. To hold otherwise is to exempt one from . . . negligence . . . on failure to take a known precaution for the safety and welfare of a patient on the ground that others in the same profession follow a similar course [11].

Not all courts are unsympathetic to hospitals, however. In another case [16], a husband and wife and their newborn infant sued for injuries suffered because of a *Staphyloccocus aureus* infection that was contracted by the baby at the Methodist Hospital in Memphis, Tennessee, and transmitted later at home to the mother and father. At the trial, the verdict of the jury was $25,000 for the three plaintiffs against the hospital. The Court of Appeals set aside the judgment entered thereon and dismissed each of the cases. The Supreme Court of the State of Washington affirmed the dismissal of the Court of Appeals, holding that the baby acquired the *S. aureus* infection in the hospital and gave it to the mother who gave it to the father, but there was no proof of negligence or proximate cause.

The medical facts in this case were that the mother entered the hospital on February 28, 1958. The baby was born that day. The mother and baby went home on March 3. When they were taken home, the father noticed some rash and pimples here and there upon the body of the infant. In the course of some days, these became worse. The mother became afflicted, and some days later the father also became afflicted.

In the last six months of 1957, staphylococcal infections appeared frequently in and out of hospitals in Memphis. As a part of a program to improve aseptic techniques, doctors and hospitals began to take nose and throat cultures from hospital personnel in the early part of 1958. After the mother in this suit was discharged, some four to eight persons in the hospital were discovered to be carriers of *Staphylococcus.* Among them was an intern, Dr. H., who had examined the mother when she entered the hospital. There was no evidence, however, that he ever came in contact with the baby.

Mrs. W., a practical nurse with duties consistent there, appeared from time to time in the hospital with a boil. When that was made known to her superior, she was at once sent home and requested to remain there until her doctor had discharged her as having been "cured." She was in the newborn nursery for only three days in more than a year at this hospital. There was no evidence that the plaintiffs' baby was exposed to her at any time or that she was in this nursery during the baby's stay there.

A trained nurse, Ms. E., testified to certain conduct in the labor section that was not in keeping with aseptic techniques. Mrs. W. likewise gave testimony to that effect. All the evidence was that these were infractions of the rules of the hospital. None of the other many employees or doctors observed these violations.

In its opinion, the Supreme Court said:

The conclusion is inescapable that the acts to which these witnesses testified were occasional violations of the rules rather than the practice in this hospital. It must be recognized that some occasional violations of the rules of a large hospital employing a large number of people will occur without regard to how strict the hospital is in the enforcement of its rules. There is no evidence that any of these violations occurred during the time Mrs. Thompson and her baby were there. . . .

[E]very doctor testifying in this case, unequivocally stated that the aseptic technique, the care, skill and diligence used by the Methodist Hospital in its newborn nursery and in its entire obstetrical department were up to the standards prevailing in any hospital in Memphis and better than in some of them. . . .

The original plaintiffs in this case concede that their case is based upon circumstantial evidence. The circumstances hereinbefore stated do not, in the opinion of this Court, furnish any evidence of negligence on the part of the hospital at the time this baby was there. . . .

The plaintiffs principally rely upon certain rules and regulations designed to lessen, insofar as they could, the obtaining of this infection. . . . These rules are entitled, "Standard and Recommendations for Hospital Care of New Born Infants, Full Term and Premature."

[T]hese rules and regulations, if they could be absolutely followed, present a hospital Utopia. . . . [N]o hospital of the usual endowments, funds and facilities could possibly comply with these rules. Nor is it necessary to do so.

By way of extreme illustration, it is shown that at the Methodist Hospital porters enter certain portions of the obstetrical department for the purpose of taking out bags of soiled linen. These bags are too heavy for the nurses to handle. One of the personnel of the hospital called as a witness for the plaintiffs was asked by the plaintiffs this: "Does the porter take a bath before he goes in every time?" meaning the entering of the delivery area from the labor room to remove the heavy cases of soiled linen. The reply . . . was that such porter "is garbed . . . in the proper things; that he puts on a cap, a mask and a gown and washes his hands when he goes in." Obviously it would be impossible in the average hospital to make such a requirement of the porter. Many other such recommendations are contained in [the] book of rules.

[S]ome eight to ten babies are born in this hospital each day. . . . [B]abies remain there for some four to five days. [I]t would mean that always there are from thirty-two to forty babies in the newborn nursery at a time. The practice in this hospital was to carry the babies for feeding six times a day in a vehicle known as a carrier. Each baby was separated from the other in this carrier by a partition which is at least several inches above the body of each baby. One of the recommendations of [the] book of regulations is that each baby should be carried separately to its mother by a nurse, who returns and washes her hands, etc. and then carries another baby to its mother, with same procedure followed each time. This would require some 240 to 300 trips the nurses would have to take each day for this one service alone. It is obviously impractical. The proof shows, without dispute, that this hospital does not have the personnel to carry out such procedure and could not obtain that many nurses, considering the shortage which exists, and assuming it could be financially afforded in the average hospital [16].

Fortunately, this court is cognizant of the practicalities of hospital life, namely, what will the personnel tolerate and what are the human limitations? Personnel are unable to follow too many restrictions.

In yet another case [15], the patient suffered a fracture of the knee in a traffic accident. He was taken to a Denver hospital, where he received emergency treatment. Later, he was taken to a private hospital, where the defendant, an orthopedic surgeon, undertook his care and treatment. Upon examination, the injury was diagnosed as a closed and partially dislocated fracture of the left femur with subluxation and fragmentation. A closed reduction of the fracture was performed and a cast applied. A few days later, roentgenographic examination revealed that the reduction was lost. The surgeon then performed an open surgical procedure in which the bone fragments were brought together with pins and screws, and a new cast was applied. Antibiotics were administered as a preventive measure for six days and then discontinued. Twelve days after the operation, a spot appeared on the cast. The cast was opened, and it was observed that the operative area was infected. Culture specimens were taken, and antibiotic therapy was instituted. The following day, a diagnosis of staphylococcal infection was made on the basis of the culture studies. Treatment was administered. About two weeks later, roentgenograms revealed osteomyelitis in the bone joint. The osteomyelitis had severely and permanently damaged the plaintiff's leg.

The plaintiff and the defendant were the only witnesses at the trial. The doctor stated that he did not know the source of the staphylococcal infection and the subsequent osteomyelitis. He also stated that such conditions are recognized complications that sometimes follow surgery even though the surgeon has followed accepted surgical practices.

The patient sued his surgeon. At the trial, the patient produced no expert witnesses and relied on the doctrine of *res ipsa loquitur*. The trial court gave judgment in favor of the surgeon. This judgment was affirmed on appeal by the Court of Appeals, which observed:

[T]he mere fact that a patient develops an infection in the area under treatment does not raise a presumption or inference of negligence on the part of the attending physician. The mere presence of infection following an operation is not prima facie evidence of negligence [15].

In another similar case [12], however, the patient prevailed against her orthopedic surgeon but not against the hospital, both of whom she had sued. The following medical facts were involved:

A hip fracture patient who claimed that a physician negligently allowed a Neufeld nail to penetrate the acetabulum won a suit against the physician in a California trial court.

The patient also alleged that during the postoperative period the physician allowed her to remain in a room with a patient who had contracted a staphylococcus infection. The woman contended that, as a result, she became infected and developed osteomyelitis of the femur. The hospital, which had also been sued, was found not liable.

The patient had sustained a severely comminuted intertrochanteric hip fracture. Her physician used a Neufeld nail and performed a displacement osteotomy to repair the hip. She alleged that the nail penetrated the acetabulum and that the physician was unable to remove the nail. After breaking two extractors, he elected to leave the nail until restoration processes occurred. The nail was later removed. The physician contended that nail penetration can occur even when due care is used.

The patient alleged that her roommate in the hospital suffered a staph infection and that she herself became infected 16 days after hip surgery had been performed. The infection allegedly resulted in osteomyelitis of the femur.

The patient claimed that, as a consequence of the alleged negligent care, she suffered a 1½ inch shortening of the right leg, severe external rotation, and knee problems.

The woman said that the physician knew the roommate was infected. She also charged that the hospital's physicians and nurses failed to follow proper sterile techniques.

Testimony indicated that the hospital was filled to capacity and that neither the patient nor the roommate could be moved. The physician and the hospital contended that when a hospital has no other available space, it is proper to place infection patients in the same room with other patients if correct isolation techniques are followed.

An orthopedist testified that the shortening of the leg was due to the nature of the fracture, that angulation was not warranted, and that ambulation was possible with a lift. He said that the patient would not need future surgery but might require physical therapy. She might have to use a cane, he commented.

The patient requested an award consisting of $8,000 for medical expenses, $10,000 for future medical expenses, and $80,000 for loss of future earnings. The jury held the physician liable for $100,000 but found in favor of the hospital [12].

Specific Problems

Medicolegal Implications of Clean-Air Systems

The question most frequently asked these days by orthopedic surgeons is whether our courts would consider it negligence in a malpractice lawsuit for a surgeon to perform a total hip-replacement operation without utilizing laminar-flow air conditioning in an operating room.

The medical problem, simply stated, is this: When a person walks, his leg articulates at the hip through a ball-and-socket joint. The "ball" is the head of the femur; the "socket" is the acetabulum that contains it. Until recent years, when a joint "froze" from arthritis or disarticulated because of fracture, dislocation, subluxation, demineralization, osteoarthritis, or whatever, orthopedic surgeons treated only the "ball" parts of the joint by removing it and replacing it with an artificial ball (e.g., stainless steel, titanium, or plastic). Except for smoothing the surface of the acetabulum, nothing was done about the "socket" half of the joint.

The first improvement in technique consisted of the use of metal sockets screwed or driven into the acetabulum, which were articulated, metal to metal, with the metal-ball prosthesis. These proved to loosen up over time, which caused articular failure. Next, plastics were used, yielding light, strong, nonirritating surfaces out of which to fashion artificial sockets. Then, acrylic resins came into use to produce glues, such as methyl methacrylate, of enormous strength that permitted a plastic cup or socket to be glued to the properly prepared acetabular surface.

The acrylic cement, however, is a foreign body, as is the plastic cup, and as such, it renders itself an "attraction" site where infection can settle. In addition, total hip-replacement surgery is complex, prolonged surgery, and there is much opportunity for the tissues to be exposed to infection. Hence, there is the apparent risk of infection; infectious agents are always present in some degree in hospitals and will localize to this site during or after surgery. Infections of this type have serious consequences, and if not carefully controlled, they can destroy the hip joint, making further surgery impossible.

The medical question is how best to control infection during total hip-replacement surgery so as to minimize this hazard of infection. The legal question, then, is: In light of this apparent and reasonably foreseeable risk, what does the duty of ordinary care require a surgeon to do to safeguard his patient against the consequences of such an apparent risk?

Medical experts—who consisted of three board-certified, very prominent, orthopedic surgeons in this area who have been performing this technique—addressed the question. The opinion of two of them is as follows:

There is no magic to laminar flow. The problem is not that the cement attracts the infection but that if you do get an infection in a patient who is undergoing total hip replacement and it settles in the cement area which as a foreign body attracts it, then you have a failure of the total hip replacement and there is nothing left to do for the patient. Accordingly, every conceivable effort must be made to hold infection to an absolute minimum.

Laminar flow is a help but it is not a necessity. What is a necessity is for the surgeon to discuss it with the engineer of the particular operating room in question, and to test that operating room at the time of surgery, to make sure that the bacterial fallout count is as low as possible. One of the things that must be done is to hold the operating time to a minimum. Another is to use all of the antiseptic devices being used in the medical community. Another is to be sure that the doors are locked and sealed so there is no movement of air about in the room. Another is to run the various bacteriological counts to make sure the fallout is zero. Another is to use an evacuation system of all exhaled air of all people in the operating room either by hooded helmets or a vacuum exhaust system. Another is to make sure the filters for filtering the air going into and out of the operating room are of excellent quality, etc.

We know of several lawsuits now pending concerning this matter. The makers of the glass cages for laminar-flow air conditioning urge that these cages be used in all cases, but the manufacturer of the methyl methacrylate cement does not say anything about this.*

In another expert opinion, Dr. C. stated† that Dr. D. of University of Z. Medical School told him that there is no proof that the use of laminar-flow air conditioning helps to reduce the danger of infection in operations and that on a recent survey throughout the country, Dr. D. found that laminar-flow air conditioning was losing its popularity among surgeons in this regard.

In December 1971, certain members of the Committee on Operating Room Environment met to consider the subject of special air-handling devices for operating rooms [1]. Various other individuals, including industrial representatives, participated in a review of opinions and data in the field. In recognition of the changing character of opinion as new data are accumulated, the committee developed the following statements with respect to special air-handling systems for operating rooms:

1.   There is no conclusive evidence at this time that laminar,‡ clean§ air flow, in itself, has a favorable influence on the incidence of surgical wound infections.

2.   At the present time, systems of air handling exist which, when properly used, may reduce the number of airborne bacteria in critical areas of the operating room.

3.   However, carefully controlled studies are required on the efficacy of clean air factors upon wound infection rates before the proper use of air handling systems for operating rooms can be defined.

4.   Therefore, all presently accepted surgical, technical, and hygienic methods of achieving surgical asepsis must be rigidly maintained regardless of the type of air systems employed.

5.   In new construction, it is advisable to give consideration to methods of air handling which may reduce airborne infection, such as the use of High Efficiency Particulate Air (HEPA) filters, air distribution, and changes per hour. This does not necessarily indicate the special equipping of one or more operating rooms for a specific type of surgery, but should be considered as standard for all operating rooms. Existing guidelines are available from a number of hospital planning agencies for this purpose.‖

6.   In existing surgical facilities, consideration should be given to the routine periodic study of the environmental bacteriology. Improvement in the bacteriologic environment does not necessarily mean the purchase of new air handling equipment. If new air handling equipment is deemed necessary, this need not necessarily include special enclosures nor laminar air systems of other types in operating rooms. Appropriate application of fundamental surgical, technical, and hygienic measures of achieving surgical asepsis may be sufficient [1].

Ordinary care toward his patient requires a surgeon who undertakes to perform total hip replacement to use that degree of care exercised by similar surgeons undertaking this procedure in the light of the foreseeable risk of infection. Clearly, such ordinary care requires careful knowledge and control of the operating-room environment to reduce this risk of infection to the minimum level acceptable to similar surgeons who employ ordinary care. Reduction of this risk to zero is not humanly possible. What must be done, however, is to take all reasonable precautions to reduce this risk to an acceptable level to a careful surgeon. This means that in terms of the benefit-to-risk ratio,

---

* Personal communication, February 3, 1972; reaffirmed September 22, 1972.
† Personal communication, June 1, 1972.
‡ "Laminar flow in surgical operating rooms is defined as air flow which is predominantly unidirectional when not obstructed" [1].
§ "Clean air in surgical operating rooms is defined as first air emitted from the final bacterial filter" [1].

‖ Center for Disease Control, 1600 Clifton Road, N.E., Atlanta, Ga. 30333; Office of Architecture and Engineering, Health Care Facilities Service, U.S. Public Health Service, 5600 Fishers Lane, Room 9-45, Rockville, Md. 20852; National Fire Protection Association, 60 Batterymarch Street, Boston, Mass. 02110.

the risk has to be reduced to that level which makes the expected benefits of the procedure worth it for the patient to take the risks left remaining. This, of course, is a matter of professional judgment; nonetheless, it must meet the standard of the law: ordinary care. Would a careful surgeon judge it so? What if different careful surgeons judge it differently? In the latter event, a court and jury must decide the benefit-to-risk ratio associated with ordinary care.

Laminar-flow air conditioning is a device designed to help reduce the risk of infection during operations and elsewhere. It is but one of many devices available to the surgeon to help reduce the risk of infection. Like all such devices, it has its proponents and its opponents. Whether to use it instead of or in addition to other such devices is—as we see it and believe the law will see it—purely a matter of professional judgment. On one hand, its use will not guarantee legal absolution; on the other, its nonuse or unavailability to the surgeon should not be a contraindication to the performance of total hip-replacement surgery. The medicolegal question is not whether or not laminar-flow air conditioning is used, but whether or not the operating surgeon uses ordinary care to reduce to an acceptable minimum the known risk of infection. What devices he employs to reduce that risk lie within the purview of sound professional judgment.

The legal danger to the doctor is that the laminar-flow air-handling system as a device to reduce the risk of infection during surgery is a procedure known to the state of the art today. If the system is available, not to use it is to run the risk, should infection later develop, of being found at fault by a court, jury, and the patient's medicolegal expert. This would seem to be a danger not worth running, unless valid reasons for not using the laminar-flow system can be substantiated. If it is as yet unavailable in a hospital, its unavailability per se should not be a contraindication to total hip-replacement surgery, provided that the surgeon can show he employed ordinary care to reduce the risk of infection to the patient to within acceptable limits by employing other devices just as reliable.

Because of the factor of hindsight (which is not the law but is, unfortunately, often the practical reality of life in the courtroom), if I were a surgeon contemplating total hip-replacement surgery, I would wish to employ all the devices now known to the state of the art, including a laminar-flow air-handling system if it is available in my hospital, unless I felt I could completely justify my failure to employ any one of these devices. The lawyer, however, becomes overcautious; "burn, bury, and cremate" is his motto. If this were to become the surgeon's motto, it might protect the surgeon in court; however, it would probably then be the patient who would be "burned, buried, or cremated," for most assuredly many such patients would die.

Surgeons should practice good medicine, not cautious law. If the surgeon has satisfied himself that he has done everything possible to know and to reduce to the absolute minimum the bacterial count in his operating room, and if, in his professional judgment, he has determined that the risk of infection has been reduced to a level acceptable in the light of the benefits hoped for (i.e., a level that would be acceptable to him if he were the patient under the same circumstances), then that surgeon is justified in proceeding with total hip-replacement surgery with or without the use of a laminar-flow air-handling system. The operation with its foreseeable risk of infection would then be, on the basis of its benefit-to-risk ratio, truly in the best interest of the patient whose only hope of becoming ambulatory again lies in total hip-replacement surgery. Furthermore, infection is only one of the risks of major surgery, all of which every patient who undergoes any major surgery, total hip replacement or otherwise, must assume. Ultimately, then, the patient's welfare is the test of good medicine. It is also the test of the law.

Medicolegal Implications of Codes and Standards

Various law bodies and professional groups promulgate standards or guidelines; some carry sanctions of their own, others are merely advisory. These codes and standards range from governmental regulations with force of law, on one hand, to mere suggestions or an institution's own self-regulating rules, on the other. A patient's attorney, if he is resourceful, will check all such regulations to see which he can attempt to enforce against the particular hospital that he is contemplating suing [13]. These may include federal laws and regulations; state laws and regulations; the regulations of the Joint Commission on Accreditation of Hospitals; the standards or suggestions of the American Medical Association, American Hospital Association, and American College of Surgeons, as well as such organizations for other specialties; and finally, all publications of the particular hospital itself, including its constitution, charter, bylaws, medical staff bylaws, nursing regulations, housekeeping regulations and rules, and so on. Any rule that he finds violated by the hospital in question is the one that he will attempt to introduce into evidence at the trial against the hospital. Accordingly, it behooves all members of the health-care team (1) not to promulgate idealistic rules that a practical hospital cannot enforce and (2) to attempt to meet at least the basic standards applicable to that hospital, which, at the minimum, include that hospital's own rules and regulations and, for an accredited hospital, the rules of the Joint Commission on Accreditation of Hospitals [10].

In handling a case involving such standards in the courtroom, the defense attorney's first line of attack is to persuade the trial court not to apply them nor to admit them into evidence on the ground that they are not admissible against the hospital for various reasons (e.g., not having the force of law, not being relevant to the particular hospital, and the like). His second line of defense is to show that they are generalized ideals that are unrelated to the practical situation confronting his hospital in its community and to explain away as best he can his hospital's failure to comply with them. In the event that the hospital has complied fully with such standards, however, the defense lawyer will want to introduce such standards into evidence to show that his hospital's compliance met the law's requirement of ordinary care [4].

How will the trial courts handle the problem of the admissibility of such standards? Although the result will vary depending upon the nature of the particular trial, the manner in which attempts are made to introduce such standards allows some basic legal observations. While all courts presumably will follow the legal requirement that the only test of the law that the defendant hospital must meet is that of ordinary care, many courts will allow the introduction of such standards into evidence for the jury to consider to show what is regarded as ordinary care in the hospital field, especially when the defendant hospital has accepted such standards either directly (as when applying for or receiving accreditation from the Joint Commission on Accreditation of Hospitals) or by implication (e.g., by belonging to an association promulgating such standards or by having key personnel, such as department heads, who do so). Such admission is based upon the tacit assumption by the court that authorities in the field of specialty favor the use of codes as a minimum duty necessary to safeguard the public and that such standards are voluntarily adopted by a professional or trade association as minimum requirements that its accepting members bind themselves to meet. Even when the particular defendant hospital has not adopted the standard in question, some courts might consider that almost universal acceptance of the standard in the trade is a basis for its admissibility. While the jury may consider all standards so admitted as evidence of what ordinary care would require, the jury is not bound thereby but may find that the duty of ordinary care requires more (or less) than what is called for by the standard. As shown in the examples previously discussed in this chapter, some courts have found some standards to be too unrealistic to be binding, although in general, the courts are apt to find such standards, when admissible, to be evidence of minimum requirements only.

Medicolegal Implications of a Hospital's Performing Surveillance for Nosocomial Infections

In the hospital's routine surveillance program for nosocomial infections, problems may arise concerning the protection of confidentiality, not only with respect to the identity of the patients involved, but also with respect to the personnel involved in the surveillance and the results of the surveillance themselves. The former problem can be dealt with by eliminating all names or other identification of the patients through the use of suitable case or code numbers when adverse hospital cases (i.e., nosocomial infections, adverse drug reactions, and the like) are reported to various agencies, for example, state health departments, the U.S. Public Health Service, federal drug agencies, or even medical-records abstracting services such as the Committee on Professional Health Activities (CPHA). The latter problem can be met to a limited extent in the same way. In addition, some states have passed laws granting confidentiality to hospital surveillance committees or their members (e.g., utilization review committees, peer review committees, tissue committees, mortality committees, and so on) and have even granted them civil and criminal immunity in connection with the proper performance of such activities. All such confidentiality, however, is subject to the balancing of the equities involved in each given case; the claimed confidentiality might be held to have to yield to the greater need for given evidence in a particular case (as, for example, executive privilege was held to have to yield to the need for evidence in a criminal trial; *United States* v. *Nixon,* 418 U.S. 683). Accordingly, any such reports of surveillance activities may become evidence in a given trial and should thus be recorded with extreme circumspection; they should never be released except upon court order, and then only after objections and argument have been presented in favor of their confidentiality.

Medicolegal Implications of Hospital Records Containing a Diagnosis of Nosocomial Infection

In the trial of a lawsuit, hospital records are important; they become the Bible of the trial. Good records help the defense, and bad records hurt the defense. For the hospital defense attorney to try to impeach his own hospital's records is a formidable task indeed. His attempts are met by his opponent's argument to the jury: "When the hospital was trying to help the doctor aid the patient in getting well, it wrote (so and so). Now that it is faced with accounting for what it wrote, it claims that its records are wrong." Accordingly, when diagnoses are written in hospital records, they should be written circumspectly and only by those fully qualified to make them. Too many lawsuits have been lost because the attorney has had to try to convince the jury that several residents' entries, such as "x-ray burn," "x-ray necrosis," "hip fracture from fall out of bed," and the like, were simply not the medical facts of what had occurred. The above rule holds especially for diagnoses that may contain an assumed answer to the medicolegal question of causation. The diagnosis "necrosis" simply tells one that the tissue has died, but the diagnosis "radiation necrosis" tells one much more: it tells not only that the patient's tissue has died but also that its death was caused by the x-ray treatment the patient was given earlier and by nothing else. To a lay jury, it virtually forecloses the hospital from thereafter disputing this causation, even though hindsight may prove that such was not the cause of the patient's necrosis. Similarly, the diagnosis of "nosocomial infection," when it is recorded and permitted to remain unchallenged by the hospital, is a finding that the patient acquired his or her infection while in the hospital. If such a finding has to be charted, it should be charted only after it is confirmed and with the understanding that if this conclusion regarding the cause of the infection should later prove to be incorrect, it will be most difficult for the hospital to prove it is incorrect to a jury in a malpractice lawsuit.

Medicolegal Implications of a Hospital's Furnishing Defective Products to Patients

If the defect in the product is such that the hospital either knew or reasonably should have known of it, then it is negligent on the part of the hospital to expose the patient to the product. In the absence of such knowledge, however, the hospital cannot insure the safety of the products it furnishes its patients and should not be held liable to the patient for harm inflicted by such products. Defects are classified as either patent or latent. A *patent defect* is one that a reasonable inspection would have disclosed; a *latent defect* is one that is not so observable. If the defect is patent, the hospital will be liable for it. If the defect is merely latent, however, the hospital should not be liable for it in the absence of notice or knowledge concerning the likelihood of the presence of such a latent defect in the product. Perhaps it should be here observed that a product that has a known potential to cause harm to a patient is not "defective," provided that this potential risk is disclosed to the patient and the patient assumes the risk. Thus, whiskey is not defective because it carries the potential harm of damaging the liver. Similarly, the possibility of acquiring hepatitis infection cannot, as yet, be excluded in all cases of blood transfusion. The duty of the hospital is to use ordinary care to select good products in the first instance, to inspect such products for patent defects after obtaining them, and to heed all warnings regarding latent defects inherent in that particular class of products. In the last case, the hospital's duty is not to use such products if it is possible to find substitutes for them, but if it is not, then the hospital must warn the patients fully about the risks involved in the use of such products for which there are no available substitutes.

Conclusion

Nosocomial infections, like death and taxes, are probably going to be with us forever, and so long as our present jury system prevails (though no one knows how long it will prevail without some drastic changes), there will be patients bringing lawsuits based upon nosocomial infections. The best defense will be to prove to the court and jury that the hospital and doctors were not negligent and that they used "due care" to minimize the potentially virulent organisms commonly transmissible within the hospital and to maximize the patient's ability to combat those organisms. The hospitals and doctors must minimize the chance and the duration of each patient's exposure to these infectious organisms and maximize the

patient's chances of recovery. If a jury can be shown that the personnel involved did all these things, the defendants should be a long way toward winning the case.

Unfortunately, certain new techniques of diagnosis and treatment that have been developed in the past ten years have increased the risk of inducing infection; the danger of iatrogenic infections is now greater. Investigators must reanalyze what is being done with these new techniques and equipment (e.g., the latest respirators, open heart-lung bypass machines, and all the rest). Is their use inducing more infection? If so, there is the duty to exercise "ordinary care" to combat this increased risk, and it will have to be met.

Also, hospitals face a dilemma regarding their rules and standards. Hospitals have to have them, but they may be used against the hospitals by patients' attorneys in malpractice cases. Thus, hospitals should be realistic about such rules and not ask more of personnel than is practical. On the other hand, good records of routine surveillance activities should be helpful in court as evidence of "good housekeeping" and thus may show that ordinary care has been exercised.

Concerning the causation of infections, the patient must prove that the alleged negligence of the hospital directly led to his infection and that without the hospital's negligent act, he or she would not have acquired it. In the future, "detective hunts" on the part of the plaintiffs and the defendants may become more sophisticated. Which is a "bad bug"? Is it masked by another "bad bug"? Is the real "bad bug" the "bug" underneath? Why does it do harm? Is the harm due to the hospital's negligence, or is it due to the patient's idiosyncrasy or to an unforeseeable, intervening event? In a recent study, for example, babies in a premature nursery were infected, and it was found that the only ones who got lung abscesses and died were on ACTH therapy [5]. The use of such therapy might not have made the difference in this case, but this study illustrates how sophisticated "detective hunts" may become regarding causation issues. Sometimes such hunts will help us, sometimes not: the more we learn, the more will be required of us.

To recapitulate, the test of good medicine is the patient's welfare; it is also the test of the law.

References

1. American College of Surgeons. Special air systems for operating rooms. *Bull. Am. Coll. Surg.* 57(5):18, 1972.
2. American Hospital Association. *Infection Control in the Hospital* (3d ed.). Chicago: American Hospital Association, 1974.
3. American Public Health Association. *Control of Communicable Diseases*. Washington, D.C.: The American Public Health Association, 1975.
4. Bledsoe, L. M. Introduction and Use of Standards and Codes for the Defendant. In Nordin, V. D., Sugarman, A. G., Rice, J. E., and Lemon, E. V. (Eds.), *Hospital Liability Law*. Ann Arbor, Mich.: Institute of Continuing Legal Education, 1968, pp. 203–212.
5. Brachman, P. S., and Eickhoff, T. C. (Eds.). *Proceedings of the International Conference on Nosocomial Infections*. Chicago: American Hospital Association, 1971.
6. Center for Disease Control. *Isolation Techniques for Use in Hospitals*. Washington, D.C.: U.S. Government Printing Office (DHEW Publ. No. 76-8314), 1975.
7. *Darling* v. *Charleston Community Memorial Hospital* (Sup. Ct. Ill., 1965), 33 Ill.2d 316, 211 N.E. 2d 253, cert. denied 383 U.S. 946.
8. *Helman* v. *Sacred Heart Hospital* (Sup. Ct., Wash. 1963), 381 P.2d 605.
9. *Jackson* v. *Muhlenberg Hospital*, 249 A2d 65.
10. Joint Commission on Accreditation of Hospitals. *Accreditation Manual for Hospitals*. Chicago: Joint Commission on Accreditation of Hospitals, 1976.
11. *Kapuschinsky* v. *United States of America* (USDC, D. So. Carolina, Charleston Div. 1966), 248 F. Supp. 732. (See also 259 F. Supp. 1 nine months later in the same year for opinion on damages.)
12. *Mershon* v. *McWhirter and Palomar Hospital* (Cal. Sup. Ct., San Diego, Co., Docket No. 309260, 1970). (Not officially reported; see *The Citation*, American Medical Association 21:182, 1970.)
13. Robb, D. A. Introduction and Use of Standards and Codes for the Plaintiff. In Nordin, V. D., Sugarman, A. G., Rice, J. E., and Lemon, E. V. (Eds.), *Hospital Liability Law*. Ann Arbor, Mich.: Institute of Continuing Legal Education, pp. 181–202.
14. *Schummer* v. *Cutter Laboratories,* et al. (Common Pleas Court of Cuyahoga County, Ohio, Docket No. 867146; unreported.)
15. *Smith* v. *Curran* (Colo. Ct. App. 1970), 472 P.2d 769.
16. *Thompson* v. *Methodist Hospital* (Sup. Ct., Tenn. 1963), 367 S.W. 2d 134.

11

Antibiotics and Nosocomial Infections

Theodore C. Eickhoff

The era of chemotherapy for infectious disease is now over 30 years old. These past 30 years have been marked by the continuous development and introduction of new and potent antimicrobial agents. Thus, the contemporary clinician has at his disposal a broad array of potent antibiotic agents of proved efficacy and sometimes significant toxicity.

During the past 30 years, significant changes have simultaneously occurred in the character of nosocomial infections. The available data strongly suggest that 30 years ago, "nosocomial infection" was generally synonymous with gram-positive coccal infection, most notably with β-hemolytic streptococci and staphylococci. During the 1950s, staphylococci—particularly those resistant to the antimicrobial drugs in common use, such as penicillin G, tetracycline, erythromycin, chloramphenicol, and streptomycin—emerged to cause epidemic infection in hospitals. For reasons that are still not understood, staphylococci subsided in importance as the major cause of nosocomial infection in the early 1960s, only to be replaced in importance by enteric gram-negative bacilli, enterococci, and funguses [26].

It is tempting to relate the changing character of nosocomial infections, so briefly sketched, to the sequential introduction of new antimicrobial agents and to impute a cause-and-effect relationship. No one can seriously doubt that antimicrobial drugs have had a profound effect in shaping the character of nosocomial infections, but such an explanation is greatly oversimplified and fails to take into account the enormous changes in the technology of medicine and the patterns of health-care delivery that have also taken place in the past 30 years.

In this chapter the way in which antimicrobial drugs are used in hospitals will be explored more fully, together with consideration of the effects of such drug usage on both the host and the microorganism. A conservative approach to the use of antibiotics for prophylaxis and therapy will be presented.

Antibiotic Usage in Hospitals

Data on the overall patterns of antibiotic usage within hospitals have appeared in the literature for little more than a decade. The general thrust of such data indicates that from one-quarter to one-third of a hospitalized population on any given day will receive systemic antibiotics.

A series of four prevalence surveys carried out at the Boston City Hospital during January or February of the years 1964, 1967, 1970, and 1973 provides interesting comparative data [54]. In 1964, 26 percent of patients in that hospital were receiving at least one systemic antibacterial agent; in 1967, the figure was 27 percent; in 1970, 34 percent; and in 1973, 36 percent of patients were receiving at least one systemic antibacterial agent. In the 1973 survey, 76 percent of patients receiving an antibiotic were considered to have an active infection at that time.

Scheckler and Bennett [73] reported on the antibiotic usage in seven community hospitals scattered throughout the United States; they employed a survey technique comparable to that used in the Boston City Hospital surveys. Twenty-four such prevalence studies carried out between November 1967 and June 1969 indicated that over 30 percent of patients were receiving one or more systemic antibiotics but that only 38 percent of patients receiving antibiotics surveyed in 1969 had recorded evidence of infection. Comparable results were reported by Roberts and Visconti [68] in a single hospital.

More recently, Kunin and co-workers [46] reported a study of antibiotic usage carried out in 1969 at the University of Virginia Hospital. During a three-month period, all antibiotic therapy given to patients on the medical and surgical services was reviewed by the infectious disease resident and staff, and the use of antibiotics in any given patient was judged to be appropriate or inappropriate according to the best judgment of the group. During the survey period, 27 percent of patients admitted to the medical service and 29 percent of patients admitted to the surgical service were given antibiotics. Among patients on the surgical service, 58 percent of the antibiotic therapy given was

for prophylaxis, whereas on the medical service, only 6 percent of antibiotic therapy given was for prophylaxis.

Inappropriate therapy was considered to include instances in which a different drug was thought to be preferable, the dose was considered inappropriate, or the administration of any antimicrobial therapy or prophylaxis was considered unjustified. In the reviewers' judgment, 52 percent of all antimicrobial therapy was considered inappropriate. On the medical service, 42 percent of all antimicrobial drug use was judged inappropriate, while 62 percent of all antibiotic therapy was considered inappropriate on the surgical service.

One might argue, of course, that the review group did not have the benefit of seeing the patients at the time the antimicrobial drug therapy was instituted or that the review group was biased against the use of antimicrobial agents. Kunin's recorded observations, however, correlate well with the day-to-day clinical experience of most infectious disease specialists. Such massive use of antibacterial drugs in hospitals, whether given for appropriate or inappropriate indications, has profound effects on both the hosts who receive these drugs and the bacteria exposed to them.

Antibiotics and Drug Resistance of Bacteria in Hospitals

Current problems of resistance of bacteria to antimicrobial drugs are in a somewhat more realistic perspective if we recall at the outset that in Paul Ehrlich's laboratory, trypanosomes became resistant to the drug p-rosaniline after repeated exposures [57]. Similarly, it was shown that pneumococci could develop "resistance" to hydrocupreine derivatives following repeated exposure [27]. In the mid-1940s, shortly after the introduction of penicillin G, it was recognized that certain strains of staphylococci elaborated a potent inactivator of penicillin and that penicillin G had no therapeutic activity in patients with infections caused by such staphylococci. This recognition surely came as a major disappointment but not as a total surprise. In the 30 years that have elapsed since that time, it has become abundantly clear that the major nosocomial pathogens are by and large those organisms that either are naturally resistant to clinically useful antimicrobial drugs or possess the ability to acquire resistance rapidly by one of several possible mechanisms. The best-known examples are the staphylococci and aerobic gram-negative bacilli, which together regularly account for the majority of nosocomial infections. Organisms that have thus far not developed significant resistance to commonly used antimicrobial agents, such as pneumococci and β-hemolytic streptococci, are occasionally the cause of focal nosocomial outbreaks; they are generally much less of a threat as nosocomial pathogens, however, at least in part a result of the fact that their drug susceptibility confers on them no particular epidemiologic advantage in the hospital environment.

Drug Resistance of Staphylococci

ORIGIN. The origin of staphylococcal resistance to penicillin G is likely to remain shrouded in mystery. It is clear, however, that penicillinase-producing staphylococci existed before the introduction of penicillin into clinical use. Eight of 13 strains of *Staphylococcus aureus* isolated from food-poisoning outbreaks before 1940, for example, were found to be resistant to penicillin G through the usual mechanism of penicillinase production [61]. Smith and Marples [79] reported the fascinating observation that penicillin was produced by a dermatophyte responsible for ringworm lesions in New Zealand hedgehogs and that penicillinase-producing strains of *Staphylococcus aureus* could be recovered from those lesions. Indeed, since penicillin is produced in nature by *Penicillium* species, it should not be a great surprise that certain microorganisms have evolved means of inactivating this compound; our recognition of this phenomenon in clinical medicine represents a relatively late event on the scale of biologic time.

TRENDS. In the case of *Staphylococcus aureus,* resistance to penicillin G appeared rapidly after the introduction of that drug, and by 1949, 40 percent of pathogenic strains of *Staphylococcus aureus* isolated at the Boston City Hospital were resistant to penicillin G [27]. By the early 1950s, 75 percent of pathogenic strains of *Staphylococcus aureus* from that hospital were resistant to penicillin G. Increasing proportions of staphylococci that are resistant to streptomycin, tetracyclines, and erythromycin were noted in succession within the first few years after each drug was introduced. By 1958, the 80/81 phage type had become predominant in many United States hospitals, and at the Boston City Hospital all these strains were resistant to penicillin; more than 80 percent were resistant to streptomycin, approximately 50 percent to tetracycline, and 10 percent to erythromycin. Of all pathogenic strains of staphylococci isolated from patients who had been in the hospital more than seven days and who had received any antibiotics, nearly all were resistant to penicillin, almost 90 percent were resistant to streptomycin, 80 percent to tetracycline, and almost 50 percent to erythromycin. In contrast, among strains obtained from outpatients or from patients at the time of their admission to the hospital, about 75 percent were resistant to penicillin, one-third were resistant to streptomycin, 20 percent were resistant to tetracycline, and less than 10 percent were resistant to erythromycin.

By the late 1960s, although the proportion of multiple-drug-resistant strains of staphylococci decreased somewhat, there was little overall change in the frequency of penicillin resistance among strains isolated from inpatients. There was, however, an increase in the frequency of penicillin resistance among strains isolated from outpatients; outpatient strains were almost as likely to be resistant to penicillin G as those isolated from inpatients [27].

Bulger and Sherris [15] reported a trend toward increasing sensitivity of *Staphylococcus aureus* over a nine-year period from 1959 to 1967 at the university hospital in Seattle. In 1959, only 15 percent of staphylococci were sensitive to penicillin G, whereas in 1967 one-third of staphylococcal strains were sensitive. In an extension of these studies, Plorde and Sherris [62] found that by 1972 the proportion of strains sensitive to penicillin G had dropped to 23.5 percent. Rather more striking, however, was the progressive reduction in the proportion of staphylococci resistant to four or more of six antibiotics. In 1959, 45 percent of

Staphylococcus aureus strains were multiple-drug-resistant as so defined, but by 1972, that proportion had dropped to 0.7 percent.

Thus, on the basis of data from both the Boston City Hospital and the University of Washington, it would appear that the frequency of multiple-drug resistance has declined among strains of *Staphylococcus aureus.* The underlying basis for these changes is not totally clear.

MECHANISMS OF RESISTANCE. In virtually all clinical settings, significant resistance to penicillin G in *Staphylococcus aureus* is due to the presence of an extrachromosomal element of DNA, a plasmid, that confers on the bacterial cell the ability to produce a β-lactamase enzyme that hydrolyzes and thus inactivates penicillin G. The evidence that staphylococcal β-lactamase is the almost universal mechanism of resistance to penicillin G is derived primarily from two readily demonstrable facts: first, small inocula of penicillinase-producing staphylococci are almost as susceptible to penicillin G as are penicillinase-negative strains, and second, penicillinase-negative segregants of penicillinase-producing staphylococci are just as susceptible as strains that apparently never possessed the ability to produce penicillinase.

Plasmid-linked resistance has similarly been demonstrated for tetracycline, chloramphenicol, kanamycin, neomycin, and erythromycin, as well as certain metallic ions. Of major clinical and epidemiologic significance is the fact that such plasmid-linked resistance may be transferable to fully sensitive staphylococci by the mechanism of transduction. Given the selection pressure of antimicrobial therapy present in a hospital setting and the ability of resistant staphylococci, under certain circumstances, to transfer plasmid-linked resistances to sensitive staphylococci via the mechanism of transduction, the scene was set for the emergence in hospitals of staphylococci that are resistant to penicillin G as well as to a variety of other drugs. That this indeed occurred is supported by the observations of Wallmark and Finland [88], who noted a direct relationship between the proportion of drug-resistant strains recovered and the type of prior antibiotic therapy of

the patients from whom those strains were recovered. Thus, the increased prevalence of resistant strains of *Staphylococcus aureus* was, at least in part, a direct result of the reduction or elimination of susceptible strains by antibiotic therapy, which permitted resistant strains not only to survive but to multiply and spread.

The mechanism of staphylococcal resistance to drugs other than the penicillins and cephalosporins is less well studied, but in some instances, the mechanism of resistance is known [47,71]. Low-level resistance to streptomycin is mediated by the production of an enzyme that catalyzes adenylation of the drug, but high-level streptomycin resistance is apparently the result of a ribosomal modification within the staphylococcal cell. Tetracycline resistance probably is a result of altered membrane permeability characteristics within the staphylococcal cell membrane. Resistance to both kanamycin and neomycin is mediated by an enzyme catalyzing the phosphorylation of the drug. Chloramphenicol resistance is mediated by the production of the enzyme chloramphenicol acetyltransferase. Resistance to erythromycin is mediated by modification of the attachment site at the level of the staphylococcal ribosome, which apparently prevents attachment of the drug.

METHICILLIN RESISTANCE. Naturally occurring methicillin-resistant staphylococci were first reported in Great Britain in 1961 [38] within a very short time after the introduction of the drug. Since that time, there have been numerous reports of the isolation of such organisms, particularly from European sources but from within the United States as well [47, 62]. Within a decade of the recognition of methicillin resistance in staphylococci, their epidemiologic and clinical importance was well established in Europe. In 1969, 5 percent of all staphylococcal isolates from eight hospitals in London were methicillin-resistant [60]. During the period 1967 to 1970, approximately 40 percent of nosocomial bacteremic strains isolated in Denmark were resistant to methicillin [37]. Kayser and Mak [41] in Zurich, Switzerland have reported that in some hospitals, up to 50 percent of staphylococcal disease is caused by methicillin-resistant organisms and that infection caused by methicillin-resistant staphylococci is almost universally nosocomially acquired.

In rather striking contrast has been the experience in the United States. Although isolated outbreaks have occurred, such as that described by Barrett and colleagues [3] at the Boston City Hospital, methicillin resistance has remained but a minor problem in the United States, and it was found in 1 percent or less of strains in this country during a survey conducted in 1970 [9]. More recently, however, beginning in 1975, there has been a disturbing increase in the frequency of identification of strains of *S. aureus* resistant to penicillin, to aminoglycosides such as gentamicin and tobramycin, and often to methicillin as well. These reports have come from the United States as well as Great Britain, and reflect both hospital outbreaks and an increased endemic level of identification [19,21,45,81,87]. Thus, there is no reason for complacency with regard to staphylococcal infection; rather, there is good reason to maintain close surveillance on antibiotic resistance patterns of this organism.

The mechanism of staphylococcal resistance to methicillin is of some interest, because there is abundant evidence that methicillin resistance is not mediated by the production of a β-lactamase enzyme [47,71]. The evidence that methicillin resistance in *Staphylococcus aureus* is not β-lactamase mediated is as follows: (1) methicillin-resistant strains produce no more β-lactamase than do most methicillin-susceptible strains; (2) the β-lactamase from methicillin-resistant strains is not different functionally or immunologically from that produced by methicillin-susceptible strains; (3) β-lactamase-negative segregants of methicillin-resistant strains are still methicillin-resistant; and (4) methicillin is not inactivated during incubation with methicillin-resistant strains.

A number of unique properties are common to virtually all methicillin-resistant strains of *S. aureus*. These include heterogeneous resistance to methicillin and all other penicillins and cephalosporins (whether the strain produces penicillinase or not), high-level resistance to streptomycin, and resistance to tetracyclines and sulfonamides. Virtually all strains can be

shown to produce enterotoxin B, and virtually all are in staphylococcal phage group III.

The precise nature of methicillin resistance is as yet uncertain, but the evidence suggests that the surface of the bacterial cell and possibly the cell wall structure are slightly different [47,71]. Evidence in support of such a mechanism includes the following: (1) methicillin-resistant cells grow more slowly than do methicillin-susceptible cells; (2) their cell size is larger; (3) they are usually resistant to many other antibiotics; (4) methicillin resistance is more easily detected at lower temperatures or at higher salt concentrations than under usual laboratory conditions; and (5) methicillin-resistant staphylococci are more resistant to lysis by lysostaphin than are methicillin-susceptible organisms.

The fact that methicillin resistance is best expressed at temperatures less than 37°C (99°F) has led Parker and Hewitt [60] to suggest that selection of methicillin-resistant staphylococci may occur in the relatively cooler environment of the skin or anterior nares. The first detection of such strains preceded the introduction of methicillin, and the prevalence of methicillin resistance does not correlate with the relative clinical usage of methicillin or other penicillinase-resistant penicillins. Thus, these investigators have suggested that other penicillins, such as penicillin V or ampicillin, might exert selective pressure in favor of methicillin-resistant strains.

PENICILLIN "TOLERANCE" IN STAPHYLOCOCCUS AUREUS. Recently, another type of penicillin resistance of *Staphylococcus aureus* has been clarified by Sabath and co-workers [72]. Such strains are inhibited by customary concentrations of penicillins, including antistaphylococcal penicillins, but are not killed except by very high concentrations of such drugs. Thus, the hallmark of "tolerance" is a wide discrepancy between the minimal inhibitory and minimal bactericidal concentrations. Tolerant strains appear to be deficient in autolytic enzyme activity. In Sabath's report, 44 percent of bacteremic strains studied demonstrated such tolerance. Many strains also showed cross-tolerance with cephalosporins and with vancomycin. The phenomenon of tolerance may prove to be a common and clinically very important type of antibiotic "resistance."

Drug Resistance in Gram-Negative Bacilli

TRENDS. The historical development of drug resistance among gram-negative bacilli is perhaps less distinctly characterized than in the case of staphylococci, but the problems are no less real. The most comprehensive studies have been those carried out at the Boston City Hospital, as reviewed recently by Finland [27]. It is apparent that there has been a progressive decrease in susceptibility to commonly used antimicrobial drugs among strains of *Escherichia coli,* the *Klebsiella-Enterobacter* group, *Serratia,* and *Proteus,* as well as *Pseudomonas.* In 1935, these organisms accounted for 12 percent of cases and 8 percent of deaths among all bacteremic infections at the Boston City Hospital, but by 1965, they accounted for fully half of all bacteremic infections and 57 percent of deaths from bacteremic infection.

A striking illustration of the development of resistance in enterobacteria occurred in the setting of community-acquired, rather than nosocomial, infections. This was the extraordinarily rapid development of multiple-drug resistance in strains of *Shigella* in Japan. The first multiple-drug-resistant strain, isolated in 1955, was resistant to the sulfonamides, streptomycin, tetracycline, and chloramphenicol. In subsequent years, the frequency of isolation of *Shigella* strains with identical or additional drug resistances increased so that by 1967, almost 50 percent of strains were multiple-drug-resistant [58].

ORIGIN AND MECHANISM. The identification of multiple-drug resistance among strains of *Shigella* in Japan, as outlined above, prompted subsequent investigations both in Japan and elsewhere to define the genetic mechanisms involved. Just as many common drug resistances among staphylococci are plasmid-linked, so, too, virtually all acquired drug resistance among aerobic gram-negative bacilli results from resistance (R) factors present as episomes, that is, microbial extrachromosomal DNAs that are capable of autonomous replication and of reversible attachment to the bacterial chromosome. Although sometimes they are spontaneously lost, R factors may be transferred by conjugation from cell to cell within individual genera, among other genera within the Enterobacteriaceae, and sometimes to related gram-negative bacilli outside of the Enterobacteriaceae. R factors are often linked, and therefore multiple resistance determinants may be transferred simultaneously.

Virtually all the resistance determinants among gram-negative bacilli are genes that code for the production of enzymes that inactivate antibiotics by hydrolysis, acetylation, phosphorylation, or adenylation. There are well-defined enzymes produced by drug-resistant gram-negative bacilli that catalyze the inactivation of penicillins, cephalosporins, chloramphenicol, trimethoprim, streptomycin, neomycin, kanamycin, spectinomycin, gentamicin, tobramycin, and amikacin.

In the ten years that have elapsed since the widespread recognition of the significance of R factors in gram-negative bacilli, several investigators have attempted to define the epidemiologic significance of the relative roles played by R-factor transfer in the human gastrointestinal tract, as contrasted to the environmental selection pressure created by antibiotic therapy, with resulting colonization of patients by resistant organisms. Gardner and Smith [29], in studying a nosocomial outbreak due to multiple-drug-resistant *Klebsiella,* concluded that colonization of patients with resistant organisms under the selective pressure of antibiotic therapy was of far greater epidemiologic significance than R-factor transfer in the gastrointestinal tract. Although there have been numerous putative demonstrations of the fact that R-factor transfer can and does indeed occur within the gastrointestinal tract, other investigators have supported the conclusions of Gardner and Smith, namely, that the selection pressure of antibiotics has been far more important epidemiologically in the drug resistance of nosocomial gram-negative rod pathogens [77].

It is difficult to put a precise figure on the proportion of drug resistance among enteric bacteria that is mediated by R factors, because of the requirement to demonstrate transferability of every antibiotic resistance from every strain studied. Evidence to date strongly suggests that the major proportion of acquired drug resistance in Enterobacteriaceae is R-factor mediated [1,64,78].

As is true of penicillin resistance in staphylococci, such evidence as is available suggests that R factors were present, though far less prevalent, in the preantibiotic era [20,30]. Thus, stool cultures from aboriginal populations unexposed to antibiotics were found to contain, in small numbers, strains of *E. coli* with R-factor-mediated resistance to antibiotics. This suggests that a small reservoir of R factors was present to take advantage of the advent of antibiotics, and that R factors were not formed more recently, de novo, after antibiotics came into common use.

Complicating the problem further is the fact that, as a characteristic property of R factors, the administration of a single antibiotic may select multiple-drug-resistant organisms, because of the linkage of multiple-resistance determinants on a single R factor. Thus, within a nosocomial setting, a prevalent R factor may be sustained by the use of any drug encompassed in its resistance package. Switching usage patterns from one drug to another, when prevalent R factors are resistant to both, may not be attended by a reduction in the frequency of multiple-drug-resistant strains having resistances to these drugs and other resistances linked with them.

Resistance of gram-negative bacilli to aminoglycoside antibiotics may be due to a decrease in permeability limiting penetration of the drug to its site of action, to alteration of the binding site, or to R-factor mediated enzymatic alteration of the drug. Aminoglycosides may be inactivated by phosphorylation, acetylation, or adenylation. A variety of such aminoglycoside-inactivating enzymes have been described [10, 19]. Typically, they vary widely in their substrate specificity. For example, gentamicin acetyltransferase I will inactivate gentamicin and tobramycin, but not amikacin; the enzyme 6^1-N-acetyltransferase will inactivate kanamycin, amikacin, tobramycin, neomycin, and part of the gentamicin complex. Thus, R factors may confer resistance to both related and unrelated antibiotics, and bacteria containing

such R factors possess a survival advantage in a hospital environment where antibiotics are widely used.

Virulence of Antibiotic-Resistant Bacteria
Evidence is conflicting regarding altered virulence—whether enhanced or diminished—of drug-resistant bacteria, in contrast to that of drug-susceptible organisms. There may prove to be no single answer to that question, the answer rather being dependent on the particular species involved, the particular drug resistance involved, the altered metabolic state of the bacterial cell as a result of the presence of genetic elements that determine drug resistance, the possible addition of other genetic elements that control other metabolic activities, and the like.

Although it is generally true that serious infection, such as bacteremic infection, caused by drug-resistant bacteria results in higher mortality rates than would be true of comparably serious infections caused by drug-susceptible bacteria, it is not at all clear whether the increased mortality is a reflection of increased virulence, or the diminished effectiveness of antibiotic therapy, or both. Jessen and colleagues [37], for example, who studied the occurrence of methicillin-resistant staphylococci and staphylococcal bacteremia in Denmark, showed that the combined effects of lysogenization, transduction, and selection not only influenced the phage type and antibiotic resistance of staphylococci, but also involved properties more directly connected with pathogenicity such as lipase production, which is thought to facilitate the development of abscesses and to affect adversely the prognosis in bacteremia. The authors could not determine, however, whether the poorer prognosis was due to the shortcomings of antibiotic therapy or to correlated bacterial properties that enhanced virulence.

Taken in totality, the available evidence does not permit a conclusion that drug-resistant bacteria of any given species are more or less virulent than their drug-susceptible relatives.

Reversal of Antibiotic Resistance
There is evidence from a number of studies that the proportion of bacteria resistant to a

given antibiotic may decrease if there is a restriction or cessation of use of the drug.

STAPHYLOCOCCI. Lepper and co-workers [49] found that after five months of intensive use of erythromycin for the treatment of all susceptible infections, three-quarters of strains were highly resistant to that drug. When all erythromycin therapy was discontinued and penicillin and tetracycline therapy was resumed, the proportion of erythromycin-resistant strains subsided, whereas the proportion of penicillin-resistant strains, which had declined while erythromycin was exclusively used, rose again rapidly. Similar results were found for tetracycline, to which resistance had increased sharply while it was used for susceptible infections and subsequently declined as its use decreased. Gibson and Thompson [31] described a similar phenomenon with staphylococci from burn wounds that had become highly resistant to tetracycline while that drug was used. When chloramphenicol was substituted for tetracycline, the proportion of chloramphenicol-resistant staphylococci rose sharply during the succeeding six months, while the proportion of tetracycline-resistant staphylococci fell. When chloramphenicol therapy was discontinued, the proportion of chloramphenicol-resistant strains dropped sharply. Bauer, Perry, and Kirby [8] reported an entirely comparable experience, and they demonstrated a correlation between the extent of resistance and the use of antibiotics. In an extensive study of staphylococci and staphylococcal infection in Great Britain, Barber and her colleagues [2] documented not only a decline in the incidence of staphylococcal infection per patient when a number of anti-cross-infection measures and a controlled antibiotic policy were put into effect, but also a sharp reversal of penicillin and tetracycline resistance of isolates toward increased susceptibility.

GRAM-NEGATIVE BACILLI. Prevailing drug resistance of gram-negative bacilli is also susceptible to alteration by restriction or cessation of use of a given drug. When kanamycin was replaced by gentamicin in an effort to control an outbreak of nosocomial infections caused by kanamycin-resistant enteric organisms, kanamycin-resistant organisms were virtually eliminated from the nursery within a month, which suggested that the selective pressure provided by the extensive use of kanamycin was a major factor in causing and propagating the outbreak. As gentamicin was increasingly used, a significant increase in gentamicin resistance of the infants' intestinal flora occurred [28].

Sogaard and colleagues [80], in studying antibiotic-resistant gram-negative bacilli in a urologic ward in Denmark, found a progressive decrease in the incidence of antibiotic resistance among enteric bacteria over a nine-year period that was coincident with a decreasing use of antibiotics in response to a restrictive antibiotic-use policy. In addition, the number of more resistant organisms, such as *Pseudomonas aeruginosa, Proteus, Providencia, Klebsiella,* and *Enterobacter,* declined during the period of study. Bulger and co-workers [14], in surveying resistance among strains of *Escherichia coli* and *Klebsiella-Enterobacter* over a ten-year period, observed a decline in the frequency of resistance to antibiotics, and they attributed their findings in part to conservative and selective use of antibiotics and in part to the development of an overall hospital infection control program.

Working in the Birmingham Accident Hospital Burn Unit, Lowbury and associates [53] studied the emergence of strains of *Pseudomonas aeruginosa* and Enterobacteriaceae that carried an R factor conferring resistance to tetracycline, kanamycin, carbenicillin, ampicillin, and cephaloridine. These strains emerged under the selective pressure of carbenicillin therapy, which was widely used on the burn unit. After the discontinuation of all use of carbenicillin and restriction on the use of tetracycline, kanamycin, ampicillin, and cephaloridine, strains of *Pseudomonas aeruginosa* and Enterobacteriaceae carrying this linked, multiple-drug-resistant pattern disappeared. Price and Sleigh [65] reported an unusually dramatic experience in attempting to control an epidemic of *Klebsiella* infection in a neurosurgical unit; the epidemic was not curtailed by radical measures for the prevention of cross-infection, and the epidemic strain disappeared only when the use of all antibiotics, both prophylactic and therapeutic, was discontinued in the unit.

CONCLUSION. The accumulated evidence therefore strongly suggests that drug-resistant organisms—whether mutants, transductants containing plasmids, or conjugants containing R factors—that are selected by the pressure of antibiotic drugs are probably at a disadvantage, however slight, in the absence of the selection pressure. If this were not so, "wild" bacteria in the community would likely be drug-resistant or would at least be represented by a mixture of sensitive and resistant cells. Although R-factor-containing bacteria acquired in the hospital do persist for a time in the community free of the selection pressure of antibiotics, only 50 percent of infants who acquired enteric organisms containing R-factor-mediated resistance to kanamycin, for example, still had the original organisms present after one year [18].

Laboratory Determination of Drug Resistance

GENERAL METHODS. Discerning readers will have already recognized the fact that in this or in other reviews of the subject of drug resistance in nosocomial pathogens, a substantial proportion of the relevant data comes from two centers in the United States, Boston City Hospital on one hand, and the University of Washington, on the other. This happenstance did not occur as a result of a carefully planned program to document patterns of drug resistance on both the east and west coasts, nor did it come about solely as a result of the fact that principal investigators in each of these centers had long-term interests in drug resistance in bacteria. Most importantly, both of these centers have maintained a methodologic approach that would permit comparison of information obtained in any given year to information previously derived from that same laboratory.

The basic methods used by these two laboratories are quite sharply different. Quantitative broth or agar-dilution susceptibility testing has been used at the Boston City Hospital, and a standardized agar-diffusion procedure has been used at the University of Washington. In both instances, however, appropriate controls were incorporated into the methods to insure the validity of year-to-year comparisons. Probably the most important of these controls has been the inclusion in susceptibility tests of appropriate laboratory control organisms, which were selected on the basis of their repeatedly documented performance in the test system being used.

Resistance to antibacterial drugs is determined in most hospital laboratories by the antibiotic disc-diffusion test [7]. A detailed review of the problems and pitfalls of this test is beyond the scope of this chapter, but a few salient features should be mentioned.

The amount of antibiotic in sensitivity-testing discs is determined by the U.S. Food and Drug Administration (FDA) and is allowed to vary within certain limits, currently set at one-third less than the labeled content to one-half more than the labeled content. Thus, a sensitivity-testing disc said to contain 10 μg of ampicillin may contain from 6.67 μg to 15 μg of ampicillin and yet fall within legally proscribed limits. This degree of variability in the content of antibiotic sensitivity-testing discs is well within tolerable limits as long as other methodologic constraints are strictly observed. These include (1) careful control of the inoculum size with a barium sulfate standard, (2) reasonable control of the amount of agar in the plate, (3) quality control of each lot of media before its use is permitted in disc-diffusion testing, and most importantly, (4) quality control of the entire procedure by the regular inclusion of control organisms whose performance in disc-diffusion testing has been repeatedly documented. Even with such controls incorporated into susceptibility testing, clinical laboratories would do well to recheck the results of disc-diffusion testing in situations in which statistically improbable results are obtained.

The use of antibiotic susceptibility testing as a means of typing organisms for epidemiologic purposes is described in Chapter 8, Part I.

METHICILLIN-RESISTANT STAPHYLOCOCCI. One special problem merits additional attention, that being the laboratory recognition of methicillin-resistant strains of *Staphylococcus aureus*. The major difficulty results from the heterogeneity of the response at 37°C (99°F): at this temperature, the majority of cells are inhibited by a very similar amount of antibiotic to that which inhibits methicillin-sensitive strains, and the resulting zone of inhibition may be interpreted as indicating a methicillin-intermediate or susceptible strain. A small proportion of the inoculum, however, is capable of multiplying in higher concentrations of methicillin and can be detected by using unusually heavy inocula, hyperosmotic culture media, or incubation for 48 hours before reading. It has now been clearly established that methicillin resistance can be fully expressed at incubation temperatures of 30°C to 35°C (86°F to 95°F), and that the disc-diffusion test is effective in detecting such strains using methicillin, oxacillin, or nafcillin discs with overnight incubation in that temperature zone [62]. Methicillin resistance can be reliably detected after overnight incubation at 35°C (95°F) using conventional methicillin discs if all strains with inhibition zones of 13 mm. or less are considered resistant. Thus, by carefully controlling the incubator temperature at 35°C (95°F) and by modifying interpretive schemes, it is possible to detect methicillin-resistant *S. aureus* reliably under test conditions that are suitable for other common clinical pathogens. Separate incubators at 30°C (86°F) and special screening procedures are not required.

The most frequent cause of apparent methicillin resistance, however, is not true methicillin resistance, but rather another potential problem in the disc-diffusion testing procedure. Methicillin discs have been found to be particularly liable to rapid deterioration under conditions other than freezer storage. Of all the penicillinase-resistant penicillins, oxacillin discs are the least susceptible to deterioration under refrigerator conditions, and thus they may be preferable to methicillin discs in representing the penicillinase-resistant penicillins. Another cause of apparent resistance is confusion of *S. aureus* with *S. epidermidis*. The latter is commonly resistant to methicillin. Thus, a report of a methicillin-resistant *S. aureus* strain should be followed by a request for a repeat coagulase test, preferably by the tube method.

A very closely associated problem is the determination of cephalosporin resistance in such strains. Most methicillin-resistant staphylococci show heterogeneous resistance to the cephalosporins as well, and there is evidence that infection caused by methicillin-resistant staphylococci often fails to respond to therapy with cephalosporins in spite of the apparent in vitro susceptibility of these organisms. Hallander and Laurell [35] as well as Plorde and Sherris [62] have found that testing with cephalothin discs under the usual circumstances is unreliable and fails to discriminate, as does methicillin, between susceptible and resistant strains. Testing with cephalexin discs, however, at an incubation temperature of 30°C to 35°C, provides good discrimination between sensitive and heterogeneously resistant strains.

Antibiotics and Host Susceptibility to Infection

Antibiotics may affect host susceptibility to infection either by a direct effect on host defense mechanisms or by an indirect effect resulting from alteration of the metabolic state of the host. Antibiotics further exert a profound influence on the nature of the host microflora, and although this selection effect may not directly influence host susceptibility to infection, it very directly influences the nature of the organisms that colonize and subsequently infect hospitalized patients.

Direct Effect of Antibiotics on Host's Defense Mechanisms

The most obvious and dramatic examples of a direct effect of antibiotics on the host's defense mechanisms are the instances of granulocytopenia or bone-marrow aplasia occasionally encountered with the use of several antibiotics, notably chloramphenicol and the sulfonamides. Adverse reactions to penicillins, cephalosporins, sulfonamides, and, less frequently, other antibiotics may take the form of a severe dermatitis, including exfoliation, and they may thus enhance host susceptibility to infection as a direct result of immunologic injury to the skin. These adverse effects of antibiotic therapy are well known and profoundly influence host susceptibility to infection.

Direct effects of individual antibiotics on the components of host defense, leukocyte function, immunoglobulin synthesis and function, and cell-mediated immune mechanisms have not been systematically studied. There is evidence in experimental systems that tetracycline, in clinically attainable concentrations, may alter leukocyte chemotaxis and mobility as well as complement activation, but these effects have not been shown to be of broad clinical significance.

Chloramphenicol, in clinically attainable concentrations, can be shown to diminish the antibody response to antigenic stimulation, but this effect has similarly not been shown to be of general clinical significance. Modulation of the host immune response to an infectious agent by specific chemotherapy—such as occurs in the treatment of rickettsial infections with chloramphenicol or tetracycline, penicillin treatment of group-A streptococcal infections, or ampicillin treatment of *Hemophilus influenzae* type-B infections—may over long periods of time alter the susceptibility of a population to a particular infectious agent, but this phenomenon probably is of little, if any, significance in the context of nosocomial infection.

Little information exists on the direct effects, if any, of antibiotics on host cell-mediated immune mechanisms. An intensively studied drug, rifampin, can be shown to reduce the number of circulating T lymphocytes, as determined by sheep red-blood-cell rosette formation, in approximately 50 percent of patients studied. Other immunosuppressive effects of rifampin on lymphocyte-macrophage systems can also be demonstrated, as well as suppression of delayed cutaneous hypersensitivity to purified protein derivative of tuberculin (PPD) in patients with tuberculosis who are receiving rifampin. These effects of rifampin therapy, however, have not yet been shown to alter host susceptibility to infection in patients being treated for tuberculosis nor to be associated with a poor therapeutic result.

Thus, there is little evidence that antibiotic therapy, as such, has a major, direct effect on host defense mechanisms, except in instances of adverse drug reactions precipitating severe dermatitis, bone-marrow depression, or the like.

Indirect Effect of Antibiotics Due to Alteration of Host's Metabolic State

Many antibiotics cause direct toxic or immunologically mediated injury to target organs regulating the metabolic activity of the host, particularly the liver, kidneys, gastrointestinal tract, and lung. The resulting dysfunction of these organs may then alter host susceptibility to infection. These indirect effects of antibiotics can in most instances be minimized or avoided altogether by the rational and careful use of potentially toxic drugs.

KIDNEYS. Interstitial nephritis has been associated with a number of drugs, notably the penicillins, including the penicillinase-resistant penicillins. Direct toxic injury to renal tubular epithelium is caused by many drugs, notably cephaloridine, all of the aminoglycosides, polymyxins, and amphotericin B. Also, glomerulonephritis has been noted shortly after rifampin therapy in persons with prior exposure to the drug. Renal failure and its resulting metabolic consequences have a direct suppressive effect on host defense mechanisms. Obviously, the therapeutic modalities used in the management of renal failure also represent added infection risk factors.

LIVER. Minor alterations of hepatic function are found frequently in the course of antibiotic therapy, but in the vast majority of instances, such alterations cannot be shown to influence host susceptibility to infection. Intrahepatic cholestasis, such as that which may occur during therapy with the sodium lauryl sulfate ester of erythromycin, similarly does not appear to represent a threat to host defense mechanisms. Overwhelming hepatic injury has been associated with both tetracycline and isoniazid therapy, but the unquestionably reduced host resistance to infection is of lesser importance than the more immediate metabolic threat to the host.

COLON. Necrotizing enterocolitis has been recognized as a complication of therapy with many antibiotic drugs, and it has most recently been associated with the use of lincomycin or clindamycin. Unlike the staphylococcal, necrotizing enterocolitis associated with tetracycline therapy (see below), the mechanism of lincomycin- or clindamycin-associated colitis is not at all clear, but it may be related to the alterations of host gastrointestinal tract flora caused by the drug. Patients who suffer this adverse effect are clearly at an increased risk of infection.

LUNGS. Immunologically mediated injury to the lungs is an occasional consequence of antibiotic therapy, particularly with penicillins and nitrofurans. It is likely that host susceptibility to infection is only mildly enhanced by such injury.

Influence of Antibiotic Therapy on Host's Microflora

Virtually all antibiotics in therapeutic doses produce marked changes in the microflora of the skin, upper respiratory tract, gastrointestinal tract, genital tract, and, indeed, any site in the host normally colonized by bacteria. Antibiotic-resistant organisms, if present or acquired, are selected out and multiply freely to replace the susceptible organisms inhibited by antibiotic therapy. In the majority of patients, these changes in host microflora are of no demonstrable consequence. As is well recognized, however, the antibiotic-resistant microflora may, on occasion, result in serious or fatal infection. It is through this mechanism that antibiotic therapy appears to exert its major influence on nosocomial infection, that is, by determining the character, rather than the frequency, of nosocomial infections.

The clearest example of an alteration of host microflora that leads directly to overgrowth and subsequent infection by antibiotic-resistant bacteria is staphylococcal enterocolitis associated with or following tetracycline therapy. Necrotizing enterocolitis in this instance appears to be a direct result of antibiotic therapy, which suppresses the normal gastrointestinal tract flora and permits rapid and uninhibited growth of drug-resistant staphylococci. If recognized promptly, antibiotic therapy directed at these staphylococci (e.g., oral vancomycin administration) is curative. Staphylococcal en-

terocolitis occurred more frequently during the period in which staphylococci were the most frequent and troublesome nosocomial pathogens, but it is only infrequently encountered at present.

A more recent and striking example is the still unfolding story of toxin-producing clostridia causing antibiotic-associated pseudomembranous colitis. This entity was highlighted by the recognition of clindamycin-associated colitis, but has also been seen in association with a number of other drugs including ampicillin, cephalexin, tetracycline, chloramphenicol, and lincomycin. There is now a substantial body of evidence implicating toxigenic strains of *Clostridium* (especially *C. difficile*) as the cause of antibiotic-associated colitis [4,6,67]. These organisms are resistant to the antibiotic administered, but have thus far been susceptible to vancomycin. In a hamster model of clindamycin-associated colitis, simultaneous administration of oral vancomycin has been completely protective [5,13].

Colonization of the gastrointestinal tract by multiple-drug-resistant gram-negative bacilli has been associated with antibiotic therapy [70,77], as has colonization of the respiratory tract. In a study at the Denver Veterans Administration Hospital, Selden and his associates [77] found that gastrointestinal colonization by multiple-drug-resistant *Klebsiella* that were acquired in the hospital was an important intermediary step in the subsequent development of disease by those organisms. Evidence has also been presented suggesting that hospital food may frequently be contaminated by multiple-drug-resistant gram-negative bacilli, and that this may be an important source of nosocomial colonization in patients whose normal gastrointestinal tract flora is suppressed by antibiotic therapy.

In a thorough study of bacterial colonization and suprainfection of the respiratory tract, Tillotson and Finland [86] showed that colonization and suprainfection were more common following high doses of penicillin and aminoglycosides or of broad-spectrum antibiotics alone. They did not, however, find a higher rate of colonization or infection by gram-negative bacilli following treatment with various semisynthetic penicillins, nor did ampicillin therapy appear to confer any additional risk beyond that observed with penicillin G. Louria and Brayton [52] found that the risk of suprainfection following penicillin treatment of pneumonia was related, at least in part, to unnecessarily high doses of penicillin.

It is, however, important to appreciate that antibiotic therapy is by no means the only factor influencing colonization and suprainfection. Johanson and his associates [39] were among the first to point out the importance of the severity of the underlying disease, independent of antibiotic therapy, in pharyngeal colonization by gram-negative bacilli. Rose and Babcock [69], studying colonization with gram-negative bacilli of patients in an intensive-care unit, observed that colonization in surgical patients appeared to be related more to the presence of indwelling tubes and the consequent colonization of multiple sites in the same patient than it was to the use of antimicrobial drugs. In medical patients, however, colonization appeared to be related primarily to antibiotic therapy. Tenney and associates at the Denver Veterans Administration Hospital [85], who also studied pharyngeal colonization in a medical intensive-care unit, found that no single risk factor for gram-negative rod colonization, such as antibiotic therapy, was associated with more than two-thirds of colonized patients and that most risk factors were present in less than one-third. The risk factors studied included, in addition to antibiotic therapy, the severity of the underlying illness, presence of acidosis, steroid therapy, mechanically assisted ventilation, tracheal intubation, and nasogastric suction, as well as others. As did Johanson and colleagues [39,40], these investigators suggested that the oropharynx is episodically or continually exposed to gram-negative bacilli and *Staphylococcus aureus,* perhaps in small numbers, and that patients vary in their ability to clear them. Pharyngeal colonization may occur only in patients whose pharyngeal clearance mechanisms are compromised by underlying disease, the patients' metabolic state, mechanically assisted respiration, or foreign bodies; in patients who are exposed to large inocula of gram-negative bacilli, for example, by contami-

nated nebulizers; or in patients in whom gram-negative bacilli are permitted to multiply more rapidly than they can be cleared, such as when antibiotic therapy suppresses normal flora. The risk of disease occurring after colonization has been established is more likely to be related to the state of host pulmonary defense mechanisms and to the virulence of the specific colonizing species than to the use of antibiotic therapy or other risk factors per se.

Sprunt and colleagues [82,83] have suggested that α-hemolytic streptococci inhibit the growth of gram-negative rods in vitro, and they have furthermore noted the disappearance of inhibitory α-hemolytic streptococci from the oropharynx in patients colonized with gram-negative bacilli. Thus, bacterial interference, with α-hemolytic streptococci acting as the inhibitory species, may be one mechanism for maintaining the normal flora of the upper respiratory tract. If these or other inhibitors are eliminated or depressed by antibiotic therapy, other drug-resistant bacteria may be able to multiply to reach detectable levels. A similar mechanism may well obtain in other areas of the body with their own flora, such as the skin and gastrointestinal tract.

In summary, there is abundant evidence that antibiotic therapy is a major determinant of alterations in host microflora and colonization of the host by drug-resistant organisms. There is also evidence, however, indicating that antibiotic therapy is by no means the only determinant involved, and that antibiotic therapy may be only one of a number of risk factors commonly encountered by hospitalized patients that facilitate colonization and often subsequent disease by drug-resistant organisms, including both staphylococci and gram-negative bacilli.

General Conclusions on the Relationship of Antibiotics and Nosocomial Infection

The interrelationships of antibiotic therapy, intrinsic or acquired resistance to antibiotics in bacteria, and nosocomial infection in the hospitalized host thus represent an extraordinarily complex equation. Considering the large numbers of other risk factors that affect patients in contemporary hospitals, it is perhaps not surprising that data simply do not exist that would permit satisfactory and valid conclusions concerning the exact role of antibiotic usage in determining either the magnitude or the frequency of hospital infection. In such instances, there are often differences of opinion, and the same is true in this instance. R. E. O. Williams has stated:

I have not referred so far to the factors so often cited as responsible for much of the trouble in hospital infection—abuse of antibiotics—because it seems important to appreciate that the secular changes that we have seen have not been wholly, or even mainly, due to alterations in the use of antibiotics or to the development of staphylococci more resistant to antibiotics [90].

In the same year, Maxwell Finland wrote:

The major factor presumed to be responsible for the changing ecology of the serious bacterial infections, and for the marked increase in their occurrence, at least at Boston City Hospital, is the selective pressure of the antibiotics so widely and intensively used in therapy, and especially for prophylaxis. Both the large number of drugs and the large doses of each used in the individual patients within the hospital are elements of this selective pressure [26].

This disagreement cannot be resolved in quantitative terms. The use of antimicrobial agents tends to promote the emergence of organisms with intrinsic or acquired resistance to those agents and predisposes patients to colonization by such organisms. With increasing use of instrumentation, increasing use of immunosuppressive drugs in therapy, and other technologic accompaniments of contemporary medical practice, resistant organisms may then emerge to cause infection. Infection resulting from multiple-drug-resistant bacteria, whether staphylococci or gram-negative bacilli, is notoriously more difficult to treat than infection by drug-susceptible pathogens, and the results of therapy in such compromised hosts are clearly less satisfactory.

Wolff and Bennett have stated the issues very succinctly:

The enhanced risks of acquiring gram-negative rod infections consequent to the proper use of antibiotics for legitimate therapeutic and prophy-

lactic purposes clearly seem outweighed by the anticipated benefits. Such risks represent undesirable but nonetheless acceptable concomitants of medical progress. Use of antibiotics for uncertain or improper indications, however, poses an unacceptable risk [91].

Principles of Chemotherapy

Space does not permit a detailed review of specific antibacterial or antifungal drugs, their mechanisms of action, indications for use, and adverse effects. It is appropriate, however, to review briefly some of the general principles of chemotherapy of infection, particularly as they relate to nosocomial infection.

Bactericidal Versus Bacteriostatic Drugs

Antibacterial and antifungal drugs are generally considered to be either *bactericidal,* if they are capable of killing susceptible bacteria at concentrations close to those required to inhibit the organism and readily achievable clinically, or *bacteriostatic,* if the action of the drug at clinically achievable concentrations is primarily to inhibit growth rather than to kill the organism. It is important to recall that the commonly used tests of bacterial susceptibility to drugs—the disc-diffusion test and the quantitative broth-dilution test—measure only the inhibition of growth by the drug being tested, and not bacterial killing.

Drugs that are generally bactericidal in their activity against susceptible pathogens include the penicillins and cephalosporins, polymyxins B and E, and the aminoglycoside drugs such as streptomycin, kanamycin, neomycin, gentamicin, and tobramycin.

Drugs that are generally bacteriostatic rather than bactericidal in their activity against susceptible bacteria include the tetracyclines, chloramphenicol, erythromycin, the sulfonamides, and lincomycin as well as its derivatives.

In general, results of therapy in serious systemic infections appear to be improved if bactericidal rather than bacteriostatic drugs are used. There are, however, only two situations in which there is substantial evidence in support of this claim. The first is the treatment of bacterial endocarditis, in which there is clear evidence that the use of bactericidal drugs results in a higher cure rate and a lower relapse rate than that of bacteriostatic drugs. The likely explanation of this phenomenon is the inability of host polymorphonuclear leukocytes to penetrate the vegetation and to ingest and kill the organisms growing therein. Thus, sterilization of the vegetation is entirely dependent on antibiotic activity.

The second example in which there is good evidence of the superiority of bactericidal drugs over bacteriostatic drugs is in treating the severely immunocompromised host, particularly the host with severe granulocytopenia (defined as less than 100 polymorphonuclear leukocytes per cubic millimeter), which may occur in drug-induced granulocytopenia, bone-marrow aplasia, or acute myelogenous leukemia. The likely explanation of this phenomenon is again to be found in inadequate host defense mechanisms.

Synergism and Antagonism
Between Antibacterial Drugs
In vitro studies of Jawetz and Gunnison [36] showed that if two bactericidal drugs were used together in concentrations in which each drug alone was only minimally effective, the bactericidal effect of the combination was sometimes markedly enhanced; this has been referred to as *antibacterial synergism.* Conversely, if a bactericidal and a bacteriostatic drug were used together in concentrations at which each of them was minimally effective, the effect of the combination was sometimes dramatically decreased, and bacterial growth, rather than bacterial killing, sometimes ensued; this has been referred to as *antibacterial antagonism.*

In general, if two bactericidal drugs are used in combination, the results may be either additive or synergistic. If either a bactericidal and a bacteriostatic drug or two bacteriostatic drugs are used in combination, the results may be additive or antagonistic but are rarely synergistic.

The best-known examples of antibacterial synergism in chemotherapy of infection are the combined action of penicillin and an aminoglycoside on enterococci and the combined action of carbenicillin and gentamicin on *Pseudomonas aeruginosa.* There is increasing evidence from in vitro studies that the combination of a penicillin and an aminoglycoside may be useful clinically against other organisms—such as viridans streptococci and staphylococci, in addition to enterococci—but there is as yet little supporting clinical evidence.

Little evidence has been presented that antibacterial antagonism is an important phenomenon at the clinical level. Antibacterial antagonism may become a clinical problem only in settings in which marginally effective concentrations of drugs occur, such as in cerebrospinal fluid.

Absorption, Excretion, Protein Binding, Tissue
Distribution, and Inactivation of Antibiotics
Potent and potentially toxic antibiotic drugs should ideally be used only when the clinician has a clear understanding of the clinical pharmacology of the drug, its absorption and routes of excretion, the appropriate dosage adjustments to be made in patients with altered renal or hepatic function, and the like. Unfortunately, our knowledge of the clinical pharmacology of antibiotic drugs is sometimes fragmentary and incomplete. Although there may be extensive knowledge of the levels of a given drug in serum following a dose, there is often relatively little knowledge of the concentration of drug delivered to the infected sites or of the effects of inflammatory exudate on the antibacterial activity of the drug.

Of the factors controlling the extravascular distribution of antibiotics, protein binding has been the most thoroughly studied, although pH, protein concentration, ionic strength, and other physicochemical factors also play a role. Among presently available antibiotics, protein binding becomes potentially significant only with the penicillins and cephalosporins. In general, the more highly protein-bound the antibiotic, the less free (i.e., microbiologically active) drug will be available to diffuse into the extravascular space.

It must be remembered, however, that protein binding is a very dynamic phenomenon, and as free drug diffuses into the extravascular compartment, some protein-bound drug in the vascular compartment is freed to maintain equilibrium, thus again increasing the diffusion gradient in favor of free drug leaving the vascular compartment. At equilibrium, the concentration of free drug in extravascular compartments would equal, but not exceed, that in the vascular compartment. The peak level of free drug in an inflammatory focus, however, will virtually never exceed the peak level of free drug in the serum.

In the clinical use of penicillins and cephalosporins, the doses used provide serum levels of free drug that are well in excess of the minimum concentrations necessary to inhibit or kill susceptible organisms. The phenomenon of protein binding is probably of little clinical significance in the treatment of infections until the extent of binding results in free concentrations insufficient to inhibit or kill susceptible organisms adequately. Competition for binding sites between antimicrobials and other substances, however, may serve to increase the free concentrations of both. This may sometimes be clinically desirable (e.g., competition between salicylates and penicillins), but it may also result in undesired toxic effects on the host; for example, competition between sulfonamides and bilirubin may enhance the risk of kernicterus in neonates.

Bacterial Persistence

The term *bacterial persistence* describes the condition in which a few, fully sensitive bacteria survive in the presence of a concentration of antibiotic that kills almost all the bacterial population. Bacterial "persisters" form only a relatively small proportion of a bacterial population, and thus may differ from the "tolerant" bacteria described previously. It is likely that these persisting bacteria are fully mature cells that happen to be relatively dormant and thus are relatively insusceptible to the action of drugs such as penicillins and cephalosporins, which exert their major antibacterial effect on rapidly growing bacterial cells. This phenomenon may account for some instances of apparent clinical relapse.

Apparent bacterial persistence may also, in some instances, be due to the formation of bacterial L forms, that is, organisms that have lost their cell walls and thus are insensitive to the action of drugs that act primarily on cell wall synthesis. Although this phenomenon has been extensively studied both in vitro and in vivo, it does not appear to be a frequent clinical phenomenon.

Of more significance is bacterial persistence within cells. This is particularly true of infections caused by intracellular pathogens such as *Brucella,* certain strains of *Salmonella,* and tubercle bacilli. Intracellular persistence may also be of significance with other pathogenic bacteria, such as staphylococci, particularly if host polymorphonuclear leukocytes are unable to kill ingested bacteria normally, as, for example, in chronic granulomatous disease. In such instances, the ultimate success of chemotherapy may be highly dependent on the intracellular penetration of antibiotics. The most commonly used bactericidal drugs—namely, penicillins, cephalosporins, and aminoglycosides—penetrate mammalian cells relatively poorly, and drugs that penetrate host cells better—such as chloramphenicol and rifampin—may offer therapeutic advantages under such circumstances.

Inactivation of Antibiotics by Host's Flora

The normal host microflora, particularly that within the gastrointestinal tract, may well contain bacteria that harbor plasmids or resistance factors mediating the production of enzymes capable of inactivating penicillins, cephalosporins, and many aminoglycosides. Similarly, bacteria present at the site of an infection or in mixed infections may contain the enzymatic apparatus necessary to inactivate drugs used against the sensitive component of the infecting flora. Thus, occasional examples are recorded of the failure of penicillin G therapy to eradicate group-A β-hemolytic streptococci from the pharynx of individuals who were simultaneously colonized with penicillinase-producing staphylococci. It is also quite possible that the inactivation of oral antibiotics by host gastrointestinal tract flora contributes, in part, to the well-known failure of drugs such as ampicillin to eradicate the gastrointestinal carrier state of certain pathogens such as salmonellae.

Cases of Failure of Chemotherapy

If an infection fails to respond to appropriate chemotherapy after a suitable interval, the reasons for a poor response can almost always be identified in the answers to the following questions:

1. Was the original clinical and bacteriologic diagnosis correct?
2. Is the pathogen that is being treated susceptible to the drug being given?
3. Is the drug being given by a route and in a dose appropriate to the clinical situation?
4. Is there an unidentified or undrained focus of infection?
5. Is a new infection superimposed on the original one?
6. Are host defense mechanisms relatively intact, or is the host severely compromised?

Chemoprophylaxis and Nosocomial Infection

It became apparent early in the antibiotic era, as hospitals were attempting to cope with nosocomial infections caused by epidemic staphylococci, that antibiotic therapy was not the long-hoped-for answer to the control of nosocomial infection. It was demonstrated in many circumstances that antibiotic therapy directed at the prevention of nosocomial infection resulted in either no significant change or an actual increase in infection rate, and its employment virtually guaranteed that the infecting pathogen was going to be resistant to the prophylactic drug used. In the past decade, the pendulum has begun to swing back from a wholly negative approach to chemoprophylaxis and rather more toward an appreciation of the fact that under certain circumstances and in certain patients, antibiotic prophylaxis may have a legitimate role in the prevention of nosocomial infection. Indications for chemoprophylaxis of hospital personnel who have been exposed to certain types of infection are beyond the scope of this chapter, which focuses on patients (see Part I, Chapter 3).

Certain underlying conceptual considerations are fundamental to an understanding of the possibilities and limitations of chemoprophylaxis in controlling nosocomial infection. One should consider first whether protection is to be provided against one specific organism or against multiple organisms and second, for what period of time such protection is to be provided. Answers to both of these questions are usually apparent from the clinical circumstances. In the newborn, the goal is to eradicate *Neisseria gonorrhoeae* from the conjunctiva; once any gonococci present have been killed, continued chemoprophylaxis directed at preventing gonococcal ophthalmia neonatorum is no longer necessary. With an indwelling intravenous catheter, the goal is to prevent local tissue invasion and septicemia caused by the skin organisms principally responsible for catheter-associated septicemia, namely, *Staphylococcus aureus, S. epidermidis,* anaerobic diphtheroids, *Acinetobacter* species, and so on; the period of risk is the length of time the catheter remains in place. In the patient with a tracheostomy, the goal is to prevent colonization and subsequent invasion of the lower respiratory tract by the organisms most commonly associated with nosocomial pneumonia, that is, staphylococci and aerobic gram-negative bacilli; the period of risk is that period during which the tracheostomy is in place and during which there is functional damage to the host defense mechanisms of the respiratory tract.

In surgical procedures involving a significant hazard of massive bacterial contamination, the goal is to protect the surgical wound against contamination as well as to provide antibiotic activity in the circulation to protect against bacteremia and metastatic infection. The organisms that are likely to cause such contamination are determined by the nature of the surgical procedure itself. The work of A. A. Miles, E. M. Miles, and Burke [56], among others, has established that the period of risk associated with an operative procedure is in fact quite short, extending to no more than several hours after an incision has been closed. Further, in a guinea pig model of staphylococcal wound infection, Burke [16] clearly established that antibiotic chemoprophylaxis should ideally be started at, or even before, the time that the experimental wound was contaminated with staphylococci and that if chemoprophylaxis was begun as little as four hours after contamination of the experimental wound, the results were very similar to giving no chemoprophylaxis at all. Thus, if chemoprophylaxis is to have any application in the prevention of surgical wound infection, the drugs must be used intraoperatively and probably need be continued for no more than several hours postoperatively.

Categories of Chemoprophylaxis
Returning to the two conceptual questions posed earlier, it is apparent that there are, in oversimplified terms, four general categories of chemoprophylaxis:

1. *Protection against one organism for a short time (1 to 72 hours).* This is generally successful as long as the organism being protected against does not develop resistance to the chemoprophylactic drug. Examples include the prophylaxis of gonococcal ophthalmia neonatorum, chemoprophylaxis of family contacts of patients with meningococcal meningitis or meningococcemia, and the prevention of streptococcal infection in family contacts.
2. *Protection against one organism for a long time (one week or more).* This can be successful only if the organism being protected against is unlikely to develop resistance to the drug used. The best example is the use of continuous penicillin administration, either penicillin G orally or benzathine penicillin intramuscularly, to prevent streptococcal infection.
3. *Protection against multiple organisms for a short time (1 to 72 hours).* Chemoprophylaxis in this category is often less satisfactory, but a few specific examples will be reviewed subsequently in which chemoprophylaxis of this type has been successfully used to prevent nosocomial infection.
4. *Protection against multiple organisms for a long time (one week or more).* There are few, if any, convincing examples of the success of chemoprophylaxis in this category. This category includes the treatment of patients with severely compromised host defense mechanisms who are subject to infection by a wide variety of gram-positive and gram-negative flora, often multiple-drug-resistant strains. Prevention of infection for extended periods by chemoprophylactic antibiotics in such patients has been notoriously unsuccessful.

Situations in which Antimicrobial Prophylaxis Is Not Indicated
Chemoprophylaxis with antibiotic drugs has been shown, or is generally considered to be, ineffective in preventing bacterial infections associated with the following circumstances:

1. *Acute viral infections.* This particularly pertains to viral infections of the respiratory tract, such as the common cold and influenza.
2. *Impaired defenses.* These are patients whose defenses are impaired permanently or for a relatively long period of time, such as by malignancies of all types, diabetes mellitus, or congestive heart failure.
3. *Foreign bodies.* These patients have foreign bodies left in place for more than several days, such as peritoneal or biliary drainage tubes, chest tubes, and indwelling intravenous or urinary catheters.
4. *Coma.* These are patients rendered unconscious as a result of drug overdosage or cerebrovascular accidents.
5. *Clean surgery.* Such patients are those who have had surgical procedures commonly regarded as being clean—such as inguinal herniorrhaphy, thyroidectomy, or mastectomy—or procedures carried out in highly vascular areas with abundant normal flora, such as tonsillectomy and adenoidectomy.

Situations in which Chemoprophylaxis Is Controversial or Equivocal
PNEUMONIA IN TRACHEOSTOMIZED PATIENTS. There has been considerable recent interest in the prevention of pneumonia in tracheostomized patients by either aerosolized or endotracheal administration of broad-spectrum antibiotics. Klastersky and associates [43]

recently studied the endotracheal administration of gentamicin and compared their results with a saline placebo in a double-blind study of 85 tracheostomized patients admitted to a neurosurgical unit. They reported that the endotracheal administration of gentamicin significantly reduced the frequency of bacteriologically proved episodes of respiratory tract infection. Seventeen of 42 placebo-treated patients developed proved pulmonary infections, whereas only 5 of 43 gentamicin-treated patients developed pneumonia. They concluded that the endotracheal administration of gentamicin to patients with tracheostomies may be a helpful adjunct in the prevention of pneumonia; they noted, however, that the organisms recovered from gentamicin-treated patients were somewhat more resistant to that drug than the organisms recovered from the control patients treated with saline.

A similar approach has been extensively studied by investigators at the Beth Israel Hospital in Boston [24,34,44]. In studying patients admitted to a respiratory-surgical intensive-care unit, they found that a polymyxin B aerosol effectively prevented an increase in colonization in patients who required controlled ventilation for at least 72 hours. In an extensive study of 744 patients admitted to the respiratory-surgical intensive-care unit in which the use of polymyxin was alternated with that of a saline placebo in alternate two-month aerosolization cycles, only three patients acquired *Pseudomonas* pneumonia during the polymyxin cycles, while 17 acquired *Pseudomonas* pneumonia during the placebo cycles. The overall mortality, however, was similar in both the placebo and polymyxin-treated groups. When polymyxin B aerosolization was carried out on a continuous basis, however, patients began to acquire pneumonias caused by polymyxin-resistant organisms. The mortality rate for pneumonia acquired under circumstances of continuous polymyxin aerosolization was greater than the investigators had noted in previous studies in which either no polymyxin or cyclic polymyxin B aerosolization was used.

It is apparent, therefore, that attempts to prevent nosocomial pneumonia in high-risk pa-

tients may, under certain circumstances, have some short-term success, but such attempts appear to carry the long-term risk of selection pressure in favor of more highly drug-resistant pathogens.

SUPPRESSION OF HOST FLORA IN SEVERELY COMPROMISED PATIENTS. Several centers have carried on investigative work during the past decade designed to identify the optimal means of protecting acutely and severely compromised hosts against infection. The majority of this work has been carried out in patients with malignancy and, in particular, in patients with acute granulocytic leukemia who are undergoing remission induction chemotherapy. Patients undergoing bone-marrow transplantation also represent an extremely high-risk, though small, group of patients.

The prevention of infection in such extremely high-risk patients has involved four basic approaches: (1) attempts to enhance the patient's host defense mechanisms through the use of vaccines, granulocyte transfusions, and, if successful, remission of leukemia; (2) limitation of invasive procedures that break natural barriers to those that are absolutely necessary for patient care; (3) protective isolation techniques to prevent acquisition of nosocomial pathogens; and (4) suppression of the host microbial flora through the use of oral, nonabsorbable antibiotics, as well as topical antibiotics and antiseptics, in order to minimize the risk of endogenous infection.

An extended discussion of this controversial and still investigational approach to the prevention of nosocomial infection in extremely high-risk, compromised hosts is beyond the scope of this chapter; readers seeking further information are referred to some recent comprehensive reviews [50,74] and to Part II, Chapters 19 and 27, of this text.

Oral, nonabsorbable antibiotic therapy to suppress the host microflora usually has taken the form of administration of vancomycin, gentamicin, and nystatin by mouth. Somewhat surprisingly, relatively little data are available on the efficacy of oral, nonabsorbable antibiotics alone in the prevention of infection or on the efficacy of protective isolation techniques using laminar air-flow rooms or life-island units alone, because most investigators have included both approaches in their studies. The data on the use of oral, nonabsorbable antibiotics alone are equivocal [42,51,66,75]. Information accumulating from the Baltimore Cancer Research Center [75] does suggest that patients treated with oral, nonabsorbable antibiotics during remission induction as part of a total program of infection control that includes protective isolation in laminar air-flow rooms as well as efforts to enhance host defense mechanisms do, as a group, have fewer total infections, fewer bacteremias, and fewer fatal infections than comparable control patients. The relative contribution to the apparent success of such regimens played by each of the component approaches, however, is by no means clear.

Not surprisingly, programs of oral, nonabsorbable antibiotic administration have some disadvantages. Patient tolerance can be a major problem because of the exceedingly unpleasant taste of the drugs; gastrointestinal intolerance manifested by nausea, vomiting, and diarrhea is sometimes sufficiently severe to require discontinuation of therapy. Furthermore, if the drugs must be discontinued, the gastrointestinal tract, with its reduced normal flora, may rapidly become repopulated with organisms relatively more resistant to antibiotics than those the patient had initially. The regimen of oral vancomycin, gentamicin, and nystatin costs over $100 per day. Finally, the selection pressure in favor of the emergence of a population of organisms resistant to the drugs being administered is enormous, and reports of sharply increased frequencies of gentamicin resistance among gram-negative rod pathogens are now appearing [33].

Thus, oral, nonabsorbable antibiotics should not be used in the management of severely immunocompromised hosts unless there is concurrently a strict program of protective isolation as part of a total infection control program. Indeed, in the absence of convincing evidence that the patients' life spans are significantly increased, this entire approach to infection prevention in severely immunocompromised hosts must still be regarded as investigational and cannot be recommended for general adoption in hospitals outside of specific investigational protocols.

Situations in which Chemoprophylaxis Has Been Shown To Be or Is Generally Regarded as Effective in Preventing Nosocomial Infections

BACTERIAL ENDOCARDITIS. It is now most unlikely, because of current sensitivities to human experimentation, that appropriately controlled studies will ever be carried out of the effectiveness of chemoprophylaxis in the prevention of bacterial endocarditis. The prophylactic regimens in use are therefore based largely on empiric or rational grounds and, more recently, on experimental animal models of the prophylaxis of bacterial endocarditis, such as recently described by Durack and Petersdorf [22]. There is a consensus that patients with rheumatic heart disease, most forms of congenital heart disease, and with intravascular prostheses should be given prophylactic antimicrobial treatment prior to a surgical procedure that may confer a substantial risk of high-grade bacteremia. Thus, such patients about to undergo dental manipulations, bowel surgery, genitourinary tract manipulations, or other invasive diagnostic procedures regularly and demonstrably associated with bacteremia should be given the benefit of chemoprophylactic therapy (see Part II, Chapter 28). Durack and Petersdorf [22] established the need to use adequate doses of bactericidal drugs, such as penicillin and an aminoglycoside, and they have shown further the chemoprophylactic ineffectiveness of bacteriostatic drugs such as tetracycline, erythromycin, and clindamycin. Chemoprophylaxis need be given only during the period of bacteremic risk. It should be evident that the particular prophylactic regimen chosen should reflect the organisms most likely to cause endocarditis at the particular site being operated upon; for example, penicillin and streptomycin provide adequate chemoprophylaxis during dental procedures, in which viridans streptococci are the most likely pathogens. In the drainage of an abscess, prophylactic coverage should include protection against staphylococcal bacteremia. For procedures on the gastrointestinal or genitourinary tract, coverage should be directed against aerobic gram-negative bacilli as well as enterococci.

BURNS. It is generally accepted that penicillin prophylaxis is indicated in an attempt to prevent streptococcal infection in burn wounds and sepsis in patients with major burns. Although it is effective in accomplishing this objective, penicillin therapy doubtlessly enhances to some degree the likelihood of colonization and potential disease caused by organisms resistant to penicillin (see Part II, Chapter 19).

Postoperative Wound Infection

Space does not permit a detailed review of the rapidly proliferating literature on the prevention of postoperative wound infections with short-term, intraoperative chemoprophylaxis. The reader is also referred to Chapters 16, 17, 18, and 22 in Part II of this text. A few specific studies in selected areas will be mentioned.

BOWEL SURGERY. Bernard and Cole [11] studied the prophylactic administration of penicillin, methicillin, and chloramphenicol intraoperatively as compared with a placebo in 118 patients who underwent abdominal operations with potential contamination. The frequency of postoperative surgical infections was 27 percent in the placebo group versus 8 percent in the antibiotic-treated group. Polk and Lopez-Mayor [63] carried out a similar study of 181 patients undergoing gastrointestinal tract surgery; they compared the administration of cephaloridine given on call to the operating room and at 5 and 12 hours thereafter with that of a placebo given on the same schedule. Twenty-eight percent of patients in the placebo group developed postoperative wound infections compared to 5 percent in the cephaloridine-treated group. Evans and Pollock [23] more recently confirmed the prophylactic efficacy of cephaloridine under such circumstances and reported comparable results. Stokes and colleagues [84] studied the effect of only two doses of either tobramycin or gentamicin plus lincomycin timed to cover the intraoperative and immediate postoperative period compared to that of a placebo in a double-blind trial in patients undergoing intraabdominal surgical procedures. Among 99 patients in the placebo

group, 8 percent developed wound infections; among 97 patients in the treatment group, 1 percent developed wound infections.

A careful study of the controversial subject of preoperative antibiotic bowel preparation was carried out by Washington and colleagues at the Mayo Clinic [89]. The study included 196 patients undergoing elective gastrointestinal surgery and who received one of three preoperative bowel preparations: (1) oral neomycin, (2) neomycin and tetracycline, and (3) placebo. Approximately 40 percent of patients in groups 1 and 3 developed wound infection, whereas only 4 percent of patients whose preoperative bowel preparation consisted of neomycin and tetracycline treatment developed wound infections.

It is apparent that patient selection is of critical importance in the studies cited and contributes significantly to the high rate of infection in the control groups. It would appear, however, that in selected instances, short-term intraoperative chemoprophylactic antibiotics or preoperative drugs directed at reducing both the aerobic and anaerobic flora of the gastrointestinal tract may play a role in reducing the frequency of postoperative wound infection endogenously acquired.

PELVIC SURGERY. There has been a similar proliferation of reports describing the efficacy of intraoperative chemoprophylaxis in reducing the frequency of postoperative infection following operations on the female genital tract, including cesarean section and vaginal hysterectomy. Among the most carefully performed of such studies is that of Ledger and associates [48], who studied 100 premenopausal women undergoing vaginal hysterectomy in a prospective double-blind fashion, utilizing intraoperative cephaloridine treatment versus placebo. Pelvic infection occurred in 34 percent of the placebo group and in 8 percent of the cephaloridine-treated group.

ORTHOPEDIC SURGERY. Boyd and associates [12] have carried out the only fully acceptable, prospective, randomized, double-blind trial of the use of prophylactic antibiotics in orthopedic patients. They studied 348 patients undergoing hip surgery. The trial compared nafcillin with a glucose placebo given before, during, and immediately after surgery. The frequency of wound infection in the placebo group was 4.8 percent as compared to 0.8 percent in the nafcillin-treated group.

CARDIAC SURGERY. There are few adequately controlled studies of the efficacy of chemoprophylaxis in cardiac surgery, and only one study has incorporated a placebo control group. Goodman and co-workers [32] studied the efficacy of preoperative and intraoperative oxacillin, penicillin-streptomycin, or placebo in 72 patients undergoing open-heart surgery. The overall incidence of infection was identical in the three study groups, but the study was terminated when two placebo patients developed fatal pneumococcal endocarditis.

Fekety and associates [25] reported the results of 191 patients who underwent cardiac surgery at the Johns Hopkins Hospital in 1963 and 1964, approximately half of whom underwent cardiopulmonary bypass. They compared prophylaxis with penicillin versus methicillin. No significant difference in postoperative infection rates was observed between these two chemoprophylactic drugs.

Conte and associates [17] carried out a prospective, double-blind study limited to patients undergoing cardiac surgery with cardiopulmonary bypass, and they compared the administration of one gram of intraoperative cephalothin with that of 20 one-gram doses of intravenous cephalothin intraoperatively and four days postoperatively. No significant differences were observed between the two groups with respect to major or minor infections or deaths. The investigators noted an increased likelihood of infection by multiple-drug-resistant organisms in the group given 20 doses of cephalothin. This investigation demonstrated clearly the lack of any additional benefit to be realized from continuing chemoprophylactic drugs after the period of risk, that is, after the surgical procedure itself is over.

SUMMARY. A proliferating literature supports the potential benefit to be realized from short-term intraoperative chemoprophylaxis in selected surgical procedures. Taken in total, these data suggest that intraoperative chemoprophylactic antibiotics are indicated if there is a high probability that host defense mechanisms will be overcome by the challenge of a surgical procedure that carries the hazard of massive bacterial contamination. The chemoprophylactic regimen used to supplement host resistance must provide the drug in sufficient concentration during the operative procedure itself, and no additional benefit is realized by continuing chemoprophylactic drugs on the first or subsequent postoperative days. In fact, such extended chemoprophylaxis can be shown to have adverse consequences as measured by the alteration of normal host flora and the selection of multiple-drug-resistant organisms.

Effects of Unnecessary Antimicrobial Prophylaxis

It must be understood that a number of undesirable consequences follow from the use of chemoprophylaxis in situations in which it is not clearly indicated. First, the individual patient is put at an unnecessary risk of a hypersensitivity or toxic reaction to the drug itself or of a bacterial suprainfection resulting from alterations in normal flora. Moreover, such unnecessary chemoprophylaxis contributes to the selective pressure in the hospital environment for the emergence and perpetuation of resistant organisms, especially *Staphylococcus aureus* and Enterobacteriaceae. The administration of any antimicrobial drug—whether indicated or not and whether for prophylaxis or therapy—has microbiologic and epidemiologic consequences that go far beyond the immediate patient at hand. Consequently, the use of chemoprophylactic drugs in situations in which there is no clear justification is not only not indicated but is, in fact, contraindicated.

Control of Antibiotic Usage

Evidence cited earlier in this chapter pointed out that approximately 30 percent of hospitalized patients receive one or more systemic antimicrobial drugs at any given time and that the use of a given antibiotic, whether for therapy or for prophylaxis, was considered by infectious disease specialists to be inappropriate approximately 50 percent of the time. Thus, there is a problem of antibiotic overuse or misuse.

A number of approaches have been suggested from time to time to control antibiotic misuse. Noone and Shafi [59] reported a reduction in sepsis and the elimination of methicillin-resistant staphylococci in a London hospital before there was a marked change in the prescribing of antibiotics and in spite of inadequate facilities for isolation. They attributed their success to efforts directed at the education of the staff and to attempts to limit the use of certain antibiotics, including the cephalosporins, by closer communication among pharmacists, clinicians, and microbiologists.

Peer review of antibiotic utilization has been instituted in some centers. In one such instance, the cost of antibiotics used within the hospital was reduced by 20 percent in one year, without an increase in infection rates or longer hospital stays for patients with infection [92].

McGowan and Finland [55] recently reviewed the amounts of certain antibiotics used at the Boston City Hospital and correlated these amounts with a requirement to justify the choice of the antibiotics. An infectious disease consultant had to concur that a given restricted drug was appropriate therapy under the circumstances. This mild restraint on antibiotic usage in hospitalized patients substantially limited the use of potentially toxic or expensive agents, and it did so without any apparent deterioration in patient care, increased length of hospital stay for patients with infection, or increased mortality due to infection.

The simple requirement that prescribing physicians must state the rationale for the antibiotics prescribed by a note in the chart or a note on the prescription form has similarly been found to exert a marked restraining influence on usage of antibiotics so restricted.

Programs or policies designed to minimize the unnecessary and inappropriate use of antibiotics, whether for chemoprophylaxis or therapy, are entirely appropriate and need to be encouraged. Experience does not yet permit a clear judgment of the best approach to this problem, whether by education, by restriction, by peer review, or by some combination of all these. Should all these fail to reverse the present trends, however, a major reevaluation will then be required of the manner in which antibiotics are used by the entire medical profession. This will include, at the very least, a reevaluation of the hallowed concept that any physician may prescribe any licensed antibiotic, and the result is likely to be either limited licensure of antibiotic drugs, limitation on the prescription of certain antibiotics to certain classes of physicians, or both. Neither of these possibilities represents ideal solutions, and it is hoped that continuous education of students, housestaff, and practicing physicians in the use of antibiotics; a strong emphasis on the desirability of infectious disease consultation in the use of antibiotics; and continuous medical audit and peer review will restore antibiotic usage in hospitals to a rational and scientific basis.

References

1. Anderson, F. M., Datta, N., and Shaw, E. J. R factors in hospital infection. *Br. Med. J.* 2:82, 1972.
2. Barber, M., Dutton, A. A. C., Beard, M. A., Elmes, P. C., and Williams, R. Reversal of antibiotic resistance in hospital staphylococcal infection. *Br. Med. J.* 1:11, 1960.
3. Barrett, F. F., McGehee, R. F., and Finland, M. Methicillin-resistant *Staphylococcus aureus* at Boston City Hospital: Bacteriologic and epidemiologic observations. *N. Engl. J. Med.* 279:441, 1968.
4. Bartlett, J. G., Chang, T. W., Gurwith, M., Gorbach, S. L., and Onderdonk, A. B. Antibiotic-associated pseudomembranous colitis due to toxin-producing clostridia. *N. Engl. J. Med.* 298:531, 1978.
5. Bartlett, J. G., Onderdonk, A. B., and Cisneros, R. L. Clindamycin-associated colitis in hamsters: Protection with vancomycin. *Gastroenterology* 73:772, 1977.
6. Bartlett, J. G., Onderdonk, A. B., and Cisneros, R. L. Clindamycin-associated colitis in hamsters due to a toxin-producing clostridial species. *J. Infect. Dis.* 136:701, 1977.
7. Bauer, A. W., Kirby, W. M. M., Sherris, J. C., and Turck, M. Antibiotic susceptibility testing by a standardized single disc method. *Am. J. Clin. Pathol.* 45:493, 1966.
8. Bauer, A. W., Perry, D. M., and Kirby, W. M. M. Drug usage and antibiotic susceptibility of staphylococci. *J.A.M.A.* 173:475, 1960.
9. Bennett, J. V. Personal communication, 1971.
10. Benveniste, R., and Davies, J. Mechanisms

of antibiotic resistance in bacteria. *Ann. Rev. Biochem.* 42:471, 1973.

11. Bernard, H. R., and Cole, W. R. The prophylaxis of surgical infection: The effect of prophylactic antimicrobial drugs on the incidence of infection following potentially contaminated operations. *Surgery* 56:151, 1964.

12. Boyd, R. J., Burke, J. F., and Cotton, T. A double-blind clinical trial of prophylactic antibiotics in hip fractures. *J. Bone Joint Surg.* [Am.] 55A:1251, 1973.

13. Browne, R. A., Fekety, R., Silva, J., Boyd, D. I., Work, C. O., and Abrams, G. D. The protective effect of vancomycin on clindamycin-induced colitis in hamsters. *Johns Hopkins Med. J.* 141:183, 1977.

14. Bulger, R. J., Larson, E., and Sherris, J. C. Decreased incidences of resistance to antimicrobial agents among *Escherichia coli* and *Klebsiella-Enterobacter:* Observations in a university hospital over a 10-year period. *Ann. Intern. Med.* 72:65, 1970.

15. Bulger, R. J., and Sherris, J. C. Decreased incidence of antibiotic resistance among *Staphylococcus aureus:* A study in a university hospital over a 9-year period. *Ann. Intern. Med.* 69:1099, 1968.

16. Burke, J. F. The effective period of preventive antibiotic action in experimental incisions and dermal lesions. *Surgery* 50:161, 1961.

17. Conte, J. E., Jr., Cohen, S. N., Roe, B. B., and Elashoff, R. M. Antibiotic prophylaxis and cardiac surgery: A prospective double-blind comparison of single-dose versus multiple-dose regimens. *Ann. Intern. Med.* 76:943, 1972.

18. Damato, J. J., Eitzman, D. V., and Baer, H. Persistence and dissemination in the community of R factors of nosocomial origin. *J. Infect. Dis.* 129:205, 1974.

19. Davies, J., and Courvalin, P. Mechanisms of resistance to aminoglycosides. *Am. J. Med.* 62:868, 1977.

20. Davis, C. E., and Anandan, J. The evolution of R factor: A study of a "preantibiotic" community in Borneo. *N. Engl. J. Med.* 282:117, 1970.

21. Dixon, R. Personal communication. August, 1978.

22. Durack, D. T., and Petersdorf, R. G. Chemotherapy of experimental streptococcal endocarditis. I. Comparison of commonly recommended prophylactic regimens. *J. Clin. Invest.* 52:592, 1973.

23. Evans, C., and Pollack, A. V. The reduction of surgical wound infections by prophylactic parenteral cephaloridine. *Br. J. Surg.* 60:434, 1973.

24. Feeley, T. W., DuMoulin, G. C., Hedley-

Whyte, J., Bushnell, L. S., Gilbert, J. P., and Feingold, D. S. Aerosol polymyxin and pneumonia in seriously ill patients. *N. Engl. J. Med.* 293:471, 1975.

25. Fekety, F. R., Cluff, L. E., Sabiston, D. C., Jr., Seidl, L. G., Smith, J. W., and Thoburn, R. A study of antibiotic prophylaxis in cardiac surgery. *J. Thorac. Cardiovasc. Surg.* 57:757, 1969.

26. Finland, M. Changing ecology of bacterial infections as related to antibacterial therapy. *J. Infect. Dis.* 122:419, 1970.

27. Finland, M. Changing patterns of susceptibility of common bacterial pathogens to antimicrobial agents. *Ann. Intern. Med.* 76:1009, 1972.

28. Franco, J. A., Eitzman, D. V., and Baer, H. Antibiotic usage and microbial resistance in an intensive care nursery. *Am. J. Dis. Child.* 126:318, 1973.

29. Gardner, P., and Smith, D. H. Studies on the epidemiology of resistance (R) factors: I. Analysis of *Klebsiella* isolates in a general hospital. II. A prospective study of R factor transfer in the host. *Ann. Intern. Med.* 71:1, 1969.

30. Gardner, P., Smith, D. H., Beer, H., and Moellering, R. C., Jr. Recovery of resistance (R) factors from a drug-free community. *Lancet* 2:774, 1969.

31. Gibson, C. D., Jr., and Thompson, W. C., Jr. The response of burn wound staphylococci to alternating programs of antibiotic therapy. *Antibiotics Annual* 1955–56:32, 1956.

32. Goodman, J. S., Schaffner, W., Collins, H. A., Battersby, E. J., and Koenig, M. G. Infection after cardiovascular surgery: Clinical study including examination of antimicrobial prophylaxis. *N. Engl. J. Med.* 278:117, 1968.

33. Greene, W. H., Moody, M., Schimpff, S., Young, V. M., and Wiernik, P. H. *Pseudomonas aeruginosa* resistant to carbenicillin and gentamicin. *Ann. Intern. Med.* 79:684, 1973.

34. Greenfield, S., Teres, D., Bushnell, L. S., Hedley-Whyte, J., and Feingold, D. S. Prevention of gram-negative bacillary pneumonia using aerosol polymyxin as prophylaxis. I. Effect on the colonization pattern of the upper respiratory tract of seriously ill patients. *J. Clin. Invest.* 52:2935, 1973.

35. Hallander, H. O., and Laurell, G. Identification of cephalosporin resistant *Staphylococcus aureus* with the disc diffusion method. *Antimicrob. Agents Chemother.* 1:422, 1972.

36. Jawetz, E., and Gunnison, J. B. Antibiotic synergism and antagonism: An assessment of the problem. *Pharmacol. Rev.* 5:175, 1953.

37. Jessen, O., Rosendal, K., Bulow, P., Faber, V., and Eriksen, K. R. Changing staphylococci

and staphylococcal infections. *N. Engl. J. Med.* 281:627, 1969.

38. Jevons, M. P. "Celbenin"-resistant staphylococci. *Br. Med. J.* 2:124, 1961.

39. Johanson, W. G., Pierce, A. K., and Sanford, J. P. Changing pharyngeal bacterial flora of hospitalized patients: Emergence of gram-negative bacilli. *N. Engl. J. Med.* 281:1137, 1969.

40. Johanson, W. G., Jr., Pierce, A. K., Sanford, J. P., and Thomas, G. D. Nosocomial respiratory infections with gram-negative bacilli: The significance of colonization of the respiratory tract. *Ann. Intern. Med.* 77:701, 1972.

41. Kayser, F. H., and Mak, T. M. Methicillin-resistant staphylococci. *Am. J. Med. Sci.* 264:197, 1972.

42. Klastersky, J., Debusscher, L., Weerts, D., and Daneau, D. Use of oral antibiotics in protected environment units: Clinical effectiveness and role in the emergence of antibiotic-resistant strains. *Pathol. Biol. (Paris)* 22:5, 1974.

43. Klastersky, J., Huysmans, E., Weerts, D., Hensgens, C., and Daneau, D. Endotracheally administered gentamicin for the prevention of infections of the respiratory tract in patients with tracheostomy: A double-blind study. *Chest* 65:650, 1974.

44. Klick, J. M., Du Moulin, G. C., Hedley-Whyte, J., Teres, D., Bushnell, L. S., and Feingold, D. S. Prevention of gram-negative bacillary pneumonia using polymyxin aerosol as prophylaxis. II. Effect on the incidence of pneumonia in seriously ill patients. *J. Clin. Invest.* 55:514, 1975.

45. Klimek, J. J., Marsik, F. J., Bartlett, R. C., Weir, B., Shea, R., and Quintiliani, R. Clinical, epidemiologic and bacteriologic observations of an outbreak of methicillin-resistant *Staphylococcus aureus* at a large community hospital. *Am. J. Med.* 61:340, 1976.

46. Kunin, C. M., Tupasi, T., and Craig, W. A. Use of antibiotics: A brief exposition of the problem and some tentative solutions. *Ann. Intern. Med.* 79:555, 1973.

47. Lacey, R. W. Antibiotic resistance plasmids of *Staphylococcus aureus* and their clinical importance. *Bacteriol. Rev.* 39:1, 1975.

48. Ledger, W. J., Sweet, R. L., and Headington, J. T. Prophylactic cephaloridine in the prevention of postoperative pelvic infections in premenopausal women undergoing vaginal hysterectomy. *Am. J. Obstet. Gynecol.* 115:766, 1973.

49. Lepper, M. H., Moulton, B., Dowling, H. F., Jackson, G. G., and Kopman, S. Epidemiology of erythromycin-resistant staphylococci in a hospital population: Effect on therapeutic activity of erythromycin. *Antibiotics Annual* 1953–54:308, 1954.

50. Levine, A. S., Schimpff, S. C., Graw, R. G., Jr., and Young, R. C. Hematologic malignancies and other marrow failure states: Progress in the management of complicating infections. *Semin. Hematol.* 11:141, 1974.

51. Levine, A. S., Siegel, S. E., Schreiber, A. D., Hanser, J., Preisler, H., Goldstein, I. M., Seidler, F., Simon, R., Perry, S., Bennett, J. E., and Henderson, E. S. Protected environments and prophylactic antibiotics: A prospective controlled study of their utility in the therapy of acute leukemia. *N. Engl. J. Med.* 288:477, 1973.

52. Louria, D. B., and Brayton, R. G. The efficacy of penicillin regimens: With observations on the frequency of superinfection. *J.A.M.A.* 186:987, 1963.

53. Lowbury, E. J. L., Babb, J. R., and Roe, E. Clearance from a hospital of gram-negative bacilli that transfer carbenicillin-resistance to *Pseudomonas aeruginosa*. *Lancet* 2:941, 1972.

54. McGowan, J. E., Jr., and Finland, M. Infection and antibiotic usage at Boston City Hospital: Changes in prevalence during the decade 1964–1973. *J. Infect. Dis.* 129:421, 1974.

55. McGowan, J. E., Jr., and Finland, M. Usage of antibiotics in a general hospital: Effect of requiring justification. *J. Infect. Dis.* 130:165, 1974.

56. Miles, A. A., Miles, E. M., and Burke, J. The value and duration of defense reactions of the skin to the primary lodgement of bacteria. *Br. J. Exp. Pathol.* 38:79, 1957.

57. Mitsuhashi, S. (Ed.). *Transferable Drug Resistance Factor R.* Baltimore: University Park Press, 1971.

58. Mitsuhashi, S. Review: The R factors. *J. Infect. Dis.* 119:89, 1969.

59. Noone, P., and Shafi, M. S. Controlling infection in a district general hospital. *J. Clin. Pathol.* 26:140, 1973.

60. Parker, M. T., and Hewitt, J. H. Methicillin resistance in *Staphylococcus aureus*. *Lancet* 1:800, 1970.

61. Parker, M. T., and Lapage, S. P. Penicillinase production by *Staphylococcus aureus* strains from outbreaks of food poisoning. *J. Clin. Pathol.* 10:313, 1957.

62. Plorde, J. J., and Sherris, J. C. Staphylococcal resistance to antibiotics: Origin, measurement, and epidemiology. *Ann. N.Y. Acad. Sci.* 236:413, 1974.

63. Polk, H. C., Jr., and Lopez-Mayor, J. F. Postoperative wound infection: A prospective study of determinant factors and prevention. *Surgery* 66:97, 1969.

64. Pollack, M., Charache, P., Nieman, R. E., Jett, M. P., Reinhardt, J. A., and Hardy, P. H., Jr.

Factors influencing colonization and anti-biotic-resistance patterns of gram-negative bacteria in hospital patients. *Lancet* 2:668, 1972.

65. Price, D. J. E., and Sleigh, J. D.   Control of infection due to *Klebsiella aerogenes* in a neurosurgical unit by withdrawal of all antibiotics. *Lancet* 2:1213, 1970.

66. Reiter, B., Gee, T., Young, L., Dowling, M., and Armstrong, D.   Use of oral antimicrobials during remission induction in adult patients with acute nonlymphocytic leukemia (Abst.). *Clin. Research* 21:652, 1973.

67. Rifkin, G. D., Fekety, F. R., and Silva, J.   Antibiotic-induced colitis: Implication of a toxin neutralized by *Clostridium sordellii* antitoxin. *Lancet* 2:1103, 1977.

68. Roberts, A. W., and Visconti, J. A.   The rational and irrational use of systemic antimicrobial drugs. *Am. J. Hosp. Pharm.* 29:1054, 1972.

69. Rose, H. D., and Babcock, J. B.   Colonization of intensive care unit patients with gram-negative bacilli. *Am. J. Epidemiol.* 101:495, 1975.

70. Rose, H. D., and Schreier, J.   The effect of hospitalization and antibiotic therapy on the gram-negative fecal flora. *Am. J. Med. Sci.* 255:228, 1968.

71. Sabath, L. D.   Antimicrobial Resistance: Mechanisms of Resistance of Gram-Positive Cocci. In Brachman, P. S., and Eickhoff, T. C. (Eds.), *Proceedings of the International Conference on Nosocomial Infections*. Chicago: American Hospital Association, 1971, pp. 70–75.

72. Sabath, L. D., Wheeler, N., Laverdiere, M., Blazevic, D., and Wilkinson, B. J.   A new type of penicillin resistance of *Staphylococcus aureus*. *Lancet* 1:443, 1977.

73. Scheckler, W. E., and Bennett, J. V.   Antibiotic usage in seven community hospitals. *J.A.M.A.* 213:264, 1970.

74. Schimpff, S. C.   Laminar air flow room reverse isolation and microbial suppression to prevent infection in patients with cancer. *Cancer Chemother. Rep.* 59:1055, 1975.

75. Schimpff, S. C., Greene, W. H., Young, V. M., Fortner, C. L., Jepsen, L., Cusack, N., Block, J. B., and Wiernick, P. H.   Infection prevention in acute nonlymphocytic leukemia: Laminar air flow room reverse isolation with oral, nonabsorbable antibiotic prophylaxis. *Ann. Intern. Med.* 82:351, 1975.

76. Schimpff, S. C., Young, V. M., Greene, W. H., Vermeulen, G. D., Moody, M. R., and Wiernik, P. H.   Origin of infection in acute nonlymphocytic leukemia: Significance of hospital acquisition of pathogens. *Ann. Intern. Med.* 77:707, 1972.

77. Selden, R., Lee, S., Wang, W. L. L., Bennett, J. V., and Eickhoff, T. C.   Nosocomial *Klebsiella* infections: Intestinal colonization as a reservoir. *Ann. Intern. Med.* 74:657, 1971.

78. Smith, D. H.   Mechanisms of Resistance of Gram-Negative Bacilli. In Brachman, P. S., and Eickhoff, T. C. (Eds.), *Proceedings of the International Conference on Nosocomial Infections*. Chicago: American Hospital Association, 1971, pp. 61–69.

79. Smith, J. M. B., and Marples, M. J.   A natural reservoir of penicillin-resistant strains of *Staphylococcus aureus*. *Nature* 201:844, 1964.

80. Sogaard, H., Zimmermann-Nielsen, C., and Siboni, K.   Antibiotic-resistant gram-negative bacilli in a urological ward for male patients during a nine-year period: Relationship to antibiotic consumption. *J. Infect. Dis.* 130:646, 1974.

81. Speller, D. C. E., Raghunath, D., Stephens, M., Viant, A. C., Reeves, D. S., Wilkinson, P. J., Broughall, J. M., and Holt, H. A.   Epidemic infection by a gentamicin-resistant *Staphylococcus aureus* in three hospitals. *Lancet* 1:464, 1976.

82. Sprunt, K., Leidy, G. A., and Redman, W.   Prevention of bacterial overgrowth. *J. Infect. Dis.* 123:1, 1971.

83. Sprunt, K., and Redman, W.   Evidence suggesting importance of role of interbacterial inhibition in maintaining balance of normal flora. *Ann. Intern. Med.* 68:579, 1968.

84. Stokes, E. J., Waterworth, P. M., Franks, V., Watson, B., and Clark, C. G.   Short term routine antibiotic prophylaxis in surgery. *Br. J. Surg.* 61:739, 1974.

85. Tenney, J. H., Hopkins, J. A., LaForce, F. M., and Wang, W-L. L.   Pneumonia and pharyngeal colonization in a medical intensive care unit: Implications for prevention. Submitted for publication.

86. Tillotson, J. R., and Finland, M.   Bacterial colonization and clinical superinfection of the respiratory tract complicating antibiotic treatment of pneumonia. *J. Infect. Dis.* 119:597, 1969.

87. Vogel, L., Nathan, C., Sweeney, H. M., Kabins, S. A., and Cohen, S.   Infections due to gentamicin-resistant *Staphylococcus aureus* strain in a nursery for neonatal infants. *Antimicrob. Agents Chemother.* 13:466, 1978.

88. Wallmark, G., and Finland, M.   Phage types and antibiotic susceptibility of pathogenic staphylococci. Results at Boston City Hospital 1959–1960 and comparison of strains of previous years. *J.A.M.A.* 175:886, 1961.

89. Washington, J. A., Dearing, W. H., Judd, E. S., and Elveback, L. R.   Effect of preoperative antibiotic regimen on development of infection after intestinal surgery: Prospec-

tive, randomized, double-blind study. *Ann. Surg.* 180:567, 1974.

90. Williams, R. E. O. Changing Perspectives in Hospital Infection. In Brachman, P. S., and Eickhoff, T. C. (Eds.), *Proceedings of the International Conference on Nosocomial Infections.* Chicago: American Hospital Association, 1971, pp. 1–10.

91. Wolff, S. M., and Bennett, J. V. Editorial: Gram-negative-rod bacteremia. *N. Engl. J. Med.* 291:733, 1974.

92. Zeman, B. T., Pike, M., and Samet, C. The antibiotic utilization committee: An effective tool in the implementation of drug utilization review that monitors the medical justification and cost of antibiotics. *Hospitals* 48:73, 1973.

12

The Relationship Between the Hospital and the Community

William Schaffner

The hospital is the place in the community where most individuals begin and many end their lives. Recognized as the most visible and identifiable health-care institution in the community, the hospital is also a major employer, frequently an educational resource, and often a focus of community pride and civic volunteer activity. This complex institution has an understandably complex relationship with the community of which it is a part.

Only recently have we begun to realize that with regard to infection control, the hospital is indeed *part* of the community and that infectious events in one may influence the character of infections in the other.

This has not always been the case. Prior to World War II and for a short period thereafter, infections that occurred within the hospital were thought to originate primarily in the community. Patients with severe community-acquired infections were admitted to hospitals for care. Nosocomial infections were recognized as an occasional problem, but for the most part, such infections were thought to be caused by microorganisms common in the community.

During the 1950s, hospitals around the world were struck with the well-known assault of nosocomial staphylococcal infections. Thus, the focus shifted to the hospital as a special, isolated environment *separate* from the community. No matter what was going around outside, staphylococcal infection was prevalent within the hospital. The dire necessity to deal with such nosocomial infections was the mother of the discipline of hospital epidemiology; this in turn stimulated intensive laboratory, clinical, and epidemiologic investigations, some of the results of which are encompassed in this volume.

The nature of nosocomial infections, however, did not remain constant. As the staphylococcal problem receded during the 1960s and others took its place, investigations began to suggest that infections that occurred within

Supported in part by USPHS Grant No. AI-03082.

hospital walls did have consequences for the surrounding population; the proverbial street was found to run both ways. Microorganisms acquired in the community continue to pose problems of spread within hospitals, but some infections acquired in the hospital only appeared after the patient was discharged or were capable of being spread from a former patient to community contacts.

Spread of Community-Acquired Infections in the Hospital

Several recent reports remind us that certain community-acquired infections continue to be capable of being spread to patients and staff in the hospital. The decline in the new case rate of tuberculosis in the community has had several effects that may have conspired to increase the occupational hazard of acquiring tuberculous infection among hospital personnel. First, the special tuberculosis hospitals are being closed, thereby requiring that general hospitals undertake the care of patients with tuberculosis. Second, hospital workers are now more apt to be susceptible (tuberculin-negative) and thus are at greater risk of acquiring infection when exposed to tubercle bacilli. Third, subtle forms of reactivation tuberculosis among the elderly may not be diagnosed for some time, resulting in the close exposure of personnel. Contemporary technology may amplify the hazard as demonstrated in the report of one patient with unrecognized pulmonary tuberculosis who infected 23 employees (physicians, medical students, nurses, aides, ward secretary, kitchen worker, and an x-ray technician), some via an unbalanced air conditioning system [4].

Pertussis is a preventable childhood disease that is not often recognized in adults. It was with some surprise that workers at the University of Colorado Medical Center discovered that two small outbreaks of pertussis had originated among children, spread to house officers and nurses, and then spread further to children in the outpatient department and to other adults [7]. The disease was prevalent in the community, and it affected medical personnel

who, in turn, infected other community contacts.

Salmonella infections are notorious for their ability to spread within hospitals. A few years ago, a pediatric ward of a midwestern hospital experienced a prolonged outbreak of salmonellosis, which was initiated when a young patient with *Salmonella* gastroenteritis was admitted. Transmission was accomplished by contact spread, most likely through the passive transfer of organisms on the hands of medical attendants. It is of special interest that the epidemic extended beyond the hospital to a foundling home and to another hospital when patients or their community contacts were admitted to those secondary facilities.

Viral infections, too, may be introduced into hospitals. This occurs regularly during the influenza season and can produce life-threatening pneumonia among patients with preexisting pulmonary disease [2]. Epidemic keratoconjunctivitis due to adenovirus type 8 is another classic example; the hands of ophthalmologists or their tonometers or solutions may transfer the virus inoculum [9]. We have recently experienced the ease with which chickenpox can spread on a pediatric ward, affecting several patients with severe burns. Numerous other examples can be cited, especially ones involving hepatitis and group-A streptococci.

Spread of Nosocomial Infections to the Community

The spread of nosocomial infections to community contacts is a phenomenon that is generally unappreciated by hospital workers, perhaps because once the patient is out of sight, he is also out of mind. Practicing obstetricians and pediatricians, however, have long been aware that staphylococcal mastitis in nursing mothers occurs after the patient has been discharged from the hospital. It is thought that the infant becomes colonized with staphylococci while in the newborn nursery and he then transmits the organism to his mother.

An examination of the antibiotic sensitivities of staphylococcal strains provides a clear example of how the microflora of hospitals can influence that of the community. For over a decade, physicians have had to cope with "hospital staphylococci" that are almost uniformly resistant to penicillin. Infections acquired outside the hospital were thought to be caused by staphylococci that had remained penicillin-sensitive. The hospital is not a cloistered environment, however, and a recent study convincingly demonstrates that most "street strains" of staphylococci are now also resistant to penicillin (68 percent and 84 percent in two populations studied) [8]. It took a little time, but those "hospital" strains have finally made it around town.

In a similar and equally disturbing vein, it has recently been established that resistance (R)-factor-carrying enteric organisms can spread from patients to their community contacts [3]. Infants who were carrying R-factor-containing enteric organisms were followed after their discharge from an intensive-care nursery. Almost half remained carriers after 12 months, and a third of their family members also had R-factor-positive strains in their fecal flora. No family members of a control group of infants were colonized with such bacilli. It would seem that some patients may act as reservoirs of hospital-derived R-factor-containing bacteria for considerable periods after their return to the community.

One would have thought that an epidemic of nosocomial sepsis due to contaminated intravenous fluid bottles would be a "pure" hospital problem, but this was not the case. A man was admitted to a hospital with an episode of bacteremia and hypotension that was related to such an outbreak [5]. He was maintained on *home* hemodialysis, and he had a supply of the implicated fluid in his home that was used for priming the dialysis apparatus. In a sense, his home had become an extension of the hospital.

Renal dialysis has provided us with yet another example of how a hospital pathogen can be spread to family contacts. It is well known that hepatitis B (hepatitis B surface-antigen-positive hepatitis) has become endemic in some dialysis centers. A patient in such a setting had a severe hemorrhage at home because his arterial shunt dislodged. Some three months later, five of nine persons who were present at the time of the hemorrhage developed hepatitis. Hepatitis B virus was implicated, an example of the nonparenteral spread of this viral agent [6]. Clearly, nosocomial infections have public health implications for the community at large.

Relationship of the Hospital to Local, State, and Federal Health Authorities Regarding Infection Control

Hospitals are developing increasingly complex relationships with health authorities at all governmental levels. The requirements of various regulatory agencies impinging on hospital construction, professional standards review, working conditions for employees, laboratory licensing, and the like may all have peripheral impact on the problem of nosocomial infection. To explore such requirements is beyond the scope of this chapter, and we will confine ourselves to more traditional concerns.

The hospital looks to health authorities for assistance in three infection control areas: consultation on the establishment of a useful program, training of personnel to carry out the program, and assistance in the investigation of epidemics.

The ability of different health jurisdictions to respond to these needs varies enormously with the resources and personnel available. Health departments and hospitals have largely gone their separate ways in our society; the one is concerned with public health, and the other, with diagnostics and therapeutics. Therefore, it is uncommonly recognized that the infection control affairs of the hospital fall within the purview of the health department. Even where such jurisdiction is acknowledged, implementation may not be possible because of conflicting priorities. Health departments must continue to discharge their traditional responsibilities of impressive diversity (ranging from monitoring the pesticide concentration of milk to supervising school health) while attempting to cope with responsibilities newly thrust upon them, including screening for sickle-cell anemia, licensing of paraprofessionals, enforcement of air pollution standards, and so on. No wonder, then, that authorities have been loathe to open the Pandora's box of nosocomial infection. Thus, one may conclude without prejudice that most local and state health departments are not currently sufficiently equipped with either expert personnel or laboratory resources to be of great aid in establishing hospital infection control programs, training personnel, or rendering epidemic assistance.

Appropriate laboratory support is essential to the investigation of all but the simplest hospital outbreaks. Most health department laboratories are reference laboratories, although they may work with primary clinical specimens in such circumscribed areas as *Salmonella, Shigella,* and gonococcal bacteriology. The techniques required to perform primary isolation of hospital pathogens from diverse clinical specimens, environmental sampling, and Kirby-Bauer antimicrobial sensitivity testing are usually not in the public health laboratory's repertoire. Even more arcane procedures—such as those relating to gram-negative bacilli (e.g., serotyping and testing for resistance transfer factor)—are becoming increasingly important in delineating nosocomial outbreaks.

Among state health departments, Virginia, New Jersey, and Iowa have led in establishing programs for the control of nosocomial infections. Other states, including Tennessee, have recently followed suit. Since it is unlikely that health departments will greatly augment their staffs in the near future, ways could be sought to amplify their influence in this area. A possible solution is for health departments to enlist the aid of infectious disease experts at university medical centers who are conversant with nosocomial infection problems. While the administrative details are formidable, states could sponsor regular training programs in the epidemiologic and laboratory aspects of nosocomial infection that employ medical center faculty. Further, some faculty members might agree to function as consultants to community hospitals in establishing an infection control program or investigating an epidemic. Whether the state or the hospital ought to pay for this consultation service would have to be arranged. An argument can be made that both parties have an interest in the results, and

thus should share in the costs. The Intermountain Regional Medical Program has demonstrated that such a cooperative arrangement is feasible [1]. With the University of Utah Hospital at its hub, consultation in nosocomial infection problems is provided to small hospitals in five states by a physician, nurse-epidemiologist, and a microbiology laboratory consultant. The life of this project has recently been threatened by the budgetary cuts of the Regional Medical Program, which emphasizes the need for stable financing for any such program.

The laboratory support for epidemic investigations remains a major problem. University hospital laboratories might be able to assist with some investigations, but it appears that if the state makes a commitment to offer increased services in hospital infection control, either directly or through the use of consultants, then state laboratories will have to acquire expertise in this area.

When the problem of nosocomial infections was increasing in magnitude and with little response possible from local authorities, it was left to federal health officials to provide leadership. The Hospital Infections Branch within the Bureau of Epidemiology at the Center for Disease Control (CDC) was established for this purpose. That program remains the most helpful of any governmental agency, and, within the constraints of its funding, it provides assistance to local hospitals and health departments in all three previously mentioned areas.

The training activities sponsored by the CDC are extensive. Brief courses (usually one or two days in length) are given across the country in cooperation with local health departments and other groups. More extensive courses lasting from one to two weeks are given at the CDC in Atlanta and are directed to nurse epidemiologists, hospital administrators, microbiologists, and the like. Although some physicians do attend these offerings, one of the obvious gaps in the national effort to deal with the hospital infection problem is that there is no training program specifically designed to educate hospital epidemiologists and chairmen of Infection Control Committees. This has led to a curious paradox: many hospitals now employ well-trained nurse epidemiologists who are more knowledgeable than their ostensible supervisors. Also clearly needed are follow-up and refresher workshops, which ideally should be held at the local level in hospitals. Sponsorship of such events might best be assumed by cooperating health departments and large community and university hospitals, whose training programs would complement, rather than duplicate, those of the CDC.

Staff members of the Hospital Infections Branch of CDC are available for telephone consultation on the wide variety of questions that arise in the day-to-day practice of infection control. If the situation warrants and if the state health department concurs, epidemic aid teams can be put into the field at short notice. In addition, the branch distributes a variety of written material describing infection control activities. Perhaps the most widely used is the manual, *Isolation Techniques for Use in Hospitals,* which is further discussed in Chapter 9 of Part I. Also useful are the quarterly reports of the National Nosocomial Infections Study. Not only do they provide a national perspective on nosocomial infections, but they also frequently contain definitive statements on particular infection control problems.

Because it is now recognized that nationally distributed products such as intravenous fluids, medications, and medical devices may on occasion not be sterile, hospital epidemiology has taken on a national as well as local dimension. The CDC's National Nosocomial Infections Study is an attempt to provide current national surveillance of infection hazards. It is anticipated that the increasing sophistication of this study will provide extremely important information both to individual hospitals and health authorities in the future.

As problems with contaminated products have received wider recognition, the relationship of hospital infection control programs to another governmental agency, the Food and Drug Administration (FDA), has been established. Hospitals are not the traditional "clients" of the FDA, and appropriate lines of communication are only now slowly being developed. Indeed, in the past the close relationship between hospitals and industry may have hampered the recognition of problems. Hospi-

tal pharmacists, for example, are more likely to contact a manufacturer's representative when a question of contaminated intravenous fluid arises than they are to contact either the FDA or CDC. Anecdotal reports also suggest that some local FDA field representatives are not familiar with hospital-related problems and thus have not been able to offer prompt and incisive assistance. There is the further difficulty of delineating the area of the FDA's responsibility vis-à-vis the CDC. Clearly, the CDC has the best perspective over the entire hospital infection arena and is the repository of the major epidemiologic expertise needed to delineate and solve problems. The FDA, on the other hand, has regulatory authority over industry and the power to recall products suspected of being contaminated. It is hoped that the evolution of the relationship between these agencies will result in greater assurances that our hospitalized patients will be at less risk of nosocomial misadventure.

Reporting of Communicable Diseases

Prevention and control of communicable disease is traditionally a primary duty of health departments. Patients with illnesses that may be a threat to the health of the community, however, are attended by scattered, individual practitioners. Therefore, it was soon recognized that a system of prompt and accurate notification of the occurrence of certain communicable diseases was a requisite to their control. In 1883 the state of Michigan adopted legislation establishing a system of communicable disease reporting, and since then all other states have followed suit. These laws have been determined not to violate the special nature of the doctor-patient relationship by the courts on numerous occasions.

The reporting system is pluralistic; both physicians and hospitals have an independent obligation to notify the public health authorities if patients with certain illnesses are admitted to their care. Concerns over possible duplication of reports should not deter reporting; health departments have the responsibility for ascertaining the best final case tally.

It is important that hospitals develop a system of disease notification for several reasons. First, by reporting such diseases promptly, hospitals can be of assistance to the public health authorities in the control of communicable diseases in their own communities. Second, by educating the staff physicians and employees as to this responsibility, the hospital becomes an advocate of good preventive medical practice. Third, the hospital's unique role enables it to be a major contributor to the state and national morbidity data-collection mechanism, which determines funding priorities for research and control activities. And last, as the medical profession's capacity to prevent disease increases, there will be a consequent, increasing need for precise information on disease occurrence. Subsequent to the widespread use of the polio vaccines, for example, there remains a continuing need to evaluate carefully all cases of poliomyelitis-like illness. A documented case may alert authorities to a population of unimmunized children or a problem with the vaccine itself. Unreported, the incident will go uninvestigated. It is likely that more reports will be required in the future. With the advent of pneumococcal vaccines, certain large community and university hospitals may be requested to provide information on the isolation of pneumococcal serotypes in order to help monitor the impact of vaccine usage. Other such examples could be given.

The list of diseases designated as reportable in Tennessee is given in Table 12-1 and is representative of such lists found in most states. Although the list appears extensive, most reporting by hospitals involves just a few diseases: hepatitis, viral meningitis, encephalitis, meningococcal infections, salmonellosis, shigellosis, and the venereal diseases, gonorrhea and syphilis. It is the responsibility of the hospital epidemiologist to establish a valid reporting mechanism. We have designed the following mechanism after consultation with our local and state authorities.

Reporting is performed weekly by the use of a standard morbidity report card that is sent to the local health department. Most reports are generated by positive culture results in the bacteriology laboratory, but the nurse epidemiologist and infectious disease faculty add re-

Table 12-1. Reportable Diseases in Tennessee

Reportable by name, address, race, sex, and age		
Amebiasis	Leprosy	Salmonellosis,
Anthrax	Leptospirosis	Typhoid fever
Botulism	Malaria	Other
Brucellosis	Measles	salmonel-
Cholera	Meningitis, viral	losis
Congenital	Meningococcal	Shigellosis
rubella	infections	Smallpox
syndrome	Plague	Tetanus
Diphtheria	Poliomyelitis,	Trichinosis
Encephalitis,	paralytic	Tuberculosis
Arthropod-	Psittacosis	Tularemia
borne	Rabies in man	Typhus fever,
Other	Relapsing fever,	Endemic
infectious	louse-borne	Epidemic
Encephalitis,	Rheumatic	Yellow fever
Postinfectious	fever, acute	
Postvaccinal	Rocky Mountain	
Hepatitis,	spotted fever	
Infectious		
Serum		

Reportable by number of cases
Influenza
Mumps
Rubella
Streptococcal infections
Whooping cough

Source: State Department of Public Health, 344 Cordell Hull Building, Nashville, TN 37219.

ports on such diseases as hepatitis and viral meningitis that would not be reflected in laboratory culture reports. The reports include the name, age, sex, race, and address of the patient. Extraordinary events, such as a patient with suspected poliomyelitis, are reported immediately by telephone. In addition, the bacteriology laboratory routinely sends subcultures of all *Salmonella, Shigella,* and meningococcal isolates to the state reference laboratory for confirmation and serogrouping.

Reporting of the venereal diseases is handled in a somewhat different manner. Regarding syphilis, all serologic results that are positive at a dilution of 1 : 16 or greater are reported immediately by telephone to the venereal disease investigator in the local health department. All other positive serologic results are reported on each Friday together with complete patient identification, including the name of the patient's physician. All isolates of *Neisseria gonorrhoeae* from patients less than ten years of age are reported immediately by telephone; others are reported on Friday. Only patients with positive cultures, not simply positive Gram stains, are reported.

In addition, the occurrence of any illness that may have public health implications is reported. Cases of suspected food poisoning seen in the emergency room, for example, are promptly reported by telephone in order that the authorities can make an investigation. During the winter months, our hospital participates in a special surveillance system for influenza organized by the state health department.

Hospitals may employ other methods of notification. Institutions that require admission diagnoses can prepare a daily list of patients admitted with suspected hepatitis, meningitis, and the like. Other institutions rely on final discharge diagnoses for reporting. The former method is less accurate, but it is of value to local health departments that give a high priority to investigation of communicable diseases. The latter method is more precise, but one loses the advantage of timeliness. The method that best suits local needs can be chosen. Some states have now included among their requirements for hospital licensure demonstrated evidence that the hospital has an approved and functioning communicable disease reporting mechanism.

Broader Influence of the Hospital Epidemiologist

As a person in the medical community with a heightened interest in preventive medicine, the hospital epidemiologist is occasionally in a position to influence decisions in areas beyond those relating just to nosocomial infections. Indeed, one of my first goals when I assumed this position at Vanderbilt University Hospital in 1969 was to convince the hospital administration to discontinue the sale of cigarettes in the hospital. As has been the case in other institutions, this was accomplished without any complaints from personnel, patients, or visitors. Unfortunately, I was unable to persuade the

administration to post signs near the vending machines explaining the policy, thereby losing an opportunity for public health education.

The Joint Commission on Hospital Accreditation recently has required that hospitals institute reviews of antibiotic usage and the use of whole blood, especially single-unit transfusions. These tasks might naturally become the province of the hospital epidemiologist.

Another area in which the epidemiologist can be of assistance is in the immediate management of community contacts of patients with certain infections. A 26-year-old married father of two children, for example, is admitted with meningococcal meningitis. Whose responsibility is it to provide antibiotic prophylaxis to his wife and children: the attending internist, the pediatrician, the local health officer, or the hospital epidemiologist himself? I believe there can be no absolute rule, but the hospital epidemiologist can act as an ombudsman to provide assurance that this essential preventive medical service is not overlooked.

It is paradoxical that hospitals, society's most visible health-care institutions, have lagged in providing preventive medical services for their employees. Hospital epidemiologists have the opportunity to persuade hospitals to provide screening programs for hypertension and other coronary-risk factors, tuberculosis, cervical cancer, and gonorrhea, as well as comprehensive immunization programs and even family planning services. If these were combined with an educational effort, hospitals, long admired for their sophisticated care of sick patients, could make a contribution to medicine's highest goal, the prevention of disease.

References

1. Britt, M. R., Burke, J. P., Nordquist, A. G., Wilfert, J. N., and Smith, C. B. Infection control in small hospitals: Prevalence surveys in 18 institutions. *J.A.M.A.* 236:1700, 1976.
2. Burk, R. F., Schaffner, W., and Koenig, M. G. Severe influenza virus pneumonia in the pandemic of 1968–1969. *Arch. Intern. Med.* 127:1122, 1971.
3. Damato, J. J., Eitzman, D. V., and Baer, H. Persistence and dissemination in the community of R-factors of nosocomial origin. *J. Infect. Dis.* 129:205, 1974.

4. Ehrenkranz, N. J., and Kicklighter, J. L. Tuberculosis outbreak in a general hospital: Evidence for airborne spread of infection. *Ann. Intern. Med.* 77:377, 1972.

5. Felts, S. K., Schaffner, W., Melly, M. A., and Koenig, M. G. Sepsis caused by contaminated intravenous fluids: epidemiologic, clinical, and laboratory investigation of an outbreak in one hospital. *Ann. Intern. Med.* 77: 881, 1972.

6. Garibaldi, R. A., Hatch, F. E., Bisno, A. L., Hatch, M. H., and Gregg, M. B. Nonparenteral serum hepatitis: report of an outbreak. *J.A.M.A.* 220:963, 1972.

7. Kurt, T. L., Yeager, A. S., Guenette, S., and Dunlop, S. Spread of pertussis by hospital staff. *J.A.M.A.* 221:264, 1972.

8. Ross, S., Rodriguez, W., Controni, G., and Khan, W. Staphylococcal susceptibility to penicillin G: the changing pattern among community strains. *J.A.M.A.* 229:1075, 1974.

9. Wegman, D. H., Guinee, V. F., and Millian, S. J. Epidemic keratoconjunctivitis. *Am. J. Public Health* 60:1230, 1970.

II

Endemic and Epidemic Hospital Infections

13

Incidence and Nature of Endemic and Epidemic Nosocomial Infections

John V. Bennett

Part I of this text emphasizes general concepts and the epidemiology of hospital infections and stresses the functions and responsibility of infection control staff. In contrast, Part II encompasses the epidemiology of specific infections and emphasizes preventive practices that directly affect patient-care practices. This introductory chapter provides explanatory material concerning the content of Part II and also provides a brief overview of nosocomial infections that may be used as a background in assessing specific endemic and epidemic infections that are discussed in other chapters.

The intended focus of Part II is primarily epidemiologic rather than clinical. Each author was requested to provide specific information concerning the incidence, sources, modes of spread, host factors, and control measures for both endemic and epidemic infections. Statistical data concerning nosocomial infections were derived from the National Nosocomial Infections Study (NNIS) and made available to authors. Descriptions of this study, its definitions of infections, and criteria for distinguishing community-acquired from nosocomial infections have been published elsewhere [1,2].

Chapters in Part II have been selected to answer specifically the most important questions about nosocomial infection problems in different sites. Infections covered by each chapter include the most common, important, serious, and communicable types of infection in each site. Occasionally, infections in certain sites have been included that do not meet these criteria but were included because their proper management is known to be a source of concern or difficulty for infection control staffs. Some sites of infection, such as deep abdominal abscesses and decubitus ulcers, have been deliberately excluded. These infections are not as effectively prevented as others by infection control measures. Such restrictions of content provide a greater specificity, which in turn, it is hoped, will improve the practical usefulness of these chapters.

General Features of Nosocomial Infections

Endemic Infections

DATA SOURCE. The following material is based upon data collected from 1971 to 1974 from acute-care hospitals that voluntarily participated in NNIS. Those data encompass 169,038 isolates from 136,912 infections. During this time, 3,957,393 patients were discharged from participating hospitals. The extent of underreporting and adherence to established criteria and definitions is unknown. Also, it is likely that some hospitals have reported service on which a patient resided at the onset of infection and others, the service of the patient at the time the infection was acquired. The accuracy of identifying microorganisms and the completeness of reporting mortality doubtlessly also varied between hospitals. Despite the above reservations, this material nonetheless represents a valuable data bank for assessing hospital infections and presents a more representative national picture than can be obtained from a summary of available publications describing individual hospital experiences.

The distribution of the types of hospitals participating in NNIS differs somewhat from the distribution of types of hospitals nationally. Data from a particular hospital category, however, can be weighted according to the proportion of acute-care admissions to each hospital category nationally, thus permitting nationally adjusted data to be developed.

INCIDENCE AND MORTALITY. The overall nationally adjusted incidence of infections, as derived from NNIS hospital reports from 1971 to 1974, is 3.8 infections per 100 patients (Table 13-1). If the reporting of nosocomial infections is 75 percent complete (a reasonable estimate based on other studies), then the overall true incidence of nosocomial infection nationally may be expected to be about 5 percent. Multiple infections (i.e., two or more infections in the same patient) constitute 5.5 percent of all infections in community hospitals with less than 300 beds and about 11 percent in university hospitals. Overall, about 7.6 percent of all nosocomial infections are multiple infections.

The adjusted national mortality rate among infected patients is 6.4 percent; such rates range from a low of 3.9 percent in university hospitals to 11.2 percent in municipal and county hospitals. These data include all deaths that occurred in patients with infection; infections were reported to be causative or contributory causes of death in 43 percent of such deaths, or about 3 percent of all infected patients. In contrast, only about 3 percent of all patients admitted to acute-care hospitals, excluding newborn services, die during hospitalization. Thus, the risk of death in those with

Table 13-1. Nosocomial Infections by Category of Hospital

Hospital category	Incidence per 100 discharges	Frequency of multiple infections	Mortality in infected patients	Estimated percentage of acute-care admissions to U.S. hospitals[a]
Municipal or county	5.4	8.4%	11.2%	23.6%
Federal	4.6	8.9%	8.2%	5.1%
University	4.3	10.9%	3.9%	21.8%
Community (300 or more beds)	3.1	5.9%	5.1%	16.0%
Community (less than 300 beds)	2.4	5.5%	5.0%	33.5%
Adjusted national estimates based on proportion of acute-care admissions	3.8	7.6%	6.4%	100.0%

[a] Based on random sample of hospitals from the 1973 *American Hospital Association Guide,* American Hospital Association, Chicago, Ill.

infection would appear to be about twice that of the overall hospital population.

There are many factors underlying the observed differences in infections among the five hospital categories: differing age and disease status of patient populations, frequency and type of procedures and therapies administered, adherence to surveillance definitions and criteria, completeness of identifying cases, effectiveness of infection control programs, physical facilities, length of hospitalization, and other factors that have not been identified.

ECONOMIC IMPACT. Given an adjusted nationwide incidence of 5 percent and 37,000,-000 acute-care admissions per year, it can be estimated that approximately 1,850,000 noso-

comial infections develop each year in the United States. Center for Disease Control (CDC) studies have indicated that the average prolongation of stay attributable to an infection is about five days and the mean, attributable, direct cost of the infection to the patient is about $700. Thus, the economic impact of nosocomial infections is over a billion dollars per year. This, however, is conservative, because no estimates have been included for indirect cost to the patient, the cost of death, time lost from productive employment, cost to the hospital deriving from adverse publicity and law suits, and cost to the community in the way of health insurance premiums; neither has the cost been included of nosocomial infections that may spread from an infected patient to community contacts to produce additional morbidity, mortality, and attendant cost.

SITE-SERVICE PATTERNS. Figure 13-1 presents nosocomial infection rates by service and site of infection and the overall relative frequency of infections in different sites. This figure has been prepared to facilitate identifying infection profiles for particular services. By scanning the material horizontally, significant divergences from the overall experience may be identified. A vertical scan, in contrast, provides a comparative profile of infections occurring on each service.

Figure 13-1. Nosocomial infection rates according to service and site. Infection rates for each site on a particular service are compared with the overall rate for that site on all services: blank spaces indicate a difference of ±1.5 times or less; dotted boxes, a difference of ±1.6 to 2.0 times; shaded boxes, ±2.1 to 3.0 times; and solid boxes, ±3 times or more. In column headings, + and − indicate above or below average rates, respectively. Secondary bacteremia rates are not included in totals; secondary bacteremia is considered to represent a complication of another infection rather than a separate infection.

Based on data from National Nosocomial Infections Study (NNIS), 1971–1974 (see text).

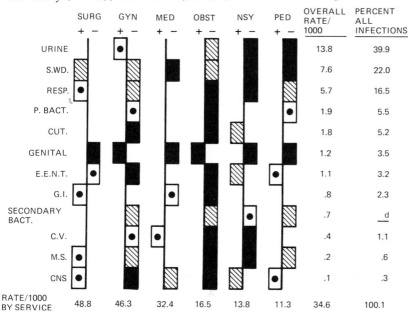

The four most frequent types of nosocomial infections are, in descending order, urinary, surgical wound, respiratory, and primary bacteremia. Their relative frequencies can be roughly approximated by an easy-to-remember rule involving twofold decrements (one-half, one-quarter, one-eighth, one-sixteenth), and collectively they account for about 80 percent of all infections.

Differences in profiles of the four most common infections by service appear to reflect the frequency with which patients on different services are exposed to particular procedures predisposing to infection. (The population at risk for surgical wound infections, for example, is primarily those hospitalized on surgery.) Host factors doubtlessly also play a role, especially in the less common infections.

If one's attention is restricted to the four most frequent types of infections (which appear in the top four rows of the figure) and to the darkened squares (solid boxes) that reflect a threefold or greater departure from overall rates, it can be seen that urinary tract infections are substantially less common on nursery and pediatric services, respiratory infections are much less common on obstetric and nursery services, and primary bacteremia is a relatively infrequent event on obstetric services. Above-average rates involving the four major sites of infection were observed for surgical wound and respiratory infections on surgical services and for urinary tract infections on gynecologic services. Other substantial differences can be determined by a careful review of the figure.

SITE-PATHOGEN PATTERNS. Figure 13-2 provides information concerning the pathogens isolated from each site of nosocomial infection and presents the overall relative frequency of occurrence of different pathogens. This information is depicted in an analogous fashion to the preceding figure. Figure 13-2 permits ready identification of the profiles of pathogens isolated from specific sites and indicates the propensity of different pathogens to produce infections in different sites.

Escherichia coli is the pathogen most frequently isolated (20 percent); it occurs more than twice as frequently as the next most common pathogen. *Staphylococcus aureus, Pro-*

teus, Pseudomonas, Klebsiella, and enterococci occur in comparable frequencies, each accounting for approximately 8 to 10 percent of all isolates. About two-thirds of the most common bacterial isolates from nosocomial infections are gram-negative rods. Anaerobic bacteria, included in the "all other" column, were doubtlessly incompletely reported by participating hospitals during the time period encompassed by the data.

Overall, 27 percent of all infections are polymicrobial (two or more pathogens reported); these ranged from a maximum of 42 percent polymicrobial infections among gynecologic infections to a minimum of 6 percent polymicrobial infections in primary bacteremia.

If one's attention is again confined to the four most important sites of infections (which appear in the top four rows of Figure 13-2) and to the darkened squares (solid boxes) that signify a threefold or greater departure from overall rates, substantial differences in the affinity of different pathogens for three different sites can be identified. Nearly all of these observations fit obvious clinical expectancies. They also probably reflect, to a certain degree, decisions of laboratory workers and infection control personnel in participating hospitals to exclude certain isolates as pathogens when obtained from certain sites. The patterns of primary bacteremia, however, are unexpected and notable; *Proteus* organisms are relatively infrequently encountered and no single organism shows a particular predominance. Many additional comparisons can be made from the data presented in this figure, and it should serve as a useful reference for those with a specific interest in less common infections.

Epidemic Infections

CLUSTERS. Computer analysis of reported infection data from collaborating hospitals has been used to detect significant increases in the monthly overall hospital rates of infection for specific site-pathogen patterns by comparison with a preceding five-month baseline period. Subsequent field investigations have suggested that about 5 percent of all nosocomial infections belong to actual clusters of disease involving patients with an average of about six

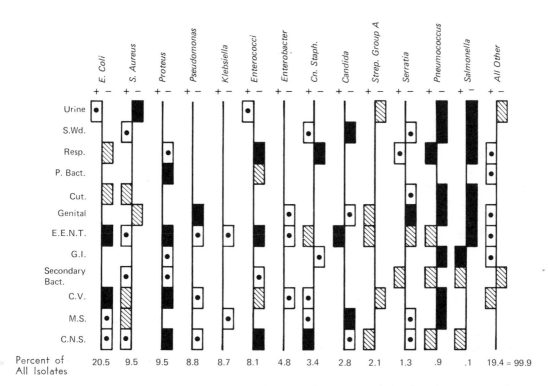

Figure 13-2. Relative frequency of pathogens in various sites. Proportion of all pathogens in a site contributed by a particular pathogen is compared with the proportion that the pathogen contributed to all pathogens in all sites: blank spaces indicate a difference of ±1.5 times or less; dotted boxes, a difference of ±1.6 to 2.0 times; shaded boxes, ±2.1 to 3.0 times; and solid boxes, ±3 times or more. In column headings, + and − indicate above or below average values, respectively.

Based on data from National Nosocomial Infections Study (NNIS), 1971–1974 (see text).

infections per cluster. If such analyses were performed for individual wards and services and if more specific markers (e.g., antibiograms) were used, clusters would be identified even more frequently. Computer analysis is very helpful in the efficient detection of such problems, because many of these clusters escape recognition by infection control personnel. Furthermore, these clusters tend to involve common organisms in common sites of infections, and they thus differ from the profile of infections associated with recognized epidemic disease. Each identified cluster, however, needs to be investigated, since it may have resulted

from cross-infection between patients or from a series of patients being exposed to the same common vehicle. In either event, potentially preventable infections must be assumed to have occurred.

These clusters are, in fact, outbreaks of a less spectacular sort than those of overtly recognized epidemics, and they often escape recognition by hospitals that do not conduct surveillance or do not subject their surveillance data to a threshold type of analysis. The detection and investigation of such clusters is thus important because they involve a large number of potentially preventable infections.

INVESTIGATED OUTBREAKS. Information on epidemic disease has been obtained from a group of outbreaks that occurred during the five years from 1970 to 1975 and were investigated by staff at the Center for Disease Control in Atlanta. Seventy-seven outbreaks of known infectious causes involving clinically recognized disease in patients in acute-care hospitals have been summarized. Only the initial investigation of those outbreaks that were attributable to contaminated commercial products has been included in these tabulations.

There are a number of difficulties in applying such data to other hospitals throughout the nation. Significant biases underlying CDC's involvement in such investigations are obviously important. Nonetheless, the above data should be of some assistance in providing the framework for assessing the epidemic potential of different pathogens. Furthermore, the presented data should provide some assistance in orienting the reader to the chapters that follow in this portion of the book.

The three most common causes of specific nosocomial epidemics during this time period were hepatitis B virus (ten outbreaks), *Salmonella* gastroenteritis (ten outbreaks), and enteropathogenic *E. coli* gastroenteritis (five outbreaks).

The gastrointestinal site was the single most common site involved in these outbreaks (19 percent), and hepatitis and bloodstream infections ranked second and third (17 percent each). Outbreaks involving the cutaneous system were fourth most common (13 percent). Infections in these sites are several times more common in epidemic disease than in endemic disease, whereas respiratory, surgical wound, and urinary tract infection sites are involved less frequently than would be expected from the endemic frequency of disease in these sites.

The common agents encountered in epidemics—hepatitis virus, *Salmonella,* and herpesvirus (varicella and herpes zoster)—are 100 times or more frequent in epidemic than in endemic infections, and both group-A streptococci and *Serratia* organisms are also encountered in substantially greater frequency (about nine and six times greater, respectively). Interestingly, *S. aureus,* Enterobacter and *Pseudomonas* occur in about the same frequency as in endemic infections. The role of enteropathogenic *E. coli* as the cause of disease is less certain in endemic than in epidemic occurrences, and similar comparisons were thus not made for this agent. The above comparisons thus indicate that the relative frequency of different pathogens involved in epidemics also differs markedly from the relatively frequency of pathogens involved in endemic disease.

References

1. Bennett, J. V., Scheckler, W. E., Maki, D. G., and Brachman, P. S.   Current National Patterns. In Brachman, P. S., and Eickhoff, T. C. E. (Eds.), *Proceedings of the International Conference on Nosocomial Infections.* Chicago: American Hospital Association, 1971.
2. Garner, J. S., Bennett, J. V., Scheckler, W. E., Maki, D. G., and Brachman, P. S.   Surveillance of Nosocomial Infection. In Brachman, P. S., and Eickhoff, T. C. E. (Eds.), *Proceedings of the International Conference on Nosocomial Infections.* Chicago: American Hospital Association, 1971.

14

Urinary Tract Infections

Calvin M. Kunin

"Urinary tract infection" is a broad term used to encompass inflammatory processes of microbiologic origin that occur in the kidney, pelvis, ureter, bladder, urethra, or adjacent structures of the urinary tract such as the prostate and urethral glands. Urine, as it is formed or passes through these structures, is readily contaminated by microorganisms that invade the tract, or it may be the medium through which various parts may become infected. Urine is normally sterile; when it is colonized with bacteria, all the structures of the tract are at risk of being invaded. Bacteriuria is the most common factor in all urinary tract infections. The presence of significant numbers of bacteria in the urine is therefore operationally equivalent to the presence of a urinary tract infection, even in the absence of symptoms of pyuria.

Urinary tract infections are of major importance not only because they are common but also because they may be the source of invasion of bacteria or their products into the bloodstream. This may lead to renal damage, disseminated infection, the syndrome of gram-negative sepsis, and considerable morbidity. More urinary tract infections, particularly in females, are of community-acquired than of nosocomial origin. The urinary tract, however, is the most common site of infection that originates during hospitalization, and urinary tract infections constitute the largest single cause of gram-negative bacterial sepsis in hospitals. Fortunately, nosocomially induced urinary infections are largely preventable by careful attention to the indications for instrumentation of the tract, by using proper procedures during the insertion of instruments, and by meticulous care of urinary drainage systems.

Urinary tract infections in hospitalized patients arise most commonly from instrumentation of the tract and, to a lesser extent, from bloodborne infection from a distant site. In addition, they may occur at times as a complication of surgical procedures or from lesions in adjacent structures that produce fistulas from the vagina, rectum, or other structures adjacent to the bladder. The most common cause of these infections, however, is the urinary catheter, particularly when the catheter remains in place for prolonged periods. For this reason, much of the emphasis in this chapter will be directed toward the problem of indwelling catheter-induced infections and their prevention.

Nature of Urinary Tract Infections

Incidence of Community-Acquired Infections

The epidemiologic characteristics of urinary tract infections have been well defined in the general population when such infections are unrelated to hospitalization. The hospital epidemiologist must be aware of this so he or she will recognize the background against which those infections that arise in the hospital must be related. In brief, the frequency of bacteriuria in the neonatal period is probably about 0.5 percent, with a slightly higher frequency in boys than in girls. The rate in preschool children is incompletely defined, but it is about 0.5 to 1.0 percent in girls and rarely seen in boys unless they have underlying structural or neurologic abnormalities of the urinary tract. In school children, the prevalence of bacteriuria is about 1.0 to 1.5 percent in girls and about 1 per 1000 in boys. Infection in males remains at very low rates until the "prostate years," beginning in about the sixth decade of life. It is at this time that catheter-associated infections pose a major problem. Urinary infections are common among adult females. The prevalence of bacteriuria rises about 1 percent with each decade. Thus, about 2 to 4 percent of sexually active women in the child-bearing years will have bacteriuria at any one time. The rate may reach 8 to 10 percent in elderly women. It must be emphasized that these data represent prevalence, that is, the frequency of infection at any one point in time. It is estimated, however, that as many as 35 percent of women will have an urinary tract infection at some time during life.

Frequency of Nosocomial Infections

The frequency of nosocomial urinary tract infections depends almost entirely on the fre-

quency of conditions in patients that lead to instrumentation of the urinary tract and the policies and procedures of the medical-care system in the hospital. The patient population characteristics differ considerably among community, university, and governmental hospitals as well as domiciliary care facilities; thus, a single estimate as to the overall frequency of the problem may poorly describe a particular hospital. Composite data from the National Nosocomial Infections Study (NNIS) indicate that about 40 percent of all nosocomial infections reported in 1971 through 1974 involved the urinary tract and that the overall rate for such infections was 1.4 per 100 hospital discharges (see Part II, Chapter 13). It can be estimated that at least two-thirds of these infections occurred in patients with catheterization or instrumentation of the urinary tract. The specific rate for catheter-associated urinary tract infections was about 1 per 100 discharges, and these accounted for about 30 percent of all nosocomial infections. Thus, the urinary tract is the site most commonly involved in nosocomial infections.

Diagnostic Criteria

Bacteria generally grow well in urine, even though it is a variable culture medium. It is now well known that most urinary tract infections will be associated with bacterial counts of 100,000 microorganisms per milliliter or more. There are exceptions to this rule, but they are distinctly unusual and make up no more than about 5 percent of cases. The major exception is in patients undergoing water diuresis or when antimicrobial agents are being used to suppress bacterial growth. Simply finding bacteria in the urine in the absence of quantitative counts is a useless exercise.

A urinary tract infection can be diagnosed when (1) 10^5 or more organisms per milliliter are cultured from a properly collected and processed midstream or catheter specimen of urine, (2) 10^2 or more organisms per milliliter are cultured from a specimen obtained by suprapubic bladder puncture, or (3) abundant neutrophils and bacteria are found on microscopic examination of the urine sediment; the last may be considered presumptive evidence of urinary infection. Other criteria include 10 or more white blood cells with 20 or more bacteria per high-powered field or pus cells with at least three or four bacteria per oil-immersion field of the Gram-stained sediment.

Classification of Infections

Classification of an infection as community-acquired or nosocomial should take into account the results of an admission urinalysis and the patient's urologic history. The infection should be considered nosocomial when culture of a urine specimen obtained from the patient during hospitalization is (1) positive, and there were normal urinalysis results on admission and no history of infection symptoms; (2) positive, but a negative culture has been obtained at a prior time during hospitalization that cannot be attributed to antibiotic suppression; or (3) positive for organisms different from those cultured at preceding times during the hospitalization.

The clean-voided method of collecting specimens should be used at all times unless the patient cannot void after being given adequate time, privacy, and clear guidance. Suprapubic taps should be considered as the next alternative if the bladder is full, particularly in infants and young children. There obviously will be emergency situations or the patient may be too ill to obtain a clean-voided specimen and a catheter must be inserted to obtain a specimen, but these must be considered as special circumstances where the need for the specimen must clearly justify the risk of catheterization.

For unknown reasons, some physicians seem to have developed the habit of requesting routine culture tests of catheter tips at the time of their removal. This makes little sense when one considers the fact that bacteria are easily detected in the urine itself and will be present in very high numbers if true contamination of the bladder urine has occurred. The tip of the catheter will be drawn through the urethra, which always contains small numbers of bacteria. These organisms usually are gram-positive and of no major concern. The deceptive nature of catheter tip cultures was recently clearly documented in an elegant study by Gross and co-workers [10].

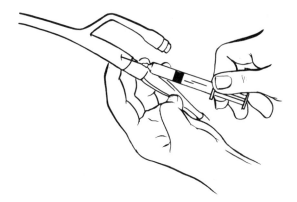

Figure 14-1. Method of obtaining urine from catheter by syringe.

Specimens may be readily obtained from patients with indwelling catheters by aspirating urine from the proximal lumen of the catheter with a syringe after carefully cleaning the site of insertion with tincture of iodine (Fig. 14-1).

Pathogens Involved in Urinary Tract Infections

General Spectrum

Most urinary tract infections are due to the gram-negative aerobic bacilli found in the gut. Anaerobic fecal flora, although present in 100 to 1000 times greater abundance in the stool, are rarely involved and do not grow well in urine. The most common organisms found in uncomplicated infections (that is, in those unassociated with major defects in the voiding mechanism) are Enterobacteriaceae. Of these, *Escherichia coli* is the most common and accounts for roughly 80 percent of infections, followed by *Klebsiella, Proteus,* and *Enterobacter.* Pseudomonads, staphylococci, and group-D streptococci account for about 5 to 12 percent of the remaining organisms in uncomplicated infection. In contrast, patients with so-called complicated or surgical urinary infection who have been treated with multiple courses of antimicrobial agents tend to be infected less often with *E. coli* and more often with the other organisms. Infections with *Pseudomonas,* indole-positive *Proteus* species, and *Enterobacter* are generally the most difficult to treat because of the refractoriness of these organisms to the commonly used antimicrobial agents and because such infections frequently are found in association with abnormal voiding mechanisms that interfere with host defenses to infection.

Organisms such as *Serratia marcescens, Acinetobacter,* and *Candida albicans* may produce disease in patients subjected to instrumentation, particularly with indwelling urinary catheters. Patients who have diabetes or who are treated with corticosteroids or immunosuppressive agents are particularly prone to be colonized with unusual organisms. Diphtheroids and microaerophilic streptococci are highly suspect as contaminants. They usually will not be isolated on repeated culture determination. They should not, however, be dismissed if repeatedly recovered under optimal conditions of collection.

E. coli, the most commonly encountered organism, can be serologically typed by over 150 different cell-wall (O) antigens and about 50 capsular (K) and flagellar (H) antigens. This has permitted detailed evaluation of the nature of recurrent infection very commonly encountered in females. The distribution of *E. coli* serotypes in urinary tract infections closely corresponds to their relative abundance in the gut.

The distribution of bacteria that colonize catheterized patients will vary depending on the selective pressure exerted by the use of antimicrobials and on the duration of catheterization. In general, *E. coli* remains the most common organism, but it will be replaced by more resistant bacteria and by yeasts when antibiotics are heavily used.

Pathogens in Catheter-Associated Infections

The distribution of bacteria found in catheter-associated urinary tract infections monitored by the National Nosocomial Infections Study conducted by the CDC in 1972 is presented in Table 14-1. These data were obtained from a large number of institutions and are subject to the problems of collecting large amounts of data from hospitals with varying degrees of expertise. The pathologic significance of some of the organisms that may be contaminants remains uncertain (lactobacilli, *Bacillus subtilis,* diphtheroids, and the like). Nevertheless,

Table 14-1. Distribution of Microorganisms Found in Urinary Tract Infections Associated with a Catheter or Other Instrument as the Predisposing Factor

Organism	Number of isolates	Percentage
E. coli	3369	33.4%
Proteus	1491	14.8%
Indole-positive	150	1.5%
Indole-negative	953	9.5%
Unknown	338	3.9%
Enterococci	1356	13.5%
Klebsiella	1002	9.9%
Pseudomonas	894	8.8%
Candida and related fungi	479	4.8%
Enterobacter	418	4.2%
Staphylococcus	429	4.3%
Coagulase-positive	136	1.3%
Coagulase-negative	293	2.9%
Serratia	142	1.4%
Others[a]	498	<1.0% each
Total	10,078	100.0%

[a] Includes streptococci (groups A through D), lactobacilli, diphtheroids, *Clostridium perfringens, Bacillus subtilis, Acinetobacter, Providencia, Citrobacter, Bacteroides, Salmonella, Shigella, Edwardsiella,* and amebae.

Data from National Nosocomial Infections Study (NNIS), Center for Disease Control, 1972.

the findings for the predominant organisms are very similar to those reported by individual investigators who have intensively studied the problem in various institutions.

Sources and Modes of Transmission

The enteric organisms that infect the urinary tract of hospitalized patients may originate from the patient's normal gastrointestinal flora, nosocomial organisms colonizing the patient after admission, or other hospital sources. The nosocomial flora of many gram-negative bacteria readily colonize the oropharynx and stool of patients, subsequently contaminate the perineal area, and then gain access to the urinary tract at the time of instrumentation. Bacteria, whether derived from the patient's flora or from other sources, may gain entrance into the bladder by the following mechanisms:

1. inadequate preparation of the periurethral area or the use of contaminated solutions in this area before catheters or other instruments are inserted,
2. insertion of instruments that are contaminated as a result of either poor aseptic technique in introducing catheters or inadequate disinfection,
3. trauma to the urethra or pressure necrosis of the meatus due to too large a catheter,
4. entry of bacteria at the junction of the catheter and the urethral meatus or urinary sinus (this is a late effect that is particularly troublesome in females),
5. contamination in the region of the connecting tube and catheter as a result of disconnection of tubes and unnecessary irrigation,
6. contamination of the collection vessel with retrograde flow of the bladder (the major factor that is eliminated by proper closed drainage), or
7. irrigation of the catheter with contaminated irrigating solutions.

Potential entry points for bacteria in urinary drainage systems are shown in Figure 14-2.

It is well established that some bacteria gain entrance to the bladder during instrumentation. The normal urethra, however, usually does not

Figure 14-2. Potential entry points for bacteria in urinary drainage systems.

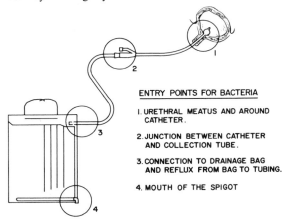

ENTRY POINTS FOR BACTERIA

1. URETHRAL MEATUS AND AROUND CATHETER.

2. JUNCTION BETWEEN CATHETER AND COLLECTION TUBE.

3. CONNECTION TO DRAINAGE BAG AND REFLUX FROM BAG TO TUBING.

4. MOUTH OF THE SPIGOT

contain large numbers of the coliform organisms commonly encountered in urinary infections. Furthermore, it is generally known that only 1 to 2 percent of healthy individuals subjected to single catheterizations acquire bacteriuria. This could not account for the fact that 90 to 95 percent of individuals with indwelling catheters attached to open drainage will develop bacteriuria within three to four days. It is therefore believed that most infections arise from the ascent of bacteria from the contaminated open collection vessel aided by the thin film of fluid that coats the drainage tubes.

The role of the periurethral route of contamination was investigated by Kass and Schneiderman [14] in three subjects with inlying catheters. They were able to document that bacteria could migrate from the perineum, around the catheter, and into the bladder urine. This phenomenon appears to be an important but late occurrence, because the simple measure of eliminating the ascending route of infection by closed drainage has markedly reduced the risk of contamination, at least during the first week or two of catheterization.

Contaminated fluid vehicles and hands of hospital personnel are the major modes of spread involved in cross-infections [13, 16, 21, 24, 28, 29]. A recent study by Maki and co-workers [21], for example, demonstrated the occurrence of cross-contamination of patients with *Serratia marcescens* as a result of carriage of the organisms on the hands of workers on the ward. Thus, all patients with catheters should be on closed drainage, and particular care must be taken by personnel who drain the system.

Outbreaks of urinary tract infections account for about 10 percent of the nosocomial epidemics investigated by the CDC; the organisms most commonly involved are *Klebsiella, Serratia,* and *Proteus.* Outbreaks tend to involve individual wards or treatment units and are often characterized by (1) crowding of catheterized patients, (2) poor catheter care (especially improper catheter irrigation), (3) multiple antibiotic resistance of cross-infecting strains, (4) transmission from patient to patient by hands of hospital personnel, and (5) unrecognized, asymptomatic bacteriuria in patients who often serve as important reservoirs that assist in propagating the outbreak. Occasionally, contaminated disinfectants or inadequately disinfected instruments are responsible for common-source outbreaks. Such sources are strongly suggested by an outbreak of *Pseudomonas cepacia* urinary tract infections, which often reflect inadequate disinfection of urinary instruments with aqueous benzalkonium chloride solutions. One should be particularly concerned about antiseptic fluids packaged with catheter insertion kits. An epidemic of nosocomial infection due to this unusual *Pseudomonas* species was traced to contaminated benzalkonium chloride packed in the kit as a germicidal cleansing solution [13].

Risks in Catheterization

Single Catheterization
In any discussion of the risks of catheterization, it is important to distinguish between single or multiple catheterizations (in which the catheter is inserted into the bladder for a short period of time) and indwelling catheters (usually with a retention balloon). One should also state the site of insertion as well, for example, single urethral catheterization, indwelling nephrostomy catheter or tube, and so forth.

INDICATIONS FOR USE. Indications for the use of single urethral catheterization include the following:

1. to relieve temporary obstruction or inability to void;
2. to obtain urine from patients who cannot give a clean-voided specimen because of weakness, obesity, or major medical problems;
3. to determine residual urine (if dye techniques or post-voiding film methods are not feasible); and
4. to permit urologic study of the anatomy of the urethra.

Urethral catheterization should not be routinely used to collect urine samples or to empty the bladder of pregnant women prior to delivery.

INFECTION RISKS. In general, single catheterizations are associated with a much lower frequency of infection than are the indwelling types. Nevertheless, a definite risk of infection exists with any form of catheterization. The benefit to be gained from the procedure must always be balanced against the harm to be accrued.

Certain groups of patients seem to be more susceptible to infection. These are women prior to delivery or post partum, the elderly or debilitated, diabetic patients, and those with significant residual urine in the bladder. In such patients, the risk that even a single catheterization will produce infection may be as high as 10 to 20 percent. This is much higher than the frequency of only 1 to 2 percent seen in otherwise healthy young adults. The most important message, however, is to avoid unnecessary instrumentation.

Indwelling Catheters
INDICATIONS FOR USE. The indwelling urinary catheter is an essential part of modern medical care. It is widely used to relieve temporary, anatomic or physiologic, urinary obstruction, to facilitate surgical repair of the urethra and surrounding structures, to provide a dry environment for comatose or incontinent patients, and to permit accurate measurement of urinary output in severely ill patients. Unfortunately, when poorly managed, the indwelling catheter may present a hazard to the very patients it is designed to protect. It is the leading cause of induced nosocomial urinary tract infections and the most common predisposing factor in fatal gram-negative sepsis in hospitals.

INFECTION RISKS. Indwelling catheters are used in about 10 percent of patients admitted to a general hospital. Most patients, even if they acquire infection, appear to do well, and they may lose their bacteriuria spontaneously or respond to appropriate therapy. Many, however, remain infected. The seemingly benign course in most patients has led some physicians to consider catheterization to be a benign procedure. The consequences of sepsis, shock, and death and the additional expense for antimicrobial therapy, prolonged hospitalization, and delayed complications must be balanced against the favorable course that is seen in the greater number of patients. It is therefore important to identify these costs of catheterization and weigh them against the benefits of preventive measures.

A rare event in a large population can result in a high overall morbidity and mortality. Perhaps the example of automobile accidents is pertinent here: very few accidents occur per million miles driven, but so many people drive that about 50,000 lose their lives each year. Some further examples may be helpful: in one study [11], data are presented indicating that in patients on catheter drainage for two to seven days, only 0.7 percent experienced subsequent clinical infections and only 8 to 10 percent had significant bacteriuria once the catheter was removed. Assuming these data to be representative, and that about 10 percent of patients admitted to acute-care hospitals are placed on catheter drainage [17, 18], and that there are 37,000,000 acute-care hospital admissions in the United States each year, we can then make the following rough estimates of symptomatic and asymptomatic infections:

1. If there are 37,000,000 acute-care hospital admissions per year and 10 percent of these patients have indwelling catheters, there will then be 3,700,000 catheterized patients.
2. If 0.7 percent develop clinical infection, there will be 25,900 clinical infections per year.
3. If 8 to 10 percent of 3,700,000 catheterized patients have significant bacteriuria, there will be 296,000 to 370,000 patients with significant bacteriuria per year who are at risk of further problems.

These calculations are presented here only to emphasize that the problem must be viewed in relation to an enormous population at risk.

Bacteremia

We have observed that about 1 percent of patients on indwelling urinary catheters in a general hospital will have a clinical episode that results in the physician obtaining a positive blood culture. The true frequency of bacteremia in patients whose urine is colonized is undoubtedly much higher. This is therefore a problem of considerable importance when one considers that the mortality in patients who are clinically ill and who have a gram-negative bacteremia ranges from 30 to 50 percent (see Part II, Chapter 29). Host factors markedly influence the outcome and death rates.

Most urinary tract infections are caused by gram-negative aerobic bacteria (see description of organisms below), which also constitute the most important group of organisms invading the bloodstream. Thus, it is worthwhile to consider the proportion of bacteremic episodes in a hospital that are associated with colonization of a urinary tract site. Fried and Vosti [8] reviewed 270 patients with gram-negative bacteremia at the Stanford Medical Center and found that 38 percent of bacteremic episodes originated in the urinary tract. An even more extensive study, reported by DuPont and Spink [7], analyzed 860 patients with gram-negative bacteremia at the University of Minnesota; 45 percent of the episodes of gram-negative bacteremia in adults arose from the urinary tract. Data from CDC's National Nosocomial Infections Study reveal urinary tract infections to be the single most important underlying site for nosocomial secondary bacteremias; 41 percent of such bacteremias were derived from urinary tract infections (see Part II, Chapter 29).

It should be emphasized that most of the studies of bacteremia are retrospective; that is, they depend on the decision of a physician to obtain a blood culture. A more detailed prospective study of the frequency of bacteremia following manipulation of the urinary tract was reported by Sullivan and associates [26]. A group of 300 patients were bled prior to and just after manipulation of the tract. Bacteria were recovered from the blood in 31 percent undergoing a transurethral resection of the prostate, 17 percent having cystoscopy, 24 percent after urethral dilation, and 8 percent with urethral catheterization. Most of the organisms were aerobic gram-negative bacilli. These were followed in frequency by enterococci, but anaerobic bacteria, which commonly colonize the urethra, were also frequently encountered. It is assumed that most of these episodes were transient, but the high rates observed in this study readily explain why we now so frequently encounter clinically important bacteremia in hospitalized patients undergoing instrumentation of the urinary tract. Similar studies report the common occurrence of bacteremia following prostatectomy and other forms of urinary instrumentation [24, 25, 27].

General Control Measures
in Urinary Tract Infections

It should be abundantly clear from all that has been stated above that instrumentation of the urinary tract must be avoided unless it is essential for patient care. The physician must always consider the benefit-to-risk relationship between the information or relief to be achieved and the relatively small yet cumulative consequences of his actions.

Systemic Antimicrobial Agents

CHEMOTHERAPY. It is well known that it is virtually impossible to render urine free of bacteria in the presence of a foreign body such as the urinary catheter. Short-term success with particularly powerful drugs such as the aminoglycoside antibiotics (gentamicin, tobramycin, or amikacin) can be accomplished, but such therapy is doomed to failure if the catheter is left in place. Sulfonamides and nitrofurantoin have no place as prophylactic agents. There also have been many trials using methenamine salts (methenamine hippurate or mandelate) combined with acidification to "suppress" infection in the presence of the catheter. Unfortunately, these methods are also unsuccessful.

Because of the above problems, antimicrobial therapy should generally be reserved for instances in which systemic spread is suspected. Systemic spread will be evidenced by fever, chills, flank pain, and signs of generalized sepsis. Under these circumstances, antimicrobial therapy may be life-saving.

It is important to attempt to eradicate any infection once the catheter is removed. The choice of drug will depend on the results of antimicrobial sensitivity tests and experience with the least expensive, least toxic drug.

CHEMOPROPHYLAXIS. Many physicians employ prophylaxis after single catheterization [3, 27]. This seems reasonable, at least for two

or three days following the procedure. We recommend nitrofurantoin or the combination of trimethoprim and sulfamethoxazole for this purpose, but many other agents should be equally effective. Penicillin and streptomycin should be used prophylactically, particularly in men with valvular heart lesions who are at risk of endocarditis. These agents are used in the hope of preventing enterococcal endocarditis, but the efficacy of such treatment is unknown. It seems reasonable, however, to maintain blood levels of both drugs in the body at the time of the procedure and for 24 hours thereafter. The dose must be a reasonable guess, such as 0.5 gm. streptomycin given twice daily coupled with a million units aqueous penicillin given every six hours intravenously (or 1.0 gm. potassium penicillin V) for the same period.

A number of studies have employed prophylactic antibiotics during prostatectomy and have reported good results. Kanamycin and gentamicin are particularly effective. One group advocates cephaloridine injection combined with closed bladder irrigation with a neomycin-polymyxin B solution [5]. Cystoscopy and transurethral surgery should be performed only after an attempt has been made to eradicate infection when present. This should reduce the frequency of disseminated infection.

Prophylactic Irrigation

Prophylactic irrigation was designed to permit continuous flow of an antimicrobial agent into the bladder to prevent an infection. No claim is made by the proponents of such systems that they will eradicate infection once the bacteria are introduced and infection is established.

ACETIC ACID METHOD. This method was designed by Kass [15] based on the knowledge that many weak organic acids are bactericidal. A solution of 0.25 percent acetic acid in physiologic saline is allowed to drip into the bladder from a bottle hung on a pole and connected to the catheter through a Y-tube. The rate of flow is generally 1 ml. per minute. The drainage tube is clamped during irrigation. Every two hours, the drainage tube is unclamped, and the bladder is allowed to empty.

This method has the advantages of low cost of materials and the ability of the agent to fill the bladder and remain long enough to kill any bacteria that may have gained entrance. The major disadvantages are confusion with ordinary intravenous fluids (this may be prevented by proper labeling and by adding colored solutions to the bottle of acetic acid), additional nursing time in adjusting flow rates and emptying the bladder, and, occasionally, irritation of the bladder by the acetic acid.

NEOMYCIN-POLYMYXIN METHOD. Martin and Bookrajian [23] have advocated this as a practical and effective method of prophylactic bladder care. In this method, a three-way catheter is used instead of a Y-tube attached to a regular Foley catheter. Continuous flow is established from a reservoir. No attempt is made to clamp and unclamp the effluent stream intermittently.

For use, 1 ml. of a solution containing 40 mg. of neomycin sulfate (equivalent to neomycin base) and 200,000 units of polymyxin B are added to 1000 ml. of isotonic saline solution. The rate of flow is adjusted to deliver 1000 ml. every 24 hours. It is recommended that the inflow rate should be adjusted to deliver 2000 ml. of solution per day if the urinary output exceeds 2 liters per day. The effluent should be attached to an effective, closed-drainage system.

This procedure has the advantage over the acetic acid method in being less complex, in requiring less nursing time, and in not causing bladder irritation. It has been shown to be at least as effective as closed-drainage methods. Neomycin and polymyxin B have not been found in the bloodstream during use. The major disadvantages are that nursing time is still required to assure proper flow rates throughout the day; the irrigating fluid only bathes the trigone, not the entire bladder; and when the system becomes contaminated, the bacteria are often antibiotic-resistant enterococci, yeasts, or gram-negative bacilli. Monitoring for bacteria is difficult in the presence of the irrigant.

This method should be recommended only after the establishment of a system of routine, good, closed drainage in the hospital. The irrigation method then can be added to improve bladder care.

Proper Use of Intermittent Catheterization

POSTOPERATIVE PATIENTS. Nurses play a critical role in being certain that the patient is adequately hydrated, is placed in a comfortable position to void, and, most important, has the privacy needed to relieve him or her of inhibition. The nurses' efforts should be encouraged by physicians. One can wait at least 8 to 12 hours before manual drainage is needed unless the patient has been overloaded with fluids. If these measures prove ineffective, intermittent single catheterization is recommended as needed. Patients who require more than two or three catheterizations, however, should be placed on continuous closed drainage, because each instrumentation presents a hazard, particularly in the older male who may have prostatic obstruction.

OBSTETRIC PATIENTS. Routine catheterization prior to delivery is no longer considered to be required and is accompanied by unacceptably high morbidity. Patients can usually empty their bladder spontaneously.

PATIENTS WITH SPINAL CORD INJURIES. Intermittent catheterization should be attempted in cases of recent injury to the spinal cord with paraplegia and quadriplegia. This procedure is useful primarily in otherwise healthy young adults who do not have obstructive lesions of the urethra. The patient will retain fluid during the first 8 to 12 hours following injury, so catheterization may be delayed until a team trained in scrupulous aseptic insertion of the catheter can care for the patient.

Guttmann and Frankel [12] have demonstrated that intermittent catheterization performed by the "no-touch" technique using meticulous control, including routine culture determinations and treatment of any positive culture, can markedly reduce the risk of urinary tract infections in patients with spinal cord injuries. This is a special group of patients who are usually young and otherwise healthy and who do not have obstructive lesions of the urethra so catheters can be passed with minimal trauma. These investigators reported that in a large series of paraplegics and quadriplegics admitted to the Stoke-Mandeville Spinal Injuries Center, 65 percent of male and 50 percent of female patients were discharged with sterile urine. It should be remembered that optimal results require an initially sterile bladder urine, easy passage of the catheter, and a well-trained team that is continuously available.

Alternatives to the Use of Urethral Catheters

CONDOM DRAINAGE. Incontinent or comatose males should be fitted with a condom catheter, provided that the bladder will completely empty spontaneously. The condom and its attached collection tube should be changed daily, and the penis should be carefully cleaned and dried to avoid maceration, which sometimes limits the duration of use of the catheter. The duration of usefulness, however, may nonetheless be sufficient to avoid urethral catheterization. There is no comparable measure for females.

Warning: Urine culture tests are unreliable when the condom is in place. The device should be removed, the penis should be carefully washed, and a clean-voided or catheterized specimen should then be obtained.

SUPRAPUBIC CATHETERS. Suprapubic drainage is beginning to become popular as an alternative to drainage through a urethral catheter. Urethral catheters drain the bladder but obstruct the urethral glands and the prostatic and ejaculatory ducts. They may produce epididymitis or prostatitis and provide a passage around the catheter for entry of bacteria into the bladder.

Most self-retaining suprapubic catheters are placed in the bladder surgically, which limits their widespread use. Several new types of plastic, disposable catheters that may be inserted through a trocar directly into the bladder have been developed. These devices have been mostly used in patients undergoing gynecologic surgery, but they may well have their use extended to more general medical patients. Preliminary results reveal them to be promising in delaying infection [22]. Physicians should become expert in their use and employ them as often as possible instead of urethral indwelling catheters.

Bacteriologic Monitoring of Patients on Catheter Drainage

Although the cost-effectiveness of bacteriologic monitoring has not been conclusively established, many believe this approach to have both clinical and epidemiologic usefulness.

Urine may be obtained by direct needle puncture at the point of junction with the collecting tube. This permits daily monitoring of the system. Daily urine culture tests can enable a hospital bacteriology laboratory to post results within 24 hours and perform antimicrobial sensitivity tests on all positive cultures. A bulletin board that lists culture results for a month is shown in Figure 14-3. This information can help the physician to ascertain the bacteriologic status of his or her patient at a glance and provide a basis for the best choice of drugs for use either during catheterization or after removal. Posting of culture results may be of value whether or not specimens are collected in conjunction with a routine monitoring system, but available data will be substantially less with the former than the latter method.

The urine culture report bulletin board should be maintained by the clinical bacteriology laboratory in a location where physicians have ready access to it. Some suggested places are the physicians' coat room, outside the bacteriology laboratory, or in the x-ray reading room. Hospitals that have automated reporting systems for the hospital chart could add this information to the form. A surcharge may be placed on catheters for the additional costs of routine monitoring services.

Spatial Dispersal of Catheterized Patients

Since the spread of organisms on the hands of personnel is an important route and infected collection-bag urine is an important source of cross-infection, it has been suggested that the dispersal of catheterized patients on patient-care units would assist in controlling cross-infections [21]. Indeed, this procedure seems to have been of considerable usefulness in controlling certain refractory infection problems caused by multiple-drug-resistant strains [20]. Dispersal of catheterized patients is of adjunctive value in controlling outbreaks transmitted

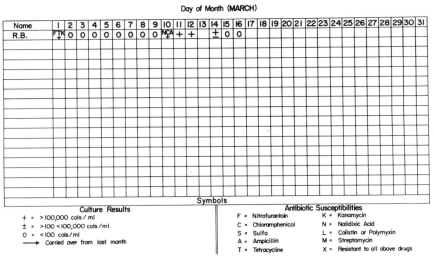

Daily Urine Culture Reports for Patients with Indwelling Urethral Catheters

Figure 14-3. The urine culture calendar to be used for daily reports on status of catheterized patients.
From Butler, H. K., and Kunin, C. M. *J. Urol.* 100:567, 1968. Reproduced with permission.

by the hands of hospital personnel, and it may also have some value as a routine preventive measure.

Catheter-Care Program
A uniform catheter-care program should be based on scrupulous aseptic technique during insertion and on aseptic, closed-drainage methods. Such techniques may be supplemented by closed antimicrobial irrigation procedures.

Catheter-Care Teams
The value of a catheter-care team approach has been emphasized by Lindan and Keane [19], who worked at a hospital devoted to rehabilitation of the chronically ill patient. There are many similar hospitals devoted to the care of the paraplegic patient in which large numbers of patients require catheter care. It seems wise to hire and train a special catheter-care team for these institutions and for large hospitals as well, because there is much work to be done and the level of care could be greatly improved by a well-motivated and specialized group. The team could be of particular help in attempting intermittent drainage for the uninfected, newly paraplegic patient, in collecting clean-voided specimens for culture, in the insertion of indwelling catheters, in monitoring and controlling infection, in decreasing cross-infection, and in providing early assistance in bladder training. The responsibilities and authorities of the team should be carefully delineated by the Infection Control Committee, and these functions should also be endorsed and supported by the chiefs of service and the hospital administration. Strong direction and support by physicians is needed. A trained physician must insert the suprapubic tubes, but the team can assist in identifying patients who might best be managed by this approach and provide necessary care after their insertion.

It seems doubtful that a catheter-care team is economically feasible for the small or medium-sized hospital unless its duties are combined with others such as intravenous administration and care. In such hospitals, indwelling catheters are used sporadically, and there simply would not be enough work to justify the expenditure. For these hospitals, the infection control nurses should be primarily responsible for in-service training and implementation of proper procedures by the staff.

Care of Urinary Catheter and Drainage Systems
Catheter Care
A number of approaches to the problem of the care of the indwelling catheter have been re-

ported to be of value. These include careful aseptic technique during the insertion of catheters, impregnation of catheters with antibacterial agents, the use of antibacterial agents instilled into the bladder or around the catheter, aseptic closed-drainage systems, continuous irrigation of the bladder with antibiotics or acetic acid, and, when possible, avoidance of the urethral route by use of suprapubic catheters. Almost all workers agree that prophylactic systemic antimicrobial therapy is of little value.

The varied nature of the busy, understaffed hospital requires a system of catheter care that is both simple to operate and effective in preventing infection. Any system, regardless of efficacy, that is too complex for routine use is inherently unsuitable to meet the problem.

Dukes' Drainage System

One of the earliest descriptions of a systematic approach to the reduction of infections associated with the use of indwelling catheters was reported in 1928 by Cuthbert Dukes, working at St. Mark's Hospital in London [6]. He was concerned with the virtually inevitable occurrence of urinary tract infections in patients on indwelling catheter drainage following excision of the rectum for cancer. Using a quantitative count of pus cells in the urine, he noted that the urine was free of infection until the second or third postoperative day. Thereafter, large numbers of leukocytes appeared in the urine with a "stream of pus" by the sixth to eighth day. He suspected that part of the cause of infection was contamination of a wooden peg customarily used to seal the catheter. This was proved when he substituted drainage into a sterile bottle. Dukes went further and developed an intermittent irrigation device (Fig. 14-4). The catheter was attached by a Y-tube to a sterile, closed-drainage bottle. Periodic irrigation with oxycyanide of mercury was used to wash the system. In addition to these measures, the catheter was fixed in place by a gauze dressing around the penis in males and by glycerine-soaked sponges abutting the vulva in females.

Dukes reported virtually complete prevention of infection during the postoperative period using this method. There can be no question that he had made a major advance in solving an important problem. It is therefore quite surprising that his method was not widely adopted as a routine measure in all catheterized patients. This, however, was not the case. During the next 30 or 40 years, catheter drainage in most hospitals remained "open." It was common to find the end of the collection tube immersed in contaminated, often foul, urine that had collected in the open bottle for several days. Only rarely did individuals become concerned with the problem even after Beeson [1] published in 1958 (30 years later) his famous editorial, "The Case Against the Catheter," in the *American Journal of Medicine.* Beeson carefully documented the dangers associated with the catheter and summarized the evidence that the ascending pathway up the drainage tube was the most likely source of contamination. No mention was made at that time of how infection could be prevented other than by avoiding unnecessary use of the instrument.

Closed-Drainage Methods

Interest in finding a solution to preventing infection arising from the indwelling urinary catheter, although pioneered by Dukes, waned until the early 1960s when Gillespie and coworkers [9] in Bristol, England, introduced closed drainage. Several American urologists, primarily Desautels [4] and Ansell, independently began to explore this approach and met with considerable success. Heretofore, virtually the entire effort was devoted to aseptic methods of inserting the catheter with amazing disregard to its continued care.

PREVENTION OF BLADDER COLONIZATION. The efficacy of closed drainage has been demonstrated in the United States as well as in the United Kingdom. These studies have pointed out that the frequency of bladder colonization in patients with indwelling catheters could be markedly reduced by measures that (1) protected the collection bottle from outside contamination, (2) insured that there was no continuity between the urine in the drainage tube and that in the collection bottle, and (3) controlled the proper positioning and sterility of the system.

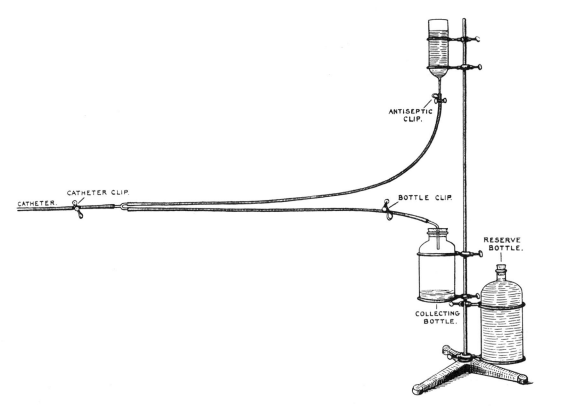

Figure 14-4. The closed irrigation method devised by Dukes in 1928.

From Dukes, C. *Proc. R. Soc. Med.* 22 (Part 1):258, 1928. Reproduced with permission.

OBJECTIVES OF CLOSED DRAINAGE. It must be emphasized that sterile, closed-drainage systems are designed for only three purposes: (1) to maintain the sterility of the urinary tract, (2) to avoid cross-contamination among patients, and (3) to reduce breakage and spills of urine. The first purpose will not be fulfilled once the urinary bladder is contaminated, but closed drainage should still be used for patient and nursing convenience and to reduce cross-contamination on the ward.

CHOICE OF SYSTEMS. The choice of a suitable closed-drainage system to be purchased should be based on the following considerations:

1. relative cost,
2. ease in positioning on the bed or during ambulation,
3. flow properties,
4. stability of construction, and
5. ease in draining the bag without producing contamination.

There are many excellent systems currently available. The ultimate decision to select a particular system should be made by the hospital's Infection Control Committee but only after trial by the nursing service to be certain that it drains well and is easy to use. It is particularly important that urologists on the staff be consulted. Surgeons are particularly concerned with careful monitoring of flow in patients with shock. This can be accomplished by somewhat more expensive units that contain flow measurement devices. These will generally not be needed on the general medical and surgical wards. It may therefore be convenient to stock two kinds of systems: one for intensive care, the other for general use. In actual practice, any system with a good drain can be used throughout the hospital. Timed urine output can readily be measured with a graduated cylinder.

Even the most expensive closed-drainage

system should be viewed as economically advantageous for the patient. The cost of antibiotics, even for one day, is usually far greater than that of a good bag, which will be left in place during the patient's hospitalization. The only reasons to change the bag are poor flow, leaks, odor, or obstruction by wetting of the air vent.

The Infection Control Committee should be aware that manufacturers may change the specifications of a particular system, often without warning to the user.

PREVENTIVE PRACTICES. It is important for the use of the closed-drainage system that several routine practices be followed. The importance of the following practices must be strongly emphasized to all personnel caring for patients with an indwelling catheter:

1. The junction of the catheter with the drainage tube must not be broken once attached after aseptic insertion of the catheter unless one suspects that the catheter is obstructed. The drainage bag should remain attached to the catheter while the patient ambulates. It should be emptied to prevent its becoming unwieldy before suspending it from a belt around the patient's waist. When the patient is being bladder-trained, the tubing should be clamped, but it should not be disconnected from the bladder.

2. Bags are drained of urine at eight-hour intervals, with care being taken to avoid contamination of the mouth of the spigot.

3. Bags may be hung on the sides of beds, chairs, and stretchers, but they must never be inverted or raised above the level of the patient's bladder unless the tubing is clamped.

4. Perineal care consists of washing with soap and water two times a day. This has not been proved to prevent infection, but it will decrease local irritation.

5. Catheters are not irrigated unless the physician suspects obstruction. Opening a closed system for this purpose may lead to contamination. The chance of infection is great and must be thoroughly considered. When it is necessary to irrigate, ster-

ile technique must be maintained. A fresh, sterile, large-volume syringe must be used with each irrigation employing sterile solution. The same syringe should never be used on more than one occasion unless it is cleaned and sterilized between uses. Irrigating solutions should be available in amounts of 100 to 200 ml.; when the required amount is used, the remainder should be discarded.

6. All indwelling catheters must be routinely attached to a closed-drainage system regardless of the planned duration of catheterization.

7. Care must be taken while turning the patient, moving the patient, or sitting him up in a chair and while the patient is ambulating to insure that good descending flow is maintained and that the tubing is arranged so that there are no kinks to obstruct flow.

8. The bag must never be allowed to touch the floor.

9. The bag should not be held upside down while emptying it.

10. Urine should flow well from the drainage tube. Obstruction should be suspected if the entire tube is filled with urine.

11. It is extremely important that periodic in-service instruction be given to all persons who are involved in catheter insertion. Aseptic technique and the risks of complications of urinary tract infection should be stressed.

Summary of the Urinary Catheter Problem

The urinary catheter is a fact of medical life. It is a valuable instrument when used for proper indications and when aseptic management is enforced. When it is improperly used, the catheter is the major source of serious gram-negative infection in hospitalized patients.

Male patients who require long-term drainage should be first tried on condom-catheter drainage if there is no obstruction to flow or significant residual urine. Condom drainage, however, may lead to severe maceration of the penis if daily changing and cleansing is not done. Indwelling urethral catheters must be attached to a good system of closed drainage, whether or not infection is present. Continuous bladder irrigation with neomycin-polymyxin solutions is a useful adjunct once closed drainage is established and working well. If the system is not carefully attended, it will not be more effective than closed drainage [30]. Suprapubic catheters are of special value for long-term use, because they do not obstruct or irritate the urethra. The development of percutaneous methods of suprapubic drainage should improve and increase the use of this method. Intermittent single catheterization is the procedure of choice in the patient with a neurologic defect of the voiding mechanism, provided that the patient is continent between procedures and the catheter can be passed without inducing trauma to the urethra.

References

1. Beeson, P. B. The case against the catheter. *Am. J. Med.* 24:1, 1958.
2. Brumfitt, W., Davies, B. I., and Rosser, E. ap I. Urethral catheter as a cause of urinary tract infection in pregnancy and puerperium. *Lancet* 2:1059, 1961.
3. David, J. H., Rosenblum, J. M., Quilligan, E. J., and Persky, L. An evaluation of postcatheterization prophylactic chemotherapy. *J. Urol.* 82:613, 1959.
4. Desautels, R. E., Walter, C. W., Graves, R. C., and Harrison, J. H. Technical advances in the prevention of urinary tract infection. *J. Urol.* 87:487, 1962.
5. Drach, G. W., Lacy, S. S., and Cox, C. Prevention of catheter-induced post-prostatectomy infection. Effects of systemic cephaloridine and local irrigation with neomycin-polymyxin through closed-drainage catheter system. *J. Urol.* 105:840, 1971.
6. Dukes, C. Urinary infections after excision of the rectum: Their cause and prevention. *Proc. R. Soc. Med.* 22 (Part 1):259, 1928.
7. DuPont, H. L., and Spink, W. W. Infections due to gram-negative organisms: An analysis of 800 patients with bacteremia at the University of Minnesota Medical Center, 1958–1966. *Medicine (Baltimore)* 48:307, 1969.
8. Fried, M. A., and Vosti, K. L. The importance of underlying disease in patients with gram-negative bacteremia. *Arch. Intern. Med.* 121:418, 1968.
9. Gillespie, W. A., Lennon, G. G., Linton, K. B., and Slade, N. Prevention of urinary infection in gynaecology. *Br. Med. J.* 2:423, 1964.
10. Gross, P. A., Harkavy, L. M., Borden, G. E., and Kerstein, M. Positive Foley catheter tip culture—Fact or fancy? *J.A.M.A.* 228:72, 1974.
11. Guinan, P. D., Bayley, B. C., Metzger, W. I., Shoemaker, W. C., and Bush, I. M. The case against "The case against the catheter," Initial report. *J. Urol.* 101:909, 1969.
12. Guttmann, L., and Frankel, H. The value of intermittent catheterization in the early management of traumatic paraplegia. *Paraplegia* 4:63, 1966.
13. Hardy, P. C., Ederer, G. M., and Matsen, J. M. Contamination of commercially packaged urinary catheter kits with Pseudomonad EO-1. *N. Engl. J. Med.* 282:33, 1970.
14. Kass, E. H., and Schneiderman, L. J. Entry of bacteria into the urinary tracts of patients with inlying catheters. *N. Engl. J. Med.* 256:556, 1957.
15. Kass, E. H., and Sossen, H. S. Prevention of infection of urinary tract in presence of indwelling catheters: Description of electro-mechanical valve to provide intermittent drainage of the bladder. *J.A.M.A.* 169:1181, 1959.
16. Kennedy, R. P., Plorde, J. H., and Petersdorf, R. G. Studies of the epidemiology of *Escherichia coli* infections. IV. Evidence for a nosocomial flora. *J. Clin. Invest.* 44:193, 1965.
17. Kunin, C. M. *Detection, Prevention and Treatment of Urinary Tract Infection* (2d ed.). Philadelphia: Lea & Febinger, 1974.
18. Kunin, C. M., and McCormack, R. C. Prevention of catheter-induced urinary-tract infections by sterile closed drainage. *N. Engl. J. Med.* 274:1156, 1966.
19. Lindan, R., and Keane, A. T. The catheter team. *Am. J. Nurs.* 64:128, 1964.
20. Lindsey, J. O., Martin, W. T., Sonnenwirth, A. C., and Bennett, J. V. An outbreak of nosocomial *Proteus rettgeri* urinary tract infection. *Am. J. Epidemiol.* 103:261, 1976.
21. Maki, D. G., Hennekens, C. H., and Bennett, J. V. Prevention of catheter-associated urinary tract infection. *J.A.M.A.* 221:1270, 1972.
22. Marcus, R. T. Narrow-bore suprapubic bladder drainage in Uganda. *Lancet* 1:748, 1967.
23. Martin, C. M., and Bookrajian, E. N. Bacteriuria prevention after indwelling urinary catheterization, a controlled study. *Arch. Intern. Med.* 110:703, 1962.
24. Moore, B., and Foreman, A. An outbreak of urinary *Pseudomonas aeruginosa* infection acquired during urological operations. *Lancet* 2:929, 1966.
25. Steyn, J. H., and Logie, N. J. Bacteremia following prostatectomy. *Br. J. Urol.* 34:459, 1962.
26. Sullivan, N. M., Sutter, V. L., Carter, W. T.,

Attebery, H. R., and Finegold, S. M.   Bacteremia after genitourinary tract manipulation: Bacteriological aspects and evaluation of various blood culture systems. *Appl. Microbiol.* 23:1101, 1972.

27. Turck, M., Goffe, B., and Petersdorf, R. G. The urethral catheter and urinary tract infection. *J. Urol.* 88:834, 1962.

28. Weil, A. J., Ramchand, S., and Arias, M. E. Nosocomial infection with *Klebsiella* type 25. *N. Engl. J. Med.* 275:17, 1966.

29. Whitby, J. L., Blair, J. N., and Rampling, A. Cross-infection with *Serratia marcescens* in an intensive therapy unit. *Lancet* 2:127, 1972.

30. Warren, J. W., Plath, R., Thomas, R. J., Rosner, B., and Kass, E. H.   Antibiotic irrigation and catheter-associated urinary-tract infections. *N. Engl. J. Med.* 299:570, 1978.

15

Lower Respiratory Tract Infections

Jay P. Sanford and Alan K. Pierce

Nature of Lower Respiratory Tract Infections

Classification

Nosocomial respiratory infections are those that develop in hospitalized patients in whom the infection was either not present or not incubating at the time of admission (see Part I, Chapter 2). Nosocomial infections are usually not manifest in the first 72 hours of hospitalization. For some lower respiratory infections, the recognition that incubating infections should not be classified as nosocomial is of importance; for example, the patient who develops influenzal pneumonia 24 hours after admission to a hospital or the patient who may have aspirated oropharyngeal materials several days before admission and who then goes on to develop a necrotizing pneumonia with community-acquired organisms after hospitalization should not be classified as having nosocomial pneumonia. Likewise, it is important to recognize that nosocomial infections may be incubating at the time of discharge from the hospital; hence, they may be initially recognized at the time of outpatient follow-up. Although the delayed appearance of disease is more frequent with infections involving other sites than the lung, such delay may occur with nosocomial respiratory infections, for example, nosocomial varicella pneumonia or tuberculosis. When the incubation period is unknown, infections are classified as nosocomial if they develop at any time after admission. An infection present on admission can be classified as nosocomial *only* if it is directly related to or is the residual of a previous admission. All infections that fail to satisfy these requirements should be classified as community-acquired.

Incidence

Standardized criteria for diagnosis (which will be reviewed subsequently) have not been employed in most of the reported studies. The fig-

The authors' studies were supported in part by Public Health Services Research Grants CC 00202 from the Center for Disease Control, HL 14187 (SCOR), and Training Grant 5T01 A10030.

ures presented represent a mixture of prevalence data and "incidence" per hospitalized patients or number of admissions; the duration of hospitalization, and hence the time "at risk," is usually not estimated. The data relate almost exclusively to rapidly growing aerobic bacterial agents that occur endemically. Data seldom are presented that include viral, fungal, or parasitic agents or that correct for the occurrence of sporadic outbreaks. The reported prevalence studies and incidences summarized in Table 15-1 should be viewed in light of these potential problems. Nosocomial pneumonia represents 8 to 33 percent of the total nosocomial infections, and the rate of nosocomial pneumonia varies from 0.5 percent to 5.0 percent of all admissions (discharges). Note that the incidence (expressed as the number of occurrences per 1000 admissions or discharges) in community hospitals [10] generally has been two to ten times lower than in university-affiliated teaching hospitals. The highest rates for university hospitals are based

on prevalence studies, however, and these measurements tend to produce higher rates than incidence studies (see Part I, Chapter 4); thus the true difference in incidence of pneumonia between community and university hospitals is likely to be less than tenfold but still higher for university hospitals. These differences may reflect social factors. University hospitals tend to be tertiary care centers to which the more sick, complicated patient is referred, support procedures may be more advanced, and university-affiliated teaching hospitals often have individuals involved in patient care who are students and who may be less knowledgeable and skilled in those aspects of care important in the prevention of nosocomial infections.

Figures derived from the National Nosocomial Infections Study (NNIS) encompass data collected from January 1970 to August 1973: among 3,456,649 discharges, there were 113,330 patients who developed infections (3.3 percent). Of these infections, 16,588 (14.6 percent) were reported as involving the respiratory tract: bronchitis, 1736 cases; lung abscess, 180 cases; lower respiratory infection (type unspecified), 3637 cases; and pneumonia, 11,135 cases. From these data, the incidence of pneumonia and lower respiratory infection (type unspecified) was 4.3 per 1000 admissions (0.4 percent).

As with most bacterial nosocomial infections, overall figures reflect composites of different patient groups who are at differing risks, depending on host factors such as age, the type of illnesses for which they are admitted to hospitals, and the like. These differences are illustrated in Table 15-2, which provides incidence figures according to hospital service.

When differences in the populations at risk are taken into account, it appears that 10 to 20 percent of nosocomial infections involve the lower respiratory tract; hence, this category of infections represents one of the major nosocomial infection problems.

Causative Agents

A large number of microorganisms have been incriminated as the causative agents in nosocomial respiratory tract infections; broadly, these include aerobic gram-positive cocci, aer-

Table 15-1. Rates of Nosocomial Respiratory Infections

Hospital	Years	All infections (percent of admissions)	Cases of pneumonia (per 1000)
Hospital for Sick Children in Toronto [44]	1959	6.5%	28
Univ. of Edinburgh Hospital [51]	1960–61	16.8%	14
Univ. of Illinois Hospital [25]	1960–62	6.5%	13
Boston City Hospital [21]	1964	13.5%	32
Univ. of Kentucky Hospital [31]	1965	6.1%	23
Johns Hopkins Hospital [54]	1965–66	4.0%	8
Boston City Hospital [2]	1967	15.5%	50
Six community hospitals [10]	1965–66	3.5%	5

Table 15-2. Incidences of Nosocomial Pneumonia and Lower Respiratory Tract Infections by Hospital Service[a]

Hospital service	No. of discharges (times 1000)	No. of infections	Incidence per 1000 discharges
General Surgery	1288	8347	6.5
General Medicine	929	5632	6.1
Pediatrics	205	346	1.7
Gynecology	227	235	1.0
Newborn Services	369	140	0.4
Obstetrics	438	72	0.2
Totals	3456	14,772	4.3

[a] Data from National Nosocomial Infections Study (NNIS), January 1970 through August 1973.

obic gram-negative bacilli, anaerobes, mycobacteria, nocardial species, and viral, chlamydial, fungal, and parasitic agents. The data on incidence relate almost exclusively to aerobic bacterial agents, because incidence figures for other classes of microorganisms are unavailable. Data reported in the literature from ten hospitals are summarized in Table 15-3. According to those data, aerobic gram-positive cocci and aerobic gram-negative bacilli each account for about 40 percent of all cases, with a combination of both accounting for another 10 percent. In studies at the University of Edinburgh Hospital, *Hemophilus influenzae* was found to cause 40 percent of all nosocomial pneumonias. These observations are in marked contrast to those in North America, where *H. influenzae* seldom is incriminated. A satisfactory explanation for this discrepancy has not been forthcoming.

Data submitted under the National Nosocomial Infections Study are summarized in Table 15-4. These data represent more recent observations than those shown in Table 15-3 and include all reported causative agents, which may account for the lower frequency of infections with coagulase-positive staphylococci (27.9 percent compared to 12.6 percent). The frequency of infections with aerobic gram-

negative bacilli is considerably higher in the NNIS data (51 percent of all causes as compared to 44% of all bacteria).

Diagnostic Criteria

Clinical Criteria

Establishing a diagnosis of nosocomial pneumonia may be difficult. The disease is most common in critically ill patients who may not be able to report symptoms accurately and in whom the primary disease may mask or simulate the occurrence of bacterial pneumonia. In the intensive-care unit setting, many patients have fever and leukocytosis from their primary disease process. Antecedent densities in the chest radiograph and purulent sputum also are common. Gram-negative bacillary pathogens are found in the sputum in a high fraction of patients with or without pneumonia. For this reason, the diagnosis of pneumonia or lower respiratory tract infection is dependent upon clinical observations, including radiographic, rather than being based solely or predominantly on microbiologic findings, although, as will be reviewed subsequently, microbiologic procedures are being evolved that will provide better correlation between clinical and microbiologic features.

Different clinicians and investigators have employed differing criteria for the diagnosis of lower respiratory tract infections. Wenzel and associates at the University of Virginia [58] have used the finding of infiltrate on chest radiography that was not present on admission and that is associated with new sputum production as a criterion for nosocomial pulmonary infections. Johanson, Pierce, Sanford, and Thomas [19] have utilized more stringent criteria and have classified infections as "definite" or "probable" according to four determinants: (1) the radiographic appearance of a new or progressive pulmonary infiltrate, (2) fever, (3) leukocytosis, and (4) purulent tracheobronchial secretions. A diagnosis of "definite" infection required the occurrence of all four determinants. A diagnosis of "probable" infection is based upon three criteria: (1) fever, (2) leukocytosis, and (3) either a new or progressive pulmonary infiltrate shown radio-

Table 15-3. Bacterial Etiology of Nosocomial Pneumonia

Bacterial species	Hospital[a] (No. of cases)						Total	
	A	B	C	D	E	F	No. of cases	Percent
Gram-positive cocci								
Staphylococci, coagulase-positive	25	109	11	9	6	45	205	27.9%
Streptococcus pneumoniae	12	0	11	8	0	35	66	9.0%
Streptococci, other	1	0	2	0	0	26	29	4.0%
Staphylococci, coagulase-negative	0	76	3	0	0	—	79	10.8%
Gram-negative bacilli								
Hemophilus influenzae	49	1	2	5	0	—	57	7.8%
Escherichia coli	24	24	9	3	2	10	72	9.8%
Klebsiella and *Enterobacter*	0	31	11	8	3	18	71	9.7%
Pseudomonas sp.	3	29	8	3	3	26	72	9.8%
Proteus sp.	5	12	1	2	4	20	44	6.0%
Miscellaneous gram-negative bacilli	4	0	0	0	0	4	8	1.1%
Serratia marcescens	0	0	0	1	0	—	1	<1%
Unknown bacterial agents	0	0	27	3	0	0	30	4.1%
Totals	123	282	85	42	18	184	734	100.0%

[a] Key to hospitals: A = University of Edinburgh [51], B = University of Illinois Research and Education Hospitals [25], C = Johns Hopkins Hospital [54], D = Boston City Hospital [21], E = Boston City Hospital [2], F = six community hospitals [10].

graphically or the presence of purulent secretions. Results of culture tests are not used in making these determinations.

The Hospital Infections Branch of the Center for Disease Control (CDC), which monitors the National Nosocomial Infections Study, utilizes the following criteria for nosocomial pneumonia. In adults, either there must be onset of purulent sputum production more than 48 hours after admission in a patient with no preceding pulmonary infection, or increased production of purulent sputum with recrudescence of fever in a patient admitted with pulmonary disease must be present. In addition, at least one of the following criteria must also be present: (1) infiltration seen on chest roentgenography or characteristic physical findings of pneumonia in the absence of a chest roentgenogram or (2) cough, fever, and pleuritic chest pain. Diagnosis of pneumonia in a child can be made in the absence of purulent sputum if both of the latter criteria are satisfied. A diagnosis of pneumonia by the attending physician is accepted even when the above

criteria are incompletely fulfilled. Other conditions that may result in similar signs or symptoms (e.g., congestive heart failure, postoperative atelectasis, pulmonary embolism, and the like) may often be differentiated from pneumonia by the clinical course of the patient.

Suprainfection of a previously existing respiratory infection may result in a new nosocomial infection when a new pathogen is cultured from sputum and clinical or radiologic evidence indicates that the new organism is associated with deterioration in the patient's condition.

While more stringent criteria may insure a higher degree of specificity in diagnosis and enable greater assurance in distinguishing between suprainfection and supracolonization, they may result concomitantly in lower selectivity. Because of this reason and because the largest data base from which comparisons and trends can be developed is that of the CDC, it would seem that their definition should be employed unless there are specific justifications in a study for not doing so. Under the latter cir-

Table 15-4. Etiology of Nosocomial Pneumonia and Lower Respiratory Infections Reported by NNIS[a]

Causative agents	No. of isolates	Percent
Klebsiella	2273	15.4%
Pseudomonas aeruginosa	1991	13.5%
Staphylococci, coagulase-positive	1867	12.6%
Escherichia coli	1627	11.0%
Enterobacter	1339	9.1%
Streptococcus pneumoniae	1187	8.0%
Serratia marcescens	294	2.0%
Influenza	10	0.1%
Mycobacterium tuberculosis	1	<0.1%
Other pathogens	4183	28.3%
Totals	14,772	100.1%

[a] Data from National Nosocomial Infections Study (NNIS), January 1970 through August 1973 (see text).

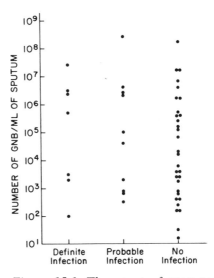

Figure 15-1. The count of gram-negative bacilli (*GNB*) per milliliter of sputum. Specimens were obtained from 22 of 26 patients with definite or probable infection at the time of diagnosis; 17 specimens contained gram-negative bacilli. These results are compared with those on specimens from 31 patients who had no clinical signs of infection.
From Johanson, W. G., et al. *Ann. Intern. Med.* 77:701, 1972.

cumstances, it is essential that the diagnostic criteria utilized be defined.

Microbiologic Criteria

Although it is usually the most readily available material for microbiologic examination, expectorated sputum is not the most satisfactory material for examination in patients with complicated pneumonia or in debilitated patients who are at risk for developing nosocomial pneumonia. Expectorated sputum is contaminated by oropharyngeal flora, which may not be representative of the cause of the pneumonia. Attempts have been made to reduce the error in diagnosis introduced by the oropharyngeal flora by means of repeated washing of expectorated sputum. This procedure, however, does not absolutely insure that the bacteria isolated from the washed sputum originated in the lower respiratory tract. In addition, the procedure places a great burden on the bacteriology laboratory. It has also been suggested that the true bacterial cause of the pneumonia can be identified by quantitative culture techniques. Our group and others have found, however, that this procedure does not necessarily identify the cause of the lung infection (Fig. 15-1).

Organisms isolated from blood, pleural fluid, lung, bronchial washings, or transtracheal aspirates in patients with clinical evidence of pneumonia should be reported as pathogens. Biopsy or postmortem specimens may be especially useful in identifying pneumonia caused by *Pneumocystis carinii* and *Aspergillus*.

The most useful diagnostic procedure is transtracheal aspiration of material for Gram stain and culture. The clinical courses of patients with pneumonia have been correlated with the results of Gram staining and culture both of expectorated sputum and of sputum obtained by transtracheal aspiration, and it has been demonstrated that the latter procedure is more likely to yield specimens that indicate the correct bacterial cause of the pneumonia. Moreover, transtracheal aspiration allows for the identification of anaerobic bacteria; this is not possible with expectorated sputum, because anaerobes are normal inhabitants of the oropharyngeal cavity. Although the incidence of serious complications is low, the procedure carries some risk, and it should be reserved for patients with complicated pneumonias and patients who are unable to produce sputum.

Even material obtained from transtracheal aspiration may contain a mixture of microorganisms on Gram stain. In addition, anaerobic bacilli may be gram negative and may thus be confused with aerobic gram-negative bacilli.

Although the value of bacteriologic study of sputum remains in serious doubt, it is likely that expectorated sputum specimens will continue to be submitted to clinical bacteriology laboratories for culture because of (1) medical contraindications to transtracheal aspiration and (2) the relative paucity of persons experienced in performing transtracheal aspiration. Therefore, a simple screening procedure for expectorated sputum would be helpful to ascertain the degree of oropharyngeal contamination. If contamination were present to a significant degree, cultures would yield a large number of different species that not only would complicate and prolong the bacteriologic procedures but also could overgrow the true causative agent. The effects of culturing oropharyngeal flora can hardly be regarded as a meaningful exercise for either the laboratory or the physician.

Bartlett [3] has proposed an objective system for evaluating the quality of lower respiratory tract secretions (see Part I, Chapter 8). Gram stains are examined under ×100 magnification after oil is placed on the slide to improve clarity. The slide is examined for the presence of neutrophils, mucus, and squamous epithelial cells. A rough quantitative estimate is made by applying a scoring system (Table 15-5). If the total score is zero or less, a report of "oropharyngeal contamination, please repeat" is rendered. Specimens with scores of +1 to +3 are cultured. Complete speciation and susceptibility testing are performed only if the number of potential pathogens isolated does not exceed the score. A score of +3, for example, signifies the absence of oropharyngeal material and the presence of mucus and abundant neutrophils.

Utilizing a similar system, Murray and Washington [33] attempted to provide bacteriologic evidence, including comparison with transtracheal aspirates, to support the criteria

Table 15-5. Criteria for Scoring the Quality of Specimens of Lower Respiratory Tract Secretions

Observation[a]	Score
More than 25 neutrophils per field	+2
10 to 25 neutrophils per field	+1
Mucus	+1
10 to 25 squamous cells per field	−1
More than 25 squamous cells per field	−2

[a] Field examined under oil at ×100 magnification (×10 objective).

From Bartlett, R. C. *Medical Microbiology. Quality, Cost, and Clinical Relevance.* New York: John Wiley and Sons, 1974.

of Bartlett. These investigators found (see Table 15-6) that specimens with more than ten epithelial cells per low-power (×100) field (groups 1 through 4) yielded similar numbers of species (4.2 to 4.4), in contrast to the smaller number of different isolates recovered from specimens showing less than ten epithelial cells (group 5) and transtracheal aspirate specimens (2.7 and 2.4, respectively). The number of leukocytes bore no relationship to the number of isolates. It is of particular note that at the time of this study, 75 percent of the sputum samples received in the laboratory were contaminated with more than ten epithelial cells per field and were judged to be unsatisfactory for culture. It is important to reserve

Table 15-6. Relationship Between Specimen Group and Mean Number of Bacterial Species Isolated

Group	Cellular composition (no./field)[a] Epithelial	Leukocytes	Specimens (no.)	Mean number of species isolated
1	>25	<10	54	4.2
2	>25	10–25	42	4.2
3	>25	>25	119	4.4
4	10–25	>25	68	4.2
5	<10	>25	99	2.7
TTA[b]	—	—	47	2.4

[a] Field examined at ×100 magnification (×10 objective).
[b] TTA = transtracheal aspirate.

From Murray, P. R., and Washington, J. A. *Mayo Clin. Proc.* 50:339, 1975.

such a screening criterion (i.e., less than ten squamous epithelial cells per field at ×100 magnification) for sputum bacteriology only. In patients with suspected mycoplasmal, viral, fungal, or myobacterial illness, the degree of oropharyngeal contamination is relatively less important.

In the event that the clinical illness does not indicate the need for, or if there are contraindications to, transtracheal aspiration, microscopic examination of sputum employing the criteria of Murray and Washington appears to be of value in determining the acceptability of a specimen for bacterial culture. The utilization of such techniques should greatly sharpen the accuracy of defining etiologic considerations in patients with nosocomial lower respiratory tract infections.

General Factors Affecting Susceptibility

The normal human respiratory tract is provided with a variety of mechanisms that act to protect the lungs from infection. The lower respiratory tract is protected by the glottis and larynx, and material passing these barriers stimulates the expulsive cough reflex. Removal of small particles impinging on the walls of the trachea and bronchi is facilitated by their mucociliary lining, and the growth of bacteria reaching normal alveoli is inhibited by their relative dryness and by the phagocytic activity of alveolar macrophages. Any anatomic or physiologic derangement of these coordinated defenses tends to augment the susceptibility of the lungs to infection. Anesthesia, alcoholic intoxication, convulsions, and disturbed innervation of the larynx depress the cough reflex and may permit aspiration of infected material. Alterations in the tracheobronchial tree leading to anatomic changes in the epithelial lining or to localized obstruction increase the vulnerability of the lungs to infection. Local or generalized pulmonary edema resulting from viral infection, inhalation of irritant gases, cardiac failure, or contusion of the chest wall provides a fluid menstruum in the alveoli for the growth of bacteria and their spread to adjacent areas of the lung. Viral infection of the respiratory epithelium with concomitant disruption of its component cells interferes significantly with the clearance of bacteria from the lungs.

Sources and Modes of Acquisition

Microorganisms may invade the alveolar level of the lung in sufficient density to produce pneumonia by one of three routes: (1) aspiration from the oropharynx, (2) suspension in inhaled gas, or (3) by way of the vasculature (lymphohematogenous spread).

Bronchogenous Spread by Aspiration of Oropharyngeal Bacteria

MECHANISMS. Most bacterial pneumonia is due to microorganisms that make up the flora of the oropharynx, and aspiration of such organisms is probably the principal mechanism underlying nosocomial pneumonia. Indirect evidence supports this hypothesis. Pneumococci instilled into the nose of unanesthetized rabbits have been noted to appear in the lung within minutes. When the bronchi of dogs were occluded with sterile cotton plugs and atelectasis was allowed to occur, pharyngeal organisms were recovered distal to the occlusion. Culture of specimens from human lungs at autopsy has revealed bacterial species similar to those cultured from the pharynx. It has been suggested that these findings are due to agonal or postmortem invasion of the tracheobronchial tree. The findings, however, are also compatible with the terminal failure of clearance mechanisms that had suppressed bacterial growth in the lungs during life. The mechanism by which bacteria spread from the pharynx to the lung during life remains unclear. The aspiration into the lung of radiopaque material instilled into the oropharynx of normal sleeping adults was demonstrated by Amberson [1] in 1937 but these findings have not been confirmed by others.

OROPHARYNGEAL COLONIZATION OF NORMAL PERSONS. The oropharynx of a normal person apparently does not provide a suitable environment for the growth of aerobic gram-negative bacilli; only about 2 percent of normal persons harbor more than occasional aerobic gram-negative bacilli at any given time. When multiple culture determinations are performed on normal persons, the cumulative percentage of subjects with at least one positive culture result increases, but previously positive persons usually are negative. This indicates that colonization is transient in normal persons, although the length of colonization has not been defined. Utilizing more sensitive broth culture media that were selective for aerobic gram-negative bacilli, Rosenthal and Tager [43] detected small numbers of Enterobacteriaceae or *Pseudomonas aeruginosa* in 18 percent of normal persons. Furthermore, massive exposure of normal persons to these organisms does not result in colonization of the upper respiratory tract. Thus, normal persons are only at slight risk (perhaps 2 percent are at risk) for developing gram-negative bacillary pneumonia by aspiration of oropharyngeal flora.

FACTORS PREDISPOSING TO COLONIZATION. Chronically or severely ill patients lose effective pharyngeal clearance mechanisms, allowing colonization with aerobic gram-negative bacilli. Exposure to such organisms from an exogenous source is evidently not necessary, because it has been found [18] that approximately 20 percent of patients sufficiently ill to be admitted to a medical intensive-care unit were colonized at the time of admission. Although previous therapy with antimicrobial drugs facilitates colonization and possibly the occurrence of pneumonia, it is similarly not a prerequisite.

As anticipated from the concentration of chronically and severely ill patients in a hospital setting, gram-negative bacillary oropharyngeal colonization is especially prevalent among hospitalized patients. There is a rapid rise in the incidence of colonization for the first few hospital days, which suggests that there is a "susceptible pool" of patients who are particularly predisposed to colonization. The patients most prone to colonization are those with features reflecting severe illness, such as coma, hypotension, acidosis, azotemia, and alterations in the leukocyte count; in such patients, the incidence of colonization approaches 75 percent. An increased prevalence of colonization among patients with respiratory disease or endotracheal intubation suggests that factors impairing lung clearance may also promote colonization. Patients who, though hospitalized, are not critically ill have a far lower prevalence of oropharyngeal colonization (approximately 30 to 40 percent).

SOURCES OF ORGANISMS. The occurrence of clusters of patients colonized with the same species of gram-negative bacilli suggests that, in part, the bacteria are transmitted from patient to patient within the hospital setting. The 20 percent incidence of colonization at the time of admission and the subsequent colonization of some patients with bacterial species not isolated from other patients in the same environment, however, suggest that many patients are colonized with organisms indigenous to each patient. The gastrointestinal tract is the most likely site from which the bacilli spread.

Ventilatory equipment may serve as a reservoir from which patients may become colonized with bacteria through several routes. Surface contamination of inhalation therapy equipment could serve as a source from which the patient's face, mouth, or nose could become colonized; such has not been demonstrated directly. The exhalation side of the circuit has received little attention; however, effluent may contaminate the patient's immediate surroundings such as bed linens. From the contaminated local environment, secondary transmission by the patient's own hands or by hospital personnel to the index patient or to other patients can occur. Of course, contamination of the internal parts of the equipment may also lead to oropharyngeal colonization. The relative importance of ventilatory equipment as a source of oropharyngeal bacteria probably varies widely among hospitals. In one observation [19] on the occurrence of colonization of the oropharynx with aerobic gram-negative bacilli, inhalation therapy was not a factor that could be significantly correlated with colonization.

Bronchogenous Spread by Airborne Organisms

MECHANISMS. Infection may be transmitted at some distance by infected small particles, or aerosols, that are generated by coughs and sneezes. Such particles range in size from 1 μ to more than 20 μ in diameter, remain airborne for long periods, may disseminate widely in the local environment such as a hospital ward, and may potentially infect large numbers of persons.

The minimum infectious dose of a number of pathogenic bacteria is less if they are delivered in aerosols of a size capable of deposition beyond the level of the ciliated epithelium. It has been estimated that at least 50 percent of 1.0 to 2.0 μ particles, when delivered to the mouth or nose of an individual, are capable of entering the bronchial tree distal to the terminal bronchioles (lowest level of ciliated epithelium), where host defense mechanisms may be overcome more easily.

The most important mechanism for the dissemination of bacteria by ventilatory equipment is the aerosolization of organisms into the stream of gas delivered by such equipment in particle sizes that are sufficiently small to be deposited in terminal lung units. Most types of nebulizers are designed to deliver aerosols in a size range of 1.0 to 2.0 μ to insure humidification or the delivery of medications to the lower reaches of the tracheobronchial tree.

Except for tuberculosis and in circumstances where individuals are receiving inhalation treatments, airborne transmission is probably of little importance in the epidemiology of nosocomial bacillary pneumonia. The bacterial density in the air, even in hospitals, is quite low.

AIRBORNE SPREAD FROM PERSONS. In controlled experiments, natural airborne transmission of coxsackievirus A21 has been demonstrated. In addition, adenovirus type 4 has been found in droplets expelled in coughs and in the air of rooms occupied by military recruits ill with adenoviral pneumonia. These observations suggest that airborne transmission is important in the transmission of these two infections and may be important in other viral infections of the respiratory tract, such as influenza. Similarly, Riley and associates [41] demonstrated the infectiousness of air on a tuberculosis ward, although they concluded that viable airborne tubercule bacilli are not very numerous and that the air of a room occupied by a tuberculous patient may not be very dangerous if it is breathed for only a short time.

ROLE OF NEBULIZATION EQUIPMENT. Since gases such as oxygen or compressed air are essentially free of water vapor, their administration without humidification results in desiccation of the upper airways and may significantly predispose the patient to infection. Hence, a method for increasing the water vapor content of administered gases is essential, even though it results in the concomitant, increased risk of bacterial contamination of the moisture source. There are two markedly differing principles utilized to increase the humidity of gases delivered to the tracheobronchial tree. The first of these involves humidification; the second, nebulization (Fig. 15-2). Definition of these terms becomes essential, because differences in terminology with resultant confusion exist in the literature.

Humidifiers are devices that saturate gas with water vapor; they do not aerosolize droplet water. Most clinical humidifiers cause the stream of gas to bubble through water, although some humidifiers used in pediatrics cause the stream of gas to be blown across the surface of the water.

In contrast, nebulizers not only saturate the gas with water vapor, but they also disperse an aerosol of droplets. Most clinical nebulizers are gas driven and operate on the venturi principle. Venturi-type nebulizers may be of small volume (5 to 30 ml.) for dispensing specific medication, or they may contain a large reservoir (approximately 500 ml.) for the adminis-

Figure 15-2. Differences in principles of operation of humidifiers and nebulizers.
From Sanford, J. P., and Pierce, A. K. In Brachman, P. S., and Eickhoff, T. C. (Eds.), *Proceedings of the International Conference on Nosocomial Infections.* Chicago: American Hospital Association, 1971. Reprinted with permission.

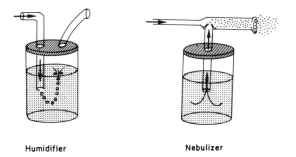

Humidifier   Nebulizer

tration of moisture. These latter nebulizers may be operated at room temperature or they may be heated. Aerosols also may be produced by dropping liquid onto the surface of a rapidly spinning disc; such nebulizers, which are infrequently used in adult medicine, also incorporate large-volume reservoirs. A third means of creating aerosols is by ultrasonic nebulizers, in which droplets are produced by a rapidly oscillating crystal.

Disinfection of each type of equipment and even different devices employing the same design principle must be evaluated independently.

In our initial observations, we demonstrated that the reservoir nebulizer was the major site that became contaminated and from which bacterial dissemination occurred. Our conclusions were based on observations derived from sampling the effluent gas with the use of an air sampler. First, it was noted that equipment that did not incorporate reservoir nebulizers into its design did not generate significant bacterial aerosols. Second, sequential disassembly of the apparatus with reservoir nebulizers demonstrated bacterial aerosols distal, but not proximal, to the reservoir nebulizer. Third, there was a correlation between both the numbers and species of organisms in the generated aerosols and those in the reservoir nebulizer fluid. The survival and multiplication of some bacterial species in the reservoir nebulizer fluid provide an effective amplification mechanism whereby even small numbers of initially contaminating bacteria ultimately may be delivered in large quantities to a patient.

There are multiple potential routes by which the fluid-containing reservoir initially may become contaminated. The relative importance of one route over another cannot be determined from the available data. The sources to be considered include at least the following (Fig. 15-3). The oxygen, compressed air, or other gas that is administered to the patient and that often drives the nebulizer may be contaminated. Room air, which usually is added through the dilutor ports to decrease the concentration of inspired oxygen, may provide another source. Personnel may contaminate the inside of the reservoir container during cleaning or replenishing of the fluid in the reservoir.

(We even have had personnel contaminate the reservoir by attempting to be more cautious than called for in cleansing procedures; they washed the jars with 3% hexachlorophene-containing soaps that were unfortunately contaminated.) The water or other fluid placed in the reservoir must be sterile. There are numerous outbreaks of pulmonary colonization and infection that have been traced to the nebulization of contaminated medications. Organisms present in secretions from the patient's nose or mouth may contaminate the fluid that tends to condense in the plastic delivery tubing connecting the nebulizer to the face mask. Bacteria have been shown to survive for considerable time in such fluid. Massive contamination may result from emptying the condensate that collects in the delivery tubing back into the reservoir. Morris [32], however, detected contamination of the condensate in only one of 96 specimens. Failure to disinfect portions of the nebulizer, such as the nebulizer jet, may occur because of entrapment of air that prevents contact with liquids if liquid disinfectants are being used. Under these circumstances, the nebulizer jet serves as a nidus from which reinoculation of the reservoir may occur.

Whichever primary mechanisms are operative, even reservoir nebulizers that are initially sterile and used by only one individual very frequently become contaminated within 24 hours of clinical use. The bacterial multiplication that then occurs results in an amplification of organisms, which can be delivered in larger numbers and in a particle size that can be delivered to the lower reaches of the tracheobronchial tree.

Lymphohematogenous Spread
Invasion of the lung through the pulmonary vasculature is possible when there is a peripheral site of infection that is causing bacteremia, such as staphylococcal pneumonia secondary to septic thrombophlebitis associated with an indwelling venous catheter, *Escherichia coli* pneumonia as a complication of pyelonephritis, and *Pseudomonas aeruginosa* pneumonia in the burned patient. In the majority of patients with nosocomial bacillary pneumonia, however, no distant locus can be identified.

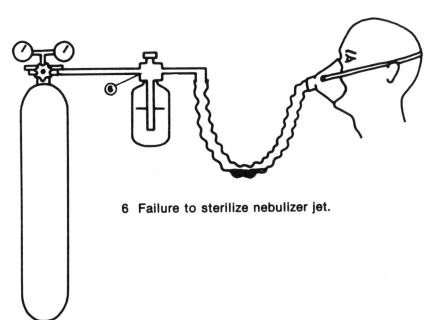

6 Failure to sterilize nebulizer jet.

Figure 15-3. Potential means by which reservoir of nebulizer may become contaminated. Key to figure: (1) Oxygen, compressed air, or other gas source; (2) room air via dilutor parts; (3) hand contact with inside of jar during refilling; 4) contaminated water used to fill reservoir; (5) organisms from patient's nose or mouth (5a) contaminated condensate (5b), which may then retroflux into reservoir; (6) failure to sterilize nebulizer jet.

Disinfection and Sterilization of Ventilatory Equipment

Several methods have been suggested for the sterilization of inhalation therapy equipment. Based on surface-culturing techniques, the mechanical ventilator, rather than the reservoir nebulizer, is frequently the focus of major concern. Although ventilators, like other hospital equipment, should receive reasonable hygienic care, they are not a major source of bacterial contamination of inspired gas. The use of bacterial filters in various positions in the stream of gas flow in ventilators also has been suggested. A filter on the driving gas of the ventilator or nebulizer eliminates only one source of potential contamination, and hence filters do not insure sterility of the effluent gas from the nebulizer. Filters interposed between the nebulizer and the patient are not practical, because they would not permit the passage of the therapeutic aerosol. Primary attention must be directed to disinfection of the reservoir nebulizer (see Part I, Chapter 6).

Definitions

In the published material on inhalation therapy equipment, varied terminology has been employed to describe the processes utilized to prevent transmission of disease. We have used the term "decontamination" for many of the procedures; however, according to common usage, this is inappropriate, and the term should be reserved for the process that renders contaminated items safe to handle with reasonable care. *Disinfection,* the more correct term, may be defined as the virtual elimination of all harmful microorganisms, except spores, in an attempt to prevent transmission of disease. *Sterilization* is the complete destruction or removal of all organisms (see Part I, Chapter 6). Objects that contact skin or mucous membranes, such as respiratory therapy equipment other than the apparatus itself, should receive at least a high level of disinfection and ideally should be sterilized before assignment to patients.

Sterilization Methods

There are three methods potentially available for the sterilization of inhalation therapy equipment: steam autoclaving, cold soaking with activated glutaraldehyde germicidal solution, and ethylene oxide gas.

AUTOCLAVING. Steam autoclaving is usually not practical, because of the sensitivity of the equipment to heat. We have utilized this procedure successfully, however, for older types of nebulizers that were constructed of cast aluminum.

GLUTARALDEHYDE. Immersion in a germicidal solution may be used to either disinfect or sterilize equipment, but ten hours submersion in activated glutaraldehyde is required for sterilization; submersion for less time results in disinfection. The greatest limitation to liquid sterilization (or disinfection) is its unreliable penetration. To sterilize an item, the active chemical must contact all bacteria-laden surfaces. Entrapment of air often prevents adequate liquid contact during treatment, and this is a particular problem with inhalation therapy equipment, because nebulizer jets are usually encased in hollow areas.

ETHYLENE OXIDE. Since gases are completely miscible with air, the ideal chemical sterilant is a gas such as ethylene oxide. Ethylene oxide denatures bacterial proteins through a process of alkylation. Moisture is essential to this reaction. Raising the temperature also hastens the reaction; sterilization is achieved six to eight times faster at 54°C (130°F) than at 21°C (70°F). Ethylene oxide is absorbed into various plastics and must be allowed to diffuse out before the plastic is used in prolonged contact with tissues to avoid its local irritant effect; this process is termed *aeration*. Aeration periods depend on several factors: the duration of exposure to ethylene oxide, the aeration environment, the type of plastic, and the intended use of the item. Although aeration may often require 24 to 48 hours, units are available to reduce all aeration periods to eight hours. The major problem of ethylene oxide sterilization is the expense of the equipment required to insure safe, prompt, effective sterilization and aeration. This technique, however,

appears to be the most satisfactory, provided it is remembered that under in-use conditions, recontamination can occur within 24 hours, even if a piece of equipment is used by only one patient.

Disinfection Methods

Many hospitals do not have the capability to sterilize all their inhalation therapy equipment with ethylene oxide. Also, it is not feasible to aerosolize the most effective liquid chemical sterilant, activated glutaraldehyde, to insure that the nebulizer jets are sterilized. Thus, various other disinfecting procedures have been employed and have been shown to be effective if rigorously applied and monitored [48]. With these procedures, it is important to cleanse the equipment mechanically. Exudates should not be allowed to dry. Equipment should be rinsed initially with cold water to avoid coagulation of protein and then washed with mechanical cleansing and detergent.

PASTEURIZATION. Heating to 75°C (167°F) for ten minutes will kill vegetative forms of bacteria, and even washing at 60°C (140°F) for two minutes destroys most bacteria. The use of hot-water "pasteurization" has been successfully employed by several groups. Roberts and associates [42] immersed equipment for a period of 15 minutes at 80°C to 85°C (176°F to 185°F), whereas Nelson and Ryan [34] processed equipment for 30 minutes at 70°C (158°F). Nelson and Ryan were concerned that jets in equipment might not be disinfected by this method, because it is questionable whether the water would enter the tiny orifices. All items with small orifices or jets were disassembled and disinfected with activated glutaraldehyde (immersion for ten minutes), rinsed in a solution of one ounce of sodium bisulfite per gallon of water, and then pasteurized and air-dried by blowing air at 38°C (100°F) over the equipment.

OTHER DISINFECTANTS. Disinfectant solutions with greater antimicrobial activity than acetic acid, such as chlorhexidine diacetate and formaldehyde, can also be nebulized. However, the potential toxicities of chlorhexidine and similar agents, when nebulized into patient areas or inadvertently into patients, have not been sufficiently defined to allow their usage without considerable study.

COPPER SPONGES. It has been reported [8] that the placing of a copper sponge in the reservoir jars of venturi nebulizers results in the nebulizer contents remaining sterile. The institution of this method of cleaning in an intensive-care unit resulted in an apparent reduction in the incidence of pulmonary infections. Although these investigators concluded that the sterility of reservoir nebulizers could be maintained for 48 hours or longer, they noted that in practice, the nebulizers and all parts distal to them were changed every 24 hours, a procedure that should have greatly improved the chances for sterility. Our own experience with this method has been limited to observations on the ability of the copper sponge to sterilize nebulizer solutions following intentional inoculation of bacteria into the nebulizer contents. We have been disappointed by the erratic ability of copper sponges to maintain sterility.

OTHER PROCEDURES. Grieble and coworkers [14] have found that the daily use of phenolic disinfectants or dilute acetic acid did not sterilize spinning-disc nebulizers. It was found that daily sterilization with ethylene oxide was necessary to prevent contamination. Since this procedure was considered impractical in their clinical setting, the use of spinning-disc nebulizers was discontinued in their hospital.

Rhoades and associates [40] have found that ultrasonic nebulizers were not sterilized either by soaking in a disinfectant solution or by the nebulization of 0.25% acetic acid for 30 minutes. However, 2% acetic acid nebulization for 30 minutes successfully removed bacteria from a nebulizer. It has also been found that 7.5% hydrogen peroxide nebulization for 20 minutes may be an effective disinfecting procedure for ultrasonic nebulizers; it is suggested that such equipment be treated at least once every 24 hours.

Dilute Acetic Acid Nebulization Regimen

METHOD. One of the most common regimens for controlling microbial contamination of reservoir, venturi-type nebulizers involves initial sterilization of the equipment with either ethylene oxide or steam autoclaving, or immersion in a disinfectant solution (e.g., glutaraldehyde or a phenolic disinfectant) in the inhalation therapy department. Daily nebulization with 0.25% acetic acid is then employed after the equipment has been assigned to a patient [37]. The details of this regimen are as follows:

1. If the nebulizer is attached to the patient, it should be turned off and the face mask (or mouthpiece) removed from the patient.
2. Remove the nebulizer jar and empty the contents.
3. Rinse the jar with sterile water.
4. Cover the fluid intake of the tube leading to the nebulizer jet with 0.25% acetic acid (approximately 200 ml. in most nebulizers).
5. Replace the jar on the nebulizer.
6. Turn on the nebulizer to a flow rate of 7 liters per minute so the acetic acid will be aerosolized. (Nebulization can be done in the room with the patient, if the patient is disconnected from the tubing, without causing unpleasant odors or the irritation of mucous membranes.)
7. Allow the acetic acid to nebulize for approximately ten minutes.
8. Turn off the gas (oxygen or air) and remove the nebulizer jar.
9. Discard the acetic acid and rinse the jar with sterile water.
10. Refill the jar with sterile water or other desired solution. (Be careful not to contaminate the inside of the jar in the process.)
11. The equipment is now ready for patient use.
12. The nebulizer fluid should be emptied and replenished every eight hours. At this time, the remainder should always be discarded from the jar to minimize any residual "inoculum."
13. Before the equipment is used on another patient, it should be sterilized or disinfected. If the use by one patient is prolonged, the equipment should be returned

and newly sterilized equipment issued every 72 hours.

RESULTS. Dilute acetic acid was chosen because it is relatively nontoxic, which enables the procedure to be performed at the patient's bedside. Acetic acid is bactericidal for only about one-third of gram-negative bacilli and gram-positive cocci. Nevertheless, significant microbiologic failure of the described regimen has not been encountered. When properly used, acetic acid treatment renders the effluent gas from most venturi nebulizers virtually sterile. It is perhaps of note, however, that when the acetic acid method was introduced from the laboratory into routine hospital use, the results were disappointing. It was found subsequently that the failure to achieve disinfection of the effluent gas from nebulizers resulted from personnel error or faulty nebulizer jets. A continuous monitoring program and the replacement of pitted nebulizer jets resulted in the effluent gas being contaminated less than 10 percent of the time while in use.

It is not possible to control contamination of all types of reservoir venturi nebulizers safely by the described regimen. Some nebulizers used in pediatric tents have been demonstrated to be resistant to this method. It has been found that such nebulizers must be sterilized at least every 48 hours; either autoclaving or ethylene oxide may be used, and acetic acid nebulization is carried out on alternate days.

During the period immediately preceding the institution of a program of culturing the effluent from inhalation therapy equipment and of disinfection employing acetic acid nebulization, the prevalence of necrotizing pneumonia was 7.9 percent [37]. Under the epidemiologic circumstances of the hospitalized patient, the histologic appearance of necrotizing pneumonia has been found to be specific enough to serve as an index of the frequency of all pneumonia due to aerobic gram-negative bacilli. The prevalence of this lesion increased from 1.8 percent of all autopsies in 1957 to 7.9 percent of autopsies in 1963. This increase was significantly correlated with the use of reservoir nebulization treatments. With a program of surveillance and disinfection, and in the face of a 9 percent increase in the use of reservoir nebulization treatments, the incidence of necrotizing pneumonia in 1966 and 1967 decreased to 2.2 and 2.1 percent of autopsies. This accompanied a decrease in the frequency of contamination of reservoir nebulizers from 84 percent to less than 10 percent. Subsequently, in a totally independent study of the occurrence of colonization of the oropharynx and the development of pneumonia in patients in a medical intensive-care unit, inhalation treatments were not significantly associated with the acquisition of aerobic gram-negative bacilli [19].

Conclusions

The information available justifies several conclusions. Inhalation therapy equipment is a potential vector of gram-negative bacilli. Not all types of equipment, however, are equally dangerous in this regard, and investigators should be more specific in their descriptions of equipment used when reporting results. Ventilators and humidifiers have a minimal potential for aerosolizing bacteria into the patient's inspired gas. Small-volume venturi nebulizers are potential disseminators of bacteria, but they evidently infrequently do so in hospital use. Large-volume nebulizers of all designs (venturi, spinning-disc, or ultrasonic) are the major source of aerosolized bacteria. The means required for sterilization differ depending on the design of the nebulizer. It has been demonstrated that contamination of most nebulizers can be controlled successfully in a clinical setting. Any system, however, requires meticulous handling by personnel and the application of some type of microbial control procedure at least once every 24 hours. No hospital can consider its own procedure satisfactory unless contamination does not exceed that of hospital air. These observations indicate the need for continuous monitoring of this form of therapy as is carried out in many other facets of patient care.

Staphylococcus aureus Infections

General Aspects

TRANSMISSIBILITY. The distribution of staphylococci in nature has probably been studied more fully than any comparable bacteriologic problem. For all practical purposes, *Staphylococcus aureus* has no significant reservoir outside of man or animals. There is general agreement that for man, the main reservoir is the human nose, specifically the squamous epithelium of the vestibule. Skin surfaces harboring staphylococci become colonized from the nose. To remain endemic, staphylococci have to pass from one individual to another; their main asset in achieving this is their ability to withstand drying. Based on prevalence studies in normal adults residing in urban areas, the average nasal-carrier rate for staphylococci is 50 percent. In sequential studies on hospital personnel, it was found that 15 percent were consistently negative, while 36 percent were persistent carriers. The persistent carriers had higher numbers of organisms, based on quantitative studies, than did individuals who were transient carriers (see Part 2, Chapter 20).

The development of staphylococcal lower respiratory tract infection may be either bronchogenous or secondary to lymphohematogenous dissemination from peripheral sites to the lung. In the former instance (which is the more common), the acquisition of staphylococci appears to be primarily through contact transmission rather than by aerosols. Once staphylococci have been established on the mucosa, spread to the tracheobronchial tree can occur through aspiration, and, provided the inoculum is sufficient, the bronchopulmonary antimicrobial defenses are compromised, or both, lower respiratory infection can ensue.

PREDISPOSING FACTORS. Staphylococcal pneumonia in infants usually occurs as a primary infection of the respiratory tract, but it may also derive by lymphohematogenous spread from the skin or from other infections. It may also occur as a complication of measles, chickenpox, influenza, or cystic fibrosis of the pancreas. The highest incidence occurs among infants.

Staphylococcal pneumonia in adults is usually associated with a prior viral respiratory tract infection, such as influenza. It may also occur as a complication of acute bacterial endocarditis or septic thrombophlebitis; septic emboli may involve the lungs.

About one-eighth to one-quarter of all nosocomial pneumonia is caused by *S. aureus* (see Tables 15-3 and 15-4).

CLINICAL FEATURES. The illness usually begins as an upper respiratory tract infection with fever, nasal obstruction or discharge, and cough associated with irritability and anorexia. The symptoms may progress rapidly or gradually to increasing cough, tachypnea, dyspnea, and subcostal retractions. Severe infections in young infants may be manifested by increasing respiratory distress, abdominal distention, pallor, cyanosis, prostration, and possibly death.

The physical findings vary with the type of pulmonary involvement. Staphylococcal infection of the lung may be followed by consolidation, abscess formation, pneumatoceles, empyema, pneumothorax, or pyopneumothorax, either singly or in combination. In children, the roentgenographic lesion is apt to appear as multiple cysts because of the characteristic pneumatocele formation. In adults, the pulmonary lesions appear as confluent areas of consolidation with rapid progression to abscess formation and cavitation.

Pneumatocele formation is a hallmark of staphylococcal pneumonia. It is thought to be an emphysematous bleb within the pulmonary interstitial tissue and is presumably produced as follows: the staphylococci invade the bronchial wall and peribronchiolar tissues, producing inflammation and abscess formation. The perforation of the bronchial wall by the abscess enables air to pass into the interstitial space. A ball-valve effect traps the air, thereby producing a cyst or pneumatocele. Thus, the bleb is a secondary manifestation of the bronchial and peribronchial infection. Pneumatoceles usually clear spontaneously within a variable period of four weeks to four months.

Pneumothorax results from the rupture of a pneumatocele. Sudden onset of severe dyspnea, cyanosis, prostration, and shock may indicate tension pneumothorax. Empyema occurs as the result of rupture of an abscess into the pleural cavity. Pyopneumothorax develops if the abscess connects with a bronchus.

The blood picture characteristically reveals an increase in the number of polymorphonuclear leukocytes. Occasionally, however, the white blood cell count is normal or low. The roentgenographic findings may reveal rapidly changing infiltrations, pneumatoceles, pneumothorax, empyema, or pyopneumothorax.

THERAPY. Since the early 1940s, the prevalence of penicillin-resistant strains of staphylococci detected in hospitalized patients has risen from between 0 and 12 percent to at least 80 percent (see Part I, Chapter 11). The occurrence of staphylococcal pneumonia represents a medical emergency, because rapid progression is typical, and the rates are high for morbidity and mortality, which ensue without therapy or with ineffective antimicrobial therapy. Initial empiric treatment should include the parenteral administration of a penicillinase-resistant semisynthetic penicillin, such as methicillin, nafcillin, or oxacillin. In the patient who is allergic to penicillin, alternatives include parenteral vancomycin or a cephalosporin (keeping in mind that a degree of cross-sensitization exists between penicillin and the cephalosporins). Additional therapy directed at maintenance of adequate oxygenation, drainage of loculated infection, and correction and prevention of fluid and electrolyte imbalance is essential, and in many patients, it is as critical as the antimicrobial therapy, especially with the development of pneumatoceles and pyopneumothorax.

Prevention of Endemic Infections

The ubiquity of staphylococci, their ready adaptability, and the nature of the parasite-host relationship make it difficult to control human staphylococcal infections.

Since there is little evidence that healthy persons carrying staphylococci in the nose are primarily responsible for transmitting infection even to premature and newly born infants (potentially the most susceptible recipients), masks are not recommended. Washing one's hands with an antibacterial detergent (e.g., an iodophor) before and after handling patients is recommended. The routine use of hexachlorophene-containing detergents is probably safe for personnel, although evidence of absorption can be demonstrated. If they are present in work areas, however, hexachlorophene-containing materials are apt to be used on newborns or in other than epidemic circumstances, where their use should be avoided.

It is most important to exclude all persons with acute staphylococcal infections of the skin or mucous membranes, who may be shedding particularly virulent staphylococci, from patient-care areas. The prophylactic use of antimicrobial agents for contacts of pneumonia cases is not recommended. Proper isolation of patients with staphylococcal pneumonia is important and will reduce risks of cross-infection by contact and airborne spread (see Part I, Chapter 9).

Epidemic Infections

INCIDENCE. Epidemics of staphylococcal lower respiratory tract infections were particularly common in the mid-1950s and early 1960s in association with outbreaks of staphylococcal skin infections in premature and newborn infants (these being associated with strains lysed by bacteriophages 80/81), and in adults following the influenza A2 (H_2N_2 [Asian] and H_3N_2 [Hong Kong]) pandemics of 1957–1958 and 1968–1970. During the 1957–1958 influenzal pandemic, though the occurrence of *Streptococcus pneumoniae* predominated in many series of patients, Hers and associates [17] demonstrated staphylococci in 69 of 103 (67 percent), Martin and co-workers [28] in 11 of 17 (65 percent), and Petersdorf and co-workers [36] in 5 of 11 (45 percent) fatal cases of pneumonia.

HIGH-RISK AREAS. The areas of highest risk are the premature and newborn nursery areas and patient-care areas in which patients with respiratory problems may be congregated, for example, respiratory intensive-care units.

SOURCES OF INFECTION. The sources and modes of spread are the same as those for endemic infections. In newborn nursery areas, transmission via the hands of personnel is the most important route. Transmission via aerosols or fomites is less important.

CONTROL OF OUTBREAKS. The prevention and control of outbreaks of nosocomial staphylococcal pneumonia mainly depend on the interruption of the transmission of *S. aureus* in newborn nurseries. The prompt control of epidemics of staphylococcal skin infections is especially important, because pneumonia as a result of lymphohematogenous spread may complicate such infections. The control of staphylococcal skin infections in neonates is described in depth in Chapter 20, Part II, of this text.

Pneumococcal Pneumonia

General Aspects

TRANSMISSIBILITY. *Streptococcus pneumoniae* are normal inhabitants of the human upper respiratory tract in 5 to 60 percent of the population, depending on the season. Most cases of pneumonia probably derive from aspiration of organisms from the oropharynx. Pneumococcal infection occurs predominantly during the winter and early spring. Morbidity and mortality rates are higher for blacks than for whites. Person-to-person transmission by droplets is undoubtedly common, but true epidemics of pneumococcal pneumonia are rare, even in closed populations. *Streptococcus pneumoniae* is responsible for about one-tenth of all nosocomial pneumonias (see Tables 15-3 and 15-4). Patients with pneumococcal infections caused by penicillin-sensitive strains need not be isolated, because the risk of cross-infection is relatively small. Proper precautions in handling the respiratory secretions of such patients is adequate.

PREDISPOSING FACTORS. Invasion of the tissues of the nasopharynx rarely, if ever, occurs, and "pneumococcal pharyngitis" is a doubtful entity. Viral respiratory infections predispose to pneumococcal pneumonia. There is generally a high incidence of pneumococcal pneumonia during epidemics of viral influenza, and a frequent clinical association is seen with sporadic viral respiratory infections.

CLINICAL FEATURES. Pneumococcal pneumonia is often preceded for a few days by coryza or some other form of common respiratory disease. The onset is usually so abrupt that patients frequently can state the exact hour that the illness began. There is a sudden shaking chill in more than 80 percent of the cases, a rapid rise in temperature, and a corresponding tachycardia.

About 75 percent of patients develop severe pleuritic pain and cough and produce pinkish or "rusty" mucinoid sputum within a few hours. The chest pain is agonizing, and respirations become rapid, shallow, and grunting as the patient tries to splint the affected side. Patients appear acutely ill; nausea, headache, and malaise are not prominent, however, and most individuals are alert. Pleuritic pain and dyspnea are the dominant complaints.

In the untreated disease, there is sustained fever of 102.5°F to 105°F (39.2°C to 40.6°C), continued pleuritic pain, cough, and expectoration; abdominal distention is frequent. Herpes febrilis (labialis) is a common complication.

Physical examination reveals restricted motion of the affected hemithorax. Tactile fremitus may be decreased during the initial day of illness but is usually increased when consolidation is fully established. The percussion note is dull. Early in the course of infection, breath sounds are diminished, but as the lesion evolves, they become tubular or bronchial in quality, and bronchophony and whispered pectoriloquy can be elicited. These findings are accompanied by fine, crepitant rales.

THERAPY. In the United States, resistance of *Streptococcus pneumoniae* strains to benzylpenicillin (penicillin G) occurs with great rarity (see Part I, Chapter 11). This situation could change abruptly, however, because in May 1977, strains of *S. pneumoniae* that were highly resistant to penicillin G, methicillin, cephalosporin, tetracycline, erythromycin, clindamycin, chloramphenicol, trimethoprim-sulfamethoxazole, and all the aminoglycosides were isolated from patients and carriers in several locations in the Republic of South Africa. These multiple-drug-resistant strains were initially susceptible to rifampin, vancomycin, bacitracin, and fusidic acid. Resistance to rifampin, however, is known to occur readily, and resistant strains have already been encountered in patients treated with rifampin and fusidic acid [5]. Strains that are resistant to the tetracyclines and, to a lesser extent, to erythromycin are clinically significant and are observed in the United States.

The antimicrobial agent of choice is benzylpenicillin (penicillin G). Optimal results have been achieved with dosages of 80,000 units

(10,000 units every three hours) of aqueous crystalline penicillin G per day. The usual recommended dose of 600,000 units of aqueous procaine penicillin G intramuscularly twice daily provides a wide margin of safety; it also minimizes the influence on the normal microbial flora and the possibility of supracolonization and suprainfection. In the patient who is allergic to penicillin, alternative agents include erythromycin (the prevalence of resistant strains is less than one percent), the cephalosporins (although a degree of cross-sensitization exists between the penicillins and the cephalosporins), and clindamycin. It should be emphasized that the aminoglycosidic antibiotics (kanamycin, gentamicin, tobramycin, and amikacin) are not effective against pneumococci in the usually recommended safe doses.

Pneumococcal pneumonia usually improves promptly when an appropriate antimicrobial drug is given. Within 12 to 36 hours after initiation of treatment with penicillin, the temperature, pulse, and respiration begin to fall and may reach normal values, the pleuritic pain subsides, and the spread of the inflammatory process is halted. In approximately half the patients, however, the temperature requires four days or longer to become normal, and a failure of the patient's temperature to reach normal in 24 to 48 hours should not prompt a change in antibacterial therapy in the absence of other indications.

Prevention of Endemic Infections
Despite 82 pneumococcal serotypes, most of the serious infections are caused by a limited number; organisms of capsular types 1 through 8 account for 60 percent of such infections in adults. The efficacy of prophylactic vaccination with 50 μg. each of the capsular polysaccharides of pneumococcal types 1, 2, 5, and 7 was demonstrated convincingly by MacLeod and co-workers [26] in 1945, and the properties of hexavalent vaccines were studied later by Heidelberger, MacLeod, and their associates [16]. Most individuals receiving such vaccines showed an antibody response to all six antigens, and half-maximal levels of antibody persisted for five to eight years following a single injection of vaccine. Preparations of pneumo-coccal vaccines were available commercially for a short period, but they were removed from the market because their use was considered unnecessary by most physicians. This view has been challenged by more recent clinical and epidemiologic studies, and vaccines of capsular types 1 through 9 and types 12, 14, 18, 19, and 23 would be especially indicated for those at high risk of infection and death. A licensed polyvalent vaccine is presently available.

Epidemic Infections
Epidemics of nosocomial pneumococcal pneumonia have rarely been reported. The above-mentioned multiple-drug-resistant strain of pneumococcus in the Republic of South Africa caused outbreaks in children hospitalized in several different hospitals [5]. Measles and prior antibiotic therapy appear to have been important conditions predisposing to pneumonia. Control of these outbreaks was achieved by cohorting infected and colonized patients, vancomycin treatment of cases and carriers, closing hospital wards housing carriers, placing carriers in isolation wards or an isolation hospital, and culturing new admissions and transferring carriers to the isolation hospital.

Streptococcus pyogenes Pneumonia
General Aspects
TRANSMISSIBILITY. Soon after birth, α-hemolytic streptococci appear in the upper part of the respiratory tract and may be isolated therefrom throughout life. Streptococci of Lancefield groups C and G and, more rarely, organisms of groups other than A may be isolated from the oropharynx of 5 percent or more of the normal population.

In general, at least 5 percent of the people of any community harbor group-A streptococci in their oropharynx. The prevalence varies and depends on the culture methods used as well as on environmental, host, and bacterial factors. Persons under 20 years of age are most likely to harbor group-A streptococci, especially if the tonsils are present.

Following either apparent or inapparent infection, the carrier state usually persists for several months and occasionally for longer periods. As the carrier state progresses, the streptococci lose their ability to produce M protein, so that by the eleventh week, about 40 percent of strains cannot be typed.

Ability to spread disease appears to be an attribute of individuals who have been infected recently. Whether such persons harbor more numerous streptococci in the nose and throat or whether the organisms are especially capable of spreading to other persons cannot be determined from the available evidence. It is established that nasal carriers of group-A streptococci are likely to spread disease. The spread of streptococci in any population group is related to the degree of exposure, and, during the winter months when people are confined to enclosed areas and are under crowded conditions, dissemination of bacteria is especially likely to occur.

Group-A streptococci naturally deposited in dust and on blankets will not produce respiratory infections in man. The evidence implicates the direct mode of transfer as being primarily responsible for the dissemination of such infections.

PREDISPOSING FACTORS. Pneumonia caused by "aerobic" streptococci accounts for less than 5 percent of all cases of nosocomial pneumonia. Except in the newborn—where group-B streptococci are a major cause of neonatal sepsis that may include pneumonia—pneumonia is almost invariably caused by group-A streptococci and may arise secondarily to an infection of the upper part of the respiratory tract. Epidemics have been observed following influenza and measles.

CLINICAL FEATURES. Primary group-A streptococcal pneumonia is rare in the absence of influenza. The onset of pneumonia tends to be abrupt, with symptoms of chills, fever, anorexia, and vomiting. Cough, sputum that is pink and thin, and chest pain are characteristic. The temperature is usually high (104°F or 40°C), and fever is intermittent. Examination reveals scattered, fine rales, but signs of lobar consolidation are rare.

A characteristic feature of group-A streptococcal pneumonia is the early development (within four days of onset of illness) of an empyema (metapneumonic).

THERAPY. All strains of *Streptococcus pyogenes* remain susceptible to benzylpenicillin (penicillin G). Strains that are resistant in vitro to the tetracyclines have been reported.

The antimicrobial agent of choice is benzylpenicillin. Six hundred thousand units of aqueous procaine penicillin G administered intramuscularly twice daily provides an adequate margin of safety and minimizes the influence on the normal microbial flora as well as the possibility of supracolonization and suprainfection. Alternative agents for treating the patient who is allergic to penicillins include erythromycin, the cephalosporins (a degree of cross-sensitization exists between the penicillins and the cephalosporins), and clindamycin. As is the case with pneumococci (see above), the aminoglycosidic antibiotics (kanamycin, gentamicin, tobramycin, and amikacin) are not effective as single agents against group-A streptococci in the usually recommended safe doses.

Control of Infections

There are no specifically recommended measures for the prevention of group-A streptococcal pneumonia per se. However, proper control of infections in other sites (see Part II, Chapters 16, 19, and 20) will reduce the chances of nosocomial acquisition of these organisms.

There are no reports of nosocomial epidemics of group-A streptococcal pneumonia.

Pneumonia Caused by Endogenous, Aerobic, Gram-Negative Bacilli

General Aspects

TRANSMISSIBILITY. *Klebsiella pneumoniae, Enterobacter aerogenes, Escherichia coli,* and *Proteus* species are aerobic, gram-negative bacilli that are commonly found among the endogenous flora of the gastrointestinal tract of hospitalized patients. Collectively, they are responsible for about one-quarter to one-third of all cases of nosocomial pneumonia (see Tables 15-3 and 15-4). In normal subjects, pharyngeal acquisition of these aerobic gram-negative bacilli is infrequent. In contrast, chronically or severely ill persons lose the ability to resist colonization of the oropharynx with this group of microorganisms [18]. Nosocomial pneumonia caused by these organisms may then occur following bronchogenous spread of the oropharyngeal organisms. This mechanism of acquisition of pneumonia is generally more common for these agents than is spread through aerosols, which may also occur.

Selden and associates [50], in the study of an endemic of nosocomial infections caused by multiple-drug-resistant strains of *Klebsiella pneumoniae* type 30, cultured these strains from stool specimens of 34 of 138 (25 percent) patients on acute-care wards, whereas only 6 of the 138 (4 percent) patients were found to be pharyngeal carriers. None of the 22 psychiatric patients was an intestinal carrier, and only one individual of 54 physician and nursing personnel cultured was a carrier. All isolates from an inanimate environmental survey were obtained from patient areas. Procedures that were significantly associated with intestinal colonization were urinary catheterization, inhalation therapy, general anesthesia, and treatment with certain antimicrobial agents (ampicillin, cephalothin, and sulfonamides). How the *Klebsiella* organisms were introduced into the patients' intestinal tract was not described, but it is assumed to be through contact with personnel who transiently picked up strains on their hands (the hands of two of eight nursing personnel on the intensive-therapy unit yielded positive cultures). In those personnel who were not on antibiotics, intestinal colonization did not follow the transient acquisition of *Klebsiella* on their hands, probably because they were not receiving antibiotics. Similarly, Story [53] observed that 76 percent of patients with nosocomial *Proteus* infections were intestinal carriers of the *Proteus* organisms.

The conditions that promote colonization of the respiratory tract with gram-negative bacilli are not known. In a previous study [19], we noted that the prevalence of colonization increased as the severity of illness increased. Indicators of the severity of illness associated with colonization in this study were coma, hypotension, acidosis, azotemia, and either marked leukocytosis or leukopenia (Table 15-7). The increased frequency of colonization

Table 15-7. Variables Associated with Colonization of the Respiratory Tract with Gram-Negative (GNB) Bacilli in 213 Patients Admitted to a Medical Intensive-Care Unit

| Variable | GNB colonization | | |
	Present (no.)	Absent (no.)	Correlation[a]
Sex:			
Men	57	66	
Women	38	52	NS
Smoker:			
Yes	56	67	
No	39	51	NS
Coma[b]:			
Yes	35	26	
No	60	92	$p < .05$
Hypotension[c]:			
Yes	19	6	
No	76	112	$p < .01$
Sputum present:			
Yes	71	46	
No	24	72	$p < .001$
Tracheal intubation:			
Yes	36	20	
No	59	98	$p < .001$
Inhalation therapy:			
Yes	88	98	
No	7	20	NS
Antimicrobial drugs:			
Yes	38	12	
No	57	106	$p < .001$
Arterial pH $\leq$ 7.31:			
Yes	33	16	
No	62	102	$p < .001$
Blood urea nitrogen $\geq$ 50 mg./ml.:			
Yes	10	2	
No	85	116	$p < .05$
White blood cell count > 15,000 or < 4000:			
Yes	37	18	
No	58	100	$p < .001$
Hemoglobin < 8 gm./100 ml.:			
Yes	2	1	
No	93	117	NS

[a] NS = not significant; p = probability.
[b] Defined as loss of consciousness with no response to commands but there may be response to painful stimuli.
[c] Systolic blood pressure less than 80 mm. Hg or requiring vasopressors for more than 4 hours.

From Johanson, W. G., et al. *Ann. Intern. Med.* 77: 701, 1972.

among patients with respiratory disease, sputum production, or endotracheal intubation suggests that conditions that impair lung clearance may also promote colonization. In contrast to our earlier findings, neither colonization nor infection was related to the use of inhalation therapy, because reservoir nebulizers had been recognized as potential sources of infection and an effective equipment-care regimen had been instituted. Although antimicrobial therapy may have played a role in some patients, our data indicate that most instances of colonization occurred independently of such therapy. Kaslow and colleagues [20] have reported cross-colonization by *Proteus* species with the occurrence of systemic infections, and they identified the catheterized urinary tract as an intermediate reservoir.

Colonization of the respiratory tract with aerobic gram-negative bacilli plays a major role in the pathogenesis of nosocomial lower respiratory tract infections [38]. In the study of Johanson and associates [19], 22 of 95 patients (23 percent) who were colonized developed infections, compared to 4 of 118 (3.4 percent) patients in whom colonization was not shown. Tillotson and Finland [54] observed that 25 percent of their colonized patients developed nosocomial infections, and Klick and co-workers [23] reported that 11 of 69 patients (16 percent) who were colonized with aerobic gram-negative organisms developed pneumonia.

From these observations, it seems reasonable to conclude that the transmission of aerobic gram-negative bacilli, especially *Klebsiella pneumoniae* and *Proteus* species, from the gastrointestinal tract of one patient to another can occur, especially if the patients are on oral antimicrobial agents. The spread between patients is probably through the hands. In the susceptible host, colonization of the oropharynx occurs, which is followed by the development of pneumonia in 15 to 25 percent of such patients.

CLINICAL FEATURES. The "classic" clinical pattern is that of acute primary *Klebsiella* pneumonia. As with pneumococcal pneumonia, the onset is usually sudden (90 percent) and associated with cough productive of sputum (90 percent), pleuritic chest pain (80 percent), and true rigors (60 percent). Early prostration is a usual feature. Occasionally, the acute onset is preceded by an undifferentiated upper respiratory infection and cough. Rarely, epigastric pain and vomiting are the initial symptoms. The characteristic sputum has been described as a nonputrid, homogeneous, thick mixture of blood and mucus, often brick-red, that is sufficiently thick to be expectorated with difficulty. This typical sputum is seen in one-quarter to three-quarters of patients. In some patients, the sputum is thin, resembling currant jelly, although in most, it is either blood-tinged or rusty. Frank hemoptysis may occur. On examination, patients appear acutely ill, febrile, dyspneic, and often cyanotic. Although temperatures are often said to be less than those observed with pneumococcal pneumonia, two-thirds of the patients have temperatures between 39°C and 40°C (102°F and 104°F). Tachycardia coincides with the fever. Chest examination typically reveals signs of pulmonary consolidation; there may be loss of lung volume as manifested by decreased size, expansion of the involved hemithorax, and diaphragmatic elevation. Auscultation may reveal suppressed breath sounds with few rales, even when advanced consolidation has occurred. Involvement of more than one lobe is frequent (occurring in two-thirds of patients), and there is a predilection for the upper lobes.

The clinical features of pneumonia due to aerobic gram-negative bacilli other than *K. pneumoniae* are generally similar to those observed in patients with *Klebsiella* pneumonia, except that hemoptysis is unusual.

E. coli pneumonia tends to present as a bronchopneumonic process in the lower lobes. The pulse is proportional to the temperature. Early findings include rales without consolidation. Empyema formation is less common than in infection with *Klebsiella* or *Pseudomonas*.

Proteus species also produce a clinical picture similar to that of *Klebsiella* infection: fever, chills, dyspnea, pleuritic chest pain, and cough productive of purulent sputum. Signs of consolidation are usual. Roentgenograms reveal dense infiltrates in the posterior segment of an upper lobe or superior segment of the right lower lobe. Progression to lung abscess formation or empyema is common.

THERAPY. The antimicrobial regimen of choice is often varied according to the gravity of the clinical situation and the extent of underlying problems. In less seriously ill patients, parenteral administration of a cephalosporin (cephalothin, cefazolin, or cephradine), kanamycin, gentamicin, or amikacin is preferable, but in patients with life-threatening infections, combination therapy (e.g., a cephalosporin and kanamycin, gentamicin, or amikacin) is usually employed. Meticulous measures directed at supportive care, the maintenance of clear airways, adequate but not excessive ventilation and oxygenation, adequate fluid and electrolyte replacement, and often the control of delirium tremens are essential.

Prevention of Infections

Because the most important mode of spread between patients appears to be through contact via the hands, the implementation of rigorous hand-washing procedures should be of major importance in minimizing the colonization of susceptible patients who are introduced into high-risk areas such as intensive-care units. In addition, restriction of antimicrobial agents may minimize the ability of resistant strains to colonize the intestinal tract. These recommendations appear rational, but are not of proved efficacy.

Utilizing a more direct approach, Klastersky, Hedley-Whyte, and colleagues [12, 22, 23] have attempted to suppress the colonization of the oropharynx and tracheobronchial tree by repeated atomization, instillation, or both, of antimicrobial agents. In their initial studies [12, 23], the use of aerosolized polymyxin B was shown to decrease the frequency of colonization of the oropharynx with sensitive strains, especially *Pseudomonas aeruginosa,* and to prevent the occurrence of pneumonia. With prolonged usage, however, polymyxin B-resistant strains of *Flavobacterium meningosepticum* were found, and these were associated with higher mortality rates than those observed with other organisms. Similarly, Klastersky and associates [22] instilled gentamicin into endotracheal tubes, a procedure that was effective

until gentamicin-resistant strains of *Providencia* species, *Pseudomonas* species, and *Klebsiella* species emerged. Subsequently, this group has utilized aminosidine (paromomycin) and polymyxin B with clinical effectiveness; however, the ultimate appearance of resistant strains, such as *Pseudomonas cepacia,* seems most likely. Regimens such as these should be considered investigational and may be hazardous.

Pneumonia Caused by Exogenous, Aerobic, Gram-Negative Bacilli

General Aspects

TRANSMISSIBILITY. Microorganisms that can survive and multiply in fluids can be readily disseminated as potentially infectious aerosols by certain types of ventilation equipment. *Pseudomonas aeruginosa, Pseudomonas maltophilia, Pseudomonas cepacia, Achromobacter* species, *Serratia marcescens, Flavobacterium meningosepticum,* and *Acinetobacter calcoaceticus* are the most common organisms found in nebulizer fluid and aerosols, and bronchogenous spread through inhalation of aerosols should be suspected when nosocomial pneumonia produced by these agents occurs. In addition, such contaminated aerosols may also result in oropharyngeal colonization. Pneumonia produced by this group of agents is more likely to derive from the acquisition of exogenous organisms than from the endogenous gastrointestinal flora of patients. These organisms collectively are responsible for about one-tenth to one-fifth of all nosocomial pneumonias.

The bacterial species isolated in our initial studies of nebulizer fluid and aerosols are tabulated in Table 15-8. Multiple species of organisms were isolated more commonly than a single species. In no samples were gram-positive organisms recovered. This general pattern has held in all subsequent studies that are based upon aerosol samples, although Nelson and Ryan [34] isolated gram-positive organisms from aerosol samples from 8 to 27 patients (*Staphylococcus epidermidis,* five isolates; *Staphylococcus aureus,* three isolates; viridans streptococci, two isolates; and hemolytic streptococci, one isolate).

Table 15-8. Results of Bacterial Cultures of Inhalation Therapy Equipment at Various Hospitals

Hospital	Source of cultures	Number of positive cultures	Bacterial species (number of isolates)								Prevalent organism
			Pseudomonas species	Flavobacterium meningosepticum	Acinetobacter calcoaceticus var. anitratus	Alcaligenes fecalis	Achromobacter species	Acinetobacter calcoaceticus var. lwoffi	Serratia marcescens	Enterobacter aerogenes	
A	Aerosol	62	32	12	20	27	15	3	3	4	P. aeruginosa
	Nebulizer fluid	44	21	7	5	22	5	3	3	4	
B	Aerosol	20	4	15	2	9	4	1	0	0	Flavobacterium meningosepticum
	Nebulizer fluid	22	9	12	0	5	1	2	0	0	
C	Aerosol	6	3	2	0	1	1	0	0	0	P. aeruginosa
	Nebulizer fluid	7	4	2	0	2	1	1	0	0	
D	Aerosol	13	3	2	11	1	2	3	0	0	Acinetobacter calcoaceticus var. anitratus (Herellea)
	Nebulizer fluid	9	1	2	8	1	1	0	0	0	
E	Aerosol	20	18[a]	5	0	2	0	1	0	0	P. species[a]
	Nebulizer fluid	19	18[a]	1	0	0	0	0	0	0	

[a] Isolates studied at Center for Disease Control and reported as *Pseudomonas* species. Isolates studied by Dr. S. G. Carey at Walter Reed Army Institute of Research were considered to resemble closely *Cytophaga johnsonae*.

Because of the failure to detect gram-positive cocci in our initial studies and because several patients had staphylococcal pneumonia at the time inhalation therapy was instituted, Reinarz and colleagues [39] studied the persistence of *Staphylococcus aureus* strain 502A, following massive contamination of a reservoir nebulizer. The reservoir nebulizer jars of three intermittent positive-pressure breathing (IPPB) machines were filled with cultures of viable *Staphylococcus aureus* strain 502A. The number of organisms varied from 1.3×10^9 to 2.5×10^9 viable units per milliliter. After flushing with sterile distilled water, viable staphylococci in the aerosols exceeded 10,000 colony-forming units per cubic foot of air. After eight hours, species of aerobic gram-negative bacilli were isolated from the aerosols generated by each of the machines. Furthermore, the number of staphylococci was less than 500 colony-forming units per cubic foot. By 24 hours, staphylococci were no longer isolated, but, in contrast, large numbers of aerobic gram-negative bacilli (*Acinetobacter calcoaceticus* var. *anitratus* and *Achromobacter* species) were isolated. This lack of persistence of staphylococci should not have been unanticipated, because McDade and Hall [29] had shown in 1963 that the survival of strains of *Staphylococcus aureus* was diminished at high relative humidity.

The ability of various microorganisms to proliferate in the fluid in the reservoir nebulizer is important in determining the organisms that predominate. Maki and Martin [27] have shown that organisms of the tribe Klebsielleae (*Klebsiella, Enterobacter,* and *Serratia*) can multiply in 5% dextrose in water, whereas pseudomonads do not. Favero and associates [11] found that "naturally occurring" strains of pseudomonads—that is, strains inoculated directly from water sources in the hospital—multiply rapidly in distilled water. Interestingly, strains precultured in broth before inoculation grew poorly. Although Sanders and co-workers [45] observed that the strains of *Serratia marcescens,* serotype 014:H4, that were isolated in an outbreak of infection due to contaminated inhalation therapy medications (especially Alevaire) would multiply in such products, intensive study of the growth characteristics of the many bacterial species associated with inhalation therapy has not been reported.

CLINICAL FEATURES. In patients with *Pseudomonas* pneumonia, apprehension, toxicity, confusion, and progressive cyanosis are characteristic. Relative bradycardia may occur. Alteration in diurnal temperature patterns, with the peak temperature occurring in early morning, was noted by Crane and Lerner [6]. The physical signs over the thorax are not characteristic. The development of empyema is common and occurs in 22 to 80 percent of cases. Roentgenograms reveal bilateral bronchopneumonic infiltrates, usually in the lower lobe, which often are nodular and may undergo necrosis, and abscesses, which may be small but are often greater than 1 cm. in diameter. A pattern of interstitial infiltration may be seen.

Serratia infections have been associated with the clinical oddity "pseudohemoptysis"; this results from the red pigment, prodigiosin, produced by some strains of *Serratia marcescens.* Other features may include abscess formation, empyema, or both.

Clinical experience with the other bacterial genera, such as *Hafnia* and *Flavobacterium,* is limited, but other characteristics suggest that the clinical features of their infections are similar to those of *Klebsiella* infections.

THERAPY. Mortality rates in the range of 80 percent are not uncommon with *Pseudomonas* pneumonia, whereas they may be lower with infections due to the other gram-negative organisms.

The antimicrobial regimen of choice may be selected according to the antimicrobial susceptibilities anticipated in a given community, but they must be confirmed by tests on the organisms infecting the individual patient. In general, *Pseudomonas aeruginosa* are most susceptible to carbenicillin, colistimethate, gentamicin, polymyxin B, tobramycin, and amikacin. In contrast, *Pseudomonas cepacia* may be susceptible only to chloramphenicol. *E. coli* is susceptible to the same agents as *P. aeruginosa,* and, in addition, most strains are susceptible to cephalothin or cefazolin. *Serratia marcescens* and the indole-positive *Proteus* species are most susceptible to gentamicin and amikacin. As with *Klebsiella* pneumonia, meticulous attention to supportive care is as important as the antimicrobial therapy in treating pneumonias caused by these other gram-negative bacilli.

Prevention of Infections

A proper disinfection and sterilization program for respiratory equipment is the major means of preventing endemic infections (see previous section, Disinfection and Sterilization of Ventilatory Equipment). Inadequate disinfection of such equipment is also the major cause of nosocomial pneumonia outbreaks, and a careful review of procedures is mandatory when an outbreak caused by these organisms is identified. In addition, the possibility of a contaminated common vehicle added directly to the nebulizers, such as a contaminated multidose medication vial, should be carefully investigated. Given the infection risks associated with use of ventilatory equipment with reservoir nebulizers, the use of such apparatus should be restricted to those clinical situations where it is clearly indicated.

Pulmonary Tuberculosis

Risk of Infection

Airborne spread of *Mycobacterium tuberculosis* is a recognized occupational hazard for persons working in hospitals, but the risk has lessened with the development of effective preventive programs and with the secular decrease in morbidity from tuberculosis [56]. Although Riley and associates [41] demonstrated the infectiousness of air on a tuberculosis ward, the average concentration of infectious particles was one per 11,000 cubic feet. Infectious particles were added at a rate of 25 to 30 particles per day. Moreover, the initiation of treatment, the presence of resistant organisms, or both, were associated with less relative infectivity; for example, if the relative infectivity of drug-susceptible organisms for an untreated patient is 100, susceptible strains from treated patients have a relative infectivity of 4, while resistant organisms from untreated patients have a relative infectivity of 28 and those from treated patients, a relative infectivity of 10.

They observed one patient with laryngeal tuberculosis, however, who produced one infectious particle per 200 cubic feet of air. From these observations, they concluded that viable airborne tubercle bacilli normally were not very numerous and that the air of a room occupied by a tuberculous patient may not be very dangerous to breathe for a short time.

Annual skin-test conversion rates are reported to be 1.6 percent and 2.3 percent in general hospital employees but may be considerably higher. Ehrenkranz and Kicklighter [9] reported tuberculin skin-test conversion in 23 employees of a general hospital that was attributed to exposure to a patient with undetected tuberculous bronchopneumonia. In an air-conditioned ward on which the patient spent 57 hours, where high-efficiency filters were not present in the ventilatory systems and where air from patients' rooms was recycled to employee areas, 21 of 60 tuberculin-negative personnel (35 percent) converted their skin tests, and two converters had evidence of active infection.

Prevention of Microbial Contamination of the Air

CHEMOTHERAPY. This is the most effective means of preventing microbial contamination of the air, since it reduces coughing due to tuberculosis (which produces droplet nuclei), the amount of sputum, and the number of organisms in the sputum. Therapy should be started at the time a presumptive diagnosis of tuberculosis is made, and it is the most important continuing means of infection control.

COVERING THE NOSE AND MOUTH. This procedure decreases the likelihood of atomized secretions becoming airborne.

MASKS. Patients may also reduce the addition of bacilli to the air by wearing masks; however, patients should generally not be required to wear masks in their rooms. To be effective, masks must filter out particles as small as 1 μ, cover the nose and mouth, fit snugly, and be discarded or sterilized after each use. Masking a coughing patient when someone enters his room may reduce the addition of bacilli to the air, but this will not completely eliminate the hazard of transmission, since the room air would already be contaminated if the patient had been coughing previously without covering his mouth.

Removal of Airborne Organisms

Air control is necessary in rooms of known or suspected transmitters and in places where persons with untreated tuberculosis might contaminate the air, for example, intensive-care units, emergency rooms, admitting areas, outpatient waiting rooms, hallways, and x-ray departments.

Any room with proper air control can be used for patients with tuberculosis. Rooms do not have to be set aside for the exclusive use of tuberculosis patients.

Mechanical ventilation and ultraviolet irradiation are methods of air control. Either method or a combination of both may be used, depending on structural and engineering factors.

MECHANICAL VENTILATION. The patient's room should have fresh air introduced through a central or window unit and have air exhausted to the outside through an individual room exhaust fan or a central exhaust system, usually through a lavatory exhaust. Preferably, such air is not recirculated, but when necessary, it should be passed through a high-efficiency filter or irradiated with ultraviolet light.

ULTRAVIOLET LIGHTS. Upper-room ultraviolet irradiation kills bacteria in the air, thus providing the equivalent of air changes, and, when properly installed and maintained, it will supplement the ventilation system.

Employee Surveillance Program

Every hospital should have an employee tuberculosis surveillance program; the specific details will vary according to the dimension of the tuberculosis problem.

INITIAL EXAMINATION. A tuberculin skin test should be provided to all employees at the time of hiring, and a chest roentgenogram should be obtained on those who have a positive reaction to the skin test.

PREVENTIVE TREATMENT. Preventive treatment should be given to infected employees, unless specifically contraindicated, to prevent

them from developing disease and infecting others. New infections among employees should be reported to the local health department so family contacts may be given skin tests, roentgenograms, or both.

REPEAT TUBERCULIN SKIN TESTS. Policies for repeating skin tests should be determined by the risk of acquiring a new infection. The following factors should be considered:

1. The number and location of tuberculosis patients admitted to the hospital indicate the relative risks of different types of employees being exposed (Table 15-9).
2. The number and location of tuberculosis patients in the community will assist in determining the risk of employee exposure in the community.
3. The number of employees already infected should be determined, so employees at risk of developing disease and infecting others can be identified.
4. The number of employees who become infected will reflect the risk of becoming infected in the hospital and in the community.
5. The flow of air throughout the hospital should be assessed in order to determine the possibility of airborne transmission of

Table 15-9. Relative Hazard of Multiple Exposures to Initially Unsuspected Tuberculosis by Occupational Category

Occupation	Percent of total occupational category with more than two exposures
X-ray technicians	38.2%
Licensed practical nurses	12.7%
Registered nurses[a]	9.2%
Attendants	5.1%
Medical students	4.8%
Physicians	4.5%
Student nurses	1.2%

[a] Emergency-room registered nurses were most at risk of multiple exposures.

From Craven, R. B., et al. *Ann. Intern. Med.* **82:** 628, 1975.

infection from one area to another (e.g., from patient areas to service areas, or vice versa).

If the risk of exposure to tuberculosis is small or infrequent, it is not necessary to repeat skin tests on a routine basis. If certain areas of the hospital and certain categories of workers have either greater exposure to diagnosed and undiagnosed cases or higher rates of new infections, however, regular tests should be repeated every six months.

Periodic chest roentgenograms of employees who have completed an adequate course of treatment or preventive treatment should be discontinued. They should be instructed to report immediately if they have any symptoms that may be due to tuberculosis.

Depending on their risk of developing disease, persons who are infected and who are unable to take preventive treatment should have a chest roentgenogram every six to twelve months. They, too, should be encouraged to report promptly any respiratory symptoms that may be due to tuberculosis. Special surveillance of these employees should be provided if they work in areas of the hospital where patients with immune deficiencies are treated, or they may be transferred to other parts of the hospital.

INVESTIGATION OF CASE CONTACTS. Careful investigations should be conducted when there is an inadvertent exposure to a "potential transmitter." Tuberculin skin tests should be immediately provided to exposed persons who previously had a negative reaction to the skin test. Those who are still negative should be retested ten weeks from the time of exposure. Preventive therapy may be necessary for some negative reactors with heavy exposure, because they may be infected even though their skin tests have not yet converted.

RECORDS. Accurate records should be kept about each employee in order to monitor infection rates and determine risks. The record should include the date of each tuberculin skin test and the method and specific antigen used; measurement of the skin-test reaction in millimeters; the date of any known exposure to

infectious tuberculosis; the date and result of chest roentgenograms of positive skin-test reactors; the dates of initiation and completion of preventive treatment; and the dates of diagnosis, initiation, and completion of treatment if disease occurs.

EVALUATION. Data should be analyzed at periodic intervals to determine and revise policies. The best index of the effectiveness of the infection control program will be the absence of new infections in employees.

Viral, Chlamydial, and Rickettsial Infections
*Nosocomial Viral Respiratory Infection:
Influenza and Respiratory Syncytial Viruses*

GENERAL ASPECTS. Although nosocomial infections caused by most viral agents have been recognized, relatively little attention has been directed toward such nosocomial viral infections that affect the lower respiratory tract. Chapters 20, 24, and 27 of Part II discuss varicella, cytomegalovirus, and other viruses that may sometimes produce lower respiratory tract infections.

During the 1957–1958 influenza pandemic ("Asian" H_2N_2), a study was implemented at the Veterans Administration Hospital, Livermore, California, to determine whether the ultraviolet disinfection of droplet nuclei in the air would block the transmission of influenza to a susceptible population during an epidemic (Table 15-10) [30]. These observations indicated a reduction in seroconversions among patients in rooms that received ultraviolet irra-

Table 15-10. "Aerial Isolation" through Disinfection of Droplet Nuclei by Ultraviolet Radiation

	Initially negative	Fourfold rise in influenza titer	
		Number	Percentage
Patients:			
Radiated	209	4	2%
Nonradiated	396	75	19%
Personnel	511	92	18%

From McLean, R. D. *Am. Rev. Respir. Dis.* 83:36, 1961.

diation. The attack rates among hospitalized patients whose rooms were not irradiated with ultraviolet light, however, are comparable to those in the community (as judged by experience in hospital personnel). More recent reports have confirmed similar attack rates for hospitalized and nonhospitalized infants and adults.

In a study that involved a pediatric ward in Great Britain [13], cross-infections from patients admitted with infections caused by respiratory syncytial virus, influenza A, and parainfluenza virus were documented (Table 15-11). The relative hazard of cross-infection was greatest for influenza A virus (nearly one cross-infection took place for each four admissions) and least with respiratory syncytial virus (one cross-infection for about 15 admissions). Another study has also documented the nosocomial acquisition of respiratory syncytial virus [15].

PREVENTION OF EPIDEMIC INFECTION. Protection against influenza A can be provided both by immunization and by the chemoprophylactic agent, amantadine or its congeners. The protection provided by amantadine, which is only effective against influenza A virus, is comparable to that afforded by an effective vaccine. Disadvantages include the necessity for twice-daily medication throughout an outbreak and the occurrence of minimal, amphetamine-like side effects in 4 to 27 percent of recipients. However, when patients at high risk of complications (such as those with underlying heart disease or chronic pulmonary disease and older patients [46]) have not been immunized and are hospitalized during an epidemic, chemoprophylaxis with amantadine hydrochloride should be strongly considered. Although isolation of patients with such infections has not been deemed necessary, precautions in handling their respiratory secretions are indicated to reduce the possibility of nosocomial transmission.

Chlamydial and Rickettsial Infections

Chlamydia psittaci, the causative agent of psittacosis, can be spread from man to man. Outbreaks involving nosocomial spread to nurses are known. In the 1943 epidemic in Louisiana, there were eight deaths among 19 recognized infections in nursing attendants, which emphasizes the potential importance of nosocomial transmission of this respiratory infection.

Q fever caused by *Coxiella burnetii* may also be mentioned, because it is often associated with respiratory symptoms and signs, and instances of its spread to hospital personnel have been recorded.

Table 15-11. Cross-Infections Related to Admissions with Virus Infections

Virus type	No. of admissions	No. of cross-infections	Ratio of admissions to cross-infections
Respiratory syncytial virus	219	15	14.6 : 1
Influenza A	61	16	3.8 : 1
Parainfluenza, type 1	55	5	11 : 1
Parainfluenza, type 2	9	0	—
Parainfluenza, type 3	56	13	4.3 : 1
Parainfluenza, type 4A	7	1	7.0 : 1
Parainfluenza, type 4B	7	0	—
Totals	414	50	8.3 : 1

From Gardner, P. S., et al. *Br. Med. J.* 2:571, 1973.

Pneumocystis carinii Pneumonia

General Aspects

Pneumocystis carinii pneumonia outside of the United States has usually been associated with endemic or epidemic focuses in nurseries for premature infants or in foundling homes. It appears as a plasma-cell pneumonia during the first year of life; symptoms appear between the sixth week and the twelfth week. Predisposing factors are prematurity, marasmus, and malnourishment. Recently, this pattern was demonstrated by the occurrence of seven cases among the 2671 Vietnamese orphans who had been airlifted to the United States.

PREDISPOSING FACTORS. In the United States, the disease occurs sporadically in patients of various ages who invariably either are suffering from a chronic disease, malignancy, or immunologic disorder or have a history of having had immunosuppressive therapy (see Part II, Chapter 27). The first large outbreak in the United States occurred at St. Jude's Children's Research Hospital in Memphis, Tennessee, where 17 cases were documented during 1968 and 1969 [35]. Subsequently, a cluster of 11 cases occurred in a three-month period in 1973 at Memorial Sloan-Kettering Cancer Center, New York [52].

TRANSMISSION. The mode of transmission and natural habitat of *P. carinii* are unknown. A few case reports with circumstantial evidence of man-to-man transmission plus the epidemic pattern in nursing homes justify the isolation of active cases from other patients who are at risk. Nevertheless, the occurrence of man-to-man transmission has not been proved [24].

CLINICAL FEATURES. The clinical characteristics of premature and newborn infants with *P. carinii* pneumonia include an average age at onset of 3.4 months and an average age at death of 4.2 months. The usual duration of illness is three to five weeks. Presenting symptoms include dyspnea in most infants (90 percent) and anorexia, cough, tachypnea, and cyanosis, each being present in about one-half of the infants. Clinical signs include dyspnea, cyanosis, and tachypnea in over 90 percent of infants, and cough, fever, and rales are each demonstrated in approximately one-quarter of infants. Radiographic findings include diffuse bilateral infiltrates in all cases, with the presence of adventitious air in about one-fifth of the patients.

THERAPY. The drug of choice has been pentamidine isethionate, but lately the combination of trimethoprim and sulfamethoxazole (TMP-SMZ) has proved effective in treating *P. carinii* pneumonia. Similarly, pyrimethamine with a sulfonamide has been given to adults and infants, but no firm conclusions can be drawn. Comparisons with pentamidine are necessary before a drug can be accepted as alternative treatment. In animals, neither immunization, pentamidine, pyrimethamine and sulfonamides, rifampin, nor clindamycin gives protection; however, TMP-SMZ has been successful in preventing the infection. Administration of sulfadoxine plus pyrimethamine reduced the incidence of *P. carinii* pneumonia in an infected orphanage in Shiraz, Iran. Although drug prophylaxis may be a means to prevention in highly susceptible patients, more work is needed before recommendations can be made. When malnutrition is the cause of susceptibility, special diets are prophylactic.

Patients need carefully monitored oxygen therapy, but oxygen toxicity must be avoided. In severe cases, ventilatory assistance with a continuous negative-pressure system, as is used in treating the respiratory-distress syndrome of newborns, has been successful. Extrapulmonary oxygenation with a membrane lung as a prepulmonary oxygenator has been employed in four very ill patients, and one recovered.

Pulmonary Aspergillosis

General Aspects

Aspergillus infection is a frequent complication of acute leukemia [47]. In recent years, the frequency of fungal infections has increased; they are reported as the cause of death in 14 percent of a large series of leukemic patients. In the series reported by Bodey [4] from the National Cancer Institute, during a ten-and-one-half-year period major fungal infections were observed in 40.6 of 100 fatalities with acute leukemia, candidiasis occurred in 29 of 100 fatalities, and *Aspergillus* was incriminated in 8 of 100 fatalities. The lung was involved in 92 of 98 patients with aspergillosis (see Part II, Chapter 27).

SOURCES. The differences in the prevalence of aspergillosis in patients with acute leukemia treated with similar chemotherapeutic regimens in different institutions suggest that major differences in environmental contamination exist that make aspergillosis a major problem in some centers and not in others. This hypothesis is supported by the observation that with the moving of patients into a new hospital at

Woods Veterans Administration Center in Wisconsin, the aspergillosis that had been common almost disappeared. Organisms are probably mainly acquired from environmental sources by airborne spread.

CLINICAL FEATURES. In 60 of 92 patients with pulmonary aspergillosis, the lung was the only site of infection. The pattern of pulmonary aspergillosis is unusual in the patient with acute leukemia. The two commonly reported primary forms—mycetoma (maduromycosis) and allergic bronchopulmonary aspergillosis—were essentially absent. The most common manifestation was that of necrotizing bronchopneumonia. All but three of the patients with necrotizing bronchopneumonia had symptoms, usually dyspnea, fever, and tachycardia. Cough commonly was nonproductive. Only three patients of 30 with necrotizing pneumonia (10 percent) had hemoptysis, and six (20 percent) had pleuritic chest pain. Roentgenographic evidence was varied; five patients (17 percent) had no x-ray evidence of pneumonia, even shortly before death.

In patients with positive chest roentgenograms, patchy pneumonitis often was first noticed in the last week of life. Hemorrhagic pulmonary infarction was found in 29 of the 92 cases with pulmonary aspergillosis (32 percent); at necropsy, each of these 29 patients had prominent vascular invasion by mycelial elements, with occlusion and thrombosis of pulmonary vessels. In this group of 29 patients, pleuritic chest pain occurred in 61 percent and was often associated with a pleural friction rub.

Fifteen patients had pulmonary lesions characterized primarily by abscess formation, and eight patients had lobar pneumonia caused by *Aspergillus* organisms. The clinical and roentgenographic findings of dense, lobar consolidation suggested the presence of specific bacterial agents, such as *Klebsiella* and pneumococci.

LABORATORY DIAGNOSIS. The diagnosis of aspergillosis in patients with acute leukemia is difficult. In the National Cancer Institute series reported by Young and associates [60], 82 percent of the patients had antemortem fungal cultures, but only 34 percent had one antemortem culture positive for *Aspergillus* and only 9 percent had more than one positive culture. In another study, Young and Bennett [59] subjected serum specimens to a battery of serologic tests; the specimens were obtained within the last three weeks of life from 15 patients with invasive aspergillosis. Using the techniques of double diffusion in agar gel, complement fixation, immunoelectrophoresis, and indirect fluorescent-antibody determinations, no antibodies to *A. fumigatus* were detected, despite subsequent histologic and cultural evidence of widespread invasive aspergillosis.

THERAPY. In view of the difficulties in reaching a definite diagnosis, initiation of treatment is often delayed. The treatment of choice is the parenteral administration of amphotericin B, which is not of proved value. Responses seem more closely related to the induction of remission in the underlying process, usually acute leukemia.

Miscellaneous Causes

Organisms other than those mentioned above may sometimes produce nosocomial pneumonia, especially in immunosuppressed patients (see Part II, Chapter 17). In addition, sporadic cases and outbreaks of nosocomial Legionnaires' disease have recently been documented [57]. Nosocomial pneumonia produced by *Legionella pneumophila* appear to be acquired mainly by airborne spread from environmental reservoirs in or near the hospital, though reactivation of latent infection may possibly occur in some instances. Environmental sources remain incompletely identified. Aerosols produced by cooling towers of air-conditioning systems from recirculated water contaminated with *L. pneumophila* appear to have been the sources for airborne organisms in some outbreaks. Person-to-person transmission, though incompletely studied, has not been documented.

References

1. Amberson, J. B. Aspiration bronchopneumonia. *Int. Clin.* 3:126, 137.
2. Barrett, F. F., Casey, J. I., and Finland, M. Infections and antibiotic use among patients at Boston City Hospital—February 1967. *N. Engl. J. Med.* 278:5, 1968.
3. Bartlett, R. C. *Medical Microbiology.* Qual-

ity, Cost, and Clinical Relevance. New York: John Wiley and Sons, 1974.

4. Bodey, G. P. Fungal infections complicating acute leukemia. *J. Chronic Dis.* 19:667, 1966.

5. Center for Disease Control. Follow-up on multiple-antibiotic-resistant pneumococci—South Africa. *Morbid. Mortal. Weekly Rep.* 27:1, 1978.

6. Crane, L. R., and Lerner, A. M. Gram-negative pneumonia in hospitalized patients. *Postgrad. Med.* 58:85, 1975.

7. Craven, R. B., Wenzel, R. P., and Atuk, N. O. Minimizing tuberculosis risk to hospital personnel and students exposed to unexpected disease. *Ann. Intern. Med.* 82:628, 1975.

8. Deane, R. S., Mills, E. L., and Hamel, A. J. Antibacterial action of copper in respiratory therapy apparatus. *Chest* 58:313, 1970.

9. Ehrenkranz, N. J., and Kicklighter, J. L. Tuberculosis outbreak in a general hospital: Evidence of airborne spread of infection. *Ann. Intern. Med.* 77:377, 1972.

10. Eickhoff, T. C., Brachman, P. S., Bennett, J. V., and Brown, J. F. Surveillance of nosocomial infections in community hospitals. I. Surveillance methods, effectiveness and initial results. *J. Infect. Dis.* 120:305, 1969.

11. Favero, M. S., Carson, L. A., Bond, W. G., and Petersen, N. J. *Pseudomonas aeruginosa:* Growth in distilled water from hospitals. *Science* 173:836, 1971.

12. Feeley, T. W., duMoulin, G. C., Hedley-Whyte, J., Bushnell, L. S., Gilbert, J. P., and Feingold, D. S. Aerosol polymyxin and pneumonia in seriously ill patients. *N. Engl. J. Med.* 293:471, 1975.

13. Gardner, P. S., Court, S. D. M., Brocklebank, J. T., Downham, M. A. P. S., and Weightman, D. Virus cross-infection in paediatric wards. *Br. Med. J.* 2:571, 1973.

14. Grieble, H. G., Colton, F. R., Bird, T. J., Torgo, A., and Griffith, U. G. Fine-particle humidifiers. Source of *Pseudomonas aeruginosa* infections in a respiratory-disease unit. *N. Engl. J. Med.* 282:531, 1970.

15. Hall, C. B., Douglas, R. G., Jr., Geiman, J. M., and Messner, M. K. Nosocomial respiratory syncytial virus infections. *N. Engl. J. Med.* 293:1343, 1975.

16. Heidelberger, M., MacLeod, C. M., and Di Lopi, M. M. Human antibody response to simultaneous injection of 6 specific polysaccharides of pneumococcus. *J. Exper. Med.* 88:369, 1948.

17. Hers, J. F. Ph., Masurel, N., and Mulder, J. Bacteriology and histopathology of the respiratory tract and lungs in fatal Asian influenza. *Lancet* 2:1141, 1958.

18. Johanson, W. G., Pierce, A. K., and Sanford, J. P. Changing pharyngeal bacterial flora of hospitalized patients. Emergence of gram-negative bacilli. *N. Engl. J. Med.* 281:1137, 1969.

19. Johanson, W. G., Pierce, A. K., Sanford, J. P., and Thomas, G. D. Nosocomial respiratory infections with gram-negative bacilli: The significance of colonization of the respiratory tract. *Ann. Intern. Med.* 77:701, 1972.

20. Kaslow, R. A., Lindsey, J. O., Bisno, A. L., and Price, A. Nosocomial infection with highly resistant *Proteus rettgeri. Am. J. Epidem.* 104:278, 1976.

21. Kislak, J. W., Eickhoff, T. C., and Finland, M. Hospital-acquired infections and antibiotic usage in Boston City Hospital—January 1964. *N. Engl. J. Med.* 271:834, 1964.

22. Klastersky, J., Hensgens, C., Noterman, J., Monawad, E., and Mennier-Carpentier, F. Endotracheal antibiotics for the prevention of tracheobronchial infections in tracheotomized unconscious patients. *Chest* 68:302, 1975.

23. Klick, J. M., duMoulin, G. C., Hedley-Whyte, J., Teres, D., Bushnell, L. S., and Feingold, D. S. Prevention of gram-negative bacillary pneumonia using polymyxin aerosol as prophylaxis. II. Effect on the incidence of pneumonia in seriously ill patients. *J. Clin. Invest.* 55:514, 1975.

24. *Lancet* Leading Article. *Pneumocystis carinii* pneumonia. *Lancet* 2:1023, 1975.

25. Lepper, M. H. Opportunistic gram-negative and pulmonary infections. *Dis. Chest* 4:18, 1963.

26. MacLeod, C. M., Hodges, R. G., Heidelberger, M., and Bernhard, W. G. Prevention of pneumococcal pneumonia by immunization with specific capsular polysaccharides. *J. Exper. Med.* 82:445, 1945.

27. Maki, D. G., and Martin, W. T. Nationwide epidemic of septicemia caused by contaminated infusion products. IV. Growth of microbial pathogens in fluids for intravenous infusion. *J. Infect. Dis.* 131:267, 1975.

28. Martin, C. M., Kunin, C. M., Gottlieb, L. S., and Finland, M. Asian influenza A in Boston 1957–1958. II. Severe staphylococcal pneumonia complicating influenza. *Arch. Intern. Med.* 103:532, 1959.

29. McDade, J. J., and Hall, L. B. An experimental method to measure the influence of environmental factors on the viability and the pathogenicity of *Staphylococcus aureus. Am. J. Hyg.* 77:98, 1963.

30. McLean, R. D. Discussion in international conference on Asian influenza. *Am. Rev. Respir. Dis.* 83:36, 1961 (Part 2).

31. McNamara, M. J., Hill, M. C., Balows, A., and Tucker, E. B. A study of the bacteriologic patterns of hospital infections. *Ann. Intern. Med.* 66:480, 1967.

32. Morris, A. H. Nebulizer contamination in a burn unit. *Am. Rev. Respir. Dis.* 107:802, 1973.

33. Murray, P. R., and Washington, J. A. Microscopic and bacteriologic analysis of expectorated sputum. *Mayo Clin. Proc.* 50:339, 1975.

34. Nelson, E. J., and Ryan, K. J. A new use of pasteurization. Disinfection of inhalation therapy equipment. *Respir. Care* 16:97, 1971.

35. Perera, D. R., Western, K. A., Johnson, H. D., Johnson, W. W., Schultz, M. G., and Akers, P. V. *Pneumocystis carinii* pneumonia in a hospital for children. *J.A.M.A.* 214:1074, 1970.

36. Petersdorf, R. G., Fusco, J. J., Harter, D. H., and Albrink, W. S. Pulmonary infections complicating Asian influenza. *Arch. Intern. Med.* 103:262, 1959.

37. Pierce, A. K., Sanford, J. P., Thomas, G. D., and Leonard, J. S. Long term evaluation of decontamination of inhalation therapy equipment and the occurrence of necrotizing pneumonia. *N. Engl. J. Med.* 282:528, 1970.

38. Pierce, A. K., and Sanford, J. P. Aerobic gram-negative bacillary pneumonias. *Am. Rev. Respir. Dis.* 110:647, 1974.

39. Reinarz, J. A., Pierce, A. K., Mays, B. B., and Sanford, J. P. The potential role of inhalation therapy equipment in nosocomial pulmonary infections. *J. Clin. Invest.* 44:831, 1965.

40. Rhoades, E. R., Ringrose, R., Mohr, J. A., Brooks, L., McKown, B. A., and Felton, F. Contamination of ultrasonic nebulization equipment with gram-negative bacteria. *Arch. Intern. Med.* 127:228, 1971.

41. Riley, R. L., Mills, C. C., O'Grady, F., Sultan, L. U., Wittstadt, F., and Shivpuri, D. N. Infectiousness of air from a tuberculosis ward. *Am. Rev. Respir. Dis.* 85:511, 1962.

42. Roberts, F. J., Cockcroft, W. H., and Johnson, H. E. A hot water disinfection method for inhalation therapy equipment. *Can. Med. Assoc. J.* 101:30, 1969.

43. Rosenthal, S., and Tager, I. B. Prevalence of gram-negative rods in the normal pharyngeal flora. *Ann. Intern. Med.* 83:355, 1975.

44. Roy, T. E., McDonald, S., Patrick, M. L., and Keddy, J. A. A survey of hospital infection in a pediatric hospital. *Can. Med. Assoc. J.* 87:531, 1962.

45. Sanders, C. V., Luby, J. P., Johanson, W. G., Barnett, J. A., and Sanford, J. P. *Serratia marcescens* infections from inhalation therapy medications: Nosocomial outbreak. *Ann. Intern. Med.* 73:15, 1970.

46. Sanford, J. P. Influenza: Consideration of pandemics. *Adv. Intern. Med.* 15:419, 1969.

47. Sanford, J. P. Aspergillosis. In Tice, F. (Ed.). *Practice of Medicine,* Vol. III. Hagerstown, Md.: Harper & Row, 1975.

48. Sanford, J. P., and Pierce, A. K. Inhalation Therapy Equipment. In DeLouvois, J. (Ed.), *Selected Topics in Clinical Bacteriology.* London: Baillière-Tindall, 1976.

49. Sanford, J. P., and Pierce, A. K. Current Infection Problems—Respiratory. In Brachman, P. S., and Eickhoff, T. C. (Eds.), *Proceedings of the International Conference on Nosocomial Infections.* Chicago: American Hospital Association, 1971.

50. Selden, R., Lee, S., Wong, W. L. L., Bennett, J. V., and Eickhoff, T. C. Nosocomial *Klebsiella* infections: Intestinal colonization as a reservoir. *Ann. Intern. Med.* 74:657, 1971.

51. Selwyn, S., McCabe, A. F., and Gould, J. C. Hospital infection on perspective of the importance of the gram negative bacilli. *Scot. Med. J.* 9:409, 1964.

52. Singer, C., Armstrong, D., Rosen, P. P., and Schottenfeld, D. *Pneumocystis carinii* pneumonia: A cluster of eleven cases. *Ann. Intern. Med.* 82:772, 1975.

53. Story, P. Proteus infections in hospital. *J. Pathol.* 68:55, 1954.

54. Thoburn, R., Fekety, R. F., Cluff, L. E., and Melvin, V. B. Infections acquired by hospitalized patients. *Arch. Intern. Med.* 121:1, 1968.

55. Tillotson, J. R., and Finland, M. Bacterial colonization and clinical superinfection of the respiratory tract complicating antibiotic treatment of pneumonia. *J. Infect. Dis.* 119:597, 1969.

56. U.S. Dept. of Health, Education, and Welfare. *Guidelines for the Prevention of TB Transmission in Hospitals.* Atlanta, Georgia: Center for Disease Control, 1974.

57. U.S. Dept. of Health, Education, and Welfare. Selected papers from the International Symposium on Legionnaires' Disease held at Center for Disease Control, Atlanta, Georgia in November, 1978. *Ann. Intern. Med.* 90: April, 1979. In press.

58. Wenzel, R. P., Osterman, C. A., Hunting, K. J., and Gwaltney, J. M. Hospital-acquired infections. I. Surveillance in a university hospital. *Am. J. Epidem.* 103:251, 1976.

59. Young, R. C., and Bennett, J. E. Invasive aspergillosis: absence of detectable antibody response. *Am. Rev. Respir. Dis.* 104:710, 1971.

60. Young, R. C., Bennett, J. E., Vogel, C. L., Carbone, P. P., and DeVita, V. T. Aspergillosis: The spectrum of disease in 98 patients. *Medicine* (Baltimore) 49:147, 1970.

16

Surgical Infections: Incisional Wounds

William A. Altemeier

The development of infection in incisional wounds continues to be one of the most serious complications that can occur in surgical patients [2, 7, 9, 16]. Surgical practice primarily depends on the healing of wounds without serious complications, and sepsis occurring in postoperative or accidental wounds and wounds of violence can have significant effects on the patient's mortality and morbidity as well as on the final result of his or her operation [5, 9, 14]. Further destruction of tissues and suppression of the process of wound healing may be caused by the infection. Tissues thus destroyed must be replaced by scar tissue, and infection therefore may cause loss of limb or may adversely affect function and cosmetic appearance. Indeed, its occurrence in wounded individuals who have been debilitated as the result of acute or chronic disease, severe or multiple injuries, or other similar factors may determine the issue of life or death.

Considerable confusion persists about the incidence, sources, causes, and nature of surgical infections that occur in incisional or postoperative wounds [3]. Many surgeons and bacteriologists had anticipated a greatly decreased incidence of postoperative wound infections after the introduction and general use of prophylactic antibiotic therapy. Such has not been the case, however, even after a third of a century of general and extensive antibiotic therapy [6]. Instead, clinical experience and laboratory studies have indicated that the overall incidence of surgical infections has not been decreased, and that the widespread use and misuse of antibiotic therapy has led to other problems such as the development of an unwarranted overdependence on its effectiveness, a de-emphasis on or disregard for established surgical principles, a relaxation of the "surgical conscience," a breakdown of isolation procedures, and the establishment of a reservoir of virulent and antibiotic-resistant bacteria concentrated in the hospital environment [6, 9, 13].

Supported by USPHS Grant 5-P01-GM15428-09.

These trends have been accentuated by the complexities of modern surgical practice and the concentration of large numbers of patients with established infections in hospitals, the extension of prolonged surgical operations and supportive procedures to an increasing number of high-risk patients, the increase of the number of individuals with severe trauma, and the growing use of drugs that decrease bodily resistance to infection [6].

It should be remembered that the possibilities for incisional wound sepsis in modern general hospital practice are numerous and ever-threatening. In addition to the reservoir of virulent and antibiotic-resistant bacteria and the potential cross-contamination and cross-infection between patients and the hospital's personnel, there are other factors contributing to this problem, such as the concentration of patients with a large variety of infections who have been admitted along with many other patients who are particularly prone to develop sepsis because of their unusual susceptibility. Another factor has been the extension of complex surgical operations, not only to aged and debilitated patients, but also to the newborn with congenital anomalies.

As surgical technology has advanced, a wide variety of new, surgically related infections have also occurred. Sufficient information is available to justify separate detailed descriptions of some of these as well as of certain other surgically related infection problems. The reader is referred to other chapters of Part II of this text that deal more specifically with these matters, in particular, Chapters 17, 18, 19, 22, 27, and 28.

Definitions

Nosocomial and Community-Acquired Infections

This chapter is concerned with infections that may occur in incisional wounds, the great majority of which are operating-room based and postoperative. All such infections are considered to be nosocomial infections, whether caused by organisms endogenous or exogenous to the patient.

Nosocomial infections other than incisional wound infections (also called operating-room-based infections) are frequently caused by antibiotic-resistant and virulent microorganisms of the hospital environment, and they may follow diagnostic and therapeutic procedures such as lower urinary tract catheterization or instrumentation, tracheostomy, continuous intravenous therapy, or arteriography. In addition, persons undergoing surgical operations are also at risk of other nosocomial operating-room-based infections.

Incisional wound infections are, by definition, unique to patients exposed to surgical procedures. However, patients hospitalized on surgical services are, in common with other patients, also at risk of other nosocomial (hospital-based) infections. Thus, overall nosocomial infection rates tend to be highest among surgical services.

There are many infections among patients on surgical services that develop spontaneously or otherwise in the home or community and consequently are considered to be community-acquired infections. Examples are acute appendicitis, acute cholecystitis, acute diverticulitis with perforation and peritonitis, acute perforated peptic ulcer with peritonitis, human or animal bite wounds, foreign bodies, and so on. As many as 30 or 40 percent of patients admitted to a busy surgical service in a general hospital may be of this type. Such community-acquired infections are not within the scope of this chapter.

Incisional Wound Infection

Microbial etiologic studies are often insufficient and unreliable because of the limited capabilities of bacteriologic laboratories, positive reports for secondary invaders or contaminants, or inappropriate sampling and culturing methods. Since it is not unusual for wound discharges to be sterile when cultured or for organisms to be recovered from wounds that are healing without clinical evidence of infection, it has been recommended that a set of clinical criteria be used to provide a better understanding, more consistent evaluation and reporting, and a more uniform and objective classification of infections by surgeons, epidemiologists, bacteriologists, and Infection Control Committees.

Any surgical wound that drains purulent material, with or without a positive culture, is considered to be the site of a nosocomial infection. Further, any wound that is diagnosed by the attending physician as "infected" should be accepted as such for epidemiologic purposes. Stitch abscesses should not be reported as an incisional wound infection unless they involve the wound itself (but they should be reported as stitch abscess). Since all wounds (infected and uninfected) are colonized by microorganisms, only bacteria isolated from purulent wound drainage should be reported as pathogens.

Microbiologic Specimens

Good laboratory support is essential to accurate and early diagnosis of surgical wound infections. In this regard, it must be kept in mind that laboratory support depends on the culture techniques employed by the clinician or technician. The physician must recognize the need for culture determinations and should utilize the proper methods and timing for the collection of the culture material in collaboration with the available laboratory personnel. When in doubt, consultation by the physician with a microbiologist or pathologist is helpful.

The following additional recommendations are suggested for the purpose of establishing an adequate microbiologic diagnosis [9]:

Collection

Representative specimens should be carefully obtained for the type of disease and organism anticipated, for example, pus, the walls of abscesses rather than their centers only, and the infected tissues near the margin of the lesion. Contact plates or punch biopsies are recommended for use in culturing burn wounds. Swab cultures are usually employed for culturing other surgical wounds, but the collection of several or more milliliters of pus from abscesses and its use in the laboratory for Gram

staining of smears as well as cultures is recommended.

Specimens should be obtained prior to the initiation of antimicrobial therapy whenever possible, and they should be obtained by means of aseptic techniques to avoid secondary contamination.

Transport

Prompt delivery to the laboratory of each specimen is important. Transportation requirements may vary with the organism involved. For cultures of suspected anaerobic infections, the obtained material should be placed in an anaerobic transport device that is used immediately after obtaining the cultures and prior to laboratory processing. Optimal handling of any culture specimen requires timely delivery of the specimen to the laboratory by a knowledgeable and responsible person, regardless of storage or transport considerations.

Processing

Aerobic and anaerobic culture techniques should be established and used for the isolation and identification of all microorganisms in specimens submitted from areas of infection or suspected infection.

Antibiotic sensitivity testing should be employed as indicated using diffusion methods or tube and agar-plate dilution techniques. The physician should familiarize himself with the limitations of the various techniques used in his hospital's laboratory.

A Center for Disease Control (CDC) study has indicated that the results of sensitivity testing—which report an organism as sensitive, resistant, or intermediate—can be carried out with a high degree of reproducibility among community hospital laboratories. This assurance is of practical importance.

Assistance from a reference laboratory, such as the CDC or a Public Health Department Laboratory, is advised in order to obtain specific typing and further study, when indicated, of pertinent pathogens isolated from infected wounds. To this end, the laboratory must be able to quick-freeze or lyophilize samples for shipment to such laboratories.

Classification of Operative Wounds

The following outline was developed in the ultraviolet-light study by the National Research Council (NRC) group and is now widely accepted as a standard classification of operative wounds [9, 11, 22]. It is recommended for use in collecting information concerning infections, relating them to sources of contamination, and estimating the degree of risk to infection as discussed in the *Manual on Control of Infections* published by the Committee on Control of Infections of the Pre- and Postoperative Care Committee of the American College of Surgeons [9].

Clean Wounds

These are nontraumatic, uninfected operative wounds in which no inflammation is encountered, there is no break in technique, and neither the respiratory, alimentary, or genitourinary tracts nor the oropharyngeal cavities are entered. Clean wounds are those that are elective, primarily closed, and undrained.

Clean-Contaminated Wounds

These are operative wounds in which the respiratory, alimentary, or genitourinary tracts are entered under controlled conditions and without unusual contamination. Wounds in which minor breaks in technique occur and those that are mechanically drained are included in this category.

Contaminated Wounds

These include open, fresh, accidental wounds, operations with major breaks in sterile technique or gross spillage from the gastrointestinal tract, and incisions in which acute, nonpurulent inflammation is encountered.

Dirty and Infected Wounds

These include old traumatic wounds with retained devitalized tissue and those that involve existing clinical infection on perforated viscera. This classification's definition suggests that the organisms causing postoperative infection are present in the operative field before operation.

Incidence of Surgical Wound Infection

International Data

A comparison of overall rates of postoperative wound infection reported from several different countries is presented in Table 16-1. The average rate for the combined group was about 10 percent.

NRC-USPHS Study

This project involved close surveillance over two-and-one-half years, beginning in 1960, of 15,613 consecutive operations carried out with support from the U.S. Public Health Service (USPHS) and under the aegis of the National Research Council (NRC) in five American university centers, including the University of Pennsylvania, Hahnemann Medical School, the University of California, Los Angeles, George Washington University, and the University of Cincinnati [22].

In this series, the overall rate of infection was 7.4 percent (Table 16-2). The average rate of infection in the 11,690 clean elective operative wounds, however, was only 5.1 percent, and the rates increased sharply as the

Table 16-1. Comparative Reports of Postoperative Wound Infection Rates

Author	Country	Number of operations or wounds	Infection rate
Clarke	England	382	13.6%
Robertson	Canada	1917	9.3%
Williams	England	722	4.7%
P.H.L.S.[a]	England	3276	9.4%
Rountree	Australia	198	14.0%
Myburgh	South Africa	(Not noted)	17.0%
NRC-USPHS[b]	United States	15,613	7.4%
Cruse and Foord	Canada	23,649	4.8%

[a] P.H.L.S. = Public Health Laboratory Service (Colindale).
[b] NRC-USPHS = National Research Council-U.S. Public Health Service study.

From Cruse, P. J. E. Fourth Symposium on Control of Surgical Infections. American College of Surgeons, Washington, D.C., November 10–11, 1972.

Table 16-2. Incidence of Incisional Postoperative Wound Infection in a Five-University Collaborative Ultraviolet Study

Type of surgical wound	Incidence of postoperative infection		
	No. of wounds	No. of infections	Infection rate
Clean	11,690	594	5.1%
Clean-contaminated	2589	280	10.8%
Contaminated and dirty	1262	277	21.9%
Not reported	72	6	8.3%
Totals	15,613	1157	7.4%

From Howard, J. M., et al. *Ann. Surg.* 160(suppl):1, 1964.

degree of wound contamination increased. The classification of wounds and their description used in this study are described earlier in this chapter.

Cruse and Foord Study

Using the categories employed in the 1964 NRC-USPHS report on wound infection and the influence of ultraviolet light cited above [22], Cruse and Foord initiated in September 1967 a prospective study of all surgical wounds at the Foothills Hospital in Calgary, Alberta, Canada, a hospital having 830 beds and ten operating rooms [18, 20]. The purposes of their study were to obtain an accurate monthly infection figure as a guide to the efficiency of function of the operating rooms, wards, surgeons, and the Infection Control Committee, to determine the factors that influence the infection rates, to obtain a statistical background for future investigations of variables, and to improve their infection rate and bed utilization.

They reported a total of 23,649 wounds, of which 1124 became infected, giving an overall infection rate of 4.8 percent (Table 16-3). As with the NRC-USPHS study, wound infection rates rose sharply as the likelihood of incisional wound contamination increased. Comparative infection rates for various surgical departments in their hospital are presented in Table 16-4.

Table 16-3. Infection Rate Related to Types and Contamination of Wounds (Cruse and Foord Study)

Type of surgical wound	Number of wounds	Number of infections	Infection rate
Clean	18,090	329	1.8%
Clean-contaminated	4106	367	8.9%
Contaminated	770	166	21.6%
Dirty	683	262	38.4%
Totals	23,649	1124	4.8%

From Cruse, P. J. E. Fourth Symposium on Control of Surgical Infections. American College of Surgeons, Washington, D.C., November 10–11, 1972.

Approximately a fivefold variation in rates for clean wounds was noted between departments with the highest (vascular) and lowest (neurosurgery) rates. Similarly, an eightfold variation in overall rates was noted between departments with the highest (urology) and lowest (neurosurgery) rates.

National Estimates

It is generally recognized that from 40 to 65 percent of the patients in general hospitals are usually surgical, and that approximately 40

Table 16-4. Comparison of Departmental Infection Rates (Cruse and Foord Study)

Department	Infection rate	
	Clean wounds	Overall
Neurosurgery	0.8%	1.2%
E.E.N.T.	0.9%	4.8%
General Practice	1.1%	2.5%
Plastic Surgery	1.2%	2.8%
Urology	1.4%	9.2%
General Surgery	1.6%	6.8%
Orthopedics	1.9%	3.9%
Gynecology	2.1%	2.7%
Vascular Surgery	3.7%	6.4%

From Cruse, P. J. E. Fourth Symposium on Control of Surgical Infections. American College of Surgeons, Washington, D.C., November 10–11, 1972.

percent of hospitalized surgical patients either have established infections at the time of admission or develop some type of infection during their hospital stay. Accurate data on the incidence of surgical wound infections throughout the United States, however, are not available [6]. The National Nosocomial Infection Study (see Part II, Chapter 13) has documented a sufficient number of infections to justify projections (more than 33,000 postoperative wound infections from data collected January 1970 to August 1973), but unfortunately, the number of operations and wound classifications for these operations are not available.

Estimates of the number of infections occurring in postoperative wounds have been made for the United States during the year of 1967 [6]. Nearly 1.4 million nosocomial surgical wound infections were estimated for the United States in 1967. This estimate was based upon the estimated number of hospital admissions (31.6 million) and operations (18.8 million) for that year [9] and multiplying the latter by 7.4 percent (the infection rate found in the NRC-USPHS study; see Table 16-2) to yield the incidence of postoperative infections projected for *operations of all types.*

Pathogens of Wound Infections

Considerable confusion has persisted concerning the microbial etiology of surgical infections [3, 6]. Particular emphasis has usually been placed on infections produced by *Staphylococcus aureus,* largely because of its epidemic potential and the ease of its identification. To a large extent, a considerable number of mixed bacterial infections and those produced by other bacteria, particularly the gram-negative bacilli, have been somewhat overlooked or deemphasized. During the past 15 years, the pattern of invasive surgical infections has changed, and a marked increase in the incidence of gram-negative bacillary infections has occurred [6, 9, 19]. In this regard, the National Nosocomial Infections Study has yielded some very interesting results concerning the etiology of wound infections (Table 16-5).

The continuing high incidence of *Staphylococcus aureus* was somewhat surprising, but the high incidence of *Escherichia coli, Pseudomonas aeruginosa,* and *Proteus mirabilis* infections was anticipated in view of the increasing incidence of gram-negative pathogens previously noted by Altemeier and others [2, 15, 21, 25]. The incidence of anaerobic pathogens, such as *Clostridium perfringens, Bac-*

Table 16-5. Postoperative Wound Pathogens Reported by National Nosocomial Infections Study

Pathogen	Service						Total	Percent
	Surg.	Gyn.	Med.	Obst.	Ped.	New-born		
Escherichia coli	4899	850	183	226	53	24	6235	18.7%
Staphylococcus aureus	5300	347	345	104	90	43	6229	18.6%
Pseudomonas aeruginosa	2612	105	166	18	46	4	2951	8.8%
Proteus mirabilis	1461	247	65	72	9	2	1856	5.6%
Bacteroides	986	203	35	55	7	0	1286	3.8%
Proteus species[a]	794	172	55	43	6	2	1072	3.2%
β-Hemolytic streptococci[b]	400	95	20	26	4	3	548	1.6%
Group-A streptococci	261	29	24	8	8	0	330	1.0%
Clostridium perfringens	324	8	14	7	2	0	355	1.0%
Other pathogens	9963	1342	579	495	104	63	12,546	37.6%
Totals	27,000	3398	1486	1054	329	141	33,408	99.9%

[a] Species unknown.
[b] Group unknown.

From National Nosocomial Infections Study (NNIS), January 1970 through August 1973.

teroides, and *Peptostreptococcus,* probably is not representative of their actual frequency, because of the problems of anaerobic cultivation and identification that prevail in many hospitals. The overall results are of broad usefulness. It must be realized, however, that the profile of most frequent pathogens varies by site of surgery and that large differences in profiles may occur in different hospitals.

Bacteria constitute the vast majority of wound pathogens, and, under the right circumstances, nearly all of them are capable of causing wound infections. Although much less common, a variety of fungi and certain viruses have also been considered responsible for incisional wound infections.

Complications of Incisional Wound Infection
Local
Infection usually develops in incisional wounds as a cellulitis associated with erythema, edema, pain, and interference of local function. There is cellular infiltration of the tissues by red blood cells, leukocytes, histiocytes, and macrophages. Liquefaction of the tissues and the formation of pus may follow with the production of an abscess. Septic necrosis of tissues and septic thrombophlebitis may also occur in the immediate vicinity of the wound.

Regional Spread
Direct extension of microorganisms along areolar, fascial, muscular, or other anatomic planes may also occur in the region of the infected wound. Lymphangitis and lymphadenitis, either suppurative or nonsuppurative, may be the result of microorganisms and their metabolic products being carried from the area of primary infection into the regional lymphatics and their related lymph nodes. Septic thrombosis may extend from the wound to produce thrombophlebitis in regional veins. Depending on the anatomic location of the surgical wound, direct regional extension may also result in peritonitis, retroperitoneal phlegmon, intraabdominal abscesses, empyema, mediastinitis, and central nervous system lesions such as meningitis and brain abscesses.

Systemic Spread
Bacteremia and septicemia are systemic infections related to the dissemination of microorganisms from a distributing focus into the circulating bloodstream. If the primary focus distributes bacteria once or intermittently, a bacteremia occurs when microorganisms transiently appear in the blood. Such bacteremia may occur without clinical signs of sepsis. If the bacterial distribution is more or less constant, septicemia is more likely to develop, and some of these cases will progress to septic shock. Bacteremia of any origin may lead to metastatic infections, and there is a danger, for example, that organisms might lodge and produce infection at the site of a recently implanted cardiac or skeletal prosthesis in a postoperative patient with bacteremia deriving from an incisional wound infection.

Role of Bacterial Enzymes
Bacterial enzymes contribute to the process of tissue liquefaction and septic necrosis [9]. Examples of such enzymes include collagenase, which produces liquefaction of collagen and aids in the dissemination of infection along fascial barriers; hyaluronidase, which is a factor favoring the spread of bacterial toxins; fibrinolysin, which is capable of dissolving fibrin and retarding the walling off of streptococcal infections; and the coagulase of *Staphylococcus aureus,* which contributes to septic thrombosis of blood vessels in and adjacent to wounds. Associated thrombophlebitis of regional veins may occur and produce septic thrombi and emboli, which gain their way into the circulating bloodstream. Microorganisms other than *S. aureus* have the propensity for producing thrombophlebitis, notably the *Bacteroides* group.

Factors Predisposing to Infection
Although the virulence, types, and numbers of contaminating bacteria are the principal factors of wound sepsis, it must be kept in mind that there are other nonmicrobial factors that are very important. The significance of these has been emphasized in an earlier publication [6].

Devitalized Tissue

The presence of dead, unhealthy, or irritated tissues in wounds enhances the growth of virulent and nonvirulent microbes, since these wounds have limited or little power of resistance to their growth and action. On the other hand, healthy tissues possess remarkable resistance and are able to withstand their effects.

Wound sepsis is more prone to develop in extensive wounds that contain large amounts of devitalized tissues, especially muscle, fascia, and bone. Such wounds furnish excellent culture material for the growth of bacteria.

Care must be exercised to prevent the development of devitalized tissue during the postoperative state. The local blood supply may be impaired by thrombosis or damage to large vessels, displacement of fractures, pressure of hematomas, tourniquets or ill-applied casts, or increased fascial tension due to swelling.

Foreign Bodies

These frequently carry large numbers of bacteria into wounds, and they increase the probability of infection by their heavy and continuing contamination and their local irritative action on tissues. Suture and prosthetic materials buried within a wound may also act as foreign bodies. Experiments in animals have shown that the required size of the infecting inoculum can be reduced several logarithmic factors in the presence of suture material.

Location of Wound

The site of the wound is of significance because various tissues in different locations in the body have varying powers of local resistance to infection. Incisional wounds of the face and neck, for example, are prone to resist infection unless they are in communication with the mouth and the pharynx. Wounds of the perineal area are more prone to become infected.

Time, Type, and Thoroughness of Treatment

These influence the development of wound infection more than is generally realized. The surgical excision and removal of all devitalized tissue and foreign bodies within the wound, preferably within four to six hours after the injury, is of primary importance in order to remove any potential pabulum before invasive bacterial growth can occur.

The multiplicity of severe wounds in one person may compromise treatment by making adequate debridement of one or more wounds impossible and thus enhancing the possibility of postoperative wound infection. If the period of time required for the patient's successful general treatment after the initial injury exceeds six to ten hours, infection may occur before local definitive wound treatment is possible.

Physical Condition of the Patient

This is another important factor that can predispose to infection. Shock, malnutrition, uncontrolled diabetes, anemia, uremia, cirrhosis, and various malignant neoplasms (e.g., leukemia) may lower the patient's resistance sufficiently to enhance the chances for bacterial growth and infection.

Remote Infection

Active infection in another site at the time of operation significantly increases the risk of an incisional wound infection. It is most important that such remote infections be properly treated and controlled, if possible, before surgical operations.

Other Factors

The following can also contribute to an enhanced risk: advanced age of the patient, marked obesity, increased length of preoperative hospitalization, increased duration of the operation, debilitating injuries, and various iatrogenic factors.

Sources and Modes of Acquisition

Infections Acquired in Operating Rooms

Most incisional wound infections probably derive from organisms that gain access to the wound at the time of operation. Adequate physical facilities and adherence to standard operating-room procedures are important in reducing the risks of intraoperative contamination of wounds. These issues are extensively discussed in Part I, Chapter 7, Section H, of this text and will not be addressed here.

AIRBORNE SPREAD. A central objective of the previously mentioned NRC-USPHS collaborative study was to establish the effect of ultraviolet irradiation of the air in operating rooms on the surgical wound infection rates. While ultraviolet light substantially reduced the number of airborne organisms, no significant reduction in wound infection rates occurred, and there was poor correlation between the types of organisms isolated from the air in operating rooms and from infected wounds. These results indicated that airborne organisms are probably of little overall importance in surgical wound infections acquired in the operating room. When the results are analyzed according to the class of wound, however, a slight (but still debated) reduction in the rates of infection of clean surgical wounds was noted among persons whose surgical procedures took place in irradiated, compared to nonirradiated, operating rooms. The importance of airborne organisms would be seen most clearly in the group with clean wounds, since the confounding influence of contamination with endogenous organisms is much less in this group.

Airborne spread sometimes appears to be an important route by which certain organisms from disseminating carriers on the operating-room staff gain access to the operative site (see later sections of this chapter).

CONTACT SPREAD. Puncture of gloves, especially at the time of closure of incisions, is probably the major mechanism of contact spread. The hands are not rendered sterile by surgical scrubs, and sweat and fluid from the sebaceous glands of the hands become entrapped within the gloves. Such fluid permits replication of residual organisms. In general, the longer the time gloves are worn, the greater the number and variety of organisms that can be cultured from their fluid contents. The incidence of glove punctures during operations has been surprisingly high in some studies (see Part I, Chapter 7, Section H).

Contaminated suture or other surgical material that directly contacts the incisional wound represents another potential mechanism by which infections may be acquired. This mechanism, however, is probably of little or no importance under the usual conditions of operations.

Organisms may also gain access to wounds by droplets from oral or nasal secretions of the operating-room staff.

ENDOGENOUS SOURCES. The principal source of organisms that produce incisional wound infections is probably the patient. Endogenous organisms are certainly a major factor underlying the rise in infection rates as wound classification progresses from clean to clean-contaminated to contaminated wounds.

Although surface organisms will be effectively removed by surgical preparation of the incision site, organisms residing within the sweat or sebaceous glands may remain in the path of the surgical incision. This mechanism might be responsible for a small fraction of incisional wound infections.

Organisms that most commonly produce incisional wound infections are also those that commonly reside on or within hospitalized patients. Some may represent community-acquired flora brought with the patient to the hospital; others may represent hospital-acquired organisms that become part of the patient's endogenous flora following admission. Such endogenous organisms, even when located at sites remote from the operative site, undoubtedly play an important role in incisional wound infections. There is evidence to support this contention, such as the substantial increase in wound infection risk associated with the presence of a remote infection in the patient and the substantially greater risk of staphylococcal wound infection in patients with *S. aureus* colonization of the anterior nares at the time of operation (staphylococcal wound infections in such persons tend to yield the same strain as that carried by the patient).

A variety of procedures and manipulations performed during the operative and immediately postoperative period, including endotracheal intubation (see Part II, Chapter 28), may produce bacteremia. Indeed, there is a surprisingly high frequency of symptomless bacteremia, even in healthy persons, that is associated with such simple procedures as brushing of the teeth. Thus, transient bacteremia with endogenous organisms may well be a mechanism by which organisms gain access to the incisional wound during and immediately following operations. Such a mechanism might also assist in explaining the somewhat puzzling lack of correlation—as seen in the NRC-USPHS collaborative study—between the identity of organisms cultured from wounds at the time of wound closure and those later cultured from wound infections.

Ward-Acquired Infections

CONTACT SPREAD. Transmission of organisms on the hands to the incision site of a recent wound at the time of wound inspection or dressing change carries a risk of producing wound infection. Surgical drains brought out through an incision offer a route for ingress of organisms from the patient's skin into the wound. Contaminated irrigating solutions represent another potential source for contact spread of wound infection.

AIRBORNE SPREAD. This route is probably of little direct importance as a source of postoperative incisional wound infection. Airborne *S. aureus,* however, may provide a means for the colonization of patients, and such organisms then become part of the patient's endogenous flora.

ENDOGENOUS SOURCES. As noted above, bacteremia with endogenous organisms (as well as exogenous organisms that may come from contaminated intravenous fluids or total parenteral nutrition fluids; see Part II, Chapter 26) poses a risk of lodging organisms in a new incisional site, and it is probably responsible for some ward-acquired wound infections. Of greater importance, organisms involved in deep wound infection may extend to involve the incisional wound in the infection process.

General Control Measures
Use of Surveillance Data
CLEAN-WOUND INFECTION RATES. Another aspect of the NRC-USPHS study was the wide variation found in the incidence of postoperative infection in clean elective wounds in the five participating medical centers. These rates ranged from 0.7 percent to 11.4 percent for the period between December 1, 1959, and February 17, 1961. Thereafter, adjustments of various operating-room technical factors, which were thought to be responsible for the variation, were made. In a group of 2288 subsequent clean elective surgical wounds studied in the same five hospitals, the differences between the extremes were decreased to between 0.8 percent and 6.1 percent. The average infection rate for the five centers during the second phase was 3.5 percent as compared to 11.4 percent for the first phase; these rates yielded an overall rate of 5.1 percent for the entire study (see Table 16-2). The incidence of infection in clean elective wounds at the Cincinnati General Hospital has continued to be 0.7 percent to 0.8 percent in subsequent determinations.

These striking results indicate that correctable deficiencies can be identified in particular institutions by comparison with peer hospitals, provided that all hospitals conduct careful surveillance and utilize the same standard criteria for infection. Such comparisons—in addition to prompting a hospital's surgical service and individual surgeons to review and correct inadequate facilities or operating-room practices—might also lead to renewed attention to gentle handling of tissues, careful hemostasis, and other time-honored principles of surgical practice. Deficiencies might also be identified by noting the changes in rates over time in a single institution.

SURGEON-SPECIFIC RATES. Comparison of wound infection rates among surgeons in a particular institution may also be of value, provided (1) comparisons are made for the same operations or for the same wound classes, (2) a sufficiently large number of procedures is included for each surgeon for whom such rates are calculated, (3) uniform surveillance using standard criteria is applied to all patients, and (4) adjustments are made for substantial differences in the susceptibility of patients. Based on the study of Cruse and Foord [18], small differences among individual surgeons might be expected.

MICROBIOLOGIC DATA. Periodic review and reporting of the culture results and the sensitivities of organisms that are causing infections are advisable, not only to help in identifying infection rates and clusters of infection, but also to permit rational selection of the initial antimicrobial therapy in life-threatening infections before culture results are available.

Chemoprophylaxis

INDICATIONS. Debate surrounding this issue has been lively. The composite findings of all appropriately controlled, prospective trials of chemoprophylaxis overwhelmingly indicate the effectiveness of chemoprophylaxis in preventing postoperative wound infection in clean-contaminated wounds [9]. Antibiotics administered to many patients with contaminated or dirty wounds, though perhaps of "chemoprophylactic" value in preventing an incisional wound infection, really represent chemotherapy directed at the established infection in deeper tissue. There is a consensus that chemoprophylaxis is not indicated for clean surgical wounds. It might be argued, however, that chemoprophylaxis has a role in preventing deep wound infection in clean surgical procedures that involve the implantation of prosthetic devices, because only a very few organisms lodging in such sites might produce infections with catastrophic consequences.

DURATION. Chemoprophylaxis should be given only in the immediately perioperative period. For greatest effectiveness, adequate tissue levels must be present at the time of operation and be maintained during the operation; treatment must then be continued for 24 hours following the procedure. It is inadvisable to begin chemoprophylaxis more than 24 hours before the operative procedure, since this may permit the outgrowth of resistant endogenous flora and predispose the patient to colonization with resistant exogenous flora. Thus, chemoprophylaxis should begin no sooner than is necessary to achieve therapeutic tissue levels, which, for most drugs, can readily be accomplished within a few hours. Similarly, it is inadvisable to continue chemoprophylaxis for more than 24 hours following the operation, because there is no present evidence that longer courses will improve effectiveness, and further therapy is likely to select more resistant strains.

CHOICE OF AGENT. The anatomic site of the operation gives an indication of the types of pathogens likely to produce wound infections. This information—coupled with ongoing information concerning the frequency of resistances of various pathogens to particular drugs or the frequency of resistances of isolates (irrespective of pathogen identity) from surgical wound infections at that site—can be used as a rational basis for selecting an agent or agents for chemoprophylaxis (see Part I, Chapter 11 for additional considerations). It is most important to realize that the most common pathogens and their resistances vary from hospital to hospital as well as within a particular hospital over time. A chemoprophylactic regimen used successfully at a particular hospital, therefore, may prove relatively ineffective in another hospital, and it may even prove ineffective at a later time in the same hospital.

Other Considerations

PROPER MANAGEMENT OF INFECTIONS. Remote infections should be treated and brought under control, if possible, before operation. Proper therapy of an established infection will reduce the numbers of pathogenic organisms potentially available for transmission to other sites and to other persons, and "no-touch" dressing technique should also be employed to minimize cross-infection risks. When indicated (see subsequent sections), patients with wound infections should be promptly and appropriately isolated (see Part I, Chapter 9).

PREDISPOSING FACTORS. Factors predisposing to infection should be identified and, if possible, corrected or controlled before operation (see Factors Predisposing to Infection, this chapter).

Staphylococcal Wound Infections
Clinical Aspects

MANIFESTATIONS. Staphylococcal infections usually have an incubation period of four to six days and tend to be localized; there is an initial area of cellulitis and subsequent swelling, pain, and central necrosis with the formation of an abscess containing thick, creamy, odorless, and usually yellow pus. Lymphadenitis or thrombophlebitis may occur, and thus they may act as distributing focuses from whence staphylococci may invade the regional lymphatics and the bloodstream and produce a bacteremia or septicemia. In closed incisional wounds, the symptoms and signs of staphylococcal infection include redness about the margins, swelling, and increasing local pain; the pain is throbbing in character and is often synchronized with the pulse beat. Fever and leukocytosis are usually present. When invasive regional or systemic infection occurs, malaise, higher fever, lymphangitis, lymphadenitis, chills, and sweats usually develop. In open wounds, a purulent discharge is the principal sign of infection. The responsible organism in the majority of instances is coagulase-positive *S. aureus*. Many of these strains are β-hemolytic, liquefy fibrin and gelatin, and produce yellow pigment in cultures.

MANAGEMENT. The treatment of staphylococcal wound sepsis primarily depends on early recognition, antibiotic therapy, and surgical drainage of the infected wound. Other methods of treatment include application of the established principles of rest, heat, elevation, and general support. Each patient with a staphylococcal infection should be considered individually and treated according to the nature of his infection, his associated diseases, and his individual characteristics. Surgical drainage of the area of infection should be temporarily delayed in the presence of acute, spreading infections and septicemia until appropriate antibiotic therapy has been started and the invasive qualities of the infection brought under control. Infected sutured wounds should first be reopened with the hemostat at the point of maximum pain, swelling, or fluctuation, and the opening enlarged to the size of the cavity. The cavity is then gently irrigated with saline solution and loosely packed open with fine mesh gauze. If pus and necrotic material are present, their removal is important.

The antibiotics recommended for treatment of patients with staphylococcal wound sepsis depend on the antibiotic sensitivities and any hypersensitivity of the patient to the available antibiotics. A penicillinase-resistant penicillin is the agent of choice in most hospitals, since a majority of strains are usually resistant to penicillin. Penicillin should be substituted for one of these, however, if the infecting strain is shown to be sensitive to it. Staphylococci that are resistant to methicillin and other penicillinase-resistant penicillins are being reported with increasing frequency in Great Britain and other European countries, but such resistances are still uncommon in the United States at present (see Part I, Chapter 11). Alternative drugs for patients with hypersensitivity to the penicillins include cephalosporins (some cross-sensitivity exists), erythromycin, lincomycin, clindamycin, and vancomycin.

It should be kept in mind that antibiotic therapy alone in the presence of infected wounds with pus formation is inadequate and incomplete; it should be supplemented by incision and drainage as indicated above. Antibiotic therapy should be started before surgical drainage, however, in order to produce bacteriostatic or bactericidal concentrations of the drug in the blood and tissues that will inhibit the growth of any bacteria disseminated by the operative procedure. In the presence of staphylococcal wound infection and invasion of the bloodstream, adequate therapy usually results in clearance of the organisms from the bloodstream within 36 to 72 hours in association with a decrease in the signs of local invasiveness. The presence of devitalized tissue, prostheses such as metal pins and plates, or other foreign bodies often limits the effect of the antibiotic therapy until such material is removed.

Epidemiologic Considerations

SOURCES. The majority of *S. aureus* strains that cause endemic postoperative incisional wound infections are derived from strains colonizing the patient, whereas outbreaks most commonly derive from a member of the operating-room staff who has active clinical staphylococcal disease or is an asymptomatic disseminating carrier.

PREVENTION AND CONTROL. The risk of *S. aureus* infection is several times higher in colonized patients, which suggests that attempts should be made to eradicate such colonization in the preoperative period. Systemic antibiotics are of limited effectiveness in eradicating the sensitive strains of *S. aureus* from their principal colonization site, the anterior nares, because of poor penetration of drugs into this area. Topical treatment is only 70 percent effective in eradicating such strains. Attempts to eradicate colonizing strains in the preoperative period are not likely to be of great value, since treatment must be given for several days, and the frequency of colonization of patients is high (at least 40 percent) while the overall rate of *S. aureus* incisional wound infections is relatively low (about 1.5 percent, i.e., about 20 percent of an overall rate of 7.5 percent). If the rate of infection in colonized patients is four times higher than that in noncolonized patients, then about 125 patients would need to be screened to identify and permit topical treatment of 50 colonized patients in order to potentially prevent one infection. Furthermore, the costs of treating all 125 persons without microbiologic screening would probably exceed the costs saved by preventing a single incisional wound infection. Limiting the preoperative stay of patients to the minimum, however, may definitely be recommended, because colonization rates increase with increasing duration of hospitalization, and strains acquired in the hospital may have enhanced virulence and a greater spectrum of resistance to antibiotics.

Isolation of infected patients and the use of "no-touch" technique for handling dressings from such infections are important in reducing the risks of staphylococcal cross-infection. Such measures also assist in preventing contact or airborne transmission of strains to preoperative patients who may become colonized by these routes. The recognition of an outbreak of infection should lead to the immediate examination of the personnel who attended the operations of the involved patients, and removal from duty and treatment are recommended for any persons with staphylococcal skin lesions. Asymptomatic disseminating carriers must be identified epidemiologically, since anterior nasal cultures per se will not differentiate disseminating from nondisseminating carriers. The most common approach is to compare the risks of wound infections with the epidemic strain (as initially defined by antibiograms)

for patients who were (1) attended and (2) not attended by each member of the entire operating-room staff (see Part I, Chapter 5). This information is then correlated with the results of anterior nasal and other cultures of persons significantly associated with the outbreak.

Disseminating carriers should be removed from duty and given a seven- to ten-day course of topical therapy with a bacitracin-containing ointment in an attempt to eradicate colonizing strains. If unsuccessful, a second course consisting of topical therapy and a systemic penicillinase-resistant penicillin should be undertaken, coupled with the use of hexachlorophene for showers or baths and the complete laundering of personal items that repetitively contact skin (e.g., clothes, towels, and the like). Such efforts sometimes merely suppress carriage during treatment, and the strain reappears shortly after antibiotics are discontinued. Long-term continuous topical antibiotic treatment may be considered for the persistent carrier. Special shedding studies should be undertaken, however, to assess whether such unfortunate persons may safely return to work.

Gram-Negative Bacillary Wound Infections
General Aspects

CHARACTERISTICS. Wound infections caused by aerobic gram-negative bacilli have become more frequent and of increasing importance during the past 15 years [1,2,8,9,15,21]. Following the discovery and general use of penicillin, secondary or superimposed infections by various gram-negative bacilli have developed during treatment and have become a serious and increasing threat in modern surgical practice. In a study of approximately 480 patients with gram-negative septicemia, the causes of this increase seemed to be related to the rapid extension of new and complex surgical operations and diagnostic procedures to elderly and other poor-risk patients whose resistance was decreased by debilitating trauma, associated chronic diseases, and leukocyte-suppression therapy.

The genera and species most frequently identified in aerobic gram-negative bacterial infections at the University of Cincinnati Medical Center are *Escherichia coli, Enterobacter aerogenes, Proteus, Pseudomonas aeruginosa,* and *Serratia.* A report of 42 patients who acquired *Serratia marcescens* septicemia from 1965 to 1970 exemplifies such infections [10]. It was noted that 80 percent of these cases were related to antecedent or concurrent antibiotic therapy, often given in large doses. This suggests either that these cases of *Serratia* sepsis were emergent, secondary infections caused by an organism of otherwise low virulence, or that the antibiotic therapy had depressed the patient's resistance and permitted invasive infections by such a microorganism.

Incisional wound infections caused by gram-negative bacilli such as *E. coli, Enterobacter aerogenes, Pseudomonas,* or *Proteus* have a longer incubation period than staphylococcal or streptococcal infections. A period of 7 to 14 days is not unusual, and periods of 30 or more days have been noted, particularly in patients undergoing antibiotic therapy.

MANAGEMENT. The treatment of purely gram-negative bacillary infections of postoperative incisional wounds includes adequate drainage, antibiotic therapy with the appropriate agents given systemically, and elevation and rest of the involved areas. The removal by sharp dissection of all necrotic tissue from these lesions is of help in their management.

The association of septic shock with gram-negative septicemia arising from wound abscesses or other deep-seated abscesses of the peritoneal cavity or abdominal viscera yields a poor prognosis. Treatment of such patients depends on early diagnosis and treatment of the sepsis and shock, as well as drainage of the obscure abscess. I have used prompt treatment with appropriate antibiotics administered intravenously, surgical drainage or excision of the source of infection, adequate supportive therapy, oxygen therapy, and the concurrent prudent use of intravenously administered corticosteroids. Failure to drain obscure abscesses or similar focuses that are contributing to the septicemia has usually resulted in death. The diagnosis of deep-seated or obscure abscesses can be made quite difficult by the masking effect of antibiotic or steroid therapy.

Epidemiologic Considerations

SOURCES AND PREVENTION. The most common organisms of this group, with the exception of *Serratia,* are also those that commonly colonize the gastrointestinal tract of hospitalized patients. Transmission of organisms from patient to patient probably takes place mainly on the hands of hospital personnel; thus, proper hand-washing is of fundamental importance in limiting transmission. (It is to be noted that *Serratia* and *Klebsiella* organisms have been found in improperly attended hexachlorophene-soap dispensers, and such contaminated equipment has been responsible for outbreaks. Further, *Serratia* may contaminate the hand lotions that are sometimes used *after* hand-washing.) Aerobic gram-negative rods may also be found in foodstuffs and occasionally have been found in oral medications. These sources probably also play some role. Airborne spread is probably of little or no importance. The use of antibiotics to which these organisms are resistant may permit successful colonization of the gastrointestinal tract by a relatively small number of organisms and lead to the emergence of resistant strains (whether endogenous or exogenously acquired) as the dominant aerobic flora. Limiting the preoperative stay and the antibiotic exposure of patients will reduce the chances of preoperative acquisition of exogenous strains. Wound and skin isolation is recommended for patients with infections that produce large amounts of purulent drainage (see Part I, Chapter 9).

Aerobic Streptococcal Infections
Clinical Aspects

MANIFESTATIONS. The majority of invasive streptococcal infections in wounds are caused by aerobic, β-hemolytic, group-A streptococci. Such infections run a relatively rapid and short course. The local process is one of diffusing cellulitis, lymphangitis, and lymphadenitis, with a large blood-filled local bleb at its primary focus. There is little tendency to form abscesses, but local breakdown or gangrene of the involved tissues can occur. The infection is thus characterized by the development of thin watery pus. Streptococcal invasion of the bloodstream is frequent and relatively early.

The systemic manifestations include chills, fever, tachycardia, sweats, prostration, and other signs of toxemia. Frequent examinations should be made to detect metastatic infectious complications as early as possible; each is treated according to its individual location and characteristics.

Surgical scarlet fever may occur rarely as a postoperative infection in a postoperative wound, and the hemolytic streptococci are associated with this lesion. The condition is characterized by spreading cellulitis with redness, swelling, and frequently bullous formation in and about the margins of the wound, as well as by a typical scarlatiniform eruption that starts at the wound and spreads peripherally over the body. The rash usually develops two to four days postoperatively.

Erysipelas, another type of cellulitis caused by a hemolytic strain of *Streptococcus,* may occur infrequently in lacerated wounds, particularly those about the face, after an incubation period of one to three days. Ushered in by chills, high fever, rapid pulse, and severe toxemia, it usually runs its course in a period of four to nine days. It is characterized by an area of advancing cellulitis with sharply demarcated, irregular, elevated, and indurated margins. The appearance of the infected skin is striking and immediately suggests the diagnosis.

Acute, hemolytic streptococcal gangrene is characterized by subcutaneous gangrene, thrombosis of the nutrient vessels, and resultant patchy slough of the overlying skin. It usually develops in the extremities, although the perineum, face, and other parts of the body may be involved.

Aerobic streptococcal infections caused by organisms other than group-A streptococci tend to be much less invasive. Group-D streptococci are commonly encountered in clean-contaminated and contaminated wounds of the gastrointestinal tract.

MANAGEMENT. The treatment of aerobic hemolytic streptococcal infections consists primarily in the control of their invasive characteristics by antibiotics, rest, elevation, warm compresses, and adequate drainage for the removal of pus and necrotic tissue. Incisions or manipulations are not advisable in streptococcal infections until the invasive characteristics have been overcome, with the exception of cases of acute, hemolytic streptococcal gangrene. Treatment of the last-mentioned depends on early diagnosis, emergency incision, and drainage through and beyond the gangrenous areas; this is in contrast to the usual, more conservative treatment used for streptococcal cellulitis. Infections caused by group-A streptococci respond very well to antibiotic therapy. Penicillin is the first choice, and erythromycin, lincomycin, and cephalothin are alternative choices. Enterococcal strains (group D) should be treated with ampicillin or a combination of ampicillin and an aminoglycoside.

In streptococcal septicemia, it is very important that the condition be diagnosed early and correctly to minimize the period of distribution of virulent bacteria to distant areas and the potential danger of forming metastatic abscesses. Prompt treatment is indicated that consists of adequate intravenous therapy with penicillin G and appropriate local treatment of the wound. If a suppurative thrombophlebitis is present in the neighborhood of the distributing infection, proximal ligation or excision should be considered. After control of the invasive characteristics of the infection is accomplished under the protection of a bactericidal or bacteriostatic concentration of antibiotic agents in the blood, pus that may have formed within the wound should be drained. General supportive therapy should be given as indicated.

Epidemiologic Considerations

SOURCES AND CONTROL. Streptococcal infections of incisional wounds are usually secondary to contamination from human sources—such as the upper respiratory tract, draining infected sinuses, other infected wounds, or contaminated instruments or dressings—or from airborne bacteria-laden particles of dust [8,11].

Several outbreaks have been traced to asymptomatic disseminators of group-A streptococci who worked in the operating room. Interestingly, the majority of these have been anesthesiologists, and rectal, rather than pharyngeal, colonization has been the source from which organisms were dispersed. Dissemination from a vaginal site has also been reported. Additional outbreaks have been traced to surgeons who continued to operate despite the presence of cutaneous streptococcal infections, which have sometimes appeared to be relatively trivial clinically. There are no reports of outbreaks resulting from streptococcal pharyngitis of surgical team members, perhaps because of the widespread accepted practice of excluding oneself from operative procedures when such an infection is suspected and the relative infrequency of group-A streptococci as a cause of pharyngitis in adults. Outbreaks should be investigated as indicated in the preceding section on staphylococcal infections, and the objectives of such an investigation are to identify and treat disseminating carriers. Penicillin, even when given in large doses parenterally, has sometimes failed to eradicate organisms in the distal gastrointestinal tract of rectal carriers, perhaps because of the penicillinase produced by other flora of the colon. Oral vancomycin, however, has proved very effective in those few circumstances where it has been used. Prophylactic penicillin administration should be considered for patients recently operated on who were attended by a person later identified to be a disseminating carrier.

Microaerophilic and Anaerobic Streptococcal Infections

Microaerophilic Streptococcal Infections

CLINICAL FEATURES. The microaerophilic hemolytic streptococci are the microaerophilic bacteria of principal importance. The hemolytic type characteristically produces burrowing sinuses that are chronic, active infections capable of penetrating any tissues in their pathway.

The nonhemolytic variety of streptococci may be associated with *S. aureus* or *Proteus* species to produce synergistic infections as the result of symbiotic metabolic activity [8,11, 24]. The most impressive of such infections is chronic progressive cutaneous gangrene, which may develop following operations for purulent infections of the chest or peritoneal cavity. The condition is caused by the synergistic action of a microaerophilic nonhemolytic *Strep-*

tococcus and an aerobic *S. aureus*. The incubation period is ten to fourteen days after operation. The wound and surrounding skin become tender, red, and edematous, particularly about stay sutures. A carbuncular infection develops within a few days about the wound margins or stay suture holes, and the central area assumes a purplish or purplish-black color. A wide area of bright red cellulitis develops around the central purplish area and central ulceration follows. This results in the characteristic appearance of the lesion, which consists of a central, enlarging area of ulceration bordered by a purplish-black, narrow margin of gangrenous skin and a large area of spreading cellulitis. Pain and tenderness are usually striking features, particularly in the region of the purplish-black margin.

TREATMENT. This infection is slowly progressive and may ultimately cause death unless specific treatment is instituted. Local excision of gangrenous margins or other conservative methods usually fail to check this process. Radical excision of the lesion with knife or cautery, followed by daily applications of zinc peroxide cream or ointment and general antibiotic therapy with penicillin if the synergistic *S. aureus* is sensitive or a penicillinase-resistant semisynthetic penicillin if the strain is resistant to penicillin, will promptly arrest the infection and permit early skin grafting and healing.

Anaerobic Streptococcal Infections

CLINICAL FEATURES. The anaerobic streptococci, or peptostreptococci, may produce a variety of severe postoperative infections with or without bacteremia, particularly after operative procedures upon the genital, intestinal, or respiratory tracts. The microorganism is difficult to grow bacteriologically, and routine cultures are frequently inadequate for detecting its presence. Careful bacteriologic studies, however, show that it is a frequent bacterial component of many infections seen in incisional wounds and deep abscesses. The pus produced by *Peptostreptococcus* infection characteristically is thick and grayish and has a fetid odor.

TREATMENT. The treatment of infections produced by *Peptostreptococcus* includes surgical drainage of abscesses, appropriate antibiotic therapy, and supportive treatment. The antibiotic of first choice is penicillin G, with tetracycline and erythromycin being alternative agents.

Other Types of Wound Infections
Surgical Diphtheria

CLINICAL FEATURES. Postoperative wounds occasionally become infected by the Klebs-Löffler bacillus (*Corynebacterium diphtheriae*) and the resultant infection usually is characterized by an acute ulceration and cellulitis with infiltration of the skin and subcutaneous tissues about the wound. A chronic, indolent ulceration of an open wound that fails to heal is another clinical type. The diagnosis is suggested by the development on the lesion of a pseudomembrane that bleeds readily when its removal is attempted. The diagnosis is proved by recovering the organism in cultures from the wound. Testing for toxin should also be done, either in vitro or in vivo (by inoculation of guinea pigs).

TREATMENT. Treatment consists of wound and skin isolation of the patient, the administration of diphtheria antitoxin, and the systemic administration of penicillin.

Mixed or Synergistic Infections

MANIFESTATIONS. A large group of wound infections that complicate surgical operations or trauma are caused by a mixed bacterial flora. This group has a polymicrobic causation; the bacterial mixture may consist of aerobic and anaerobic, gram-negative and gram-positive microorganisms whose origin most often is a lesion or perforation of the gastrointestinal, respiratory, or genitourinary tracts. The aerobic and anaerobic bacteria often relate to each other in symbiosis [4], and their synergistic action determines the characteristic nature of these septic processes. The process spreads, producing abscess formation, thrombosis of neighboring vessels, and extending necrosis, particularly of the areolar tissue. Crepitation of the infected tissue may develop as a result of the bacterial action of the clostridia, anaerobic streptococci, or associated aerogenic or aerobic bacilli.

MANAGEMENT. Successful treatment depends on early diagnosis and adequate surgical drainage of the infected wound if it is closed. Roentgenograms for soft tissue detail may be helpful in showing the presence of progressive gaseous infiltration and may aid in the diagnosis of associated crepitant cellulitis or abscess. Bacterial necrosis of tissue may be excessive, particularly in postoperative abdominal wounds. Antibiotic therapy with penicillin G and an appropriate broad-spectrum antibiotic is recommended. Gentamicin, tobramycin, tetracycline, cephalothin, clindamycin, lincomycin, and minocycline are agents to be considered for this purpose. The associated impairments of wound healing and intestinal ileus may lead to wound dehiscence. Septicemia with one or more bacteria may occur during the progress of this lesion.

Gas Gangrene and Clostridial Wound Infections

GENERAL FEATURES. Clostridial infections are particularly serious complications of incisional wounds that are most likely to occur in the presence of extensive damage to muscle masses, impairments of regional blood supply, gross contamination by dirt and other foreign bodies, and significant delay in adequate surgical treatment.

They are relatively infrequent in modern clinical practice, but when they occur, they are usually spectacular in their development and are associated with serious morbidity and mortality.

The microorganisms that cause such infections are anaerobic, and the most important type is *Clostridium perfringens*. It is recognized as the most important cause of gas gangrene in 56 to 100 percent of various series of patients studied by McLennan [23], Weinberg and Seguin [26]; and by Altemeier and Fullen [12]. Other clostridia—such as *C. novyi, C. sporogenes, C. septicum, C. histolyticum,* and *C. sordellii*—may occur alone or in combination with *C. perfringens*. Less frequently, clostridial infections may be caused by only one of this latter group without the association of *C. perfringens.*

Clinical forms of infection other than gas

gangrene include cellulitis, synergistic infections, tetanus, and wound botulism. Only gas gangrene will be considered here.

MANIFESTATIONS OF GAS GANGRENE. Gas gangrene is a spreading clostridial myositis, which may occur as the crepitant, edematous and noncrepitant, mixed, or profoundly toxemic types. It is primarily an infection of the muscles that spreads rapidly and involves to a lesser degree the neighboring connective tissues. The accumulation of edema and gas in fascial compartments produces an expanding pressure that aids in the lateral and longitudinal spread of the infection and contributes to further necrosis of the muscles. In this manner, groups of muscles, an entire limb, or large areas of the body may become successively involved.

The muscles become hemorrhagic and friable during the early stages of the process and noncontractile and disclosed later, and they exude a brown, watery, foul discharge that frequently contains bubbles of gas.

Occasionally, localized lesions of clostridial myositis that are crepitant or noncrepitant are seen. This type of lesion is less severe and does not have the ability to spread rapidly and to produce the progressive toxemia. Bloodstream invasion by the clostridia is relatively infrequent, and its occurrence is a particularly bad prognostic sign.

PREVENTION. The most effective way of preventing gas gangrene and other clostridial infections is early and adequate surgery of wounds with removal of contaminated foreign bodies, devitalized tissue, or both. Most experimental and clinical evidence indicates that antibiotic therapy alone cannot be relied upon to prevent the occurrence of clostridial infections. Prophylactic administration of gas gangrene antitoxin has been of little or no practical value in the prevention of gas gangrene. The evaluation of the prophylactic use of hyperbaric oxygen therapy has not been completed, and experimental studies in animals have shown equivocal results.

MANAGEMENT. In the treatment of established gas gangrene, success depends upon early diagnosis and the institution of prompt emergency operative treatment that includes multiple incisions and fasciotomy for decompression and drainage of the fascial compartments, excision of the involved muscles, and open amputation when necessary. Early and adequate surgery is the most reliable and effective primary treatment. Antibiotic therapy with penicillin in large doses intravenously and tetracycline in doses of 250 to 500 mg. intravenously every six hours or during the operative treatment has been effective. Erythromycin is another alternative agent. There is evidence to indicate that the tetracyclines are the antibiotics of choice in the treatment of clostridial infections. Antibiotic therapy has been most effective when used as an adjunctive treatment to the operative procedures.

Polyvalent gas gangrene antitoxin administered pre- and postoperatively is also of equivocal value in treating established gangrene. Many surgeons doubt its efficacy; others use it in an effort to prevent death from toxemia, allowing additional time for surgery and antibiotic therapy to bring the infection under control. Other supportive treatment should be considered, such as the administration of blood plasma, electrolytes, and steroids in certain patients with overwhelming toxemia and septic shock.

The use of hyperbaric oxygen in the treatment of gas gangrene and other clostridial infections was introduced by Brummelkamp and co-workers [17] in 1961. Numerous favorable reports have appeared that indicate there is rapid, dramatic, clinical improvement within the first day, whereas others have found hyperbaric therapy without the use of surgical debridement or radical incision ineffective. At this time, it would appear that no type of chemotherapy, serotherapy, or hyperbaric oxygen therapy has replaced early and adequate surgery in the treatment of clostridial infections.

Tuberculous Infections of Wounds
Postoperative wounds may occasionally become infected by the tubercle bacilli, particularly following operations upon known or unknown tuberculous lesions. This complication should rarely occur in modern surgical practice if antituberculosis agents are used. The infection may be apparent as a cold abscess, an indolent ulceration, one or more chronically draining sinuses, or a granuloma-

tous lesion with ulceration. The diagnosis is suggested by its appearance and proved by biopsy or demonstration of the organism by smear, culture, fluorescent microscopy, or animal inoculation. Treatment consists of the usual therapy for tuberculosis, including two or more antituberculosis chemotherapeutic agents.

Actinomycotic Infections

Actinomycotic infections, usually caused by *Actinomyces israelii,* may develop in wounds made in the presence of deep-seated actinomycosis, such as ileocecal or thoracic lesions, for example. This fungal infection is characterized by the development of a chronic, stony-hard, granulomatous mass, usually in the cervicofacial, thoracic, or abdominal areas. It subsequently breaks down to form central abscesses and multiple sinuses, which discharge a peculiar seropurulent fluid containing "sulfur" granules. There is adherence of the mass to the overlying skin, which then assumes a bronze or purplish-red color. The diagnosis is suggested by the appearance of the lesion and is proved by demonstration of the ray fungus in the pus or biopsied material by microscopic examination of the culture.

The lesion may be resistant to therapy. Antibiotic therapy over a prolonged period of several months or more may produce excellent results, however. Penicillin with or without sulfadiazine, a tetracycline, or erythromycin is the antibiotic treatment of choice for this infection.

Other Mycotic Infections

It is impossible to give here a description or illustration of all types of mycotic infections that may occur in incisional wounds. Numerous causative agents other than *Actinomyces* may cause infections of various types of wounds, including *Candida, Blastomyces, Coccidioides, Sporotrichum, Mucor, Aspergillus, Fusarium,* and *Nocardia.*

The *Candida* group of organisms have become serious problems, and they are the most frequent mycotic agents found in infected wounds, particularly in burn patients, patients under intensive antibiotic therapy, and those under immunosuppressive therapy. Long-term infusion or hyperalimentation has been incriminated as a factor leading to the development of yeast infections in a wide variety of surgical conditions. When the organism is identified in wounds, it has often been discounted or considered to be of little clinical significance. Disseminated candidiasis likewise may be easily missed, because the organism may be poorly stained with hematoxylin-eosin, and special techniques may be necessary to demonstrate the presence of the yeast organisms within the tissues. On the other hand, the presence of *Candida* organisms, as demonstrated by smear of the wound, generally has not been considered to be an indication for therapy unless hyphal forms are demonstrated in the tissue and the patient is not doing well clinically. If candiduria is demonstrated, nystatin should be orally administered, and if a Foley catheter is present, it should be removed. For active established *Candida* infections, treatment with the intravenous administration of amphotericin B is recommended.

Viral Infections

Herpesvirus, varicella, poxvirus, and cytomegalovirus are rare causes of incisional wound infections. Other viral agents also have the potential for causing nosocomial wound infections.

Summary

Surgical infections occurring in incisional wounds are a continuing, complex, and changing problem in hospital practice. Unfortunately, the overall incidence of such infection has not been reduced by the general and widespread use of antibiotic therapy. As some infections have been successfully controlled, other types have taken their place, and the struggle has continued.

The opportunities for microbial contamination and infection of wounds by a large number and variety of microorganisms are legion. The sources of these causative agents are several, and they include direct contact from exogenous sources, direct contact from endogenous sources, sedimentation from environmental air, and endogenous bacteremic sources. Various experimental studies indicate that contamination from endogenous sources is of the greatest importance, and operations involving transection or resection of bacteria-laden organs of the alimentary, respiratory, or genito-urinary tracts have a significantly higher incidence of postoperative wound infection. The importance of controlling this type of microbial contamination pre- and intraoperatively should be stressed.

In addition, the importance of a large number of nonbacterial factors in the causation of wound sepsis has been brought into sharper focus by the reports of Howard and associates [22] and of Altemeier. These factors have been enumerated, defined, and described in some detail in this chapter. A more purposeful and thoughtful incorporation of surgical techniques and surgical practice to overcome these factors is needed for improved control and prevention of infections in incisional wounds.

References

1. Altemeier, W. A. Bacteriology of Surgical Infections. Clinical and Experimental Considerations. In *Vingt-quatrième Congrès de la Société Internationale de Chirurgie*. Moscow, 1971, pp. 53–70.
2. Altemeier, W. A. Bodily response to infectious agents. *J.A.M.A.* 202:1085, 1967.
3. Altemeier, W. A. Control of wound infections. *J. R. Coll. Surg. Edinb.* 11:271, 1966.
4. Altemeier, W. A. The pathogenicity of the bacteria of appendicitis and peritonitis. *Ann. Surg.* 114:158, 1941.
5. Altemeier, W. A. Postoperative infections. *Surg. Clin. North Am.* 25:1202, 1945.
6. Altemeier, W. A. The significance of infection in trauma. *Bull. Am. Coll. Surg.* 57:7, 1972.
7. Altemeier, W. A., Barnes, B. J., Pulaski, E. J., Sandusky, W. R., Burke, J. F., and Clowes, G. A., Jr. Infections: Prophylaxis and management—A symposium. *Surgery* 67:369, 1970.
8. Altemeier, W. A., and Berkich, E. J. Wound Sepsis and Dehiscence. In Hardy, J. (Ed.), *Critical Surgical Illness*. Philadelphia: W. B. Saunders, 1971.
9. Altemeier, W. A., Burke, J. F., Pruitt, B. A., and Sandusky, W. R. (Eds.). *Manual on Control of Infection in Surgical Patients*. Philadelphia-Toronto: J. B. Lippincott, 1976.
10. Altemeier, W. A., Culbertson, W. R., Fullen, W. D., and McDonough, J. J. *Serratia marcescens* septicemia. *Arch. Surg.* 99:232, 1969.
11. Altemeier, W. A., Culbertson, W. R., and Hummel, R. P. Surgical considerations of endogenous infections—sources, types, and methods of control. *Surg. Clin. North Am.* 48:227, 1968.
12. Altemeier, W. A., and Fullen, W. D. Prevention and treatment of gas gangrene. *J.A.M.A.* 217:806, 1971.
13. Altemeier, W. A., and Levenson, S. Trauma Workshop Report: Infections, immunology and gnotobiosis. *J. Trauma* 10:1084, 1970.
14. Altemeier, W. A., McDonough, J. J., and Fullen, W. D. Third-day surgical fever. *Arch. Surg.* 103:158, 1971.
15. Altemeier, W. A., Todd, J. C., and Inge, W. W. Gram-negative septicemia: A growing threat. *Ann. Surg.* 166:530, 1967.
16. Altemeier, W. A., Todd, J. C., and Inge, W. W. Newer aspects of septicemia in surgical patients. *Arch. Surg.* 92:566, 1966.
17. Brummelkamp, W. H., Hogendijk, J., and Boerema, I. Treatment of anaerobic infections (clostridial myositis) by drenching the tissues with oxygen under high atmospheric pressure. *Surgery* 49:299, 1961.
18. Cruse, P. J. E. Prospective Study of 20,105 Surgical Wounds with Emphasis on Use of Topical Antibiotics and Prophylactic Antibiotics. In *Fourth Symposium on Control of Surgical Infections*. American College of Surgeons, Washington, D.C., November 10–11, 1972.
19. Cruse, P. J. E. Surgical wound sepsis. *Can. Med. Assoc. J.* 102:251, 1970.
20. Cruse, P. J. E., and Foord, R. A five-year prospective study of 23,649 surgical wounds. *Arch. Surg.* 107:206, 1973.
21. Finland, M., Jones, W. F., and Barnes, M. W. Occurrence of serious bacterial infections since introduction of antibacterial agents. *J.A.M.A.* 170:2188, 1969.
22. Howard, J. M., Barker, W. F., Culbertson, W. R., Grotzinger, P. J., Iovine, V. M., Keehn, R. J., and Ravdin, R. G. Postoperative wound infections: The influence of ultraviolet irradiation of the operating room and of various other factors. *Ann. Surg.* 160 (Suppl.):1, 1964.
23. MacLennan, J. D. Anaerobic infections in Tripolitania and Tunisia. *Lancet* 1:204, 1944.
24. Meleney, F. Differential diagnosis between certain types of infectious gangrene of skin with particular reference to hemolytic streptococcus gangrene and bacterial synergistic gangrene. *Surg. Gynecol. Obstet.* 56:847, 1933.
25. Roger, D. E. A changing pattern of life-threatening microbial disease. *N. Engl. J. Med.* 261:677, 1959.
26. Weinberg, M., and Sequin, P. La gangrène gazeuer. *Monogr. Inst. Pasteur.* 8:444, 1918.

17

Infections of Cardiac and Vascular Prostheses

John P. Burke

The development of synthetic materials that are chemically inert and durable enough to retain their geometric and other physical properties over many years has made possible the wide application of reconstructive operations on the heart and blood vessels. Devices that are commonly implanted in the cardiovascular system include cardiac total-valve prostheses, patches for repairing congenital heart defects, arterial grafts, permanent cardiac pacemakers, and external arteriovenous shunts for performing hemodialysis. Ventriculoatrial shunts for treating hydrocephalus are discussed in Part II, Chapter 28, and will not be specifically addressed in this chapter.

Nature of Infections

Incidence

Patients who receive cardiovascular implants are predisposed to a variety of nosocomial infections. The overall frequency of infections following open-heart surgery has ranged from 8 to 44 percent in various reports. The highest rates of infection have been found when special efforts have been made to identify asymptomatic and mild infections. The most common sites of infections are the respiratory and urinary tracts and the surgical wound.

The frequencies of intravascular infections associated with the different prostheses vary widely [2,5,9,10,15]. Table 17-1 shows the approximate ranges of these rates for each of the major types of prostheses. It is not possible to give an accurate incidence of infection for each device, because the duration of follow-up in most reports is either variable or unspecified. The highest rates of infection are associated with appliances, such as external arteriovenous cannulas, that are continuously exposed to skin flora. Endocarditis occurs more often with aortic ball valves than with other intracardiac prostheses. Similarly, the risk of infection is

Supported in part by a training grant 3T01 AI00039-15 from the National Institute of Allergy and Infectious Diseases.

Table 17-1. Frequencies of Cardiovascular Pros-thesis-Associated Infections

Type of prosthesis	Percent of patients with infections
Cardiac:	
Valve prosthesis	0.2%–9.5%
Patch repair	0.1%–2.7%
Vascular:	
Arterial graft	1%–6%
Permanent pacemaker	1%–11%
Arteriovenous cannulas	2.5%–26.6% [a]

[a] Rate per 100 patient-months.

greater with a prosthetic cardiac valve than with a patch repair of a congenital heart defect.

Infections at the site of a prosthetic implant account for a minuscule proportion of the entire spectrum of nosocomial infections. Among 113,330 infections in nearly 3.5 million patients included in the National Nosocomial Infections Study (see Part II, Chapter 13) from January 1970 to August 1973, only 30 infections of cardiac and arterial prostheses (including pacemakers) were reported. Nonetheless, the economic cost of these infections is high in relation to that of many other types of nosocomial infection, and for patients with infected cardiac valve prostheses, the mortality is as high as 75 to 80 percent.

The small numbers of reported cases, the anecdotal nature of many reports, and the lack of centrally coordinated national surveillance of patients who receive prosthetic implants each contribute to an astonishing paucity of epidemiologic data. No prospective data have yet been published that might help to establish a baseline level of endemic infections associated with these prostheses. Therefore, all cases should be thoroughly investigated to identify possible irregular procedures, sources of contamination, or improper techniques.

Only a few outbreaks of infections in cardiovascular surgery units have been described. An "outbreak" of four cases of *Aspergillus* infections associated with cardiac prostheses that occurred in a three-year period in one hospital and two cases of *Penicillium* endocarditis in another hospital, for example, were traced to environmental contamination [6,8]. These experiences emphasize that epidemics may be recognized by the occurrence of infections due to an unusual pathogen, rather than from an analysis of the overall infection rate. A few *Mycobacterium chelonei* infections deriving from intrinsic contamination of porcine aortic valve prostheses have also been reported [3]. These organisms appeared to withstand the glutaraldehyde disinfection regimen used by a company to prepare the valves. Modifications of the disinfection regimen appear to have reduced the risk of such intrinsic contamination.

Pathogens
A wide variety of bacterial, fungal, mycobacterial, and rickettsial species have been recovered from infections associated with cardiovascular prostheses (Table 17-2). Organisms that have been judged to be of low virulence are often recovered from these infections and cannot be easily dismissed as contaminants in blood cultures. *Staphylococcus epidermidis* and *S. aureus* are involved most often in prosthetic-valve endocarditis; *Candida, Aspergillus,* diphtheroids, and a variety of enteric gram-negative

Table 17-2. Causative Agents of Infections Associated with Cardiac and Arterial Prostheses

Pathogen	Number of cases	
	Cardiac prosthesis[a]	Arterial prosthesis
Staphylococcus aureus	9	1
Staphylococcus epidermidis	5	1
Group-D streptococci	0	1
Diphtheroids	1	0
Herellea-Mima	0	1
Enterobacter	0	1
Serratia	1	0
Proteus species	1	0
Pseudomonas aeruginosa	1	1
Candida	0	1
Nocardia	1	0
Other or unknown fungi	0	2
Unknown	2	0

[a] Includes pacemakers.

From National Nosocomial Infection Study (NNIS), January 1970 to August 1973 (see text).

bacilli are also commonly found. The patterns of microbial species reported from infections associated with cardiac pacemakers and patch repairs for congenital heart defects are similar to those from prosthetic-valve infections.

Although gram-negative bacilli predominate in most nosocomial infections, this has not been true of prosthetic-valve endocarditis. Gram-negative bacilli were the most common pathogens in one report of infections associated with arterial grafts, however, and they are especially common in retroperitoneal prostheses contaminated from the gastrointestinal or genitourinary tract. *Staphylococcus aureus* and *Pseudomonas* species are the pathogens most frequently responsible for infections at the sites of external arteriovenous shunts for hemodialysis [9].

Classification of Infections

Existing guidelines for determining the presence of infection and for classifying it, as developed by the Center for Disease Control (CDC) in Atlanta, can be applied to nosocomial infections related to intravascular prostheses [7]. In many instances, however, these definitions are not entirely satisfactory and require further interpretation. A diagnosis of prosthesis-associated intravascular infection requires confirmation by the attending physician, because some patients may have bacteremia or fungemia from a focal infection without involvement of the prosthesis, and others with prosthesis-associated infection may not have positive blood cultures.

Infections related to prosthetic cardiac valves have been classified according to the time of onset of symptoms as either *early* (less than 60 days after operation) or *late* (more than 60 days). These two groups differ from each other in their epidemiologic and clinical features; early infections are considered to arise most commonly from operative contamination, and late cases from bacteremias such as those associated with dental, urinary, or other manipulations. Infections associated with other cardiovascular prostheses should also be classified as either early or late in onset by the same (60-day) criterion.

The incubation period of postoperative in-fections related to prosthetic materials is often uncertain and probably varies within broad limits, perhaps depending on such factors as the virulence of the organism, size of the inoculum, prophylactic use of antibiotics, and host resistance.

Infections that become apparent within 60 days after placement of a cardiovascular prosthesis should be classified as nosocomial. In addition, intravascular infections with onsets during hospitalization that are secondary to focal infections in sites such as the urinary or respiratory tracts should be considered nosocomial, even though their onset may occur more than 60 days postoperatively. A patient who enters the hospital with an intravascular infection for which he receives a vascular graft or prosthesis and who later develops postoperative infection with the same organism involving the implanted material is also considered to have a nosocomial infection.

The clinical onset of infection related to an intracardiac prosthesis may be delayed until weeks or months after the operative procedure and discharge from the hospital. The majority of late infections should be considered to be community-acquired, however, because the causative agents recovered from them are usually those seen in classic infective endocarditis in patients without prosthetic devices. It is unknown which, if any, of these late infections may originate from operative contamination or bacteremia while the patient was hospitalized.

Diagnostic Criteria

The sudden appearance of a regurgitant murmur or cardiac failure, the disappearance of the distinct click of the prosthetic valve, or an abnormal tilting motion of the valve demonstrated fluoroscopically are each virtually diagnostic of endocarditis in patients with prosthetic cardiac valves and positive blood cultures. Similarly, patients with vascular grafts who have positive blood cultures may be considered to have almost certain involvement of the graft if bleeding, clotting, or other clinical evidence of malfunction of the graft occurs.

In the presence of clinical findings of infection, the discovery of microorganisms by microscopy or culture in vegetations or pus removed from completely intravascular prostheses at either repeat operation or autopsy is evidence of active infection. A positive culture from a removed arteriovenous cannula or an extruded cardiac pacemaker in conjunction with the recovery of the same organism from a blood culture obtained from a different site is also evidence of intravascular infection. In all other instances, the diagnosis of infection at the site of a cardiovascular prosthesis is indirect and is based on the presence of either typical clinical findings, repeated positive blood cultures, or both.

Predisposing Factors

Postoperative endocarditis occurs more often following open-heart surgery that requires the implantation of foreign material than following other open-heart procedures. The foreign-body effect of these implants is poorly understood, but it is probably related to the persistence of microorganisms in sites inaccessible to the inflammatory response.

The risk of infection is also greater in procedures involving the placement of a prosthesis in a high-pressure system with turbulent blood flow, such as an aortic ball valve. The relative risks of infection have not been determined for various models of the available cardiac valve prostheses or for synthetic prostheses as compared to transplants of valves of animal origin.

Cardiopulmonary bypass appears to alter the defense mechanisms of patients as well as to increase the opportunities for operative contamination.

Concomitant infection in other sites—such as the urinary and lower respiratory tracts, the surgical wound, and venous and arterial catheters—provides a source for direct contamination during the operative procedure and also predisposes to bacteremia with seeding of the prosthetic device. The risk of infection at the site of a femoral-popliteal arterial graft is increased by open, infected lesions on the legs at the time of operation.

The most important single factor shaping the character of postoperative endocarditis and other infections related to cardiovascular prostheses is the use of antimicrobial agents before, during, and after operative procedures. The extensive preoperative use of antibiotics may increase the risk of postoperative endocarditis when an intracardiac prosthesis is implanted. The reasons for this are not clear, but they may be related to the replacement of "normal flora" by antibiotic-resistant species and the overgrowth of certain microbial flora of the skin, mucous membranes, or gastrointestinal tract. The use of prophylactic antimicrobial agents during and after operations has been responsible for shifting the patterns of infecting agents to a more antibiotic-resistant group of pathogens, including *Staphylococcus epidermidis,* the diphtheroids, and various fungi.

The overall risk of infection is probably greater with longer than with shorter courses of chemotherapy, both pre- and postoperatively. When a major break in aseptic technique occurs during the operation, however, prophylaxis merges with early treatment, and a prolonged course of high-dose chemotherapy may be desirable.

Certain patients have other risk factors that are commonly associated with nosocomial infections. Serious underlying illnesses (e.g., congestive heart failure, rheumatoid arthritis, and diabetes mellitus) and the use of medications (e.g., steroids and indomethacin) are associated with decreased host resistance and often with defective inflammatory or immune responses, which thereby increase the risks both of intravascular infection and of other focal infections.

Specimens

Collection

Isolation of the pathogen from blood cultures is the essential laboratory procedure for the diagnosis and effective treatment of intravascular infections. The techniques for obtaining specimens are far more important than the use of special media or the ability of the laboratory to isolate unusual microbial species (see Part II, Chapter 29).

The best time for obtaining blood cultures is thought to be about two hours before the patient's temperature begins to rise, if this is feasible based on the regularity and predictability of the fever. The bacteremias accompanying intravascular infections related to such prostheses have not been studied with quantitative blood cultures during the untreated course of the disease, as were those of natural infective endocarditis in the preantibiotic era. Since the source of the infection is an intravascular lesion, organisms are probably present in the blood at all times. In urgent clinical circumstances, five or six blood cultures can be obtained at ten-minute intervals and antimicrobial treatment given without delay.

In adults, a total blood volume of 50 to 60 ml. should be obtained for culture in order to detect bacteremia with very few circulating microorganisms. The sample obtained from a single venipuncture, however, should not be divided among several different culture bottles, because potential contaminants may be assigned clinical importance if all the cultures are positive. The yield from additional blood cultures is small when five or six samples taken at different times are negative.

The microorganisms that are the most common contaminants in blood cultures (e.g., *S. epidermidis* and diphtheroids) are also often responsible for infections associated with cardiac and vascular prostheses. The rate of false-positive cultures will depend on the aseptic precautions used in obtaining specimens; calculation of this rate in one's own hospital is helpful for interpreting reports of cultures and for stimulating efforts to improve the techniques of collection. The chance that a single blood culture is falsely positive should not be more than 2 percent.

Use of alcohol (70% to 95% isopropanol or 70% ethanol) for skin cleansing followed by tincture of iodine (2%) is preferred for preparing the skin for venipuncture. Solutions of benzalkonium chloride and other quaternary ammonium compounds should not be used for skin disinfection, because these agents are relatively inactive against gram-negative bacilli and may become contaminated with such organisms. The skin should not be touched after cleansing. In adults, the smallest amount of blood taken for culture on each occasion should be 10 ml.; 1- to 5-ml. samples are often taken from young children. The sample is then inoculated into a culture medium that is at least ten-

fold greater in volume in order to dilute the antibacterial substances of the whole blood. Organisms from the deeper layers of the skin may adhere to the outside of the needle used for venipuncture. Therefore, the needle must be removed and replaced with a sterile needle before the blood is inoculated from a syringe into the culture bottles. The diaphragm top of the bottle should be wiped with alcohol or tincture of iodine before the needle is inserted. Alcohol may be used to remove residual iodine on the skin after the blood culture is collected.

If the patient has been receiving a penicillin or cephalosporin, penicillinase may be added to the medium. When this is done, however, a sample of penicillinase should be cultured as a control to detect any contamination of the enzyme preparation.

Direct communication between the physician and laboratory personnel is necessary for evaluating these serious infections. The physician should be responsible for insuring that a colony of any microorganism recovered is placed in a holding medium and not discarded by the laboratory as a "contaminant." A separate colony from each positive culture should be preserved for later typing by either biochemical reactions, antibiotic sensitivity patterns (antibiograms), phage typing, or serologic methods when these results may be useful for determining whether the organisms are pathogens or contaminants. The isolation of identical organisms from two or more blood cultures obtained on separate occasions is, of course, strong evidence of bacteremia and possible intravascular infection. Specimens of the isolated microorganism itself will also be necessary for later tests to insure the effectiveness of antibiotic treatment.

When the clinical findings suggest intravascular infection and the conventional blood cultures are negative, special procedures should be employed to recover potential pathogens. Blood cultures that are initially reported sterile, for example, may become positive if they are held for two to four weeks. Special procedures for recognizing cell wall-defective bacterial variants (L forms) may be performed in research laboratories.

Negative blood cultures may be found in

patients with intravascular infections that due to *Chlamydia,* rickettsia, *Aspergillus, Candida,* and certain other fungi. If embolism to a major artery occurs, the embolus should be removed and later examined and cultured to detect the presence of fungi. Blood cultures are also occasionally negative when the infection involves the right side of the heart.

Transport of Specimens

Because antibacterial substances and antibodies in whole blood may interfere with bacterial growth, blood for culture must be inoculated into the medium at the bedside. Many commercially available blood culture media also contain substances (e.g., polyanethol sulfonate) that inhibit such antibacterial activity. No special precautions are necessary for the transport of the culture bottle, which may be kept at room temperature. Refrigeration of the culture bottle will delay bacterial growth.

Specimens of the prosthetic apparatus or tissues obtained from operations and autopsies should be immediately delivered to the laboratory in sterile containers, rather than in formaldehyde solutions.

Clinical Aspects of Intravascular Infections
Manifestations

GENERAL FEATURES. The symptoms and signs of intravascular infection related to prosthetic materials are, with some important differences, similar to those of classic infective endocarditis. The intravascular location is the feature that all these infections have in common and that is responsible for their protean manifestations. The specific clinical features are determined by the type and location of the prosthesis, the nature of the responsible microbial agent, and the presence of underlying chronic illness, especially uremia.

The most common symptoms are nonspecific ones such as fever, malaise, and weakness, Indeed, a surprisingly high proportion of these patients appear entirely well at the time of the first positive blood culture. Fever and other signs of infection may be suppressed by injudicious antibiotic treatment, or they may not occur in the presence of chronic illness such as

uremia. In patients whose illness begins early in the postoperative period, the dominant symptoms may be ones of associated infection, such as pneumonia and wound infection.

VALVULAR PROSTHESES. In patients with prosthetic cardiac valves, the occurrence of regurgitant murmurs and severe cardiac failure as a result of the separation of sutures from the valvular annulus is highly suggestive of endocarditis. These infections are frequently accompanied by embolic phenomena and sometimes produce ventricular and aortic aneurysms. The valve itself may become occluded by a thrombus. Other findings usually associated with endocarditis—such as anemia, hematuria (macroscopic or microscopic), Roth's spots, subungual hemorrhages, conjunctival petechiae, and enlargement of the spleen—help to direct attention to the possibility of intravascular infection. Over 50 percent of patients subjected to open-heart surgery with cardiopulmonary bypass develop conjunctival petechiae postoperatively that are unrelated to infection, however. Thus, this sign may be falsely interpreted as evidence of intravascular infection.

Prediction of the tempo of the clinical course cannot be based reliably on knowldege of the responsible microbial species. Rapid destruction of the valvular annulus may occur in prosthetic-valve infections due to organisms such as *S. epidermidis* that have been judged to be of low virulence as well as in infections due to *S. aureus.*

Fungal endocarditis with unusually large and friable vegetations is often complicated by embolic occlusion of the large arteries, especially those in the lower extremities. The complications of uveitis or endophthalmitis are especially suggestive of infection due to *Candida* species.

OTHER VASCULAR PROSTHESES. In endocarditis following Teflon patch repair of a congenital heart defect (e.g., a ventricular septal defect), the only evidence of infection may be fever, either low-grade or spiking. Separation of the patch with or without subsequent embolism may occur.

Inflammation at the operative site may be found in patients with infected arterial grafts, subcutaneous cardiac pacemakers, and arteriovenous shunts. Common signs of infections related to arterial grafts are bleeding, clotting of the prosthesis, a localized abscess, a chronic draining sinus, and peripheral septic emboli with secondary abscesses. Arteriovenous shunts may also show instability of the Teflon cannula, oozing of blood, repeated clotting, or a local abscess.

Management

INITIAL TREATMENT. The management of infections associated with intravascular prostheses requires the use of high doses of microbicidal agents intravenously and a consideration of the removal and possible replacement of the prosthesis. The principles of antimicrobial therapy are similar to those for the treatment of infective endocarditis with natural heart valves [13, 14]. Full bacteriologic study of the sensitivity of the pathogen is necessary for optimal treatment of these intravascular infections. Nonetheless, chemotherapy must be begun before the results of sensitivity tests become available. The selection of antimicrobial agents at that time is based on consideration of the usual sensitivities of the specific pathogen and the antimicrobial agents previously used for that patient. The pathogen should be assumed to be resistant to the prophylactic antibiotics used for open-heart surgery. Postoperative infections commonly occur, however, with organisms that are fully sensitive to the prophylactic antibiotics, especially in prosthetic-valve endocarditis due to *S. epidermidis*.

If, because of fulminant illness, it is necessary to begin treatment before the responsible pathogen is isolated, the selection of specific antimicrobials should be influenced by consideration of the types and sensitivities of pathogens isolated from similar patients in that hospital. Even in such urgent circumstances, however, it is possible to obtain five or six blood cultures before treatment is begun. A penicillinase-resistant penicillin or cephalosporin, directed at the possibility of staphylococcal infection, should be included in the antibiotic regimen while one is awaiting culture results.

TREATMENT FOR SPECIFIC PATHOGENS. Specific drugs of choice cannot be listed for many pathogens, in part because of the chang-ing and unique patterns of antibiotic resistance in different hospitals. However, guidelines for the selection of antimicrobial agents with activity against important pathogens can be given.

A penicillinase-resistant penicillin or cephalosporin is used for infections due to staphylococci. Cross-resistance between the penicillinase-resistant penicillins and cephalosporins has been found for *S. aureus* but not for *S. epidermidis*. Therefore, a cephalosporin may be preferred for initial treatment of infection due to *S. epidermidis* when a penicillinase-resistant penicillin has been previously used for prophylaxis. Special care is required when disc sensitivity tests are used to detect resistance to penicillinase-resistant penicillins (see Part I, Chapters 8 and 11). Apparent resistance of staphylococci should be confirmed by tube-dilution tests.

Most patients who are allergic to penicillin can be safely treated with cephalosporins, although some patients are allergic to both. A cephalosporin can be used if the reaction to penicillin was mild or the history is vague. Vancomycin is a suitable alternative for patients with a history of a life-threatening reaction to either a penicillin or cephalosporin, as well as for those with infection due to a staphylococcal strain that is later shown to be resistant to both of these groups of agents.

Every effort should be made to use a penicillin or cephalosporin, because they are the most effective antimicrobials in treating intravascular infections due to susceptible organisms. Skin tests are useful for predicting more severe penicillin reactions, but they are not yet widely available. Hyposensitization to penicillin may be attempted for selected patients when the results of antibiotic sensitivity tests are available.

Intravascular infections due to viridans streptococci, enterococci, or diphtheroids may be treated with combined penicillin G and streptomycin. The addition of streptomycin, while not strictly necessary for infections due to viridans streptococci, may provide a more rapid bactericidal effect. Some strains of enterococci and diphtheroids are resistant to this combination, and early sensitivity testing is mandatory.

Infections due to gram-negative bacilli nearly

always require early operative intervention. Failure of treatment with antibiotics is a major problem, in part because the antimicrobial agents that are most active against gram-negative bacilli have either prohibitive toxicity for the high-dose therapy needed, poor diffusibility in tissues, or merely bacteriostatic properties. Initial therapy must always include at least two antimicrobial agents that are likely to be effective against recent nosocomial isolates of that species in one's own hospital. At the present time, gentamicin, tobramycin, and amikacin are likely to possess the widest spectrum of activity against gram-negative bacilli from nosocomial infections. One of the antibiotics selected should be either a "broad-spectrum" penicillin (ampicillin, amoxicillin, carbenicillin, or ticarcillin) or cephalosporin.

Pseudomonas infections associated with intracardiac prostheses are a special problem and may require treatment with three agents: polymyxin B, gentamicin or tobramycin, and carbenicillin or ticarcillin. The results of antimicrobial therapy—even with in vitro demonstration of the sensitivity of the organism to the antimicrobial agent used—are dismal, and removal of the prosthesis may be life-saving.

Yeast and fungal infections, which are usually due to either *Candida* or *Aspergillus* species, require removal of the prosthesis and systemic treatment with amphotericin B.

The effectiveness of chemotherapy is most conveniently monitored by determining the antibacterial activity of the patient's serum against the organism recovered from the blood (or from the prosthesis itself) with a serial, twofold dilution test. Blood specimens for this test are obtained within 30 minutes after the intravenous injection of the antibiotic and again just before the next dose. It is most desirable to maintain a bactericidal (not merely a bacteriostatic) effect of 1:8 or higher in the "trough" specimen. A single specimen may be obtained regardless of time if the antimicrobial agent is being given by continuous intravenous infusion. Intermittent, rather than continuous, intravenous infusion is preferred, however.

Antibiotic assays are a suitable substitute for serial, twofold dilution tests of the patient's serum when the infecting organism is known to be sensitive, and such assays can assist in preventing toxicity from excessive drug levels. Serum concentrations should be maintained within acceptable therapeutic ranges. Assays are probably preferable in monitoring therapy with antibiotics that are highly protein-bound or very sensitive to pH changes, since erratic results sometimes occur with the serum dilution method.

The optimal duration of antibacterial treatment has not been determined. Therapy should generally be continued for at least four weeks. Most experts recommend longer treatment for intracardiac prosthesis-associated infection than for natural-valve endocarditis.

REMOVAL OF PROSTHESES. Vigorous antibiotic therapy will cure some of these infections. In others, antibiotics may suppress the systemic signs and symptoms while the infection persists at the site of the prosthesis. Antibiotic therapy of prosthetic-valve endocarditis fails more often in those cases with an early postoperative onset than in those with a late onset. In order to detect antibiotic failure at the earliest possible time, it is useful to obtain blood for culture periodically during treatment and, especially, in the weeks and months after the completion of treatment, irrespective of the lack of fever or other signs of infection.

Removal of an intracardiac prosthesis is necessary when antibiotic therapy has failed to clear the bacteremia. Other indications for the removal of a prosthetic valve, in addition to uncontrolled infection or the resistance of the organism to available bactericidal chemotherapeutic agents, include dysfunction of the valve (as manifested by a regurgitant murmur, abnormal angulation of a partially detached valve as shown by roentgenograms or fluoroscopy, or severe cardiac failure), major systemic embolism, and suspected yeast or fungal infection. Similar considerations apply to other intravascular prostheses.

Furthermore, it seems advisable to recommend removal of the prosthesis if a single adequate course of appropriate antimicrobial treatment has failed to eradicate the infection. In the presence of indications for the removal of the prosthesis, temporizing for more than a few days with antibiotic therapy does not appear to reduce the risk of relapse. The presence of active infection is not a contraindication to cardiac surgery in these patients, but antibiotics should be continued for a total of four to five weeks postoperatively.

Dysfunction of the prosthetic valve or systemic embolism will often be the only evidence of involvement of the prosthesis when blood cultures are negative. Fungi are responsible for many of these infections, and removal of the prosthesis is necessary for cure.

Epidemiologic Considerations

Sources and Prevention

In general, nosocomial infections at the site of a prosthetic implant may arise either from direct contamination at the time of operation or from bacteremic seeding of the prosthesis secondary to another nosocomial focal infection. Appropriate preoperative care and aseptic surgical technique may lessen the risk of the former; those practices described elsewhere in this book relating to the prevention of urinary, respiratory, wound, and intravenous catheter-associated infections will assist in the control of the latter.

PATIENT-CARE PRACTICES. Many operative procedures to implant cardiac or vascular prostheses are semielective, thereby allowing for meticulous preoperative care. Special attention should be given to the preoperative diagnosis and treatment of focal infections and conditions such as asymptomatic bacteriuria. Some surgeons recommend washing the patient's skin with a 3% hexachlorophene emulsion several times a day for several days before the operation. No special precautions or techniques for shaving the operative site have proved advantageous, but shaving should be done immediately before the operative procedures rather than the night before surgery.

Many procedures to implant a cardiovascular prosthesis are so complex and lengthy that eventual breaks in aseptic technique are almost inevitable. Punctured gloves, for example, occur with nearly every sternotomy. In relation to the many opportunities for contamination of the operative field, the low infection rates observed suggest that infections may be caused by either uncommonly massive contamination, unusually virulent microorganisms, or especially dangerous personnel shedders. Nonetheless, firm discipline in the operating room, the avoidance of unnecessary traffic and talking, and the exclusion of personnel with overt skin infections should assist in the control of infection [4].

The development and maintenance of the professional skills of the nursing and technical staff are especially important. The Inter-Society Commission for Heart Disease Resources has recommended guidelines for the clinical and physical environment in which cardiovascular surgery may be performed most effectively [11].

The measures for the prevention of arteriovenous shunt-associated infections are similar to those for the prevention of intravenous catheter-associated infections (Part II, Chapter 25). Because the cannula is exposed on the surface of an extremity, the site is continually subject to microbial contamination from the patient's own flora as well as from external sources, including the dialysis fluid and equipment. The surgically created subcutaneous arteriovenous fistula is used more often than the Silastic-Teflon cannula in most hemodialysis centers, in part because there is a lower risk of infection with the internal shunt.

A topical antimicrobial agent, such as neomycin-polymyxin-bacitracin, and a dry sterile gauze dressing may be placed over the external shunt, which is then covered with an occlusive bandage. The dressing should not be disturbed between dialysis periods. Aseptic technique during dialysis should be used in the care of the external shunt. Personnel who handle the shunt should wear gloves, and both patient and nurse should wear face masks whenever the dressing is removed.

ENVIRONMENTAL FACTORS. The majority of nosocomial infections associated with cardiovascular prostheses are thought to occur as a result of direct contamination of the prosthesis in the operating room. Blood in the heart-lung bypass machine appears to be an important source for this contamination. The fact that the most common microbial species recovered from blood cultures obtained from various sites during bypass are the most common pathogens found in cases of postoperative prosthetic-valve endocarditis has been cited as evidence of the role of contamination of the bypass machine. Indeed, positive cultures of pump-oxygenator blood are associated with an increased risk of later infection. Furthermore, the predominance of gram-positive organisms recovered from these cultures is cited to justify prophylactic treatment of the patient with penicillin, a penicillinase-resistant penicillin, or cephalosporin.

Blood in the operative field is returned by suction tubing to the pump oxygenator for recirculation. These suction lines have been found to yield the highest frequency of positive blood cultures when samples are obtained from several different sites during heart-lung bypass procedures. Nearly 25 percent of blood cultures from this site may be positive. Direct contamination from operating-room air at the site of the turbulent blood-air interface is, of course, suspected. One possible means of partially reducing this source of contamination is clamping the suction tubing when it is not in use.

The instruments and equipment for bypass procedures should be thoroughly cleaned of debris, autoclaved, and assembled under aseptic conditions before use. The use of disposable bubble oxygenators has done much to simplify the problems of sterilization. Many centers use a bacterial filter in the oxygen supply line, because the oxygen itself and the junction between the nonsterile oxygen tank and the oxygenator may be sources for potential contamination.

The operating-room air should have a slight positive pressure in relation to the surrounding areas, and the doors must be kept closed. U.S. Public Health Service standards require at least 12 complete changes of operating-room air each hour, with five changes coming from outside air [12]. There are no controlled data showing a reduction in the incidence of surgical wound infections by laminar airflow systems. Nevertheless, there is heavy pressure for the installation of such equipment in operating rooms where prosthetic orthopedic, cardiovascular, and neurosurgical devices are implanted. The development of clean-room technology and laminar (or unidirectional) airflow systems that are capable of reducing the microbial concentration to less than one organism per cubic foot has provided a research tool for the investigation of the relation of airborne bacteria to wound infection (see Part 2, Chapter 18). Conventional air-conditioning systems, however, are capable of reducing the microbial concentration in operating-room air to between one and three organisms per cubic foot. Nonetheless, it seems advisable to protect protheses from prolonged exposure to operating-room air before their insertion in the patient. The American College of Surgeons issued a statement in 1971 recommending periodic study of airborne contamination in existing surgical facilities and advising continued use of more conventional air-handling systems [1].

A variety of other unproved measures have been recommended to reduce environmental contamination in operating rooms. A few—such as regular cleaning of the operating-room floor with a phenolic disinfectant and the use of disposable, waterproof, paper draping material and surgical gowns—are both reasonable and in widespread use; others—such as changing shoe covers at the entrance to the operating room and passing all traffic over disinfectant-soaked blankets—appear irrational and useless. All such measures should have a secondary role to attention to proper aseptic techniques, hand-scrubbing, and minimizing the number of personnel and traffic within the operating room (see Part I, Chapter 7, Section H).

Inadequate sterilization of the prosthesis before insertion has also been suspected as a cause of subsequent infection. Prosthetic materials that cannot be autoclaved are frequently sterilized by ethylene oxide. Intrinsic contamination is more likely for materials treated with ethylene oxide. Neither of these techniques is used for porcine valves, which are treated with glutaraldehyde. When sterilization is undertaken by a hospital, the process should be monitored with bacterial spore strips. Many surgeons have resorted to soaking the device in an antibiotic-containing solution just before insertion, with the hope of killing any surviving organisms in the interstices of the fabric of the prosthesis. Contamination of the prosthesis could occur from soaking it in a nonsterile antibiotic solution, however, and patients who are allergic to the antibiotics used may be inadvertently exposed to serious reactions by this practice.

PROPHYLACTIC ANTIBIOTICS. The major preventive measure held to be effective by cardiovascular surgeons, and the source of considerable controversy, is the use of prophylactic antimicrobial agents in the perioperative period. Several prospective controlled studies have failed to document a beneficial effect of prophylactic antibiotics, and these studies have shown that infections of sites other than the prosthetic implant are associated more often with antibiotic-resistant pathogens in patients who receive the prophylactic regimen. On the other hand, many large, nonrandomized studies have documented much lower rates of infections at the sites of prosthetic appliances in groups of patients who receive prophylactic antibiotics compared to groups who do not receive prophylaxis.

In the former studies, the low rates of postoperative endocarditis and the small numbers of patients preclude firm conclusions about the effectiveness of prophylaxis, and it appears unlikely that a study that does include enough patients will ever be completed. The latter studies are, of course, uncontrolled and cannot account for the possible effects of improved aseptic technique and superior operative skill, as well as other differences, in the groups with the lower rates of infection.

Antibiotic prophylaxis that is directed at specific pathogens known to be sensitive to the drug will probably be effective. Thus, prophylactic treatment with penicillinase-resistant penicillins probably reduces the incidence of postoperative infection with *S. aureus* and other sensitive pyogenic cocci. This use of antibiotics is well established and will not change unless, or until, infections with antibiotic-resistant microorganisms become recognized with increasing frequency. The task of the hospital epidemiologist is to document and analyze the occurrences of infection so that obsolete or inappropriate prophylaxis will be recognized at the earliest possible time.

The optimal duration of prophylactic treatment has also been controversial: some advocate short perioperative courses, whereas others claim that at least ten days of treatment are required for the prevention of these infections. Longer courses of treatment are considered to increase the risk of infection by some. Since the doses of prophylactic antimicrobial agents used are inadequate to treat established intravascular infection, prolonged periods of chemoprophylaxis appear unnecessary.

Management of Outbreaks

SOURCES AND MODE OF SPREAD. In order to apply control measures for an outbreak of such infections, it is necessary to identify the source and mode of spread of the pathogen. The few reported outbreaks of these infections are inadequate to establish the sources and modes of spread of pathogens responsible for epidemic, as compared to endemic, infections. Postoperative infections of various types due to *Pseudomonas* species in patients undergoing extracorporeal circulation have been associated with the use of quaternary ammonium compounds for "cleaning" mechanical pump oxygenators. The epidemic of *Aspergillus* infections previously mentioned was attributed to defects in the ventilating system of the operating room and postoperative recovery room.

METHODS OF INVESTIGATION. A line-listing of the cases is prepared. Although only a few cases may have occurred, a detailed listing of the clinical and epidemiologic circumstances of each case is made, and each feature shared by two or more cases is expressed as a ratio. The listing should include the dates of onset and the outcome of the infections. Additional factors might include the ages and sexes of the patients, underlying diseases that predispose to such infections, dates of operations, types and suppliers of the prostheses, methods of sterilization and handling of prostheses before insertion, numbers of the operating rooms, names of surgeons and other members of the surgical teams, results of cultures and antibiograms of isolates, prophylactic antimicrobial agents used, and presence of other focal infections. The latter data should also be collected from a group of patients who underwent comparable surgical procedures during the same time period but who did not develop infections associated with their prostheses. Analysis of these data may suggest certain factors associated with the cases that will set directions for the investigation (see Part I, Chapter 5).

Recent operating-room records should be reviewed to determine the total number of operative procedures of a similar nature that have been performed. These procedures should be tabulated separately for periods before and during the epidemic for use in determining changes in the infection rate. At the same time that these data are being collected and analyzed, a review of aseptic techniques, methods for disinfecting equipment, and the mechanics of the ventilating system in the operating room may reveal a productive area for special bacteriologic study.

The pathogen recovered from each case should be saved, whenever possible, both for serum inhibition tests to be used in evaluating treatment and for later laboratory study to characterize the "epidemic strain." Review of the susceptibilities to antimicrobial agents of the pathogens will help to determine whether a single or multiple strains are involved, and such susceptibility data may lead the epidemiologist to recommend changes in prophylactic antibiotic usage.

While the investigation is proceeding, the epidemiologist should recommend a protocol for collecting prospective data from new patients. For example, culture of blood from the bypass machine after each operation, if it is not already being done, will help to establish the frequency of contamination from this source. If such cultures have been routinely performed, an immediate review of the results from pre-epidemic and epidemic periods is useful. Prospective cultures of prostheses just before insertion might also be undertaken, especially when the epidemic strain is an organism that is more likely than others to resist sterilization, or the prostheses are subjected to disinfecting rather than sterilizing procedures. Diphtheroids, staphylococci, and spore-forming bacilli, for example, are more difficult to sterilize than gram-negative bacilli, and mycobacterial species appear to be relatively resistant to certain disinfectants. The temptations to obtain nasopharyngeal or other swabs for culture from personnel and environmental cultures from the operating room should be resisted until the foregoing tasks have been completed. Because the pathogens from these infections are ubiquitous, positive cultures from such human and environmental sources have limited meaning and may be misleading. Cultures should be obtained when a source is found to be epidemiologically relevant, and isolates of appropriate identity should be fully characterized and compared with isolates of the "epidemic strain" from cases.

CONTROL. The measures taken to control an epidemic are determined by the urgency of the problem. In an outbreak with a high attack rate that is recognized as a grave threat to the safe conduct of such operations, it may be necessary to close the operating room temporarily and suspend further procedures. In less urgent circumstances (i.e., usually when the outbreak is insidious and protracted), thoughtful investigation may precede the application of control measures.

Available data should be reported to local and federal health authorities. Pooled data from multiple institutions may be necessary to establish low-frequency, intrinsic contamination of commercially distributed prosthetic materials conclusively.

If the investigation fails to uncover the source of the outbreak, the operating room should be temporarily closed and thoroughly cleaned. The importance of hand-washing and aseptic technique should be stressed to personnel. In some circumstances, discontinuation of the use of ineffective prophylactic antibiotics alone may control the outbreak, even if the source is not found. Prompt removal or elimination of a possible source that is suggested by the epidemiologic investigation, even when the data are inconclusive, will allow the epidemiologist to evaluate his hypothesis through well-planned, continuing surveillance.

References

1. American College of Surgeons. Special Air Systems for Operating Rooms. *Bull. Am. Coll. Surg.* 57:18, 1972.

2. Brewer, L. A., III (Ed.). *Prosthetic Heart Valves.* Springfield, Ill.: Charles C Thomas, 1969.

3. Center for Disease Control. Follow-up on mycobacterial contamination of porcine heart valve prostheses—United States. *Morbid. Mortal. Weekly Rep.* 27:92, 1978.

4. Clark, R. E., Amos, W. C., Higgins, V., Bemberg, K. F., and Weldon, C. S. Infection control in cardiac surgery. *Surgery* 79:89, 1976.

5. Finland, M. Current problems in infective endocarditis with special reference to cases acquired in hospital or after cardiac surgery. *Mod. Concepts Cardiovasc. Dis.* 41:53, 1972.

6. Gage, A. A., Dean, D. C., Schimert, G., and Minsley, N. *Aspergillus* infection after cardiac surgery. *Arch. Surg.* 101:384, 1970.

7. Garner, J. S., Bennett, J. V., Scheckler, W. E., Maki, D. G., and Brachman, P. S. Surveillance of Nosocomial Infections. In *Proceedings of the International Conference on Nosocomial Infections,* Center for Disease Control, August 3–6, 1970. Chicago: American Hospital Association, 1971.

8. Hall, W. J. *Penicillium* endocarditis following open heart surgery and prosthetic valve insertion. *Am. Heart J.* 87:501, 1974.

9. Kaslow, R. A., and Zellner, S. R. Infection in patients on maintenance haemodialysis. *Lancet* 2:117, 1972.

10. Lemire, G. G., Morin, J. E., and Dobell, A. R. C. Pacemaker infections: a 12-year review. *Can. J. Surg.* 18:181, 1975.

11. Scannel, J. C. (Chairman). Optimal resources for cardiac surgery—Report of Inter-Society Commission for Heart Disease Resources. *Circulation* 44:A-221, 1971.

12. U.S. Public Health Service. *General Standards of Construction and Equipment for Hospital and Medical Facilities.* Washington, D.C.: U.S. Government Printing Office (USPHS Publ. No. 930-A-7), revised February 1969.

13. Weinstein, L., and Rubin, R. H. Infective endocarditis—1973. *Prog. Cardiovasc. Dis.* 16:239, 1973.

14. Weinstein, L., and Schlesinger, J. Treatment of infective endocarditis—1973. *Prog. Cardiovasc. Dis.* 16:275, 1973.

15. Willwerth, B. M., and Waldhausen, J. A. Infection of arterial prostheses. *Surg. Gynecol. Obstet.* 139:446, 1974.

18

Infections of Skeletal Prostheses

Jorge A. Franco and
William F. Enneking

Plastic and metal skeletal prostheses have been used by orthopedic surgeons in the treatment of many clinical problems (principally fracture repair and partial joint replacement) for several decades. In the past decade, prostheses capable of totally replacing the hip, knee, and finger joints have reached the clinical level, and others are now on the surgical horizon. Patients who have been in constant pain and unable to walk or take care of themselves can now be successfully rehabilitated by the insertion of such prosthetic devices. Unfortunately, not all these efforts are successful. The leading cause of surgical failure in skeletal implants is infection in or around the prosthetic device. Such infections inevitably lead to compromise or loss of function of the prosthesis and occasionally have led to the death of the patient.

Since total hip replacement (THR) has been studied more extensively from the standpoint of infection than operations involving any other skeletal prosthesis, the ensuing discussion will center about this particular procedure and device. The principles enumerated, however, pertain to all implantable skeletal devices.

Classification of Infections

Wound infections are classified according to their onset into early and late infections.

Early (Acute) Infections

Early infections are defined as those that occur during the first postoperative month. As a general rule, all such infections should be considered to be nosocomial. Early infections are subdivided according to whether they are superficial or deep to the fascia lata.

Suprafascial (superficial) infections are the most common of all the surgical infections in THR, and they possess the characteristics of incisional wound infections (Part II, Chapter 16). Since superficial infections have a good prognosis compared to deep infections, they

In part supported by Clinical Research Center Grant 5-M01-RR00082-12.

are usually omitted in the majority of reports dealing with THR complications.

Deep wound infections include all infections extending deep to the fascia lata. In large series, these infections are much less common than the late, deep infections. This difference appears to be related to increasing awareness by surgeons that has resulted in stricter aseptic discipline in the operating room.

Late Infections

As the name indicates, these are the infections that present after the patient has resumed painless function. Such deep infections are noted some months or even years after apparently successful THR, and they represent a mixture of nosocomial and community-acquired infections. Insufficient information exists to permit reliable differentiation of these.

Incidence

The incidence of surgical wound infections involving the use of skeletal prostheses varies widely according to the type of prosthesis used.

Infection rates range from approximately 6 percent in prosthetic knee replacement [6] in patients undergoing correction of scoliosis with Harrington instrumentation [7] to about 2 percent in patients undergoing prosthetic hip replacement (Table 18-1). This variation in the infection rate is not completely understood, but it could be related to factors such as the different anatomic site, selection of patients, experience with the procedure, and so on.

The rate of deep infections following THR varies among institutions, but it is recognized that the usual, expected wound infection rate is from 1 to 3 percent. Table 18-1 displays the major series of deep wound infection associated with THR that have been reported in the literature. The composite mean wound infection rate for the entire series of published reports is 2.1 percent (see Table 18-1).

Pathogens

The principal pathogenic organisms reported in a composite of publications on deep wound

Table 18-1. Rates of Deep Wound Infection in Total Hip Replacement Surgery

Author(s)	Country	Number of operations	Deep wound infection rate	Duration of follow-up
Bentley and Duthie [10]	England	229	2.3%	1 to 4 years
Bergstrom et al.[a] [10]	Sweden	283	4.9%	—
Buchholtz and Noack [10]	W. Germany	3205	2.3%	1 to 5 years
Chapchal et al. [10]	Netherlands	340	0%	3 months to 4 years
Charnely[b] [3]	England	5600	1.6%	>2 to 10 years
Eftekhar and Stinchfield [10]	U.S.A.	700	0.4%	6 months to 3.5 years
Fitzgerald et al. [5]	U.S.A.	658	1.1%	>18 months
Freeman et al. [10]	Scotland	360	3.6%	6 months to 6 years
Johnston [10]	U.S.A.	360	3.6%	—
Lazanski [10]	U.S.A.	501	0.8%	6 months to 5 years
Leinbach and Barlow [10]	U.S.A.	700	1.0%	6 months to 4 years
Moczyuski et al.[a] [10]	U.S.A.	237	9.7%	—
Murray [10]	U.S.A.	808	1.5%	3 months to 4 years
Nicholson [10]	New Zealand	1666	2.5%	1 to 2 years
Ring [10]	England	887	0.7%	1 to 8 years
Wilson et al.[c] [12]	U.S.A.	436	9.8%	—
Total		16,970	2.1%	

[a] Authors have reported a decrease in infection rate to less than 2.5 percent in their latest cases.
[b] Author has reported a decrease in infection rate to less than 1 percent in later cases.
[c] Superficial infections and deep infections were not separated.

infections following THR are listed in Table 18-2. In practice, isolation of suspected microorganisms from an infected prosthetic hip is not always easy. In some large series of THR, the microbial cause of deep wound infections has not been documented in at least 12 percent of the cases [3]. Because of this problem, surgeons tend to consider the isolation of any organisms from deep tissue as conclusive evidence of infection. This is compounded by the fact that a normally saprophytic organism, *Staphylococcus epidermidis,* is one of the leading causes of wound infection in THR.

Staphylococcus aureus

Coagulase-positive *S. aureus* causes about one-half of all deep infections following THR (Table 18-2). This species is seen much more frequently among early than late infections. For additional microbiologic, clinical, and epidemiologic features, the reader should refer to Part II, Chapters 16 and 20.

Staphylococcus epidermidis

The term "coagulase-negative staphylococci" is used by most clinical laboratories to encompass all members of the family Micrococcaceae other than *S. aureus.* The majority of clinical microbiology laboratories do not distinguish *S. epidermidis* from other Micrococcaceae species; hence, the relative frequency of these two groups of organisms in reported infections is not known, and potentially important clinical and epidemiologic differences among these organisms remain undisclosed. We will refer to coagulase-negative staphylococci as *S. epidermidis.*

S. epidermidis has assumed the role of a major pathogen in implant surgery, and it causes approximately 29 percent of all infections following THR (see Table 18-2), including approximately 21 percent of the early acute infections and "mixed" infections, and approximately 41 percent of the late infections. The true incidence of infection due to *S. epidermidis* is very difficult to calculate. There has been a tendency to consider its mere presence as infection. Therefore, the infection rate of 29 percent due to these organisms may be somewhat inflated, especially in early infections. Undoubtedly, *S. epidermidis* is a bona fide pathogen in late infections after THR operations, but the reported incidence is probably elevated because of the ubiquity of this organism.

Aerobic Gram-Negative Rods

These organisms are responsible for a much smaller proportion of THR infections than other surgical wound infections (see Part II, Chapters 13 and 16). Gram-negative rods are isolated from about one-fifth of early, deep THR wound infections and from only about one-tenth of late infections (see Table 18-2).

Anaerobes

Anaerobic surgical wound infections are receiving increasing attention. In THR patients, anaerobic infections have seldom been reported, and anaerobes have been infrequently recovered from the wound at the time of surgery. Whether this really represents a low incidence of anaerobic infections, a lack of proper anaerobic techniques in specimen collection and transport, or a lack of adequate facilities to isolate strict anaerobes is not clear at this moment. It is conceivable that some of the "sterile" wound infections are due to anaerobic organisms.

Microbiologic Diagnosis

Microbiologic findings can only be considered as supportive evidence in the diagnosis of hip infections. Clinical diagnosis obviously is of

Table 18-2. Bacterial Etiology of Deep Wound Infections Following 17,170 THR Operations

Organism	Early infections	Late infections	Total
Staphylococcus aureus	58%	39%	50%
Staphylococcus epidermidis	21%	41%	29%
Gram-negative rods	17%	10%	14%
Others[a]	4%	5%	7%
Overall	60%	40%	100%

[a] Includes group-D streptococci, group-A streptococci, *Peptococcus,* group-B streptococci, *Peptostreptococcus,* and anaerobic *Corynebacterium.*

primary importance, but the identification of the pathogenic organisms involved is highly valuable, especially for choosing the appropriate antimicrobial therapy.

The following points should be kept in mind when collecting specimens or interpreting the result of cultures:

Swabs and Liquid Specimens

A superficial (skin) swab of the wound is not a suitable specimen, because in most cases, it is impossible to determine whether the isolates are members of the normal skin flora or the causative agents of the infection. These swab specimens are also not adequate for the recovery of anaerobic organisms.

When pus is present, it should be aspirated with a needle and immediately taken to the laboratory. This is the best specimen (short of a tissue biopsy) for recovering both anaerobic and aerobic organisms. If possible, such a specimen should be collected before starting antibiotic therapy.

Biopsy Specimens

When tissue from biopsy is sent to the laboratory for culture, deep tissue should be used in order to minimize contamination; the specimens should be handled as cautiously as possible to avoid excessive contamination of the tissue with gloves, gown, and the like. The presence of one or two colonies in a tissue specimen must be interpreted with caution. *S. epidermidis,* diphtheroids, micrococci, and some streptococci are ubiquitous organisms in the surgical theatre, and airborne contamination with these organisms is a possibility.

A negative Gram stain of a tissue section is not to be interpreted as indicating the absence of infection, since a small number of bacteria might not be detected by this technique. The appearance of inflammatory cells is probably a better indication of the presence of infection, but it must be kept in mind that the occurrence of some granulomatous tissue may be directly related to the presence of the acrylic cement, the prosthesis itself, or both. As a part of exploratory surgery in a clinically suspected, infected hip without microbiologic evidence of infection, multiple specimens

should be submitted to the laboratory, including pieces of deep tissue, cement, pseudocapsule, and so on. Recovery of the same organisms from several areas is important in that such data should rule out specimen contamination.

Specimens for Anaerobes

For the best recovery of anaerobic organisms, the laboratory must be provided with a proper specimen. All liquid specimens should be collected in syringes to maintain anaerobic conditions. Transport tubes for tissue or swabs must be oxygen-free; these tubes are now commercially available under a variety of brand names. Finally, the laboratory must have appropriate anaerobic isolation and identification equipment.

Predisposing Factors

Operative Factors

It has long been recognized that bacteria produce necrosis of the bone, when an infection occurs, by destroying the tenuous blood supply in the marrow spaces or haversian canals. Bacteria in this environment are relatively inaccessible to host defense mechanisms and antibiotics. Thus, the presence of necrotizing organisms in bone leads to persistent infection until such time as the necrotic sequestrated bone is spontaneously extruded or removed.

The insertion of a prosthetic device compromises the blood supply of the microenvironment about the implant. Bleeding from bone cannot be controlled in the usual surgical fashion; therefore, all skeletal implants are surrounded by a hematoma. In addition, the use of exothermal plastics for skeletal fixation of skeletal implants produces thermally induced necrosis in the microenvironment of the implant. The presence of necrosis and hematoma provides favorable growth conditions for microorganisms.

THR surgery is associated with the implantation of two large foreign bodies. It has been established experimentally that fewer *S. aureus* organisms are needed to establish an infection in the presence of a foreign body.

Finally, a large wound is exposed to contamination for a relatively long period of time (two or three hours) in technically difficult cases or in the hands of inexperienced operators.

These factors conspire to produce a high risk of infection. This risk, coupled with the serious disability from infected implants, has led to major efforts to prevent postoperative sepsis associated with these procedures.

Previous Hip Surgery

A large percentage of THR patients with infection have had previous hip operations. It is well known that the incidence of infection in refined, clean cases is lower than that in those operated on previously [8]. Approximately one-third of THR operations are now being done after the failure of other types of implants. These "idiopathic" painful hips are quite often due to occult infection. Despite negative preoperative cultures, the incidence of infection in THR is twice as high in such cases compared to the incidence in previously unoperated hips. Most surgeons prefer to remove such suspect devices, carefully obtain culture and biopsy specimens from the wound, and close it. If subsequent studies indicate that occult infection is not present and if the wound is well healed, subsequent THR might be contemplated with relative safety. Others prefer to rely on Gram-stained smears, frozen sections, and gross inspection to reach an intraoperative decision.

In cases where clinically obvious, occult, deep infection has compromised a previous implant, the safest management is implant removal, wound drainage or suction irrigation, appropriate antibiotic treatment, and a delay of one to two years with no signs of inflammation prior to undertaking THR. Some advocate implant excision, radical debridement, antibiotic lavage, and THR with massive antibiotic treatment. This aggressive approach has brought about better functional surgical results in some cases, but these are counterbalanced by disastrous exacerbation in others.

Other Factors

Another factor contributing to infection is obesity. Conclusive data are not available, but circumstantial evidence points out that obese patients are more prone to develop superficial wound infections than are nonobese patients. This difference appears to be related to the heavy retraction required on the subcutaneous tissue, which leads to necrosis and difficulty in closing the subcutaneous space in obese patients.

A large number of patients receive steroid therapy for rheumatoid arthritis. It has been shown by Charnley [3] that these patients are at a higher risk of infection than other candidates for THR.

General Control Measures

Orthopedic surgeons involved in THR operations have gone to great lengths in an attempt to control surgical wound infections. The pioneers in THR experienced an initial infection rate of 8 to 10 percent. As noted in Table 18-1, the infection rate has decreased in the last decade to approximately 2 percent. Although some surgeons have emphasized antibiotic prophylaxis, others are advocates of "clean-room" surgery employing either a unidirectional airflow system (UAFS) or the use of ultraviolet (UV) lights. In all the series reported in Table 18-1, prophylactic systemic antibiotics, clean-air rooms, or both were used except in those of Chapchal and associates [10], Nicholson [10], and Bucholtz and Noack [10]. The last authors used gentamicin mixed with the methylmethacrylate.

Surgical Techniques

An awareness of the infection problem in THR has led to the "rediscovery" of strict discipline in the operating room, with emphasis on meticulous aseptic surgery, double gloving, double masking, and the use of hoods and body-exhaust systems that employ relatively impermeable gowns. Such techniques have been accepted as routine procedure in THR surgery. Preparation of the skin before surgery is done meticulously because of the closeness of the surgical area to the perineum. Proper draping of the incision is important to avoid endogenous contamination. The use of self-sealing plastic drapes about the perineum has been of particular help in decreasing wound contamination with perineal flora.

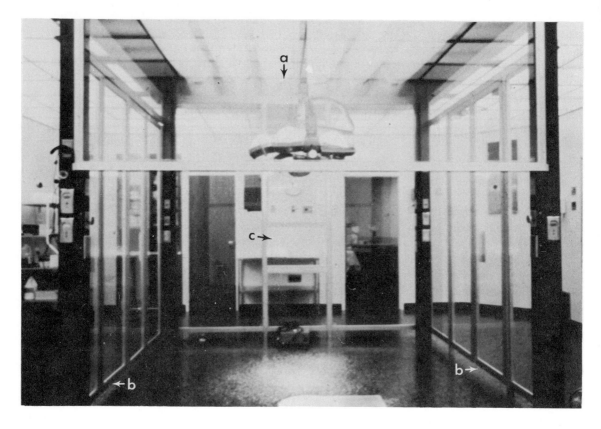

Figure 18-1. A vertical unidirectional air-flow system. Air enters from the ceiling of the enclosure through HEPA filters and flows downward (*a*) to exit beneath the enclosing walls (*b*). A pass-through window (*c*) serves for instrument exchange. The opening for the patient in the foreground is sealed by a plastic drape that leaves the patient's head and neck and anesthesia personnel outside the enclosure.

An improvement in skin closure techniques has been suggested by Charnley [3], who recommends the use of the retention (pull-out) sutures for wound closure after THR. Lazansky [10] has shown a statistically significant reduction in the incidence of superficial wound infections using this technique.

Clean-Air Room System
The "clean-air" room has become very popular among orthopedic surgeons, mainly because of the enthusiastic support of Charnley, Nelson, and others. The clean-air room usually has a unidirectional air-flow system (UAFS) installed in a plexiglass or glass enclosure to

which only the surgical personnel are allowed access. In most clean-air systems, the surgeons and the supportive personnel inside the enclosure also wear body-exhaust suits.

UAFS equipment is capable of delivering a high volume of unidirectional air that has been filtered by high-efficiency particulate aerosol (HEPA) filters capable of removing more than 99 percent of particles greater than 3 μg in size. This equipment provides an air volume sufficient to exchange the air of a room at a rate of up to 300 changes of room air per hour (Fig. 18-1).

Body-exhaust suits consist of a helmet attached to a vacuum pump that is capable of sucking out all the expired air of the surgeons, thus controlling the microbial fallout from the head, neck, and other body surfaces of the surgeons.

The surgical enclosure unit usually consists of a series of transparent panels with dimensions of up to 10 feet by 20 feet. In addition to providing particulate-free air, the enclosure insures restriction of traffic about the operating table. Furthermore, the body-exhaust suits impose both discipline and close surgical teamwork. Many consider these side benefits as significant as the "clean" air, but feel they can be achieved without the inconvenience and expense of the system. The efficacy of such systems in reducing airborne particulate and microbial contamination at the periphery of the wound has been established in many studies. Whether or not this reduction in contamination significantly influences wound infection rates is unknown. The data available for clean-room surgery have not established that there is a significant decrease in the number of wound infections.

The experience of the authors with a clean-room system is that the air is indeed "cleaner" in terms of particles and bacteria. When serial, quantitative wound cultures were done in a large series of cases, however, there was no significant difference between the clean room and a conventional room in either the quantity or the types of bacteria recovered from the wound itself.

These results suggest that airborne wound contamination in a conventional room with adequate air handling (7 to 12 changes of room air per hour) is not significantly higher than in a clean room if strict surgical technique is followed. The question of whether or not a clean-air system is really a necessity in controlling sepsis in THR cannot be answered in absolute terms. It would appear that the wound infection rates under optimal conventional surgical conditions with thoughtful antibiotic therapy and proper patient selection are approximately the same as they are when the surgical conditions are modestly improved with clean-air systems without antibiotics. Whether to use a clean room would then seem to require an institutional judgment based on local conditions, rather than a decision based on a universal rule.

Prophylactic Antibiotic Therapy

A national survey showed that 87 percent of orthopedic surgeons used antibiotic prophylaxis in total joint replacements [9]. This figure is not surprising, because the use of prophylactic antibiotics in THR has been widely advo-

cated. Whether or not prophylactic antibiotics are necessary to maintain a low infection rate is not definite at this time. Double-blind studies have shown that in an institution with an unusually high incidence of *S. aureus* infection, the use of cloxacillin reduces the infection rate significantly [4]. Prophylactic antibiotics would appear to be indicated when there is an unusually high institutional infection rate or when the patient is believed to be at an exceptionally high risk of infection, that is, patients undergoing THR in a previously suspected, infected hip or patients undergoing exploratory or corrective surgery following active hip infection. Whether antibiotics are indicated in low-risk situations depends on the balance between the modest reduction to be expected in infection rate weighed against the undesirable effects of such prophylaxis. Reports of undesirable side effects following the use of prophylactic antibiotics, the emergence of antibiotic-resistant organisms, alteration of the normal flora, allergic side effects, and so on, abound in the literature, and the surgeon must be aware that the routine use of prophylactic antibiotics in the absence of a "real" indication may be more dangerous to the patient than beneficial (see Part I, Chapter 11).

S. aureus, as previously mentioned, is the leading cause of infection in THR surgery. If prophylactic antibiotics are to be used to prevent *S. aureus* infection, a semisynthetic, penicillinase-resistant penicillin (e.g., methicillin) should be given. The timing of the dosage is critical. It has been established both clinically and experimentally that if optimal results are to be expected from prophylactic antibiotics, the antibiotic concentration in the tissues must be high at the time of surgery (when inoculation with organisms occurs) or very shortly thereafter. Prophylactic antibiotics should be parenterally administered, beginning one hour prior to surgery or at the time of anesthetic induction, and they should be continued for the remainder of the first postoperative day. In patients who are allergic to penicillin, lincomycin could be substituted. Most surgeons recommend continuing the administration of prophylactic antibiotics for a longer period than the one mentioned above. There is no clinical evidence supporting the use of prolonged prophylactic antibiotics in THR, however, and experimental evidence indicates that prolonged treatment is unnecessary [1,3]. Furthermore, prolonged antibiotic prophylaxis may create serious complications.

Early Deep Wound Infections
Clinical Features

MANIFESTATIONS AND MANAGEMENT. The prompt clinical diagnosis of postoperative wound infections following THR surgery is very important, because the earlier the treatment is started, the better the chances are of salvaging the prosthesis.

Acute, deep infections present two to five days following surgery, and they are associated with fever, leukocytosis, and red-hot inflammation. Frequently, pus drains from the wound. Such infected patients should initially be treated vigorously with high doses of the appropriate antibiotics and incision and drainage of the wound. In most instances, subsequent removal of the device is required to achieve closure of the draining sinuses. As long as such preliminary steps contain the infection, the removal of the prosthesis should be delayed until it is certain that removal is inevitable. This state is manifested by either recurrent dislocation or gross loosening of the device. Once it is clearly established that an early, acute infection is superficial to the fascia lata, it must be decompressed to prevent deep extension. These infections cause little systemic toxicity, and when evacuated, they show no deep communication with the device. Should drainage persist an unusual length of time, communication must be sought assiduously by fluoroscopy and arthrography.

ANTIBIOTIC THERAPY. Therapy should be directed toward the organisms involved, and it should be based on the antibiogram of the pathogenic organism. If an infection is suspected and the culture results are not available, antibiotic treatment should be started immediately in order to prevent the involvement of the prosthesis. *S. aureus* is responsible for about 60 percent of these infections (see Table 18-2); therefore, an antistaphylococcal drug

such as methicillin is the antibiotic of choice. *S. epidermidis* causes about 20 percent of acute, deep infections, and methicillin will effectively treat sensitive strains. Resistance of *S. epidermidis* to methicillin and similar penicillins, however, is frequently found in some hospitals, and a cephalosporin antibiotic, rather than methicillin, might be chosen for initial therapy in these circumstances (see Part II, Chapter 17). An aminoglycoside antibiotic should be given in addition, because about 17 percent of acute infections are caused by gram-negative organisms (see Table 18-2). As soon as the laboratory results are available, the antibiotic therapy should be adjusted according to the type of organisms found.

In most hospitals in the United States, methicillin-resistant strains of *S. aureus* are rare, but they have been reported in Europe. In England and Germany, there are increasing problems with methicillin-resistant *S. aureus,* which point out the importance of performing adequate antibiotic susceptibility tests (see Part I, Chapter 11). If an antibiotic must be chosen in the absence of susceptibility testing, the physician should use antibiotics that are most effective against the organisms that have been isolated from acute, deep infections in his hospital. Updated information regarding susceptibility patterns of organisms in the hospital should be routinely available through the clinical microbiology laboratory or the hospital epidemiologist.

Sources and Modes of Acquisition

The sources and modes of acquisition of organisms that produce surgical wound infections are systematically described in Part II, Chapter 16. Only those features especially pertinent to infected THR prostheses will be described in the following section.

GLOVE PUNCTURES. Direct contact spread by hands of personnel likely plays a prominent role. Puncture holes in the surgical gloves at the time of surgery is a common finding, especially in orthopedic surgery, where surgeons handle hammers, saws, power tools, sharp wires, and the like. It has been shown by Wise and colleagues [13] that up to 1.8×10^5 organisms can be cultured from inside the gloves after a surgical procedure. Ninety-eight percent of the gloves cultured were positive for microorganisms, and 14 percent of them were positive for *S. aureus*. The implication of this study is simply that when gloves are punctured during surgery by a surgeon who is a heavy carrier of *S. aureus,* the wound will be inoculated with a sufficiently large number of organisms to cause wound infection.

POSTOPERATIVE HAND TRANSMISSION. Transmission from the hands of personnel after surgery (i.e., in the wards, intensive-care units, or wherever) is a more controversial subject, but it is doubtful that it plays a significant role in THR patients, because the wound is covered at the time of surgery and the dressings are not usually removed for five to seven days. This is sufficient time for the skin to seal; therefore, the opportunity for infection to enter from the "outside" appears to be remote.

S. aureus SHEDDERS. *Staphylococcus aureus* resides in the skin as well as in the anterior nares of many of the surgical personnel and patients. Desquamated skin loaded with *S. aureus* is released in the air and can settle into the open wound. It is conceivable that these organisms may cause a wound infection in this type of high-risk procedure. Of course, this will require that a member of the surgical team is able to disseminate large numbers of *S. aureus* into the environment. It has been our experience that when personnel demonstrated to be "shedders" are present on a surgical team that is using clean-room techniques, *S. aureus* has not been recovered from the air, and no *S. aureus* infections attributable to such shedders have developed. This has prompted us to study the role of *S. aureus* disseminators in surgery, and a prospective study is currently under way.

It should be said that the importance of "shedders" is open to controversy. Many experienced orthopedic surgeons consider this the most important component in implant wound infections. As a consequence, many orthopedic surgeons are carefully evaluating the use of clean-room technology in order to control this potential mode of spread.

AIRBORNE SPREAD. Airborne spread from sources other than the patient and surgical personnel that leads to wound contamination and infection does not appear to be an important component in the epidemiology of early, deep, surgical wound infections. Filtration of the air and improved air-conditioning systems have controlled the spread of organisms from the outside as well as from adjacent wards.

ENDOGENOUS SOURCES. These are clearly a source of infection in many surgical wounds, and skeletal implants are no exception. The number of infections of endogenous origin, as compared to other sources of contamination, has not been clearly established. It is highly probable that some of the acute implant infections and a larger proportion of the late infections are endogenous.

Prevention

CLEAN-ROOM SYSTEM. Obviously, an institution with a high acute infection rate, in which surgical conditions are less than optimal, and in which drug-resistant organisms are prevalent, would do well to consider seriously the use of a "clean room." The system does not make up for poor surgical technique any more than antibiotics do. Of necessity, it does impose a discipline on personnel who, in many hospitals, are not within the direct control of the surgeon. Certainly the benefit of a clean room is minimal in institutions where the surgical and microbiologic conditions are adequate.

INVESTIGATION AND ATTACK OF CAUSES. When the infection rate is above the expected range of 1 to 3 percent, the situation deserves a thoughtful approach. If there is such an infection rate, a blind, injudicious rush to institute control measures should be avoided. Rather, attempts first should be made to find out why the infection rate is high. The first steps are to review the surgical techniques and to conduct epidemiologic studies of the infections (see Part II, Chapter 16, and Part I, Chapter 5).

Carriers (i.e., shedders) that disseminate *S. aureus* into the environment may be responsible for surgical infections, but the mere presence of a carrier on the surgical team is not enough to consider this person as a dangerous source of staphylococcal infections. If staphylococcal strains from a carrier have the same characteristics, including antibiograms, as those recovered from infected wounds, however, this should be sufficient to incriminate the carrier presumptively as a dangerous shedder. Epidemiologic incrimination of such a carrier requires the demonstration of a significantly higher risk of infection with the "epidemic strain" among patients whose THR operations are attended by the carrier than there is among patients whose THR procedures are not attended by the carrier. Such carriers should be managed as indicated in Part II, Chapter 16.

If surgical personnel are the sources of sporadic *S. aureus* infections, special efforts—such as the use of UAFS, body-exhaust suits, impermeable gowns, and the like—may be employed in order to minimize shedding. If the strains are usually traced to the patients (i.e., are endogenous), the method of preparation of the surgical area before surgery should be reviewed, and antibiotic prophylaxis should be considered.

Late Deep Wound Infections

Clinical Features

MANIFESTATIONS. It is necessary to emphasize the importance of the supplementary use of acrylics in implant fixation and its relationship to late deep wound infections. In order to fix the prosthesis to the bone, the acrylic is used as a "cement." Loosening of the prosthesis is one of the universal symptoms of late infections. A few bacteria causing bone resorption at the interface between the bone and the acrylic are sufficient to cause surgical failure. *S. epidermidis* is of special importance in this regard, since it is a very frequent contaminant in surgical wounds. Even though these organisms are considered to be of relatively low virulence, they are capable of causing bone resorption with subsequent loosening of the prosthesis. *S. epidermidis* is about twice as frequent in late infections than in early infections, and it slightly surpasses *S. aureus* as a cause of late deep infections (41 percent versus 39 percent, respectively; see Table 18-2). Gram-negative rods are uncommon causes of late infections.

Late deep wound infections present months or years after surgery. Due to their usually in-

sidious nature, a high index of suspicion is necessary in order to establish the diagnosis at the earliest possible time. Early warnings are continuous pain in the hip area and a slightly elevated erythrocyte sedimentation rate (ESR). Fever and leukocytosis are usually absent. The first suggestive sign of the presence of late infections is loosening of the prosthesis, which is usually detected roentgenographically. Periosteal, new bone formation about the femoral stem-acrylic complex is usually associated with loosening, and this may be the initial sign of deep, occult infection. Prosthetic loosening is considered by many surgeons to be due almost exclusively to latent infections. Mechanical loosening of the prosthesis can also occur as a late complication in the absence of infection, and its appearance on roentgenograms will be similar to that of "infective" loosening.

All late infections are not insidious, and some present with the typical characteristics of acute, deep wound infections, namely, fever, leukocytosis, abscess formation with or without sinus tracts, inflammation, and so on.

MANAGEMENT. In general, the late deep wound infections resolve only after the prosthesis is removed. In a few instances, hip function may be salvaged by the removal of the loose device, debridement of the surrounding infected tissue, suction, irrigation, and the administration of antibiotics. Led by Bucholtz [10] in West Germany, many surgeons recommend the insertion of a new prosthesis using antibiotics (e.g., gentamicin or, in some cases, erythromycin) mixed with the fixing methylmethacrylate. There are insufficient data at the present time to determine whether or not this approach is useful. Experimental studies [11] have shown that the activity of gentamicin incorporated in methylmethacrylate is detectable for more than 70 weeks. Further research in this particular area is needed to determine the usefulness of such an approach for the treatment, prevention, or both, of infection following THR surgery.

ANTIBIOTIC THERAPY. Antibiotic treatment in patients with infections of insidious onset can be postponed until the identification of the microorganisms and their antibiotic sensitivity patterns are established. This postponement is possible because by the time the infection is diagnosed, extensive involvement is present. When the culture reports are negative and a clinical diagnosis of infection is strongly suspected, the following factors should be taken into consideration in choosing an antibiotic: Late infections are almost always (about 80 percent) due to staphylococci, either *S. aureus* or *S. epidermidis*. Negative culture results may be obtained because of a failure to isolate strict anaerobic organisms; Gram stains have been known to be positive and wound cultures negative. In such cases, guidance in choosing appropriate antibiotics may be provided by the morphology and staining characteristics of the organisms; gram-negative organisms are rarely involved in late infections.

In summary, an antistaphylococcal agent will usually be the drug of choice; preferably, one may be used that will be adequate for coagulase-negative staphylococci (see earlier comments about therapy of early infections). When anaerobes are suspected, clindamycin seems to be a good choice, and *S. aureus* and *S. epidermidis* may also be susceptible to this drug. The choice of therapy for *S. epidermidis* infection should depend, whenever possible, on the antibiogram of the isolated pathogen. Choosing an antibiotic in the absence of laboratory results is difficult, because *S. epidermidis* strains vary greatly in terms of their antibiotic susceptibility patterns.

Diagnostic Considerations

The following systematic approach is useful in evaluating the presence of latent deep infection about a skeletal prosthesis in a patient with a history of continuous pain accompanied by an elevated erythrocyte sedimentation rate.

ROENTGENOGRAPHY. Roentgenograms should be evaluated to determine whether or not the following indications of infections are present:

Loosening of the prosthesis is a common sign, but it is not diagnostic of infection. This diagnosis may require both fluoroscopy and arthrography. The arthrograms are performed to find out whether or not the injected dye can be seen in the interface between the acrylic cement and the bone; this test is sometimes positive even when the roentgenograms show no apparent loosening (Fig. 18-2). Arthrograms are also valuable to visualize abscess cavities and to determine whether sinus tracts communicate with the prosthesis. Periosteal reactive bone formation is another common finding in infection. Bone resorption about the cement, if present, will facilitate the diagnosis of osteomyelitis, and it is the most reliable roentgenographic sign of infection about a prosthesis (see Fig. 18-2).

JOINT ASPIRATION. The aspiration of a prosthetic hip joint to obtain material for microbiologic examination is technically difficult. The pseudocapsule must be entered with the needle; therefore, an arthrogram may be needed to determine the position of the needle.

RADIONUCLIDE SCINTIMETRY. The use of this technique has been suggested in the diagnosis of hip infections. Scintimetric results may be positive in the absence of positive roentgenographic findings. Scintimetry may also occasionally sharply delineate whether the acetabular component, the femoral component, or both are involved. Care should be taken in the interpretation of bone scintimetric results, however, because high scintimetric values may be due to periarticular bone formation rather than infection.

BIOPSY OF THE CAPSULE. Frequently, the definitive diagnosis of infection requires examination of a biopsy specimen from the capsule. Biopsy specimens are usually obtained as part of the surgical procedure to remove the prosthetic device when it must be removed because of loosening. The material obtained should be from the deep tissue or bone in order to minimize contamination. The material should be sent for microbiologic culture and for histologic examination (see Microbiologic Diagnosis, above). It is important to realize that chronic granulation of tissue is normally found about the prosthesis. This lining tissue is covered by a fibrinous membrane, and by itself is not a diagnostic sign of an infective process.

Sources and Modes of Acquisition

The sources of organisms that cause late infections are puzzling. It has been previously felt that they are acquired at the time of surgery and remain dormant until the infection is de-

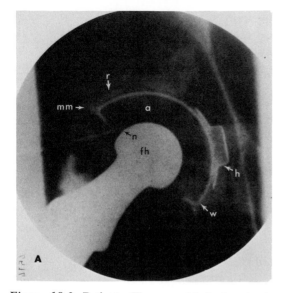
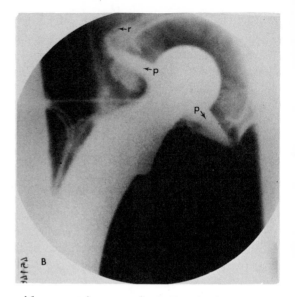

Figure 18-2. Patient, 67 years old, had pain for two months following 14 months of pain-free function. After THR, there were no systemic or laboratory manifestations of infection. Cultures obtained during the procedure showed no growth.

A. An AP view of the prosthesis. The tip of the needle (*n*) is in the articulation of the metallic prosthetic femoral head (*fh*) and the radiolucent polyethylene acetabular component (*a*). The methylmethacrylate used to bond the polyethylene socket to the adjacent bone is made radiodense by adding barium to it (*mm*). The circular wire (*w*) marks the junction between the plastic socket and the bonding methylmethacrylate. The wire "hat" (*h*) restrains methylmethacrylate from entering the pelvis. There is a distinct line of bone resorption (*r*) between the bone-methylmethacrylate interface that suggests loosening.

B. After aspiration, an injection of opaque dye outlines the cavity about the prosthetic joint (*p*). Dye can be seen in the zone of resorption (*r*), which positively indicates loosening of the prosthesis and is highly suggestive of indolent infection. Culture of the aspirant yielded coagulase-negative staphylococci.

tected. Alternatively, the organisms may be seeded into the area via the bloodstream from distant focuses; for example, brushing the teeth may cause transient bacteremias.

Charnley [3] and Ericson and associates [4] have shown a reduction in the incidence of late infections when control measures were instituted in the surgical theater. Their results suggest that at least a portion of the late infections are acquired at the time of surgery. Further

evidence against a principal role for endogenous sources of late infections may be provided by the profile of causative agents, since this profile differs markedly from that of naturally occurring bacterial endocarditis (mainly viridans streptococci), and the latter infections clearly derive from bacteremic "seeding."

Controversy continues as to whether these late infections are mainly acquired at the time of surgery (i.e., are nosocomial) or are due to hematogenous spread months or years after surgery (i.e., are community-acquired). There is not enough evidence at this time to determine which is the most important route of infection. It seems clear, however, that endogenous sources and acquisition by direct and indirect contact at the time of surgery are each responsible for some infections.

Finally, in reference to endogenous infection, it is worth pointing out that many patients become colonized with *S. aureus* after admission. This colonization may be the source of a subsequent "endogenous" infection. Persistent colonization may be important, because a number of the THR patients require bilateral hip replacements involving two different periods of hospitalization.

Prevention

Prevention of infections with *S. epidermidis,* the most common cause of late infections, appears to be a very difficult task because of the large numbers of *S. epidermidis* organisms in the environment. The number of *S. epidermidis* organisms needed to establish a wound infection in a system including acrylics, polyethylene, metal, and bone is not known. Studies are presently under way to determine the size of inoculum needed to cause such infection in experimental animals. If a large inoculum is needed to initiate an infection (more than 100 organisms), then preventive measures such as clean-air systems (e.g., UAFS) may be helpful in reducing the number of organisms settling in the wound during THR operations (with UAFS, less than five microorganisms are calculated to settle in a wound per hour).

The use of prophylactic antibiotics to reduce the likelihood of endogenous contamination may be important if there is a significantly large number of endogenous infections. Prophylactic antibiotic administration for THR patients undergoing procedures that are likely to result in transient bacteremia might well be justified, and a controlled study of the effectiveness of this approach might provide further insights into the relative importance of endogenous sources.

For infections that are acquired at the time of surgery, remain dormant, and subsequently cause late wound infection, all the preventive measures described above for the prevention of early infections should be used. "Clean" rooms or prophylactic antibiotics at the time of surgery should be useful in the prevention of such infections.

In many institutions, careful microbiologic wound monitoring is now taking place. Correlation of these data with the microbiologic data from late infections could provide a clue to the route of infection. The scant data available at this time suggest no correlation between wound contamination at the time of surgery and the occurrence of late infection in well over half the cases so studied.

Conclusion

The advent of total hip replacement (THR) has focused attention on the disastrous effect of wound infections upon skeletal implants. Studies of such problems have brought to light clinical and microbiologic information applicable to all skeletal implants. THR surgery has also displayed some unique problems related to such implants, but it has provided a model for gathering data of general importance to all surgical endeavors.

References

1. Bowers, W. H., Wilson, F. C., and Green, W. B. Antibiotic prophylaxis in experimental bone infections. *J. Bone Joint Surg.* [Am.] 55:795, 1973.
2. Burke, J. F. The effective period of preventative antibiotic action in experimental incision and dermal lesions. *Surgery* 50:161, 1961.
3. Charnley, J. Postoperative infections after total hip replacement with special reference to air contamination in the operating room. *Clin. Orthop.* 87:162, 1972.
4. Ericson, C., Lidgren, L., and Lindberg, L. Cloxacillin in the prophylaxis of postoperative infections of the hip. *J. Bone Joint Surg.* [Am.] 55:808, 1973.
5. Fitzgerald, R. H., Jr., Peterson, I. F. A., Washington, J. A., II, Van Scoy, R. E., and Coventry, M. C. Bacterial colonization of wounds and sepsis in total hip arthroplasties. *J. Bone Joint Surg.* [Am.] 55:1242, 1973.
6. Kettelkamp, D. B., and Leach, R. B. Total knee replacement. *Clin. Orthop.* 94:2, 1973.
7. Lonstein, J., Winter, R., Moe, J., and Gaines, D. Wound infection with Harrington instrumentation and spine fusion for scoliosis. *Clin. Orthop.* 96:222, 1973.
8. National Academy of Sciences–National Research Council. Postoperative wound infections: The influence of ultraviolet irradiation of the operating room and of various other factors. *Ann. Surg.* 160(Suppl.):1, 1964.
9. Operating-Room Survey. Operating room survey finds most orthopaedic surgeons use antibiotics regularly. *Orthop. Rev.* 3:156, 1974.
10. Stinchfield, F. E. Statistics on total hip replacement. *Clin. Orthop.* 95:2, 1973.
11. Wahlig, H., Hameister, W., and Grieben, A. Über die freisetzung von gentamycin aus polymethylmethacrylat. I. Experimentelle untersuchungen *in vitro. Langenbecks Arch. Chir.* 331:169, 1972.
12. Wilson, P. D., Salvati, E. A., Aglietti, P., and Kutner, L. J. The problem of infection in endoprosthetic surgery of the hip joint. *Clin. Orthop.* 96:213, 1973.
13. Wise, R. I., Sweeney, F. J., Jr., Haupt, G. J., and Waddell, M. A. The environmental distribution of *Staphylococus aureus* in an operation suite. *Ann. Surg.* 149:30, 1958.

19

Infections of Burn Wounds

J. Wesley Alexander and
Bruce G. MacMillan

Nosocomial infections have been more prevalent following major burns than perhaps any other condition in medicine. From the earliest recordings concerning this type of injury, infection has been the leading cause of death. Even now, the development of life-threatening nosocomial infection remains the major obstacle to successful therapy, despite recent improvements in care that have led to opportunity for survival for some patients with 90 percent burns or even more.

Nature of Infections

It is sometimes difficult to determine the presence and degree of infection in burn wounds, since they are invariably contaminated with microbes. This problem has led to the establishment of several guidelines for more exacting evaluation, but all fall short of their intended goal. To compound the problem, multiple organisms are often involved in infections of the burn wound, and it is not rare to find two or more organisms associated with septicemia or other types of invasive infection.

Incidence

The incidence of serious infections in the burned patient varies with the size of the burn. With current methods of topical chemotherapy, serious infections are not expected in otherwise healthy patients with burns involving less than 30 percent of the total body surface area. A progressive increase in the incidence of serious infection, however, is seen as the size of the burn increases, necessitating constant vigilance and repeated evaluation. The extent of the problem is shown in Figure 19-1, which is constructed from admission data from the Cincinnati General Hospital Burn and Trauma Unit and the Cincinnati Shriners Hospital during the decade 1964 to 1973. These admissions are broken into two five-year periods to emphasize the improvement in prevention of in-

Supported in part by the Cincinnati Shriners Burns Institute and USPHS Grant 5-P01-GM 15428-06.

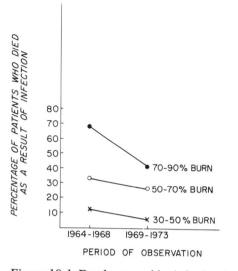

Figure 19-1. Deaths caused by infection in a major burn unit. There is a clear association with the size of the burn injury (see text).

fectious complications during this decade. The data shown involve only patients with 30 to 90 percent burns who survived for at least five days after admission. This excluded a few patients who were admitted with terminal sepsis or who died with preexisting disease as a major contributing cause. Although overall mortality caused by infection in these patients dropped from 22.7 percent in the 1964–1968 period to 16.5 percent in the 1969–1973 period, the rate of nonseptic deaths remained relatively constant, being 6.8 percent in the earlier period and 6.4 percent in the later period. Of all the patients who died from 1964 to 1968 with burns of greater than 30 percent, 76.9 percent died of infections, compared to 73.2 percent who died with infection in the period 1969 to 1973. The fact that nearly three-quarters of all patients with burns of greater than 30 percent who die following burn injury die as a result of infection underscores the complexity and seriousness of the continuing problem.

Septic problems were even worse in the preceding decade. In a review of 1049 patients treated at the U.S. Army Surgical Research Unit between January 1953 and December 1962, there were 228 deaths that occurred after the first five days following admission, and 184 (80.7 percent) were caused by septicemia [19].

The important relationship of the age of the patient and the size of the burn to the risk of infection has been emphasized by many authors and was especially well documented by Thomsen [28]. Suffice it to say that the incidence of infection increases with age (dramatically so in patients over the age of 60) and with size of the burn (infection affects nearly all patients with more than 40 percent burns).

Pathogens

Nowhere in medicine and surgery has the changing parade of pathogens been more evident than in burns (Fig. 19-2). Before the availability of penicillin and the sulfonamides, hemolytic *Streptococcus pyogenes* was the pathogen most frequently recognized. The clinical course of such infections was often dramatic; an invasive streptococcal cellulitus would spread rapidly to become a fulminating infection with generalized toxicity, and early death of the patient would ensue. In 1933, Aldrich [1] reported that all severe burns at the Johns Hopkins Hospital were colonized with streptococci within the first day. In 1935, Cruickshank [8] noted that two-thirds of patients in Glasgow had hemolytic streptococci on their wounds three to six days after admission, and in 1941, from the same institution, an incidence of 83 percent acquisition of hemolytic streptococci was found within a few days of admission. By 1945, however, Colebrook and Lond [7] noted that significant group-A streptococcal infections had almost been eliminated by the use of penicillin.

As a cause of burn wound infection, both *Staphylococcus aureus* and gram-negative bacteria were coming into prominence by 1943, when Meleney [17] reported bacteriologic studies from 347 burns associated with military injuries early in World War II. Hemolytic streptococci were very frequent in the wounds, but he noted that staphylococci were the most numerous of the pathogens in persistent infections, and the gram-negative aerobic bacilli were close in contention. Many of those patients were treated with local or systemic sulfonamides. During the 1950s, *S. aureus* emerged as the predominant organism, and in the study of Moncrief and Teplitz [19], *S. aureus* was re-

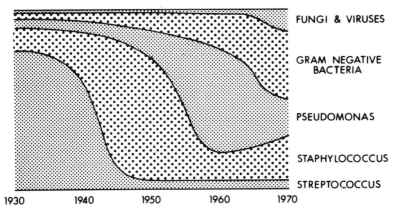

FUNGI & VIRUSES

GRAM NEGATIVE
BACTERIA

PSEUDOMONAS

STAPHYLOCOCCUS

STREPTOCOCCUS

1930   1940   1950   1960   1970

Figure 19-2. Major pathogens causing nosocomial infections in burn patients during four decades. The relative importance of each pathogen, rather than their incidence, is emphasized. Before antimicrobial agents were available, streptococcal infections dominated. With improved control of each major pathogen, others have arisen to assume greater importance.

covered from the blood in 75 percent of the patients who died of septicemia in 1954. By the early 1960s, however, *Pseudomonas aeruginosa* had surpassed *S. aureus* in frequency. Many advances in the control of *P. aeruginosa* resulted in a sharp decline in the rate of fatal infections, but it still continues to be an important pathogen. Data from the National Nosocomial Infections Study (see Part II, Chapter 13), which were collected from January 1970 to August 1973, revealed that *P. aeruginosa* was the predominant organism recovered from cultures of the burn wound, with *S. aureus* running a close second (Table 19-1). Other gram-negative organisms—including *Klebsiella, Enterobacter, Proteus, Escherichia, Providencia,* and *Acinetobacter*—formed another important group that came into increasing prominence in the late 1960s. Of more recent concern has been an increase in the number of infections that has resulted from a variety of yeasts and fungi. Currently, it would seem that virtually any organism can become a lethal pathogen in the seriously burned patient.

The changing pattern of flora in the burn wound often reflects changing methods of therapy more than any other factor, and although the ecology of the burn wound flora can be al-

tered by therapy, the burn wound cannot be sterilized. All too often, the administration of antimicrobial agents merely provides an environmental pressure for a change in the burn wound flora to more resistant organisms. To further complicate the picture, there is ample evidence that depression of numerous immune resistance factors in seriously burned patients contributes in a major way both to proliferation of microbes on the burn wound and to their systemic invasion.

The incidence of recovery of significant pathogens from the blood, burn wound, sputum, and urine at the Cincinnati Shriners Burns

Table 19-1. Distribution of 1457 Pathogens Recovered from Infected Burns in the National Nosocomial Infections Study

Pathogen	Total	Percentage
Pseudomonas aeruginosa	336	23.1%
Staphylococcus aureus	321	22.0%
Escherichia coli	135	9.3%
Klebsiella	131	9.0%
Proteus	112	7.7%
Enterobacter	109	7.5%
Candida	67	4.6%
Providencia	28	1.9%
Acinetobacter	22	1.5%
β-Hemolytic *Streptococcus*	9	⎱ 1.1%
Group-A *Streptococcus*	7	⎰
Unspecified fungi	12	0.8%
Aspergillus	4	0.3%
Mucor	1	0.1%
Other or unspecified	163	11.2%
Totals	1457	100.1%

Data from National Nosocomial Infections Study (NNIS), January 1970 to August 1973.

Table 19-2. Incidence of Recovery of Pathogens from Patients at the Cincinnati Shriners Burns Institute[a]

Site	Blood	Wound	Sputum	Urine	Totals
Streptococcus					
1969	4	63	13	49	129
1971	4	49	15	34	102
S. aureus					
1969	12	71	10	28	121
1971	3	63	10	27	103
P. aeruginosa					
1969	4	47	3	28	82
1971	4	59	9	30	102
Klebsiella					
1969	2	40	3	28	73
1971	0	44	8	35	87
Acinetobacter					
1969	1	13	0	6	20
1971	0	21	0	2	23
E. coli					
1969	2	40	2	36	80
1971	3	47	2	40	92
C. albicans					
1969	5	23	4	16	48
1971	1	36	5	26	68
Yeast					
1969	7	53	3	29	92
1971	0	28	3	15	46
Fungus					
1969	0	32	0	4	36
1971	0	16	2	4	22
Totals					
1969	37	382	38	224	681
1971	15	363	54	213	645

[a] There were 76 acute admissions in 1969 and 83 acute admissions in 1971.

Institute is shown in Table 19-2. The relative incidence of pathogens may vary remarkably from that reported from other institutions because of differences in therapy and institutional microbial ecology, which, as mentioned before, are often brought about by pressures related to antibiotic therapy.

Community-Acquired versus Nosocomial Infections

Infections of burn wounds or skin grafts placed at a burn site should be considered nosocomial if the onset of the infection occurs during hospitalization. Infection of burn wounds on initial admission should be classified as community-acquired; these are most likely to be encountered among persons with minor burns whose injury did not initially require hospital care.

Clinical and Microbiologic Classification of Burn Wound Infections

Unfortunately, infections of the burn wound often fail to segregate into neat categories that facilitate accurate classification. Several factors contribute to the problem; for example, the wounds themselves differ considerably in extent and depth. Occasionally, burns on one portion of the body may become massively infected, while other areas remain relatively unaffected. To further complicate matters, wounds that appear to be uninfected sometimes heal poorly, whereas others that have a heavy purulent discharge may heal without incident. There are often associated infections of the urinary tract or respiratory tract, and infections may occur as a complication of the use of intravenous lines or other instrumentation. These conditions are considered elsewhere in Part II of this text and will not be discussed in this chapter except to emphasize their relatively high frequency in the burn patient.

Unfortunately, there is no universal agreement for definitions of infection associated with burn injury. The complex physiologic derangements associated with the burn, the necessity for intensive therapeutic manipulation, and the marked overlapping between microbial infections and microbial contamination all contribute to the numerous exceptions that invalidate any inflexible rule. We feel that it is nevertheless useful to categorize infections of burn wounds (excluding specific complicating infections of secondary sites) into three admittedly overlapping divisions: (1) noninvasive infections of the burn wound, (2) invasive infections without bacteremia, and (3) invasive infections with bacteremia. To facilitate consistent surveillance of nosocomial burn infections, noninvasive infections with heavy exudation of purulent material and all invasive burn infections should be reported. All burns with large numbers of organisms in the eschar, however, represent potentially important sources of cross-infections, and these must not be ignored in epidemiologic investigations of infection problems.

Noninvasive Infections

Infection occurs to some extent in virtually all burn wounds, and colonization with one microorganism or a mixture of microorganisms is universal. Usually, when careful cultures are made of the wound, there is a predominant organism with other bacteria and fungi occurring in lesser numbers. The numbers of bacteria in the exudate or in the dead eschar vary from as few as 10 to up to 10^{10} organisms per gram without evidence of invasive infection. Heavy colonization of the wound is unusual within the first few hours, but it is seen more regularly after several days have passed. When surface proliferation reaches a critical number for the interaction between the particular microbe and the immune system of the host, it is followed by invasive infection.

During the second and third weeks after the burn, a layer of granulation tissue develops at the interface between the viable and the nonviable tissue of the burn wound. Associated with the increased vascularity and reactivity of this layer of granulation tissue, resistance to invasion by microorganisms increases progressively. Healthy granulation tissue can resist invasion by extraordinary numbers of bacteria placed on its surface. The dead eschar begins to separate during this same time, the separation resulting in part from enzymes associated with the granulation layer and partly from degradative enzymes produced by microbes in the eschar. Being a dead tissue that is exposed to varying degrees of external contamination, the eschar is an excellent pablum for microbial proliferation. Control of this proliferation is the basis for successful treatment of significant burn injury. When there are large numbers of bacteria in the eschar, hydrolysis occurs at a more rapid rate, and microbial products that are capable of causing systemic responses in the patient also diffuse across the granulation barrier.

The clinical criteria for noninvasive infection of the burn wound vary somewhat with the age, size, and depth of the wound. In general, the clinical picture of noninvasive infection is characterized by the rapid separation of the eschar and an increased or heavy exudation of purulent material from the burn wound.

Cultures of the eschar or drainage usually show 10^6 organisms or more per gram of material. Incisive biopsies into healthy tissues, however, usually reveal less than 10^5 organisms per gram of tissue and, on frozen section, do not show bacteria invading normal tissue. Systemic manifestations of infection are mild to moderate and include a low-grade but spiking fever and a mild to moderate leukocytosis without a marked shift to immature forms of granulocytes. The patient remains alert and responsive. One of the great benefits of recognizing noninvasive infection of the burn wound is to prevent its progression to invasive infection.

Invasive Infections without Bacteremia

Such infections occur more commonly with some organisms (e.g., *Streptococcus pyogenes*) than with others (e.g., *Candida albicans*). In the host with marked depression of immune resistance, however, all microbes can seemingly become pathogens. The lack of quantitative measurements in clinical observation has led to the performance of quantitative bacteriology to establish and confirm the extent of colonization and invasion. In general, quantitative cultures of specimens from incisional biopsies into viable tissues of the burn wound that yield counts of 10^5 or more organisms per gram of tissue are considered to represent invasive infection. Counts of 10^{10} or 10^{11} organisms per gram of tissue are often found with invasive infections. Correlation between such counts and the clinical status of the patient varies considerably with individual strains of organisms as well as with their genus and species.

In invasive infections of the burn wound, the once-healthy appearance of the granulation bed deteriorates with the invasion of organisms into viable tissue. Invaded tissues become edematous and pale and do not bleed briskly from abraded surfaces. As the infection progresses, the surface may become dry and crusty, and in very advanced infections, the wound may become frankly necrotic. Unless the process is halted very early, invasion of a partial-thickness wound can quickly convert it into a full-thickness injury that later requires grafting [22]. "Conversion" of partial-thickness injuries occurs not only because of damage to the vestiges of epithelial structures by the organisms, but also because of progressive thrombosis of the blood supply of the affected wound, which results in extension of necrosis into the subcutaneous tissues.

Frozen sections of incisive biopsy specimens of the burn wound may show microbes within formerly healthy tissue. The diagnosis of fungal infection by the identification of hyphae is particularly facilitated by this technique.

The onset of invasive burn wound sepsis may be rather sudden, but the clinical picture is more often superimposed in a patient who already has a purulent drainage, spiking temperatures, and leukocytosis. Early and moderately severe cases usually show an augmentation of the fever, a further elevation in the white blood cell count, and a decrease in the ratio of segmented to nonsegmented neutrophils. In more severe cases of burn wound sepsis, the temperature may fall to subnormal levels, and the peripheral white blood cell count may be depressed. However, there is nearly always a moderate to marked decrease in the ratio of segmented to nonsegmented neutrophils. The cheerful and alert patient usually becomes less responsive, and his or her condition may progress to coma in very severe cases. In some patients, such a picture can be present in the absence of bacteriologic confirmation of septicemia; this was originally pointed out by Moncrief and Tepletz [19], who noted toxemia and death in their patients from *P. aeruginosa* infection without confirmed bacteriologic proof of septicemia. The diffusion of toxins from certain bacteria through the burn eschar to the systemic circulation seems to play an important role. It is much more frequent, however, for bloodstream invasion to occur as a concomitant complication of invasive burn wound infection.

The occurrence of burn wound sepsis always requires vigorous treatment for successful outcome.

Invasive Infections with Bacteremia

Both colonizing and invading bacteria may enter the lymphatics and traverse into the systemic circulation, and direct invasion of bacteria into blood vessels can also occur. Thus, when repeated blood culture specimens are taken on a routine basis in patients with large burns, it is not infrequent to recover organisms. Recovery of organisms by blood culture in a burn patient sometimes occurs without clinical evidence of systemic infection, and, as mentioned before, septic death can occur without septicemia. Furthermore, bacteremia and septicemia in burn patients may derive from other sites of infection, and these may be caused by the same organisms as those isolated from the burn wound. Because of this, some burn centers have placed decreasing emphasis on monitoring burn sepsis by repeated blood cultures. Although it is true that both false-negative and false-positive blood cultures can be obtained, there is nevertheless a very good correlation between clinical evidence of septicemia and the presence of positive blood cultures. It is our strong feeling that differentiation between bacteremia, septicemia, and burn wound sepsis should not be too rigid, and that the entire clinical and bacteriologic picture must be taken into account in the frequent and critical reevaluation of infections in these patients.

It is apparent that the clinical manifestations of invasive infection of the burn wound associated with septicemia and bacteremia are really not much different than those without bacteremia. The former deserves separate classification, however, because of the objective nature of the diagnosis. In cases of invasive burn wound sepsis with septicemia and bacteremia, it is not unusual to recover more than one organism from the blood culture, which indicates that such patients have a generalized lack of resistance to infection. In our experience, the large majority of patients with burn wound sepsis also have associated bacteremia.

Microbiologic Specimens

Routine bacteriologic monitoring is an essential component of any well-run burn unit.

There are considerable differences in the techniques and practices used, however, based upon economic consideration and individual preferences. Practices vary from taking occasional culture specimens of the burn wound with a dry swab to regular, almost daily, incisive biopsies of the burn wound under local anesthesia for quantitative cultures. There is almost universal agreement that methods to quantitate the number of bacteria on the surface of the wound do not accurately reflect the degree of invasion into normal tissue. Incisive quantitative cultures of the wound obviously provide a more objective assessment of the degree of infection in the burn wound than surface cultures can ever hope to provide [24]. Routine qualitative cultures of the burn wound also provide information concerning the types of bacteria on the wound and their antibiotic sensitivity patterns. Coupled with careful clinical monitoring, surface cultures can provide a useful guide for the choice of antimicrobial agents in patients who require treatment on a clinical basis. It is the practice in our unit to culture wounds after cleansing, either at the time of dressing change and debridement or following hydrotherapy. It is advisable to culture more than one area.

We have found that the most practical technique for routine use in our unit is to sample a moistened wound area using a sterile swab; the swab is immediately placed into transport media and promptly processed. It has not been helpful to perform routine quantitative culturing on the burn surface, and quantitative incisive biopsies have been too expensive for routine monitoring. Incisive biopsies, however, may be extremely helpful in the evaluation of selected patients, particularly in the diagnosis of invasive fungal infection. The presence of mycelia on frozen sections of biopsy specimens from viable tissue is diagnostic of invasive fungal infection.

Defects in Immune Response and Burn Wound Infections

Virtually every measurement of immune response has been found to be abnormal at some time following burn injury [2]; these include depression of circulating immunoglobulin G (IgG) and complement levels, especially in association with hemodilution and protein loss during the first week following injury; abnormalities of complement function; depressed response of circulating antibody to certain antigens, especially in large burns after the fifth day following the burn; a decrease in chemotactic activity of leukocytes; lymphoid depletion in both primary and secondary lymphoid organs, especially in relation to the T-cell population of lymphocytes; altered T-cell function; abnormal response to antigens that cause delayed hypersensitivity reactions (e.g., tuberculin, streptokinase, and the like); prolongation of allografts; depressed response to nonspecific stimuli; and abnormalities of the antibacterial function of neutrophils. Undoubtedly, any of these could contribute in a significant way to the development of nosocomial infections in burn patients. Clinical and laboratory correlative studies from our unit, however, have suggested that abnormalities of neutrophil function and of the opsonic proteins are foremost among those factors that predispose to infection in burn patients. We do not believe that abnormalities of lymphoid function are of primary concern in seriously burned individuals.

General Control Measures
Patient-Care Practices

Perhaps nowhere else in medicine are patient-care practices more important in controlling infection. Of most importance is the principle emphasized by Aldrich in 1933: "It must be stressed that there is no way to heal a burn and adequately care for the patient without constant supervision and interest" [1].

DEBRIDEMENT. Since the burn wound is a nonviable tissue that is continuously exposed to the external environment, common sense has dictated that the removal of this dead tissue should decrease infection by limiting bacterial growth in the eschar. When the portal of entry is closed by autograft or suitable biologic dressings, a further advantage can be achieved.

Progressive debridement of all nonviable tissue as it begins to separate from the viable interface followed by autografting is the time-honored method of treatment. Debridement should be vigorous, and the burn wound should be continually monitored for the development of infection. Daily care is required for successful management. The use of enzymatic debridement has received repeated evaluation during the past several years, but at the present time, it appears that more potential harm can be done by enzymes than can be gained with their use [10].

Surgical excision is another means of early removal of the burn eschar. Full-thickness excision by either cold knife, electrocautery, or laser has been quite helpful in the management of both small and large burns. Another technique, tangential excision, also has considerable value in both second- and third-degree injuries. One of the reasons for improved survival in patients with very large burns during recent years is the introduction of the technique of excision of large areas of third-degree burns on admission with immediate autografting; this procedure can modify the injury to one of lesser severity.

NUTRITION. With the pain, inanition, marked fluid loss, interruption of daily routine by therapeutic measures and physical therapy, and repeated trips to the operating theater, the patient is apt to become deficient in caloric intake. In addition, losses from the burn wound and the marked increase in the catabolic rate (which can be almost double that of normal individuals) magnify the problem and can precipitate a marked nutritional deficit. In patients with large burns, this nutritional deficit cannot be managed by regular dietary regimens. In the past, it was not uncommon to see loss of body weight of 20 percent or more following a large burn. Sepsis was a frequent accompanying factor. In order to correct these deficiencies, regimens of intravenous hyperalimentation were begun, but even when the caloric intake was improved to meet metabolic demands, the incidence of septic complications was not diminished [23]. Because of the central intravenous catheter problems (see Part II, Chapter 25) that are associated with parenteral hyperalimentation, a program of oral hyperalimentation was instituted at the Cincinnati Shriners Burns Institute in 1971. Concurrent with this program

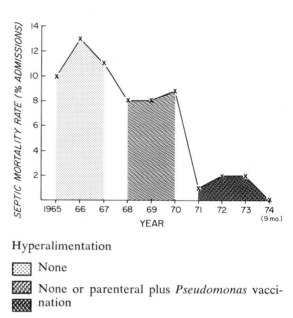

Hyperalimentation

▨ None

▨ None or parenteral plus *Pseudomonas* vaccination

▨ Oral plus *Pseudomonas* vaccination

Figure 19-3. Improvements in septic mortality in patients admitted to the Cincinnati Shriners Burns Institute during the last decade. In 1968, *Pseudomonas* vaccination was begun, and in 1971, a program of oral hyperalimentation was instituted.

was an associated improvement in patient mortality and a marked decrease in deaths related to septicemia. Emphasizing this change has been the fact that there were no septic deaths in 1974 (Fig. 19-3). The effect of oral hyperalimentation is confounded by the simultaneous change in other variables, but nonetheless appeared to be an important factor. An analysis of the variables that might have contributed to this abrupt and outstanding improvement in our septic problem showed that the patients who received oral hyperalimentation regimens had a marked improvement in neutrophil function compared to previously studied patients who did not receive oral hyperalimentation. Since a direct correlation exists between the ability of circulating neutrophils from burn patients to kill bacteria in vitro and the incidence of septic complications in such patients [3], this improvement seems critically important. From analysis of the data it would appear that either alimentation by the oral route with improved hepatic metabolism or the added administration of vitamins and mineral supplements were the most important contributing factors [12].

Environmental Control

BURN UNITS. Before the concept of burn-unit care, the transfer of invasive organisms from adjacent patients was a crucial problem. Even within modern, controlled burn units, the essential importance of regulating environmental factors to control nosocomial infections needs to be repeatedly emphasized. New burn units should be planned and constructed to permit patient care to be delivered in a protected environment with reduced microbial contamination within the area of patient care. Access to the patient-care area should be limited to those personnel concerned with the care and support of the patients. Any visitors to the unit should comply with the rigid rules followed by personnel, including wearing caps, masks, shoe covers, and operating-room attire. Reverse isolation techniques should be used on all patients with exposed wounds, with strict attention to mandatory hand-washing and the use of disposable materials whenever possible. Dirty areas should be contained. At our institution, color-coding techniques greatly assist in containment. Conventional air-handling equipment can be used, and laminar-flow units and patient-care isolators are not essential. Special attention should be given to measures for control of fomites and the care of supporting equipment such as respirators and nebulizers. Additional environmental control may be necessary for certain patients, such as those harboring group-A streptococci, who should usually be placed in strict isolation (see Part I, Chapter 9).

MacMillan [15] has recently emphasized that in a rigidly controlled burn-care unit, the most common nosocomial reservoirs, in order of decreasing importance, were found to be the patients themselves, the personnel, sinks, floors, diet, soaps, respirators, warming and cooling equipment, and hydrotherapy equipment. The most common organisms recovered from these areas have been *P. aeruginosa* and saphrophytic gram-positive and gram-negative organisms. *Staphylococcus aureus,* α-hemolytic streptococci, *Proteus,* and *Candida albicans* were less frequently isolated. The strains of *Pseudomonas aeruginosa* isolated from environmental sources were invariably rough strains, whereas those isolated from patient sources were invariably smooth strains.

In a highly controlled burn unit, environmental factors contributing to the development of nosocomial infections in burned patients can be minimized, but without control, such variables may assume major significance. The techniques necessary for general environmental control are discussed in Part I, Chapter 6, and elsewhere in this book.

HYDROTHERAPY EQUIPMENT. Conventional hydrotherapy equipment poses a significant risk of transmitting organisms from patient to patient. Such equipment, however, can be modified by removing the agitator and using plastic liners in which tubes are incorporated for compressed air. When such tubes are punctured in appropriate areas, the compressed air leaving these vents agitates the water and helps in the debridement of the burn wound. When physical-therapy personnel protect themselves with plastic gloves and plastic aprons, burn patients can be treated in these facilities without running the risk of becoming contaminated from the burn wounds of other patients who have utilized the same area [16].

Antibiotic Therapy

Prophylactic and therapeutic antimicrobial regimens have played an important role in the control of infection in burn patients.

TOPICAL THERAPY. Topical therapy was tried intermittently after the introduction of the antimicrobial agents, but it was not very successful until 1964 [18]. It is now a routine component in the management of any serious burn injury. Topical agents merely control the numbers of bacteria sufficiently to prevent invasive infection. With any antimicrobial drug, resistant strains may arise, and it is for this reason that the burn wound must be carefully monitored and the topical agent changed if infection becomes obvious. The use of ointments as a vehicle for the application of topical drugs has largely been replaced by that of water-soluble creams or solutions. The preferred primary agent at the present time is silver sulfadiazine cream. Mafenide (Sulfamylon) is also an extremely useful agent, but it has the disadvantage of aggravating metabolic disorders and pulmonary complications in many patients with burns exceeding 50 percent. It also has the disadvantage of causing significant burning on application, particularly over second-degree injuries. Silver nitrate does not penetrate into the burn wound, and this agent has not been used in our unit as a topical agent since 1968. It is still used extensively in a few centers, however, particularly because of its lower cost. Povidone-iodine ointment and gentamicin ointment should generally be reserved as secondary agents; an iodofor is particularly useful to control overgrowth of *Candida* in the burn wound, and gentamicin will control overgrowth of *Pseudomonas* or *Staphylococcus*. Gentamicin should not be used as a primary agent, because of the emergence of resistant pathogens. Routine sequential testing for the effectiveness of topical agents permits early change of the agent when resistant organisms arise.

SYSTEMIC CHEMOPROPHYLAXIS. For several decades, penicillin has been used prophylactically to prevent the occurrence of acute, invasive, streptococcal infections of the burn wound (see Part I, Chapter 11). With the extensive use of topical antimicrobial agents, however, streptococcal infection in burns is now a rare event. Penicillin causes the emergence of resistant organisms and a deleterious change in the ecology of the burn-wound flora [15]. Thus, we recommend careful monitoring of the burn wound and nasopharyngeal flora for beginning signs of infection or colonization and delaying specific therapy until there is clinical or bacteriologic evidence of streptococcal infection or colonization. Other prophylactic systemic antibiotics clearly encourage the emergence of antibiotic-resistant pathogens in the nosocomial environment and should not be used in burn patients.

Group-A *Streptococcus pyogenes*
General Aspects
TRANSMISSIBILITY. Group-A *Streptococcus pyogenes* is a highly transmissible organism

that can cause rapidly lethal infections in the burn patient.

CLINICAL COURSE. The clinical course is characterized by an abrupt deterioration in the wound that is associated with an increase in wound pain, redness, induration, and swelling. Redness extending from the margin of the burn wound is perhaps the most significant sign of streptococcal infections, which characteristically invade into normal tissues. Within hours of the onset of the more fulminant infections, systemic symptoms occur, characterized by a high, spiking fever, rapid tachycardia, and flushing of the face. Untreated, the condition can progress rapidly to death. Leukocytosis with a marked shift to the left is characteristic. Shock usually does not occur until terminally. Most streptococcal infections are seen within the first week following burn injury, and invasive infection of healthy granulation tissue by *Streptococcus* rarely occurs. It is for this reason that penicillin has been used so extensively for prophylaxis during the early burn period.

The freshly grafted wound and fresh donor site are other sites that frequently become infected with group-A *Streptococcus pyogenes*. The clinical course is usually less abrupt, and of more concern is the loss of grafts from infection or the conversion of a donor site to a full-thickness injury.

PREDISPOSING HOST FACTORS. These are not different from those of other types of bacterial infection in burn patients, but from the available data, it would appear that a decrease in serum opsonic activity during the first 10 to 15 days after injury is especially important. Perhaps of more significance as a predisposing factor is carriage of the organism by the patient, because those who carry streptococci in oropharyngeal sites are at a much higher risk.

THERAPY. Fortunately, group-A *Streptococcus* infection almost always responds to penicillin therapy. For those individuals allergic to penicillin, alternative drugs include erythromycin, vancomycin, and the cephalosporins. Patients with penicillin allergy tend to be sensitive to cephalosporin as well, and cephalosporins should probably not be used in those with a history of severe penicillin reactions. Streptococci are exquisitely sensitive to vancomycin, and this is the drug of choice in treating serious life-threatening infection in a patient with penicillin allergy. It is well to remember that gentamicin, while having a broad spectrum of activity against most staphylococcal organisms, is relatively ineffective for streptococcal infections.

Endemic Infections

INCIDENCE. Despite the high transmissibility, endemic infections are much more common than epidemic infections in well-run burn units. Positive cultures from burn wounds for group-A *Streptococcus* are found in 5 to 10 percent of all admissions to the Cincinnati Shriners Burns Institute. Clinical infections became evident in only a few of these individuals, however, and such infections are relatively minor. Only one life-threatening infection with group-A *Streptococcus* has occurred during the last decade, and this was in a patient with a reconstructive orthopedic procedure.

SOURCES. The major source of the group-A streptococci that cause endemic infection is the nasopharynx of the patient. The patient's wounds can also be an important source, however, particularly the small, chronically draining wounds in ulcerated burn scars or burn sites that are slow to heal. Fomites and other environmental sources do not seem to play a prominent role in endemic infections.

MODES OF SPREAD. Spread is usually from the patient to himself, either from the nasopharynx or from open areas to recently grafted sites. Less common but very important is spread by nursing and supporting personnel from one patient to another.

PREVENTION. Prevention of endemic infections by group-A streptococci is best accomplished by bacteriologic monitoring of the patient and his wound. Every patient should have a nasopharyngeal culture as well as culture tests of all wounds upon admission to a burn unit. Such cultures should be repeated on a routine, periodic basis during his hospital stay. Those individuals who have or who develop a positive culture for group-A *Streptococcus* should be isolated immediately and treated with systemic penicillin therapy until the cultures are negative. Any patient with positive cultures in the recent past that required operation or debridement should be given prophylactic penicillin therapy to protect against invasive infection by hemolytic *Streptococcus*. We feel that it is not indicated to give penicillin prophylactically to patients for most reconstructive procedures or for debridement or grafting in patients with negative cultures. We also feel that the routine administration of penicillin during the first five days after the burn injury is not necessary in well-controlled burn units. While it has been claimed that penicillin does little harm, data from our unit would suggest that the microbial flora of the wound can be adversely shifted to a more resistant population in patients who have received prophylactic penicillin on a routine basis [15].

Epidemic Infections

INCIDENCE. With good environmental control and bacteriologic monitoring, epidemic infections should be exceedingly rare. However, most older, experienced burn surgeons have observed the devastating consequences of such outbreaks in the pre-penicillin era. In our unit, such an outbreak has not occurred in over 20 years.

HIGH-RISK AREAS. Both open wards and intensive-care units can pose high risks in hospitals that treat burns in such areas. The enhanced risk is related mostly to a high density of patients with susceptible wounds, which in turn results in inadequate protective isolation of the burn patient.

SOURCES. In epidemic infections, nursing and supporting personnel must be highly suspected, but initial infections may come from the patients or visitors (see Part II, Chapters 16 and 20).

MODES OF SPREAD. In contrast to endemic infections, spread is usually by contact from carriers or from personnel who transmit the infection from patient to patient.

CONTROL OF OUTBREAKS. Strict isolation procedures should be used to control any acute β-hemolytic streptococcal burn infection. All patient-care personnel and patients should have cultures of the nares, oropharynx, and wounds, and epidemiologic studies should be undertaken to identify potential disseminating carriers (see Part I, Chapter 5, and Part II, Chapters 16 and 20). Patients with positive cultures should be isolated and treated with penicillin. Personnel with positive cultures must be removed from patient-care duties either until they are treated and have negative cultures or until their strains are shown to be different from the epidemic strain on the basis of M and T typing. Strict attention to "no-touch" technique is essential to the control and prevention of outbreaks, and gloves and masks should be worn anytime there is contact with the wound. One important aspect of the prevention of such outbreaks is to prohibit visitation by persons with upper respiratory tract infections.

Staphylococcus aureus
General Aspects

TRANSMISSIBILITY. *S. aureus* is an organism of moderate virulence that is easily transmissible. The extremely large numbers of organisms that may colonize or infect burns are accompanied by significant risks of transmission by contact and airborne routes. Because they survive even in the dried state, staphylococci can become airborne on dust particles and desquamated epithelial cells, but contact is by far the most important mode of their transmission in burn patients.

CLINICAL FEATURES. Patients who develop invasive infections of the burn wound with *S. aureus* have an insidious course; two to five days often elapse between the earliest symptoms and the full-blown infection. These patients have early dissolution of granulation tissue in the burn wound, become hyperpyretic with a leukocytosis, develop disorientation that is often severe, and often develop a prominent gastrointestinal ileus. Shock is not infrequent and is often accompanied by renal failure.

PREDISPOSING HOST FACTORS. The most important host factor that predisposes to staphylococcal infections appears to be an abnormality of the antibacterial function of the neutrophils. Serum factors seem to be less important in the control of this microorganism than they are in other infections.

THERAPY. Fortunately, many antimicrobial agents are effective against *S. aureus*. Although penicillin is effective against some strains, the high incidence of penicillin resistance makes it mandatory that other antibiotics be chosen as a primary agent. In our unit, systemic methicillin and nafcillin have proved to be valuable drugs. Antibiotics should only be administered when there is evidence of invasive infection of the burn wound. Because of the problem of superinfection, therapy should be restricted to relatively short time intervals. To reverse a tendency to administer the antistaphylococcal drugs too long, we recommend a thorough reassessment of the need for their continuation after each five days of therapy. Generally, *S. aureus* cannot be eradicated completely from a burn wound until it is covered by graft or replaced by another pathogen.

Endemic Infections

INCIDENCE. *Staphylococcus aureus* is one of the most important organisms causing infection in burn patients [29]. Approximately 60 percent of all patients become colonized with *S. aureus* on their burns, and it is the leading cause of septicemia in our burn unit at the present time. With the availability of effective antimicrobial agents for the treatment of systemic infections, however, mortality from staphylococcal infection in our unit is rare.

SOURCES. Environmental sources are probably much more important for *S. aureus* than for most of the organisms encountered in the burn unit. Indeed, the organism is almost ubiquitous. Furthermore, patients colonized in the anterior nares may spread the organisms to their burns. The greatest source of endemic spread is the nosocomial reservoir. For this reason, it is extremely important to develop rigid environmental control techniques, as mentioned above.

MODES OF SPREAD. Staphylococcal carriers among personnel can be an important source, but the most important mode of spread is usually via personnel from patient to patient in an environment that is not closely controlled. Fomites and even food are occasionally implicated.

PREVENTION. Environmental control is of utmost importance in preventing endemic infection by *S. aureus;* these measures have already been outlined. In addition, the restrictive use of systemic antibiotics favors easier control of this infection. Among the topical agents, povidone-iodine (Betadine) and mafenide (Sulfamylon) appear to give reasonably good control for *S. aureus* infection.

Epidemic Infections

Epidemic infections with *S. aureus* occur at a low incidence, even in high patient-density areas such as intensive-care units. When they do occur, epidemiologic studies and bacteriologic surveys of personnel for carriers should be performed. If carriers are epidemiologically associated with the outbreak, they should be temporarily excused from duty, and attempts should be made to eradicate the colonizing strain (see Part II, Chapters 16 and 20).

Pseudomonas aeruginosa

General Aspects

TRANSMISSIBILITY. *P. aeruginosa* is an organism of low pathogenicity that rarely causes infections in immunologically normal individuals. However, it grows well in moist environments, especially in open wounds; it is resistant to most commonly used antibiotics; and it invades frequently in immunodepressed individuals.

CLINICAL FEATURES. Invasion of the burn wound by *P. aeruginosa* may occur either abruptly or slowly. In a typical case, the burn wound develops a heavy, green-pigmented, foul-smelling discharge over a period of two or three days. In rapidly advancing and invasive infections, the eschar may become dry, and previously healthy granulation tissues develop a shaggy, green exudate and later progress to form patchy, black areas of necrosis. In certain cases, however, the granulation tissue may not show necrotic areas and may not have a greenish exudate. Gangrene in non-burned areas (ecthyma gangrenosum) is often seen before death in patients with septicemia. Patients usually become hypothermic and have a depressed white cell count and clinical ileus, but they are usually not disoriented until terminal.

PREDISPOSING HOST FACTORS. Predisposing host factors are extremely important in the de-velopment of infections with *P. aeruginosa*. In burn patients, these are related both to abnormalities of the antibacterial function of neutrophils and to deficiencies in serum opsonins, namely, specific natural or immune antibody and components of the complement system. With heavy colonization of the burn wound, a selective consumption of specific antibody can occur that renders the patient increasingly susceptible to the organism on the burn wound (Fig. 19-4).

THERAPY. In the treatment of established septicemia in the burn patient, polymyxin B and colimycin are relatively toxic and almost totally ineffective. In recent years, certain aminoglycoside antibiotics—especially gentamicin, tobramycin, and amikacin—have been the antibiotics of choice in the treatment of *Pseudomonas* septicemia. Simultaneous administration of carbenicillin has been useful in selected cases, especially in overwhelming infections. One alarming observation has been a marked increase in the numbers of bacteria in some hospitals that have been found to be resistant to gentamicin, carbenicillin, and even the newer aminoglycosides.

Such increases in antibiotic resistance patterns emphasize the need for a continued immunologic approach to therapy. At the Cincinnati Shriners Burns Institute, 14 patients with *Pseudomonas* burn wound sepsis and septicemia that failed to respond to gentamicin and carbenicillin therapy have been treated with hyperimmune anti-*Pseudomonas* γ-globulin. All but two of these patients have recovered from their *Pseudomonas* sepsis; one had an organism that was not reactive with the specific immunoglobulin mixture administered, and the other patient had an established *Pseudomonas* sepsis at the time of admission.

Endemic Infections

INCIDENCE. As indicated before, it is difficult to establish the incidence of infection by any one organism in burn patients because of the spectrum between colonization and frank sepsis. In a survey in the Cincinnati Shriners Burns Institute, over half of all admitted patients became colonized with *P. aeruginosa* on their burns during their hospital stay (Fig. 19-5).

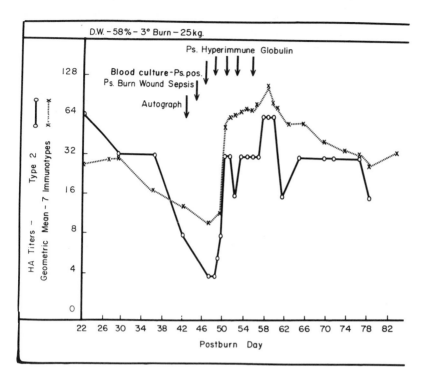

Figure 19-4. Selective consumption of type-specific anti-*Pseudomonas* antibody by surface infection of the burn wound with the corresponding immunotype. Invasive infection and septicemia occurred when antibody levels became very low. Antibody levels were restored by the passive administration of hyperimmune globulin, and the infection was aborted.

During this same period, approximately 6 percent of immunized patients with burns of greater than 20 percent of the body surface area developed *Pseudomonas* septicemia, which is in contrast to 18 percent who developed such infection before the use of the *Pseudomonas* vaccine described below.

SOURCES. A survey in our intensive-care unit demonstrated that the major source of *P. aeruginosa* on a patient's burn wound was the patient himself, predominantly via the gastrointestinal tract [16]. This observation has been emphasized by others [9,27]. Nosocomial acquisition of *P. aeruginosa* in the gastrointestinal tract is common among seriously ill hospitalized patients. *P. aeruginosa* was found in a number of environmental areas, but these were felt not to be reservoirs for pathogenic organisms, since the organisms were invariably of the rough, nonpathogenic type that were not found on patients. Other reports relating to *Pseudomonas* in hospital environments, however, have indicated that fomites (including flowers), mop buckets, sink traps, faucet aerators, respirators, nebulizers, hospital food, and contaminated oral medications may be reservoirs for *P. aeruginosa* [13,14]. The first two items are probably of little or no importance as proximate sources of infective organisms.

MODES OF SPREAD. The predominant mode of spread within burn units is transference by personnel who have direct patient contact. Another important mode of spread in some burn units is via whirlpool and Hubbard tank units, especially when extensive decontamination and aseptic procedures are not followed properly.

PREVENTION. Colonization of the burn patient by *P. aeruginosa* is extremely difficult to prevent. General control measures are important in preventing the spread of this organism, and topical therapy has been beneficial in limiting its growth in colonized patients. Perhaps of equal or greater importance in preventing invasive infection in our burn unit has been the administration of an effective *Pseudomonas* vaccine (Pseudogen) to all patients with a burn

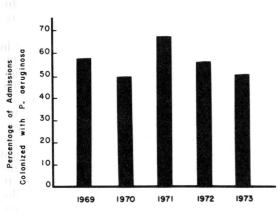

Figure 19-5. Colonization rate with *Pseudomonas aeruginosa* at the Cincinnati Shriners Burns Institute.

Table 19-3. Experience with an Immunization Program against Pseudomonas aeruginosa *at the Cincinnati Shriners Burns Institute and the Cincinnati General Hospital Burn Unit*[a]

Phase and time of study	Number of patients	Mortality from *Pseudomonas* infection
Antecedent controls (Jan. 1967–Mar. 1968)	75	14.7%
Initial low dose trials (Mar. 1968–Feb. 1969)	40	12.5%
Optional vaccination (Feb. 1969–Jul. 1970)	96	3.1%
Optional vaccination plus hyperimmune globulin for patients developing bacteremia (Jul. 1970–Nov. 1974)	379	0.0%

[a] All patients were included in the study who had burn injuries of 20 percent or more and who survived in the initial five days after admission without developing evidence of *Pseudomonas* sepsis.

injury of greater than 20 percent of the total body surface area. In association with an effective vaccination program with Pseudogen during a six-year period, the incidence of *Pseudomonas* septicemia has dropped from 18 to 6 percent in this selected population (i.e., those who have lived for at least five days after admission), and mortality from *P. aeruginosa* has been virtually eliminated by the use of vaccine combined with hyperimmune globulin in patients who develop bacteremia (Table 19-3). Other significant changes in the care of burn patients occurred during this time, but we believe the vaccine has been mainly responsible for these changes.

Numerous dosages, routes, and schedules of administration of *Pseudomonas* vaccine have been evaluated. The most effective one has been to administer 25 micrograms per kilogram of body weight intramuscularly initially, at 48 hours, and at 96 hours; this dosage is continued weekly thereafter until the burn wound is covered by an autograft. Provided that the immunization schedule is begun within the first five days after burn injury, the antibody response is characteristically good, and there is associated protection from invasive infection [4].

Epidemic Infections
Epidemic infections with *P. aeruginosa* are practically nonexistent in a well-controlled

environment. Outbreaks traced to contaminated hydrotherapy equipment have occurred, and this source should be carefully evaluated if an outbreak develops.

Other Organisms Causing Burn Infections
Candida albicans

CLINICAL COURSE. Invasive infection caused by *Candida albicans* is not frequently seen; it occurs commonly in only those patients who have extensive and debilitating burn injuries. Such patients have usually received broad-spectrum antibiotics for relatively long periods of time for the treatment of other infectious complications. Clinically, the granulating wound usually becomes dry and flat with a yellow or orange color. There is a gradual, downhill course, during which the patient's temperature and white blood cell count usually remain unchanged.

PREDISPOSING HOST FACTORS. The mechanism for defense against *Candida* infections are essentially the same as those for bacterial infections, although delayed hypersensitivity mechanisms seem to be more important and antibody-mediated immune reactions less important for ridding the host of these pathogens.

Such agents infrequently cause primary infections, but they are troublesome opportunistic invaders in patients with abnormalities of host resistance such as occur in some immunologic deficiency diseases or during immunosuppressive therapy. An improvement in the survival rate for the extensively burned patient has contributed to the rise in the incidence of serious yeast and fungal infections. *Candida* often becomes the predominant organism of mucosal surfaces and of burn wounds when the usual bacterial flora have been destroyed by antibiotic therapy, and superinfections not infrequently follow successful treatment for systemic bacterial sepsis. Among mycotic agents, *Candida albicans* is the most frequent cause of both local and systemic infections as a secondary invader, probably because of its normal occurrence in the gastrointestinal tract.

The presence of *Candida* on burn wounds is of little clinical significance in the majority of cases. Occasionally, colonization precedes invasion, which may herald the occurrence of *Candida* septicemia and systemic mycosis. In this instance, biopsies of the burn wound can be of great help, because the demonstration of pseudohyphae deep in viable subcutaneous tissue by wound biopsy can alert the clinician to the danger of possible *Candida* septicemia and systemic candidiasis [21]. Systemic candidiasis can also be suspected by the demonstration of *Candida* organisms in the urine. Krause and co-workers [11] have demonstrated candiduria in a human promptly after swallowing a pure culture of *Candida albicans,* and they have shown that invasion from the gastrointestinal tract can be effectively controlled by the use of oral nystatin (Mycostatin).

Colonization of the burn wound depends on several predisposing factors, including antibiotic therapy. Nash and associates [20] have shown a tenfold increase in the occurrence of fungi on burn wounds following the use of mafenide acetate cream as a topical antibacterial agent at the U.S. Army's Institute of Surgical Research. Seelig [26] has noted the development of candidiasis in patients receiving multiple, systemic, broad-spectrum antibiotics. Williams, Chandler, and Orloff [30] have noted an increase in the incidence of candidiasis in association with certain therapeutic measures, namely, the use of blood transfusions, central venous pressure lines, and intravenous hyperalimentation therapy.

THERAPY. Local colonization of *Candida* in the burn wound can be controlled by the incorporation of nystatin (Mycostatin) in the appropriate topical antibacterial agent. Systemic spread from the gastrointestinal tract can be effectively controlled by the use of oral nystatin. Early, invasive candidiasis should be treated by the discontinuation of systemic antibiotic therapy whenever possible, the removal of intravenous and urinary catheters, and the intravenous administration of amphotericin B.

ENDEMIC AND EPIDEMIC INFECTIONS. Colonization of burn wounds by *C. albicans* in patients treated at the Cincinnati Shriners Burns Institute has increased from 30 to 50 percent during the early 1970s. This increase paralleled a steady rise in the incidence of disseminated candidiasis, and systemic candidiasis became the major cause of septic deaths in this unit for a short while. Endemic colonization on the wounds of burn patients can be minimized by the limited and selective use of antibiotic therapy, including, whenever possible, the avoidance of broad-spectrum agents such as tetracycline, nutritional support by the oral route, the use of intravenous hyperalimentation only in those patients who are suffering from a superior mesenteric artery syndrome, and the administration of intravenous fluids for short periods through butterfly (scalp vein) needles. Consideration might also be given to the prophylactic use of oral nyostatin in units experiencing high rates of *Candida* infection.

Epidemic infections of candidal organisms are rarely seen in well-controlled burn units. The major source of cross-infection with fungal organisms in the burn unit has been the inappropriate use of hydrotherapy equipment. This mode of dissemination can be eliminated by the use of protective liners on hydrotherapy equipment.

Other Mycotic Infections
GENERAL ASPECTS. With improved control of burn wound sepsis caused by gram-negative and gram-positive bacteria, increasing numbers

of mycotic infections of the burn wound have been reported. One study from the Institute of Surgical Research in 1971 reported 30 cases of invasive infection with funguses of the *Phycomycetes* or *Aspergillus* species [5]. Nine of the 30 patients died from invasive fungal infections, and of the 15 surviving patients, seven required amputation to eradicate their disease. Of the cases of infection, 8 cases were caused by *Aspergillus,* 19 by *Mucor,* and 2 by *Rhizopus.* The incidence of clinically significant fungal burn wound infections was approximately 3 percent of patients treated for thermal injury. Other fungal organisms recovered from burn wounds included isolated species of *Geotrichum, Rhodotorula, Cephalosporium, Penicillium, Trichosporum, Trichophyton, Fusarium,* and *Fonsecaea* [6], but these did not seem to invade. Little is known about their transmissibility, sources, and modes of spread within burn units.

CLINICAL OBSERVATIONS. The mycotic infections cited above were most frequently seen between days 9 and 15 after the burn, and the majority of patients had burns of greater than 30 percent. Clinical signs included fever, swelling, and conversion of the burn wound. The most frequent manifestations were ulceration, induration, edema, tenderness, early separation of the eschar, and muscle necrosis. Hyphal invasion of viable tissue is diagnostic of fungal burn wound infection. Invasion may be identified by microscopic examination of frozen sections from incisional biopsy specimens.

Hyphal invasion of viable tissue very often extends laterally to involve unburned subcutaneous tissues beneath unburned skin, and hyphae often invade through the fascia and into skeletal muscle. Thrombosis and vascular necrosis of the tissue are common because of invasion of the blood vessel walls. The vascular invasion is also responsible for dissemination of organisms into the abdominal and thoracic organs and the central nervous system. At the Cincinnati Shriners Burns Institute, we have had only one death caused by these agents (a disseminated *Mucor* infection). In this patient, there was rapid invasion of normal tissue followed by general dissemination and death within a short time after the diagnosis.

PREDISPOSING HOST FACTORS. Little is known about the host factors that predispose to invasive fungal infections of this type in burned patients. Such infections, however, have been seen with increasing incidence in other disorders associated with decreased host resistance, particularly in patients with malignancies of the lymphoid and reticuloendothelial systems and in those with diabetes mellitus, especially when acidosis is present.

THERAPY. Effective therapy of invasive fungal infections in burn patients must be instituted promptly. Therapy consists primarily of radical excision of the involved area [5]. Immediate histologic examination of the excisional margins is a helpful adjunct to excisional therapy in order to document complete removal. Following surgical excision, frequent examination of the remaining wound to detect areas of incomplete excision is necessary. Amputation may be necessary to eradicate the disease. Amphotericin B should be reserved for those patients who are suspected of disseminating the organism or in whom radical surgical debridement or amputation cannot completely eradicate the disease.

Other Aerobic Gram-Negative Bacteria

PATHOGENIC AGENTS. Gram-negative enteric bacteria other than *Pseudomonas aeruginosa* have become increasingly important in infections occurring in burn patients. These organisms include *Escherichia, Klebsiella, Proteus, Enterobacter, Providencia, Acinetobacter,* and *Alcaligenes. Salmonella* and *Shigella* species do not seem to cause infections of the burn wound. The gram-negative organisms generally appear on a burn wound as a consequence of contamination from the endogenous flora of the patient or the environment, but the most important factor in their becoming pathogenic is the selective elimination of competing gram-positive organisms from the burn wound by antibiotic therapy. Another problem of special importance is that these organisms can be controlled on the burn wound, but they can rarely be eliminated by antibiotic therapy. When antibiotic-resistant strains begin to appear, the transfer of resistance (R) factors to nonresistant strains occurs (frequently even to different genera), which leads to the accumulation and proliferation of antibiotic-resistant organisms within the nosocomial environment of the burn unit [25].

TRANSMISSIBILITY. Most of the gram-negative bacteria of enteric origin have low pathogenicity, and most infections occur because the host is immunologically compromised. Cross-colonization of the gastrointestinal tract of hospitalized patients is facilitated by the use of antibiotics to which prevalent nosocomial strains are resistant.

CLINICAL FEATURES. Invasive infections may show deterioration of healthy granulation tissue, which becomes edematous and pale. Classical ecthyma gangrenosum is rare with gram-negative organisms other than *Pseudomonas,* but progressive thrombosis of vessels extensively invaded can occur and result in conversion of partial-thickness injuries to full-thickness injuries. The clinical picture of systemic infections with these gram-negative organisms in burn patients is similar to that of gram-negative septicemia in other patients. Systemic infection is usually heralded by an initial elevation in temperature, which may be followed by hypothermia in later stages. Hypotension is not uncommon. Either leukocytosis or leukopenia may be present, but there is usually a marked shift in the differential count to immature forms.

PREDISPOSING HOST FACTORS. Abnormalities of complement, natural antibody, and neutrophil antibacterial function have all been shown to be important in the development of systemic invasion with these organisms.

THERAPY. Systemic gentamicin has been our drug of choice for initial treatment of gram-negative sepsis before specific antibiotic-sensitivity patterns are established, but therapy should be altered if so indicated by specific sensitivities. Usually, it is also wise to switch to another topical antimicrobial agent when burn wound sepsis appears. In our unit, we have usually started initial topical therapy with either silver sulfadiazine or mafenide (Sulfamylon) cream and have switched to gentamicin ointment in occlusive dressings if there is evidence of the development of invasive infections by gram-negative bacteria. During the last two years, the selection of the alternative topical

therapy has usually been based upon sensitivity tests.

PREVENTION. Most infections caused by gram-negative bacteria are endemic, and there is a relatively high incidence of superinfections following therapy for infections with gram-positive organisms. The usual source of the gram-negative agents is the gastrointestinal tract of the patients themselves. Hyperendemic disease caused by one or more of the pathogens may occur from time to time within particular burn units, and it probably results from the establishment of a large reservoir of a particular strain. Such strains are usually multiple-drug-resistant and are selected by the continuous use of particular, popular, antibiotic regimens. They are usually found in the patients and environment of the burn unit, and continual cross-colonization and infection of new admissions take place. Parental antibiotic therapy in burn patients should thus be restricted to situations with clear indications, and periodic shifts in popular drug regimens, when possible, might also be considered. Hands of personnel and contact with contaminated hydrotherapy units can spread these organisms. The prevention of such infections depends on excellent care of the burn wound and strict attention to those general control measures mentioned earlier in this chapter.

Anaerobic Bacterial Infections
Anaerobic infections following burn injury are surprisingly infrequent, possibly because of the aerobic environment of the burn wound in most instances. However, early contamination with clostridial species, including *Clostridium perfringens* and *Clostridium tetani,* is relatively common. In very deep burns, such as can occur with electrical injuries in which muscle necrosis is often associated, prevention of gas gangrene and tetanus should be of great concern, and early debridement or excision of dead tissue is advisable. Tetanus in the burn patient is a potential hazard in almost every case, but it can be easily prevented by current active and passive immunization procedures. In present practice, both gas gangrene and tetanus are exceedingly rare. Other types of anaerobic infections, such as those caused by *Bacteroides*

species, are likewise very uncommon and cause no particular problem.

References

1. Aldrich, R. H. The role of infection in burns: The theory and treatment with special reference to gentian violet. *N. Engl. J. Med.* 208: 299, 1933.
2. Alexander, J. W. Infections in the patient with severe burns. In Nahmis, H. J., and O'Reilly, R. J. (Eds.). *Immunology of Human Infections,* vol. I. New York: Plenum Publishing. (In press)
3. Alexander, J. W., and Meakins, J. L. A physiological basis for the development of opportunistic infections. *Ann. Surg.* 176:273, 1972.
4. Alexander, J. W., and Fisher, M. W. Immunization against *Pseudomonas* in infection after thermal injury. *J. Infect. Dis.* 130:S152, 1974.
5. Bruck, H. M., Nash, G., and Pruitt, B. S., Jr. Opportunistic fungal infection of the burn wound with phycomycetes and *Aspergillus*. *Arch. Surg.* 102:476, 1971.
6. Bruck, H. M., Nash, G., Stein, J. M., and Lindberg, R. B. Studies on the occurrence and significance of yeasts and fungi in the burn wound. *Ann. Surg.* 176:108, 1972.
7. Colebrook, L., and Lond, M. B. The control of infection in burns. *Lancet* 1:6511, 1948.
8. Cruickshank, R. The bacterial infection of burns. *J. Pathol. Bacteriol.* 31:367, 1935.
9. Haynes, B. W., Jr., and Hench, M. E. Hospital isolation system for preventing cross-contamination by staphylococcal and pseudomonas organisms in burn wounds. *Ann. Surg.* 162:641, 1965.
10. Hummel, R. P., Kautz, P. D., MacMillan, B. G., and Altemeier, W. A. The continuing problem of sepsis following enzymatic debridement of burns. *J. Trauma* 14:572, 1974.
11. Krause, W., Matheis, K., and Wulf, K. Fungemia and funguria after oral administration of *Candida albicans*. *Lancet* 1:598, 1969.
12. Lennard, E. S., Alexander, J. W., Craycraft, T. K., and MacMillan, B. G. Association in burn patients of improved antibacterial defense with nutritional support by the oral route. *Burns* 1:95, 1975.
13. Lowbury, E. J. L. Infection of burns. *Br. Med. J.* 1:994, 1960.
14. Lowbury, E. J. L., and Fox, J. The epidemiology of infection with *Pseudomonas pyocyanea* in a burns unit. *J. Hyg.* (Camb.) 52:403, 1954.
15. MacMillan, B. G. Burn wound sepsis—A ten-year experience. *Burns* 2:1, 1975.
16. Macmillan, B. G., Edmonds, P., Hummel, R. P., and Maley, M. P. Epidemiology of *Pseudomonas* in a burn intensive care unit. *J. Trauma* 13:627, 1973.
17. Meleney, F. L. The study of the prevention of infection in contaminated accidental wounds, compound fractures and burns. *Ann. Surg.* 118:171, 1943.
18. Moncrief, J. A. The development of topical therapy. *J. Trauma* 11:906, 1971.
19. Moncrief, J. A., and Teplitz, C. Changing concepts in burn sepsis. *J. Trauma* 4:233, 1964.
20. Nash, G., Foley, F. D., Goodwin, M. N., Bruck, H. M., Greenwald, K. A., and Pruitt, B. A., Jr. Fungal burn wound infection. *J.A.M.A.* 215:1664, 1971.
21. Nash, G., Foley, F. D., and Pruitt, B. A., Jr. Candida burn-wound invasion. A cause of systemic candidiasis. *Arch. Pathol.* 90:75, 1970.
22. Order, S. E., Mason, A. D., Jr., Walker, H. L., Lindberg, R. F., Switzer, W. E., and Moncrief, J. A. The pathogenesis of second and third degree burns and conversion to full thickness injury. *Surg. Gynecol. Obstet.* 120:983, 1965.
23. Popp, M., Law, E., and MacMillan, B. G. Parenteral nutrition in the burn child: A study of 26 patients. *Ann. Surg.* 179:219, 1974.
24. Pruitt, B. A., Jr., and Foley, F. D. The use of biopsies in burn patient care. *Surgery* 73: 887, 1973.
25. Roe, E., and Jones, R. J. Effects of topical chemoprophylaxis on transferable antibiotic resistance in burns. *Lancet* 1:109, 1972.
26. Seelig, M. The role of antibiotics in the pathogenesis of *Candida* infections. *Am. J. Med.* 40:887, 1966.
27. Shooter, R. A., Walker, K. A., Williams, V. R., Horgan, G. M., Parker, M. T., Asheshov, E. H., and Bullimore, J. F. Fecal carriage of *Pseudomonas aeruginosa* in hospital patients. Possible spread from patient to patient. *Lancet* 2:1331, 1966.
28. Thomsen, M. The burns unit in Copenhagen. VI. Infection rates. *Scand. J. Plast. Reconstr. Surg.* 4:53, 1970.
29. Thomsen, M. The burns unit in Copenhagen. VIII. Bacteriology. *Scand. J. Plast. Reconstr. Surg.* 4:126, 1970.
30. Williams, R., Chandler, J., and Orloff, J. J. *Candida* septicemia. *Arch. Surg.* 103:8, 1971.

20

Selected Infections of the Skin and Eye

Walter E. Stamm, Allen C. Steere,
and Richard E. Dixon

Nature of Infections

This chapter discusses selected common infections of the skin and eye that do not occur at sites of previous surgery and do not involve decubitus ulcers or burns. Such infections occur at an approximate rate of 2.6 per 1000 discharges (Table 20-1) and represent about 5 percent of all nosocomial infections. In descending frequency, infections of the skin and eye combined follow urinary tract, surgical wound, and respiratory tract infections and are about equal in frequency to primary bacteremia. In addition, superficial nosocomial infections (along with lower respiratory infections) have a greater propensity for causing secondary bacteremia than urinary tract or surgical wound infections (see Part II, Chapter 29). Skin infections due to smallpox, measles, rubella, and cytomegalovirus are discussed elsewhere (see Part II, Chapter 24).

Incidence

The incidence of superficial infections varies considerably with the hospital service (Table 20-1). Newborn patients are particularly susceptible to superficial infections, especially omphalitis, conjunctivitis, and pyoderma. Adult patients have a considerably lower incidence of superficial infections, with the most common manifestations being pyoderma and eye infections.

Pathogens

Staphylococcus aureus causes approximately 34 percent of superficial infections. This organism predominates as the causative agent for furunculosis, omphalitis, and for maternal mastitis; it also plays an important role in eye infections. *S. aureus* infections occur on all hospital services, but they are particularly important in newborn and pediatric patients.

Taken collectively, gram-negative organisms account for about 40 percent of superficial infections. These organisms are less important than *S. aureus* as a cause of pyoderma in newborns, but they are often isolated from infants

Table 20-1. Nosocomial Superficial Infections: Incidence by Hospital Service[a]

Site	Rates of infection per 10,000 discharges[b]						
	Nursery	Med.	Surg.	Pediat.	Obstet.	Gynec.	Totals
Skin	60.5	21.3	16.8	13.2	1.6	3.3	19.5
Eye	22.1	2.4	1.3	3.8	0.2	0.1	3.6
Umbilicus	15.5	0.2	—	0.8	—	—	1.6
Breast	0.9	—	—	0.1	1.8	0.1	0.4
Overall	80.0	24.7	18.7	18.3	4.5	3.6	25.6

[a] Data from National Nosocomial Infections Study (NNIS), July 1974–November 1976. Data are based on 2,797,911 discharges.
[b] — equals rate of infection less than 0.1 per 10,000 discharges.

with omphalitis or eye infections. Gram-negative organisms predominate as the most frequent causative agents for all forms of superficial infections in adult patients.

Streptococci were responsible for approximately 6.5 percent of the superficial infections reported to the National Nosocomial Infections Study (NNIS) (see Part II, Chapter 13); these organisms usually infected newborn or pediatric patients. A wide variety of other bacterial, viral, and fungal agents occasionally cause nosocomial superficial infections (Table 20-2).

Classification of Infections
The development of purulence in superficial tissues after hospital admission can generally be

Table 20-2. Percentage Distribution of Pathogens Causing Nosocomial Superficial Infections[a]

Pathogen	Percentage
Staphylococcus aureus	34.0
Escherichia coli	8.7
Pseudomonas aeruginosa	6.4
Coagulase-negative staphylococci	5.6
Proteus species	5.5
Klebsiella species	4.9
Enterobacter species	3.9
Other streptococci	3.8
Enterococcus species	2.7
Candida species	1.6
Other	22.9
Total	100.0

[a] Data from the National Nosocomial Infections Study (NNIS), July 1974–November 1976.

used to define a nosocomial infection, whether cultures of the lesion are positive, negative, or not taken. In patients who have skin infections on admission, a change in the type of pathogens cultured from the infected site also indicates a nosocomial infection if continued purulent drainage is due to the new pathogen(s). Cellulitis and certain other cutaneous infections are often not accompanied by purulence, and cultures may not yield the pathogenic organism; in such instances, clinical judgment must be used to determine the presence or absence of infection. Cellulitis that is not present on admission is considered nosocomial in origin.

Skin lesions such as decubitus ulcers or dermatoses (psoriasis, eczema, and others) are usually superficially colonized with several bacterial species; thus, simple isolation of an organism from such a lesion should not be equated with infection. Purulent drainage from such lesions that begins during hospitalization, however, constitutes a nosocomial infection, even though microorganisms were present in the lesion upon admission.

The clinical manifestations of many superficial infections, particularly in newborns and other patients hospitalized for a short time, often do not occur until after the patients leave the hospital. Cutaneous infections that have their onset within ten days of a previous hospitalization are usually nosocomial in origin, but clinical judgment and an evaluation of the epidemiologic circumstances are usually necessary to decide whether a superficial infection that occurs after recent hospital discharge is community-acquired or nosocomial. Although they are occasionally indicative (see following sections), incubation periods for most common superficial infections vary considerably and hence are of little assistance in classifying infections as nosocomial or community-acquired.

Diagnostic Criteria
Clinical
Characteristic clinical manifestations of superficial infections (Table 20-3) generally provide an adequate basis for their diagnosis, even without additional microbiologic data. Specific clinical syndromes are detailed in subsequent sections.

Microbiologic
Numerous microorganisms normally reside either temporarily or permanently on the skin

Table 20-3. Diagnostic Clinical Findings in Nosocomial Superficial Infections

Type of infection	Clinical criteria for diagnosis
Pyoderma	Cutaneous or subcutaneous collections of pus, usually in multiple, discrete lesions and often associated with erythema
Omphalitis	Presence of purulent drainage from the umbilical cord, or presence of nonpurulent drainage associated with periumbilical erythema or pustules
Cellulitis	Presence of red, warm, and often tender and edematous skin without initial evidence of purulence; may have associated lymphadenitis and lymphadenopathy
Dermatitis	Superinfection of a noninfectious skin lesion such as psoriasis or eczema, usually characterized by redness, tenderness, swelling, and mucopurulent drainage
Mastitis	Marked tenderness, redness, and induration of the breast, often associated with fever, leukocytosis, and superficial pustules; may progress to abscess formation
Conjunctivitis	Conjunctival redness associated with hyperemia, drainage of mucopurulent material, and often photophobia or the sensation of a foreign body in the eye

and may obscure the bacteriologic diagnosis of superficial infections. *Staphylococcus aureus,* group-A streptococci, and gram-negative rods can all be recovered from healthy skin, particularly that of hospital patients, and isolating them from the skin does not necessarily imply that they have a pathogenic role. In addition, permanent cutaneous residents such as *Staphylococcus epidermidis,* micrococci, or *Propionibacterium acnes* often grow in cultures obtained from skin.

Cultures from superficial infections most often yield the causative microorganism when purulent material can be obtained. If present, such material usually contains the pathogenic agent in high numbers and should always be Gram stained and cultured. When purulence is not present (as in cellulitis), skin cultures are less likely to yield the causative organism, and interpretation of culture results is often difficult. Cultures obtained from nonpurulent dermatoses or from large, open wounds such as decubitus ulcers are rarely useful as a guide to therapy, because they generally harbor many species of microorganisms that may change from day to day.

Collection and Transport of Specimens
Purulent material, if present in sufficient quantity, should be aspirated into a sterile syringe and taken directly to the laboratory for Gram staining and inoculation into aerobic and, if clinically indicated, anaerobic media. When immediate transport to the laboratory is not possible, the material should be inoculated into the appropriate transport media. Swabs premoistened in culture media can be used to obtain cultures from lesser amounts of purulent material, from serous skin discharges, or from dry skin lesions. Scrapings of superficial crusts or vesicles can also be obtained for viral culture. Intradermal injection and subsequent aspiration of sterile saline may yield the agent that is causing cellulitis. Finally, punch or excisional biopsy specimen of ulcerative skin lesions can be cultured. All material for culture should be Gram stained for examination and, if indicated clinically, examined by other special methods, such as a potassium hydroxide

preparation, acid-fast staining, or the Tzanck preparation when herpes or varicella-zoster infection is suspected.

Patients with conjunctivitis or keratitis may have a purulent or serous discharge that can be sampled with a premoistened swab. Corneal scrapings, however, more often contain the causative agent, particularly in the absence of purulence. Material obtained by either method should be examined using Gram stain, acid-fast smear, and potassium hydroxide wet mount, and it should be inoculated into appropriate culture media. All ophthalmic cultures should be obtained prior to the use of a topical anesthetic, since these compounds have antimicrobial activity.

General Control Measures

Prevention of superficial infections involves recognizing and removing animate reservoirs of infecting microorganisms, interrupting person-to-person spread, and, to a lesser extent, reducing airborne transmission of microorganisms.

Patient-Care Practices

Although the skin cannot be sterilized, transiently acquired skin flora can be removed by regular, thorough washing with soap and water; both transient and resident skin flora can be reduced in number by the use of topical antiseptic agents. Appropriate skin antisepsis should precede any procedure that disrupts the integument, such as venipuncture, biopsy, or intramuscular injection. Strict aseptic technique should be observed by personnel carrying out these procedures.

Since many nosocomial pathogens reach the skin of hospitalized patients via the hands of hospital personnel, the importance of employee hand-washing cannot be overemphasized as a measure for preventing both superficial colonization and infection. A 15 to 30 second vigorous scrub using soap and running water should be done before and after each patient contact; in the nursery, in intensive-care units, and in special isolation areas, an antiseptic agent should be used for hand-washing [43].

Separation of infected and uninfected patients frequently reduces the spread of cutaneous microorganisms from one patient to another. This may be accomplished either by the actual isolation of infected patients or by the "cohorting" of groups of patients, as is described in the next section (see Endemic Infections, Prevention, under Staphylococcal Infections).

Hospital personnel who become colonized with staphylococci or streptococci may serve as important reservoirs for these organisms. When clusters of infections occur in patients or employees, disseminating carriers must be sought, identified, and removed from work while appropriate treatment is undertaken.

Environmental Factors

Crowded conditions, open wards, and high patient-to-staff ratios encourage person-to-person transmission of microorganisms and should be avoided, particularly in nursery or intensive-care areas. A sufficient number of sinks for hand-washing should be available. Appropriate environmental disinfection and adequate air control may also reduce skin colonization with potential pathogens.

Therapy

Appropriate antimicrobial therapy (in addition to surgical drainage when necessary) not only treats the infected patient but also reduces the hazard of transmission to other persons. Identification of the infecting pathogen and antimicrobial susceptibility testing should serve as a guide to therapy. Topical antimicrobial agents can be used to treat milder skin infections. Treatment of streptococcal or staphylococcal carriers is discussed in subsequent sections of this chapter.

Staphylococcal Infections
General Aspects

Staphylococci that coagulate plasma in vitro (coagulase-positive strains) cause the bulk of staphylococcal disease and, by convention, are called *Staphylococcus aureus*. Staphylococcal strains that do not coagulate plasma are designated *S. epidermidis* (formerly *S. albus*); these organisms are universal inhabitants of normal skin but rarely cause cutaneous infections. The following discussion applies to *S. aureus* only.

Superficial infections due to these strains rank among the most important of all nosocomial infections, particularly in newborns and pediatric patients [11,30]. Historically, nursery outbreaks caused by staphylococci in the 1950s and 1960s first focused widespread attention upon nosocomial infections and fostered efforts for developing preventive measures.

TRANSMISSIBILITY. Anyone may acquire transient, superficial carriage of *S. aureus* on the skin and mucous membranes through contact with other persons who harbor the microorganism or with the environment. Carriage may lead to colonization where the agent persists and multiplies on skin or mucosal surfaces. In asymptomatic adults, the nasal vestibule is the major reservoir for *S. aureus.* Colonization at other skin sites rarely occurs when the anterior nares are free of staphylococci, but *S. aureus* can often be isolated from numerous other body sites when the nares become colonized. Repeated culture specimens of the anterior nares obtained over a prolonged period show that at least 80 percent of normal adults are colonized with *S. aureus* on occasion. In most individuals, periods when no staphylococci can be isolated alternate with other periods when a single strain is present for weeks to months. However, up to 25 percent of colonized adults have sustained carriage of a single strain, while another 10 to 15 percent of adults resist colonization with *S. aureus,* and the agent will not be isolated from them, even with repeated samplings. The factors responsible for these differences in susceptibility to colonization are incompletely understood but probably include the presence or absence of other cutaneous flora (which can be influenced by antibiotic therapy), underlying host defense mechanisms, and the intensity of exposure to staphylococci. Several studies have found higher colonization rates in persons exposed to the hospital environment. Colonization rates among patients increase with increasing duration of hospitalization, but increases among personnel have generally been small except when staphylococcal infection was frequent in the institution.

Neonates rarely become colonized by maternal staphylococci at birth, but colonization develops in the first few days of life, either in the hospital nursery or in the home. Infants may be first colonized at the umbilicus, in the nose, or at wounds such as circumcision sites, but colonization at any of these sites usually leads to colonization at all sites within several days. Therefore, in testing for colonization, the highest yield is obtained if several sites are sampled; if only one site is to be sampled, the umbilicus has had the highest relative yield in most studies.

Most colonized persons do not effectively transmit staphylococci, although any individual who harbors staphylococci may theoretically serve as a source for subsequent transmission to others. Occasionally, however, an individual colonized with *S. aureus* is the source for an outbreak of disease. Several factors have been thought to facilitate the dissemination of staphylococci in this circumstance. Persons with large numbers of staphylococci in the nares transmit staphylococci more readily, as do colonized persons who have dermatitis. Viral upper respiratory tract infections may also be associated with enhanced dissemination. This mechanism has been one proposed explanation for the "cloud baby" phenomenon [10], a situation where apparently asymptomatic babies shed large numbers of staphylococci into their immediate environments. Finally, tetracycline treatment of a staphylococcal carrier appears to increase the risk of transmission when the colonizing strain is resistant to this drug, but this phenomenon may not apply to other antibiotics. Doubtless other factors that are not well understood at present also influence the likelihood of staphylococcal shedding during colonization. Some colonized individuals, called "dangerous disseminators," shed staphylococci from all body surfaces (usually in greater numbers from the perineum) and readily transmit the organisms to other persons or the environment. They constitute only a small proportion of all people colonized with staphylococci. Unfortunately, no reliable, simple measure exists to screen staphylococcal carriers for their ability to spread the organism. Persons who are repeatedly positive for the same strain at multiple sites, however, are more likely to be disseminators, and many disseminators give a history of recurrent staphylococcal skin infections.

Persons with active staphylococcal infections are a major reservoir for the organism. Obvious sources include lesions with extensive purulent drainage (e.g., burn, traumatic, or surgical wounds) and infections that produce copious contaminated secretions (e.g., staphylococcal pneumonia or enterocolitis). Staphylococcal outbreaks have also been traced to hospital staff with minor staphylococcal pyodermas, paronychia, or styes. Neonates with staphylococcal pyodermas markedly increase the risk of colonization and disease among other exposed infants, hospital personnel, and family members [15,22,32].

Only rarely have contaminated environmental objects been considered an epidemiologically important reservoir for staphylococci in the hospital. Although persons harboring staphylococci readily contaminate their environment, the level of environmental contamination declines rapidly in the absence of human carriers.

In most circumstances [27], hand transmission is a more important means of spreading

staphylococci than the airborne route (Fig. 20-1). Transmission of organisms from the hands of hospital employees to patients is more often the proximate cause of clinical infection than other routes of spread. Airborne transmission seemingly plays a minor role in the spread of staphylococci that directly cause patient infections, but few investigators doubt that airborne staphylococci may inoculate the nares of personnel and patients, establish colonization, and subsequently result in infection via contact transmission. Airborne spread therefore results in the transmission of infections via several indirect routes (see Fig. 20-1), but it accounts for fewer direct infections than hand transmission.

Several factors may explain the apparent paradox that large numbers of airborne staphylococci may be isolated in the hospital yet they seldom seem directly responsible for disease. First, droplet nuclei, dust, and skin squames capable of airborne dissemination carry few microorganisms compared with contaminated hands or the droplets that are responsible for contact transmission. Second, airborne microorganisms settle slowly; most remain suspended for prolonged periods and therefore have a low

Figure 20-1. Important routes of staphylococcal transmission involved in nosocomial infection and disease.

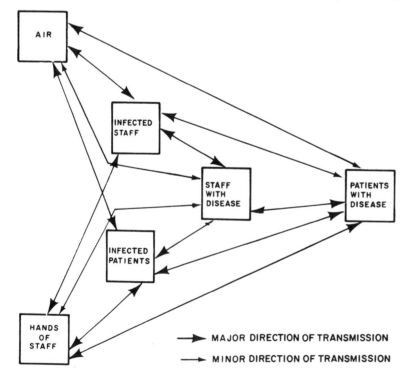

probability of implanting on a susceptible tissue surface. Finally, staphylococci in the inanimate environment may be less virulent because of drying or other environmental stresses.

CLINICAL MANIFESTATIONS. Several clinical syndromes suggest staphylococcal infection, but carefully obtained specimens for culture are necessary to confirm the cause of a particular infection. Even without culture determinations, however, a typical skin lesion occurring in association with a documented staphylococcal outbreak should be considered presumptively staphylococcal for purposes of initial treatment, isolation, and epidemiologic analysis.

Staphylococcal pustulosis may arise by primary or secondary infection of existing vesicles or pustules. Large pustules arising in hair follicles are termed "furuncles" and commonly occur about the nose and in intertriginous or macerated areas. They begin as firm erythematous nodules, progress over several days to form fluctuant pustules, and then discharge a necrotic core. Multiple furuncles may become confluent to form a deeper, more extensive, subcutaneous abscess, a "carbuncle." Involvement of the hair follicles and sebaceous glands of the eyelid produces a painful "stye" (hordeolum). Paronychia are painful, inflammatory infections of the tissue surrounding the fingernail, which usually progress to abscess formation. These superficial pyodermas usually produce no systemic signs of infection.

Although staphylococci often secondarily colonize impetiginous lesions, most impetigo in children and adults is caused by group-A streptococci (see later section). Primary staphylococcal impetigo does occur, however. Clinical differentiation between streptococcal and staphylococcal impetigo is difficult, but the streptococcal infection tends to have a golden crust, systemic manifestations of infection, and regional lymphangitis, whereas staphylococcal impetigo is more localized and has a gray-white crust.

One form of impetigo, bullous impetigo, is typically caused by *S. aureus*. In adults, the localized form of this disease is usually seen: large (1 to 10 cm.), flaccid bullae, instead of the small vesicles characteristic of streptococcal impetigo, form upon an area of pyoderma. When the disease remains localized and occurs in an area of preceding pyoderma, the bullous fluid contains large numbers of white cells and staphylococci. After the bulla bursts, extensive crusting occurs. Generalized rather than local bullous impetigo may occur in newborns (see below).

Staphylococcal mastitis in adults almost exclusively affects mothers who nurse infants colonized or infected with *S. aureus;* it is characterized by onset three to eight weeks after delivery, fever, leukocytosis, and marked tenderness, erythema, and induration of the breast. Fissuring of the nipple may predispose to infection. Superficial pustules on the breast are sometimes seen, and staphylococci can be isolated from these lesions or from breast milk. If not treated promptly, mastitis often progresses to breast abscess. Such conditions may be the first recognized manifestations of a nursery-associated staphylococcal outbreak; in fact, they rarely occur in the 1970s, but they were common in association with outbreaks due to phage type 80/81 staphylococci in the decade beginning in the mid-1950s.

Staphylococci also cause a variety of infrequent nosocomial superficial infections in adults, including infections of decubitus ulcers, conjunctivitis, subcutaneous abscesses (usually associated with a foreign body), and, rarely, cellulitis. Additional very rare superficial staphylococcal infections in adults include pyomyositis, which is an indolent, destructive process involving muscle [23], and necrotizing fasciitis [35], a rapidly progressive, deep cellulitis that is more often associated with group-A streptococci or anaerobic organisms (see Part II, Chapter 16).

Most nosocomial superficial staphylococcal infections involve neonates, with pustular lesions occurring most commonly (48 percent; see Table 20-4). Omphalitis—characterized by local inflammation and purulent drainage from the umbilical stump—also occurs frequently (27 percent). Both lesions are commonly associated with staphylococcal purulent conjunctivitis (21 percent). In the 1950s and early 1960s, these lesions were most often caused by the staphylococci that are lysed by group I phages, especially phage types 80 and 80/81, and they

Table 20-4. Distribution of Superficial Staphylo-coccal Infections[a]

Service	Rate per 10,000 discharges	Predominant forms of infection[b]
Nursery	18.8	P (48%), O (27%), E (21%)
Pediatric	7.2	P (39%), E (33%), O (21%)
Medicine	2.1	P (50%), E (27%), C (18%)
Surgery	1.4	P (51%), E (33%), C (10%)
Obstetrics	0.3	M (77%), P (15%)
Gynecology	0.2	P (40%)
Overall	3.6	P (47%), E (25%), O (18%)

[a] Data from the National Nosocomial Infections Study (NNIS), 1970–1973. Data are based on 3,456,649 discharges.
[b] P = pyoderma, O = omphalitis, E = eye infection, C = cellulitis, M = maternal mastitis.

were often complicated by disseminated infection, including pneumonia, osteomyelitis, and meningitis. Although uncomplicated pyodermas still occur frequently, disseminated staphylococcal infection secondary to pyoderma occurs less often in the 1970s.

Although disseminated staphylococcal disease has become less common in neonates, exfoliative staphylococcal pyodermas appear to have become more common. When this disease is mild, a localized pyoderma is followed by a tender, sandpaper-textured, scarlatiniform rash that may be either localized or generalized. In three to five days, large sheets of epidermis desquamate (in contrast to the small flakes of desquamation seen following streptococcal infection). Bullous impetigo is a more severe form of the disease, and it also may be either localized or generalized. Generalized bullous disease —known as toxic epidermal necrolysis (TEN), Ritter's disease, Lyell's TEN, or the "scalded skin" syndrome—is seen rarely. In this syndrome, a local pyoderma precedes the sudden appearance of generalized erythema, low-grade fever, and leukocytosis. Within several days, large, flaccid bullae form over much of the body and subsequently burst, leaving large areas of raw, erythematous skin resembling a second-degree burn or scalded skin. In this generalized disease, microorganisms usually cannot be isolated from intact bullae. Staphylococci lysed by type 71 phage or by other phages in group II usually cause this group of diseases, although other strains have also been associated. Approximately 40 percent of group II strains produce a protein exotoxin that appears to be responsible for intraepidermal cleavage and bulla formation [26].

Infant mastitis was frequently seen when phage types 80/81 were prevalent, but it occurs less often now (0.5 percent). Suppurative cervical lymphadenitis caused by staphylococci is also quite uncommon now; a long, asymptomatic, incubation period (20 to 80 days) may occur before the onset of disease.

MICROBIOLOGIC DIAGNOSIS. Staphylococci are usually identified on the basis of colonial and microscopic morphology and the catalase reaction. They characteristically appear as gram-positive cocci arranged in clusters, although single organisms, pairs, short chains, and tetrads may be seen on Gram stain of clinical specimens. Staphylococci are catalase-positive, whereas streptococci are catalase-negative. *S. aureus* is usually differentiated from *S. epidermidis* by coagulase production and mannitol fermentation. Production of coagulase (as measured by the tube test) should be performed to identify *S. aureus*. The slide coagulase test is more difficult to read and requires fresh human plasma (commercially available lyophilized rabbit plasma can be used in the tube test); negative results obtained in the slide test should be confirmed using the tube test. Care must be taken to use pure isolates, since mixed specimens may cause false-positive tube tests. With either test, concurrent controls, including saline controls in the slide test to detect autoagglutinins, are recommended. Many clinical laboratories label all coagulase-negative strains as *S. epidermidis,* although this reaction is also shared by *Sarcina, Gaffkya,* and other micrococci. The clinical and epidemiologic value of routine species identification of coagulase-negative strains is uncertain. However, microorganisms that are involved in outbreaks and that have atypical antimicrobial suscepti-bility patterns, uncertain coagulase reactions, or other unusual characteristics may be differentiated by their ability to ferment mannitol and other sugars aerobically and anaerobically as well as by their susceptibility to lysostaphin.

Other methods to differentiate *S. aureus* and *S. epidermidis* are not reliable. Although coagulase-negative staphylococci are usually more resistant to antibiotics than *S. aureus,* susceptibility patterns alone cannot differentiate between species. Most coagulase-positive staphylococci produce golden-hued colonies on culture, and most coagulase-negative strains have white colonies. Pigment production, however, does not reliably predict virulence, because nonpigmented strains, if coagulase-positive, produce typical staphylococcal disease. Similarly, β-hemolysis typifies *S. aureus* and is usually absent with *S. epidermidis,* but some coagulase-negative strains also produce β-hemolysis.

S. aureus phage typing is of value epidemiologically in comparing strains from different patients and potential carriers. It offers little information that is useful clinically or for the evaluation of sporadic disease, and it should not be done routinely. Antibiograms may provide a rapid and useful means of typing staphylococci if an unusual pattern is recognized.

CLASSIFICATION OF INFECTIONS. Nosocomial staphylococcal disease may become clinically evident during hospitalization or after discharge. Since the incubation period of cutaneous infection varies considerably, arbitrary intervals for separating community-acquired and nosocomial infections cannot be sharply defined. As a general rule, however, infections with an onset of more than 24 hours after admission and all neonatal staphylococcal infections with an onset prior to hospital discharge are considered nosocomial. Since the median incubation period for most neonatal pyoderma syndromes is seven to ten days, the onset of most infections in term infants occurs after discharge. Any neonatal staphylococcal infection occurring shortly after hospital discharge should be presumed nosocomial.

Antimicrobial susceptibility patterns or phage typing are generally not reliable in differentiating nosocomial and community staphylococcal strains.

SPECIMEN COLLECTION AND TRANSPORT. Material for staining and culturing should be obtained by aspiration or incision of pustules or abscesses. When pus cannot be obtained for culture, superficial crusts of pyoderma lesions should be lifted off and the base of the lesion sampled with a cotton or Dacron swab moistened in sterile saline or nutrient broth. If swabs are planted promptly on culture media, carrying media are not required.

Staphylococcal colonization of adults may be demonstrated by swabbing the anterior nasal vestibule with a sterile swab that has been premoistened in saline. Throat and nasopharyngeal cultures have a lower yield. Since occasional individuals do not show nasal colonization but have colonization at other sites, intertriginous and perineal samples should be obtained from persons suspected epidemiologically of being carriers.

PREDISPOSING HOST FACTORS. Little is known about the factors that predispose to clinical staphylococcal infection. Certainly, colonized individuals have a much greater risk of developing disease than noncolonized patients, but only a minority of those colonized actually develop overt disease (the colonization-to-disease ratio usually exceeds 20 to 1). Host defense mechanisms clearly play a role, because infants seem universally quite susceptible but later become relatively resistant to disease. Furthermore, neonates develop disseminated infections more often than adults. Some individuals appear to have lifelong susceptibility to recurrent staphylococcal pyoderma. Despite these observations, specific factors that determine susceptibility to staphylococcal disease have not been identified. Humoral antibodies against many staphylococcal components are found after infection, but none has been shown to protect against subsequent infection.

Patients with diabetes mellitus, particularly if they are insulin-dependent, suffer more frequent and severe staphylococcal infections than nondiabetics. Skin defects also increase susceptibility to staphylococcal pyoderma. A local foreign body such as a silk suture reduces by

1000 times the number of staphylococci necessary to produce a cutaneous abscess.

TREATMENT. All but the mildest staphylococcal cutaneous infections require systemic antibiotic therapy. Parenteral therapy should be administered if the patient is toxic, but well-localized and drained lesions usually respond to oral agents. Since penicillinase-producing strains cause the majority of infections, a semisynthetic penicillin should be used initially. If the infecting strain proves susceptible to penicillin, the semisynthetic agent should be discontinued and penicillin substituted. Nafcillin has greater activity against streptococci than do other semisynthetic penicillins, and it should be used for mixed infections or when the identity of the causative agent is uncertain.

A patient with penicillin allergy or one infected with a methicillin-resistant strain may be treated with a cephalosporin. Cross-reactions between the penicillins and cephalosporins occur, however, and individuals with a history suggesting that an immediate hypersensitivity reaction might occur should probably be given an alternative agent, such as vancomycin, erythromycin, or clindamycin. In addition, strains that are resistant to methicillin also tend to be resistant to the cephalosporins. Thus, vancomycin (a bactericidal agent) may be preferable for treating overwhelming infections. Erythromycin, while only bacteriostatic, is also effective in treating most milder staphylococcal infections. Gentamicin and kanamycin show in vitro activity against most staphylococcal strains, but they are clinically less effective than the agents listed above. Tetracycline should not be used for serious staphylococcal infections.

Topical therapy is a useful adjunct in treating staphylococcal pyoderma and in eradicating asymptomatic colonization. Minor pyodermas respond to local cleansing with soap and water. Topical bacitracin has activity against *S. aureus* strains and is useful when applied after cleansing. Other topical antimicrobial agents are of uncertain value, and topical hexachlorophene (HCP)—as noted below—may be harmful under some circumstances.

A variety of regimens have been used to eradicate staphylococcal colonization in adults who have been implicated as a source of nosocomial infections. Topical bacitracin ointment applied to the nasal vestibule four times daily for ten days usually eradicates staphylococcal carriage at the nasal as well as untreated skin sites. Simultaneous administration of an appropriate systemic penicillin may increase the eradication rate, but systemic antimicrobials are usually not effective if used alone. On occasion, colonization recurs after treatment, because of either recolonization or relapse. If recolonization with the same strain occurs, persisting hospital or family reservoirs must be identified and concurrently treated. Suppression of strains that cause relapse following treatment may require HCP hand-washing, limited HCP bathing, and frequent changing and cleaning of clothing, linens, and other fomites, in addition to topical and systemic antimicrobial therapy (see Part II, Chapter 16).

Until recently, 3% HCP in a detergent base was generally considered both effective and safe. Hexachlorophene has been demonstrated to reduce neonatal staphylococcal colonization and disease in controlled clinical studies [15, 32], and despite occasional reports to the contrary, the majority of published studies provide convincing evidence of its efficacy. In the late 1960s, however, heavy HCP exposure among adults with skin diseases (extensive burns or dermatitis) was linked to convulsive-seizure disorders and other neurologic symptoms; several of these patients examined at autopsy had unusual cystic degenerative changes in their central nervous system white matter. Studies of infant experimental animals also associated these neuropathologic lesions with topically applied HCP [24]. Retrospective studies have suggested that similar neuropathologic changes occur more frequently in human infants (particularly premature infants) bathed with HCP than in infants without HCP exposure [33, 39]. Clinical symptoms of neurologic dysfunction, however, have not yet been convincingly shown to result from traditional HCP bathing procedures in nurseries, and data suggest that these neuropathologic changes are reversible after discontinuation of HCP exposure. Nevertheless, it is generally agreed that HCP should not be used *routinely* to bathe either premature or term neonates. We believe, however, that in-hospital infant bathing with HCP should be used in conjunction with other control measures when high rates of staphylococcal disease occur in the nursery. In this circumstance, the potential benefits outweigh any documented risks.

Several other topical antiseptic agents have been used to reduce neonatal staphylococcal colonization. Bacitracin applied topically to umbilical stumps and circumcision sites appears to be as effective as HCP in limited trials [14], and it has no obvious toxicity. Alcohol applied to umbilical stumps may also be of value. Several centers have applied triple dye (an aqueous mixture of brilliant green, proflavine hemisulfate, and crystal violet) to umbilical stumps [7] and have reported decreased colonization, but the safety of this compound and its effectiveness in preventing infection have not been well studied. Neither the safety nor the efficacy of other agents, such as iodophors or quaternary ammonium compounds, has been appropriately evaluated.

Finally, the implantation of less virulent staphylococcal strains has been used as a means of interfering with colonization by virulent strains [38]. The penicillin-sensitive 502A strain of *S. aureus* has usually been used, and it has been effective on occasion in preventing colonization of infants and adults by other strains. Failures to abort epidemics with this approach have been reported [2], however, and this strain has produced cutaneous or occasionally disseminated infection and death [18]. The risk of infection following colonization with strain 502A seems comparable to that of infection with other nonepidemic strains of *S. aureus,* and thus, implantation of strain 502A might only be expected to show therapeutic efficacy when this strain replaces strains more virulent than itself.

Endemic Infections

INCIDENCE. Cutaneous staphylococcal infections occurred in 1242 of approximately 3.5 million hospitalized patients in hospitals included in the NNIS during 1970 to 1973. Rates of infection were much higher in newborn and pediatric patients than among adults (see Table 20-4). Pyoderma was the most common type of infection on all services except obstetrics, where mastitis constituted more than three-quarters of reported superficial staphylococcal infections. Approximately a quarter of the infections among newborns and children were omphalitis.

SOURCES. Staphylococci that cause sporadic infections come from the patient's autogenous flora, from other patients or personnel, or from the environment. As noted above, persons with clinically active infections, especially those with draining lesions, are very important sources of *S. aureus.* Asymptomatic carriers, particularly dangerous disseminators, also constitute a nosocomial reservoir. The inanimate environment is a less important source of staphylococci when usual hygienic standards are maintained, but it can facilitate the colonization of patients with hospital strains that, under the right conditions, may cause infection.

MODE OF SPREAD. Colonization and infection may be acquired by direct and indirect contact spread from infected and colonized persons. Airborne transmission probably plays a less important role in spread of staphylococci.

PREVENTION. Hand-washing by personnel before and after each patient contact is probably the most important measure to prevent staphylococcal disease. In the newborn nursery or other high-risk areas, an antiseptic hand-washing agent such as HCP, chlorhexidine, or an iodophor should be used.

Hospital personnel with staphylococcal infections should not provide patient care. Because of the high prevalence of asymptomatic staphylococcal colonization among personnel and the relative infrequency that such personnel cause disease, programs to identify and treat asymptomatic employee carriers are not warranted unless there is evidence of transmission of infection.

Standard environmental sanitation (Part I, Chapter 6) is adequate to render the inanimate environment safe. The effects of ultraviolet light and laminar airflow on staphylococcal skin infections have not been adequately studied. However, adequate dilution, filtration, and direction of hospital air probably reduces the risk of patients and personnel being colonized with nosocomial strains.

Measures to prevent contact transmission of staphylococci should be employed. Highly susceptible patients, such as those with extensive dermatitis, may benefit from protective isolation precautions, and all patients with suspected staphylococcal infections should be appropriately isolated. In the nursery, crowding should be avoided, and a cohort admission system, which further reduces the opportunity for person-to-person transmission, should be used. In the cohort system, all infants admitted during a 48-hour period are placed in a single room. Infants are not transferred to other units unless they require special care, and personnel movement between different cohort rooms is minimized or avoided entirely. At the end of the 48-hour period, no further infants are admitted to the room. After all infants in the cohort have been discharged and the room thoroughly cleaned, it is then reopened to accept a new cohort of infants. Modified or strict rooming-in of infants with mothers may also minimize the risk of staphylococcal colonization.

Because of the potential toxicity of HCP, it should not be used for routine bathing in nonepidemic situations (see above).

Epidemic Infections

Since many staphylococcal skin infections have their onset after hospital discharge, even a few recognized infections in hospitalized patients should arouse suspicion that an epidemic may be occurring. In fact, two or more simultaneous skin infections in a nursery or a single case of breast abscess in a nursing mother or infant should be considered presumptive evidence of an epidemic [1].

INCIDENCE. Hospital epidemics of staphylococcal skin infections infrequently occur in adults except among burn patients (see Part II, Chapter 19) and on dermatology wards. Small outbreaks of staphylococcal pyodermas have been reported on pediatric services.

In contrast, although their actual incidence is not known, staphylococcal epidemics among newborns occur quite commonly and are among the most frequently recognized nosocomial outbreaks. The incidence of such epidemics can be estimated using data reported to the

NNIS. In a one-year period (1971) before most hospitals discontinued routine HCP bathing of neonates, 36 NNIS hospital nurseries had 19 outbreaks; thus, each hospital had an approximately 50 percent chance of an outbreak each year. Overall, a baseline endemic rate of approximately one staphylococcal infection per 1000 live births was noted in these hospitals.

HIGH-RISK GROUPS. Neonates are at the greatest risk of epidemic staphylococcal disease because of the absence of flora that compete with staphylococci for colonization, the presence of cutaneous wounds (umbilical and circumcision), the many opportunities for contact spread of microorganisms in the nursery, and their enhanced susceptibility to staphylococcal infection. Adults with dermatoses, particularly extensive dermatitis, are also at increased risk.

SOURCES. Often the initial source of an epidemic staphylococcal strain cannot be defined. Many outbreaks have been attributed to hospital personnel with minor skin lesions (paronychia, styes, or pustulosis), while others have been attributed to asymptomatic patient or personnel carriers. Parturient mothers have seldom been documented as sources for nursery outbreaks. Once infection becomes established in a population, infected patients themselves serve as a reservoir for ongoing transmission. As with endemic infections, inanimate surfaces, fomites, and the air seem to play minor roles as reservoirs of pathogens that may cause outbreaks, although such sources may amplify the colonization of patients and personnel.

MODES OF SPREAD. Contact transmission was responsible for the spread of staphylococci in most epidemics where the modes of transmission have been carefully studied. The single most important mechanism has been carriage of staphylococci on the hands of hospital personnel. Less often, airborne spread contributed directly or indirectly to colonization, and only rarely have outbreaks been traced to an inanimate common source.

CONTROL OF OUTBREAKS. When a staphylococcal outbreak is recognized in a patient-care unit, all infected patients must be identified promptly, isolated appropriately, and treated with systemic and, when indicated, topical antimicrobial agents. Hospital personnel should be examined for staphylococcal disease, and infected personnel should be removed from direct patient care and treated.

An epidemiologic investigation should be initiated promptly in order (1) to identify the original source of the epidemic strain and to determine whether exposure to individual staff members is associated with patient disease, (2) to define existing staphylococcal reservoirs, (3) to assess the patient-care practices that might facilitate transmission, and (4) to define the population at risk of disease. To define the reservoir, culture surveys of patients and personnel may be necessary, and colonized patients should be isolated from susceptible ones. Personnel carriers of the epidemic strain should be removed from the direct care of susceptible patients, but they may care for patients who are already infected if the personnel are under appropriate treatment for colonization and if personnel shortages would result from their removal from work. Colonized personnel may return to work after treatment has been initiated and their culture specimens are negative for *S. aureus.* Follow-up cultures after discontinuation of therapy should be obtained to insure eradication of colonization. Since phage-typing results may not be available immediately, staphylococci isolated from patients and personnel should be considered the epidemic strain if they have the same antimicrobial susceptibility patterns as the strains causing disease.

Factors that encourage staphylococcal transmission (e.g., patient crowding, inadequate hand-washing, insufficient numbers of nursing personnel, and failure to isolate infected patients promptly) should be corrected. Prompt discharge of uninfected patients should be encouraged, and elective admissions to the affected unit should be curtailed. The cohort admission system very effectively interrupts the transmission of staphylococci to susceptible patients. In nursery populations, a staphylococcal epidemic may justify the use of a topical agent to inhibit staphylococcal colonization of infants. Short-term, prophylactic, HCP bathing

of susceptible infants (preferably limited to infants over 2000 gm.) should be instituted; HCP should be rinsed off thoroughly after each use and efforts should be made to expose no infant to more than two baths. Topical applications of bacitracin ointment to umbilical stumps, anterior nares, and circumcision wounds four times daily and after bathing may also be beneficial. We believe the risks outweigh the potential benefits of employing bacterial interference with the 502A strain of *S. aureus.* On occasion, it has been necessary to close a unit to control a staphylococcal epidemic. It must be stressed that if a member of the staff is a dangerous disseminator of staphylococci and remains undiscovered or untreated, the unit remains at risk to recurrent disease when it is reopened.

Streptococcal Infections
General Aspects
Skin infections caused by group-A β-hemolytic streptococci include (1) impetigo, a superficial pyoderma that usually occurs after a minor or unrecognized break in the skin; (2) cellulitis, a deeper skin infection that often follows more significant trauma to the skin; (3) erysipelas, a characteristic, raised, sharply marginated cellulitis that is limited to the corium; and (4) omphalitis [8,45]. Of these, cellulitis and omphalitis occur most commonly as nosocomial infections, whereas impetigo ordinarily is community-acquired. Group-A streptococci also cause secondary pyodermas in hospitalized patients who have eczema, varicella, burns, or other skin lesions.

TRANSMISSIBILITY. About 10 percent of healthy adults and 10 to 20 percent of healthy children in the community carry group-A β-hemolytic streptococci in their upper respiratory tract. Asymptomatic carriage at other sites (skin, vagina, or rectum) is uncommon except during an epidemic, after intense exposure, or when associated with an acute streptococcal infection. Organisms spread readily from persons colonized or infected with streptococci to noncolonized individuals. In the community, epidemics of streptococcal skin infections occur commonly (particularly in warm climates, in overcrowded areas, or where hygiene is poor), and secondary attack rates in families are often high. Persons with active streptococcal infections of either the skin or the respiratory tract, nasal carriers, and, on occasion, perineal carriers appear particularly prone to disseminating the organism.

CLASSIFICATION OF INFECTIONS. A very short incubation period (6 to 48 hours) characterizes streptococcal cellulitis, whereas impetigo or streptococcal pyodermas generally have a longer incubation period (up to ten days). Streptococcal infections that have their onset more than 24 hours after hospitalization should be classified as nosocomial, even though colonization of the skin may have taken place before hospitalization. Streptococcal skin infections that occur in newborns either during hospitalization or within ten days of discharge are considered nosocomial.

CLINICAL MANIFESTATIONS. Impetiginous lesions often involve the lower extremities, begin with small vesicles that rapidly become pustular, and eventually develop thick, honey-colored crusts. Fever, malaise, and regional lymphadenopathy frequently accompany lymphatic spread, while local spread follows scratching and the release of infected vesicle fluid.

Acute inflammation (warmth, tenderness, redness, and swelling) with little necrosis or suppuration characterizes streptococcal cellulitis, which is often accompanied by lymphangitis, lymphadenitis, fever, and malaise. In erysipelas, one sees a red, indurated, expanding area of severe cellulitis that often involves the face and is sharply demarcated from adjacent unaffected skin.

The duration of streptococcal skin infections ranges from weeks to months, and bacteremia may complicate these infections, particularly cellulitis. Ten to fifteen percent of patients who have skin infection with a nephritogenic strain develop acute glomerulonephritis, but skin infections are not followed by acute rheumatic fever [8,21,45].

MICROBIOLOGIC DIAGNOSIS. Group-A β-hemolytic streptococci cause the majority of streptococcal skin infections. These organisms are best isolated using a pour-plate method with sheep blood in an infusion agar base that is free of fermentable carbohydrate and has a final pH of 7.3 to 7.4. Gram stain, characteristic β-hemolysis, absence of catalase activity, and sensitivity to the bacitracin differential disc allow presumptive identification of most group-A streptococci. Even if culture results are negative, about 90 percent of patients have elevated anti-DNase B titers following streptococcal skin infection. Only about 50 percent of patients with skin infections have positive antistreptolysin O titers.

The group-A streptococci are divided into over 50 specific types by a precipitin test for M protein or by an agglutination reaction to the T protein. During an outbreak of streptococcal skin infections, M and T typing may assist in epidemiologically identifying a carrier and related cases. M types 2, 12, 49, 55, and 57 have all been frequently associated with epidemics of streptococcal skin infections followed by nephritis.

COLLECTION AND TRANSPORT OF SPECIMENS. Streptococci can usually be isolated from vesicular fluid or from the base of lesions under a crust. In impetigo, cultures are more often positive early in the course of the disease; later in the disease, staphylococci are also frequently isolated but these probably play a secondary role. Streptococci usually cannot be isolated from areas of cellulitis. However, one may inject and then withdraw sterile saline from the margin of the lesion and sometimes isolate the organism. Most laboratories place specimens suspected of containing streptococci in a Todd-Hewitt enrichment broth. If shipping is required, the swab may be placed in a silica-gel packet and then transferred to Todd-Hewitt broth after transport.

PREDISPOSING HOST FACTORS. Although streptococci colonize normal skin, they rarely invade unless the skin surface is broken by abrasions, insect bites, or other trauma. Most nosocomial streptococcal skin infections occur in children, particularly in newborns. Immunity resulting from these childhood infections lasts for as long as 30 years and may explain why they are less common in adults. Geriatric patients, however, are also prone to streptococcal skin infections.

THERAPY. Intramuscular benzathine penicillin or oral penicillin V is the treatment of choice for streptococcal skin infections; erythromycin can be used in penicillin-allergic patients. Mild streptococcal skin infections may sometimes be successfully treated by removing the crusts and bathing the lesions with soap and water, but antibiotics should be given to prevent poststreptococcal glomerulonephritis. Hexachlorophene has not been found effective in treating streptococcal skin infections in several controlled trials; in addition, its application to denuded skin may be dangerous. Other topical antimicrobials such as bacitracin, however, have been successfully used in treating mild streptococcal skin infections.

Endemic Infections

INCIDENCE. According to data from the NNIS, 0.3 nosocomial streptococcal skin infections occurred per 10,000 hospital discharges. The rate of infection was approximately four times greater in newborns than in adults. The majority of neonatal infections were omphalitis, while pyoderma was the manifestation most often seen in adults.

SOURCES. Hospitalized patients or hospital employees with major or minor streptococcal infections of the skin or respiratory tract constitute the most important nosocomial reservoir for streptococci. The importance of asymptomatic cutaneous colonization remains unclear [45]. Apparently because of the bactericidal action of certain fatty acids on streptococci, most strains do not survive on healthy skin for longer than 24 hours. Therefore, pharyngeal colonization or infection with streptococci was thought to be the important reservoir from which organisms subsequently infected open lesions on the skin. Several studies have now shown, however, that healthy skin may become colonized with certain strains of streptococci several weeks before infection takes place [9]. The majority of these patients do not have prior pharyngeal colonization, although about one-third subsequently develop it. Thus, although skin lesions infected with streptococci constitute the most important hospital reservoir for these organisms, colonized skin may also play a role. The importance of asymptomatic

perineal carriage of streptococci as a source of organisms causing endemic nosocomial infections is unknown. Fomites such as bed clothes and sheets used by infected patients sometimes contain large numbers of streptococci, but these do not appear to be an epidemiologically important reservoir within the hospital. In contrast to other streptococcal skin infections, erysipelas often follows a prior pharyngeal infection.

MODES OF TRANSMISSION. Although the mode of transmission of streptococci that cause pharyngeal infections clearly seems to be contact with droplets expired from the pharynx of an infected patient, the modes of transmission of the streptococci that cause skin infections are less clear. Most often, organisms are probably spread by direct contact from a patient with an infected lesion to a patient with healthy skin. The skin of the recipient, however, usually must be broken before infection occurs. It is uncertain how important either contact with droplets from pharyngeal carriers or airborne spread from cutaneous, pharyngeal, or perineal carriers might be in the transmission of endemic nosocomial streptococcal disease. Fomites do not appear important in the transmission of streptococci.

CONTROL MEASURES. Patients with streptococcal skin infections should be treated and placed on wound and skin precautions (see Part I, Chapter 9).

Epidemic Infections

INCIDENCE. The incidence of epidemic streptococcal skin infections in the hospital is unknown. Outbreaks in the community occur most frequently in the late summer and early fall, and a warm climate, overcrowding, and skin trauma all contribute to epidemics. Nosocomial epidemics have nearly always been related to a patient or employee who is infected or, less often, colonized with skin strains of streptococci.

SOURCES. As in endemic infections, patients or personnel with streptococcal skin lesions are usually the source of streptococci during outbreaks. Anal and vaginal carriers have been described as reservoirs for streptococci that cause wound infections [36,42], and pharyngeal carriers may sometimes be a source (see Part II, Chapter 16).

MODES OF TRANSMISSION. Direct contact with lesions infected with streptococci is probably the most important mode of spread, although contact with droplets from pharyngeal carriers may also occur. Epidemics of omphalitis in the nursery have most often been related to personnel with skin lesions. They have also been related to infants with streptococcal infections acquired at birth who serve as a source for subsequent cross-infection of other infants. Epidemics of streptococcal bacteremia have been related to personnel with streptococcal skin infections who have started patients' intravenous lines [5]. Patients with extensive burns infected with streptococci and asymptomatic perineal carriers may shed streptococci via the airborne route.

CONTROL OF OUTBREAKS. In nosocomial outbreaks, epidemiologic investigation should seek to identify a patient or employee who is a carrier of streptococci. Suspected individuals should be examined for skin lesions, and, if present, specimens from such lesions should be cultured. If no lesions are apparent, nose, throat, vaginal, and anal cultures should be obtained from persons who have been epidemiologically implicated as suspected carriers. Personnel with positive cultures should be treated with penicillin and should not work until repeated cultures are negative. Since respiratory carriage of streptococci is usually not important in causing skin lesions such as omphalitis, it is not recommended that routine nose and throat cultures be performed on nursery personnel. Patients with streptococcal skin infections should be placed on wound and skin precautions (Part I, Chapter 9), and those with extensive burns should be placed on strict isolation. In the nursery, infants with streptococcal omphalitis should be treated with penicillin and separated from noninfected infants. Each group should have its own nursing staff.

Infections Due to Herpesvirus Hominis
General Aspects
With the recent advent of improved serologic and virologic techniques, infections with her-

pesvirus hominis (HVH) have been more frequently recognized [28,29,31]. These viruses cause a wide spectrum of illness, ranging from localized, recurrent, mucocutaneous infection to disseminated disease, encephalitis, and death. The differentiation of two antigenic types (HVH type 1 and type 2) and the distinction of primary infections from recrudescences have permitted better description of the epidemiology of herpetic infections. Nosocomial infections due to HVH cause particular concern in that they often occur in neonates or immunosuppressed patients susceptible to disseminated infection.

TRANSMISSIBILITY. Serologic surveys suggest that the majority of adults in the United States have experienced symptomatic or asymptomatic infection with HVH. Primary infection with HVH type 1 (HVH-1) usually occurs between six months and four years of age, and it most often involves the oral cavity. Approximately 1 to 15 percent of this population have symptomatic gingivostomatitis and an additional 20 percent excrete HVH-1 asymptomatically. The prevalence of antibodies to HVH-1 increases rapidly between ages one and four and less rapidly thereafter; the prevalence of antibody in the general adult population is 30 to 50 percent in upper socioeconomic groups and 80 to 90 percent in lower socioeconomic groups. Type 1 infections in older patients are usually recurrent rather than primary, and they tend to involve the lips, skin and eye.

Primary HVH type 2 (HVH-2) infections generally occur in sexually active young adults. Antibody to HVH-2 is uncommon before age 12, increases rapidly in prevalence after age 15, and can be found in 10 to 60 percent of adult populations, depending on socioeconomic status and sexual habits.

CLINICAL MANIFESTATIONS. The clinical diagnosis of cutaneous HVH infections depends mainly on the characteristic skin lesions and a history of recrudescent symptoms. Local erythema, sometimes preceded by hyperesthesia or burning, is usually the first manifestation noted. Characteristic, thin-walled, grouped vesicles then form on an erythematous base and frequently proceed to pustule formation, crusting, or ulceration. Although either primary or recurrent infections may be asymptomatic, primary cutaneous lesions usually involve a larger skin area and are more often associated with fever, constitutional symptoms, and lymphadenopathy.

Dermatitis caused by HVH may involve any portion of the body, but it frequently occurs at sites of abrasion or other wounds. Type-1 HVH generally causes lesions above the umbilicus, whereas type-2 HVH usually infects skin below the umbilicus. Cutaneous infections of the extremities (hand and fingers, primarily) are approximately half HVH-1 and half HVH-2. Eczema herpeticum, an extensive cutaneous infection, occurs in compromised hosts, in burn patients, and in patients with atopic eczema or other skin disorders.

MICROBIOLOGIC DIAGNOSIS. Fresh vesicles may be unroofed and scrapings from the base of the vesicle stained with Giemsa or Wright's stain to demonstrate the multinucleated giant cells with intranuclear inclusion bodies that are typical of both HVH and herpes zoster skin infections. Viral isolation requires one to four days, and it is accomplished by placing fresh vesicle fluid in tissue culture. A large number of biologic techniques (e.g., cytopathologic effects, plaque appearance in tissue culture, pock size on egg chorioallantoic membrane) and serologic techniques can be used for viral subtyping.

Demonstration of humoral antibodies to HVH type 1 and HVH type 2 can be accomplished using neutralization, complement-fixation, passive-hemagglutination, and indirect-immunofluorescence methods. In patients with previous HVH infections, however, complete differentiation between type 1 and type 2 infections may not be possible. In some situations, quantification of HVH antibody in specific immunoglobulin fractions may prove useful (i.e., IgM HVH antibody in a newborn would suggest infection in utero).

CLASSIFICATION OF INFECTIONS. The tendency of HVH to cause symptoms episodically often makes distinction between nosocomial and community-acquired infections difficult. If the onset of a primary HVH infection occurs during hospitalization, the infection should certainly be classified as nosocomial. In addition to the patient's history, both the incubation period (two to eighteen days, an average of six days) and the presence of an antigenic response (a rise in circulating antibodies to type 1 or type 2 HVH one to four weeks after infection) may help to distinguish a primary infection from a recurrence. Because recurrences of infection cannot always be distinguished from primary infection, however, we recommend classifying all herpetic infections with onset during hospitalization as nosocomial, realizing that some such episodes represent reactivation of latent virus.

Neonates acquire herpetic infections during passage through an infected birth canal or in the postpartum period (see Sources, under Endemic Infections, below); thus, neonatal herpetic infections should be classified as nosocomial. Intrauterine infections may rarely occur.

SPECIMEN COLLECTION AND TRANSPORT. Fluid from fresh vesicles should be obtained for viral isolation. Swabs or fluid can be placed in either Leibovitz-Emory or Stuart media at ambient temperature for transport to an appropriate laboratory.

PREDISPOSING HOST FACTORS. Patients with atopic eczema and other dermatoses (seborrheic eczema, Darier's disease, pemphigus, and Wiskott-Aldrich syndrome) tend to develop extensive HVH dermatitis (Kaposi's varicelliform eruption), and such cases may progress to viremia and disseminated infection. Other patients who are predisposed to developing viremia and disseminated or central nervous system disease include newborns, patients with native or iatrogenic immunologic defects, and patients with protein malnutrition or severe infectious diseases. Up to 90 percent of patients who undergo nerve root section for trigeminal neuralgia manifest oral or circumoral HVH lesions in the postoperative period.

TREATMENT. The large number of therapeutic modalities used to treat mucocutaneous HVH infections reflects the fact that none is very effective. Autoimmunization, interferon induction, vaccinia immunization, immunization with inactivated HVH vaccines, and photoactivation therapy have been employed but without success. Adenine arabinoside (ara-A), available as a topical ointment, has recently been shown to be effective in treating herpetic keratitis and is relatively well tolerated. Topical idoxuridine (IDU) has also been successfully used to treat herpetic keratitis, but unfortunately, it does not prevent recurrences. Topical IDU is less effective for treating mucocutaneous HVH infections, but it may be beneficial when used in higher doses with dimethylsulfoxide. Adenine arabinoside is the first antiviral agent with effectiveness demonstrated in well-controlled trials for treatment of HVH encephalitis and may also be effective for other systemic infections. Cytosine arabinoside and IDH have also been used to treat disseminated HVH infections but are relatively toxic and seem to be less effective than ara-A. The potential role of ara-A in other HVH infections is being evaluated, but, at present, no agent is proved to be safe and effective for mild cutaneous infections.

Endemic Infections

INCIDENCE. Accurate estimates of the incidence of nosocomial HVH infections in adult patients are not currently available, but these infections seem to be rare. The absence of clinical symptoms or the trivial nature of these infections in most patients, the difficulty in distinguishing a recurrence from a new infection, and the lack of microbiologic confirmation of HVH infections in most hospitals all obscure their true incidence. Herpetic paronychia occurs sporadically in hospital employees, but the incidence of this infection is also unknown.

In contrast to the asymptomatic infections commonly seen in adults, HVH infections are clinically evident in most neonates. Further, such infections are clearly nosocomial rather than recurrent. Approximately one to five HVH infections occur per 10,000 live births, with cutaneous involvement present in half. Premature infants have a greater incidence of HVH infection than term infants.

SOURCES. Human beings appear to be the only important reservoir for HVH; acquisition of disease from a contaminated inanimate object has been demonstrated only after accidental laboratory inoculation. Surveys in the community and within hospitals indicate that 1 to 10 percent of hospitalized patients and employees have symptomatic or asymptomatic infection with HVH [12,28]. These infected persons constitute potential sources of infection for other hospitalized patients or employees. In particular, three groups of patients have an increased likelihood of transmitting HVH to other patients or personnel: (1) neurosurgical patients (and probably other patients with infected oral secretions who require tracheostomy or intubation), (2) patients with eczema herpeticum or other extensive cutaneous HVH lesions, and (3) patients with disseminated HVH infection.

Although occasional cases of neonatal HVH infection have been related to postnatal exposure to hospital personnel with mucocutaneous HVH infections [4,20,29], most neonates acquire HVH by passage through their mother's infected genital tract. The incidence of maternal genital infection at delivery varies between 5 and 100 infections per 10,000 mothers, depending on their socioeconomic status, but only 20 to 30 percent of these women have characteristic symptoms or clinical lesions. Transplacental transmission of HVH has not been conclusively demonstrated in human beings; it clearly occurs in rabbits and mice, however, and transplacental transmission of other viruses (cytomegalovirus and varicella-zoster) does occur in humans. Infection of infants via breast milk has not been demonstrated.

MODE OF TRANSMISSION. Transmission of HVH requires direct contact with infected skin or secretions in most instances. Skin abrasions, burns, or other epithelial defects may facilitate infection. HVH-1 usually spreads by nonvenereal contact and generally involves nongenital sites (the mouth, lips, and skin above the waist), whereas HVH-2 most often spreads venereally. Newborns nearly always acquire either HVH-1 or HVH-2 by passage through an infected birth canal.

Herpetic paronychia illustrates the direct-contact transmission of HVH that affects hospital personnel exposed to patients with infected oral secretions [44]. After administering oropharyngeal care to such patients (many of whom have no obvious clinical lesions), a vesiculobullous paronychia develops following an incubation period of three to seven days. This infection commonly involves young hospital personnel, most of whom lack circulating antibodies to HVH-1 or HVH-2. Paronychia caused by HVH-2 follows direct contact with infected genitalia.

Neither the indirect-contact spread of HVH via skin squamae, fomites, or aerosolized droplets nor the airborne transmission of HVH has been demonstrated.

PREVENTION. Hospital personnel who have frequent contact with oropharyngeal secretions of patients (i.e., nurses and respiratory therapists in neurosurgical or intensive-care units) should wear gloves and observe sterile technique when inserting, manipulating, or aspirating oropharyngeal or tracheal catheters. Particular caution must be observed when hospital personnel have skin abrasions or cuts. Similarly, gloves should be worn by nurses, physicians, or others who directly contact herpetic genital or cutaneous lesions. Patients with eczema herpeticum or multiple HVH skin lesions and patients with disseminated herpetic infection should be placed under wound and skin precautions to prevent transmission to personnel or other patients.

Of particular concern are neonates, immunosuppressed patients, or patients with chronic dermatoses, all of whom appear more likely to develop severe cutaneous or disseminated disease if infected with HVH. At the present time, the risk of nosocomial HVH infection has not been demonstrated to be of sufficient magnitude in such patients to recommend protective isolation. These patients, however, should not be exposed to other patients with eczema herpeticum or disseminated HVH infection. Although no definite evidence exists to substantiate the practice, it seems prudent to exclude temporarily staff members with active herpetic lesions from directly caring for these patients. At present, no evidence exists to support the exclusion of asymptomatic herpetic carriers from nursery or obstetric staff.

Recognition and treatment of maternal genital infections prior to term would theoretically reduce neonatal HVH infections. Unfortunately, an efficacious form of therapy is not currently available. Delivery by cesarean section has been advocated when maternal genital HVH infection is recognized at term, particularly when this procedure can be performed within six hours of membrane rupture or when amniocentesis does not show multinucleated giant cells in amniotic fluid. Although controlled studies have not been conducted, the use of cesarean section appears to reduce the likelihood of neonatal HVH infections in such circumstances. Although infant-to-infant transmission of HVH within the nursery has not been conclusively demonstrated, infected infants or infants born to mothers with genital HVH infections should be placed on wound and skin precautions (Part I, Chapter 9) and should preferably be segregated from other infants [12]. Infected mothers should not be allowed in the nursery and should not handle other infants.

Epidemic Infections

Clusters of HVH infection have occurred in medical personnel. Most commonly, nonimmune personnel develop herpetic paronychia after exposure of their ungloved hands to infective oropharyngeal secretions of patients while suctioning or providing oral hygiene. Outbreaks have also occurred in institutional populations (orphanages and dormitories) and among members of athletic teams such as wrestlers or rugby players. Nosocomial outbreaks among patients, however, have not been recognized to date.

Varicella-Zoster Infections
General Aspects

Varicella-zoster (V-Z) virus produces two clinical syndromes: varicella, a generalized exanthematous illness, and zoster, which is characterized by painful, discrete vesicles in the distribution of a sensory dermatome [17,25]. Varicella results from primary infection with V-Z virus and usually affects children, whereas zoster is ordinarily seen in adults and follows the reactivation of the latent virus in an individual with partial immunity derived from a preceding varicella infection. The facts that zoster does not increase in incidence during winter and spring as varicella does and that zoster patients usually have antibody titers characteristic of an anamnestic response support this hypothesis. Outbreaks of apparent zoster have occurred, however, which suggests that exogenous reinfection can also cause this syndrome [3,34].

TRANSMISSIBILITY. V-Z virus can be isolated from the oropharynx of persons with varicella and from the vesicular lesions of patients with either varicella or zoster. Varicella usually follows exposure to another person with varicella, although occasionally it may follow exposure to a person with zoster. An incubation period of 16 days (range of 10 to 23 days) precedes the onset of symptoms. Persons with varicella are most infectious one to four days before the onset of the rash and rarely transmit the virus after the third day of the rash. Immunosuppressed patients, however, may shed the virus for longer periods.

Unlike persons with varicella, most patients who develop zoster do not have a history of recent exposure to V-Z virus [6]. Furthermore, transmission of V-Z virus from patients with zoster to susceptible individuals does not occur as readily as it does from varicella patients, and such transmission has been demonstrated only when active vesicular lesions are present. The enhanced transmissibility of V-Z virus from patients with varicella probably results from (1) the fact that they have more vesicles; (2) the presence of lesions on the oral mucous membranes of varicella patients, a site from which the virus may be easily aerosolized; and (3) the ability to cover the more localized lesions of zoster patients.

Maternal varicella infection in the last weeks of pregnancy may cause transplacental infection of the infant. Vesicular lesions usually develop ten days after birth. Transplacental varicella infection during the first trimester has been postulated to have teratogenic effects on the developing fetus [41].

CLINICAL MANIFESTATIONS. Fever and maculopapular lesions of the skin and mucous membranes characterize early varicella. In three to five days, vesicles, pustules, and then crusts develop; new crops of lesions appear so that within two to four days, lesions of all stages are present. The disease usually lasts one week, although scabs may remain for two or three weeks. Pneumonia or encephalitis may complicate the usually self-limited clinical course.

Neuralgic pain and vesicles localized to two or more sensory dermatomes characterize herpes zoster. Few systemic symptoms are noted. The majority of cases involve thoracic dermatomes, with cervical dermatomes next most often involved; 10 to 15 percent of patients have fifth cranial nerve involvement and may develop conjunctivitis if the ophthalmic division is affected. The cutaneous lesions of zoster begin as macules and papules and progress over the next one to three days to form vesicles that then become crusted. New lesions may appear for up to a week, and crusted lesions may persist for one to six months. About 2 to 5 percent of patients develop disseminated zoster with marked constitutional symptoms, high fever, malaise, and severe pruritus; this syndrome may be difficult to differentiate from varicella. Disseminated zoster without constitutional symptoms or with an unusual distribution of skin lesions is sometimes called atypical zoster.

MICROBIOLOGIC DIAGNOSIS. Varicella and herpes zoster can usually be diagnosed clinically, and microbiologic diagnosis is rarely necessary. When smallpox, generalized herpes simplex, or hypersensitivity reactions cannot be excluded, however, fluid or scrapings from vesicles should be obtained. To differentiate smallpox from varicella, vesicular fluid may be Giemsa stained and examined immediately; giant cells with folded nuclei characterize both V-Z and HVH infections but not smallpox. Electron microscopy has also proved useful as a rapid diagnostic procedure to differentiate V-Z virus and smallpox virus.

For isolation of V-Z virus, primary or diploid human tissue-cell cultures should be used. Presumptive identification is based upon typical cytopathologic effects. HVH and cytomegalovirus (CMV) cause similar effects, but they can be distinguished from V-Z by using other cell lines. Fluorescent-antibody (FA) or complement-fixation (CF) techniques can specifically identify V-Z virus.

A fourfold rise in CF or FA antibody titers to V-Z virus from acute to convalescent serum in the absence of a fourfold rise to herpes simplex antigen (a third of individuals with HVH infections show a typical antibody response to V-Z antigen) is diagnostic of recent V-Z virus infection. In varicella, antibody titers become elevated about seven days after the appearance of the rash and peak one to two weeks later. In zoster, antibody titers usually begin to rise by the third day of the rash and may reach levels fourfold higher than those usually observed in varicella. A titer of 1 : 128 or higher suggests recent infection with V-Z virus.

COLLECTION, SHIPMENT, AND STORAGE OF SPECIMENS. Vesicular fluid and cellular scrapings should be collected aseptically within three to seven days after the appearance of the lesions. Vesicles should be first washed with sterile saline; the fluid is aspirated or swabbed and is then placed into 1 to 2 ml. of nutrient broth tissue-holding medium (buffered tryptose phosphate broth with gelatin) that contains salt and protein at a neutral pH. The base of the opened vesicle may be scraped gently and the cellular material placed in the medium with the vesicular fluids. Fluids or swabs in holding medium should be stored at $-70°C$ ($-94°F$) until processed in the laboratory, and if shipped, they should be surrounded by dry ice to maintain this temperature.

CLASSIFICATION OF INFECTIONS. Varicella is usually a community-acquired infection, and herpes zoster is nearly always an endogenous reactivation of infection in a patient with partial immunity to V-Z virus. Nosocomial varicella infections most often occur when a child admitted to a pediatric service is incubating varicella and transmits it before the onset of symptoms to other susceptible children on the same ward. The incubation period for varicella (10 to 23 days, mean of 16 days) may be helpful in distinguishing nosocomial from community-acquired cases. Several outbreaks of zoster have occurred in hospitals, which suggests that patients may rarely acquire this disease exogenously as a nosocomial infection. Reactivation of zoster during hospitalization in a patient who has had previous episodes of this disease should be considered a nosocomial infection.

HOST FACTORS. V-Z virus infects 70 to 90 percent of exposed, susceptible persons, and by age 20, 70 percent of the population has a history of having had varicella. Life-long immunity usually follows this primary infection, except in severely immunosuppressed children,

who may suffer reinfection. Corticosteroids given during convalescence from varicella may cause a second eruption.

Herpes zoster occurs when aging, serious underlying diseases, corticosteroid administration, radiation therapy, or trauma partially compromises immunity to V-Z virus. Patients with Hodgkin's disease are particularly predisposed to zoster. Patients with other lymphomas, leukemias, and solid malignancies, especially those involving the brain, also have a higher incidence of zoster than normal individuals, but this incidence does not approach that observed in patients with Hodgkin's disease [16,25,37].

THERAPY. Varicella ordinarily requires only supportive therapy. However, children with lymphomas, leukemias, or other malignancies, children receiving steroid or antimetabolite therapy, newborn infants, or susceptible adults may develop severe infections. In such patients, zoster immune globulin (ZIG) has been shown to prevent varicella if a 2 ml. dose is given within 72 hours of exposure; benefits are less clear if ZIG is given after varicella has developed [13]. Limited supplies of ZIG prevent its use in all but high-risk children.

Patients with herpes zoster usually require only pain medications and tranquilizers. In older patients, however, postherpetic neuralgia may be severe, and in immunosuppressed patients, zoster may be fatal. A variety of antiviral agents have been employed for the treatment of localized or disseminated zoster. None has been shown effective [19], although adenine arabinoside appears promising. Patients at high risk of developing V-Z infection (e.g., an immunosuppressed host with no prior history of varicella and no serologic evidence of previous infection) may be treated with ZIG, which may be efficacious in preventing exogenously acquired zoster.

Endemic Infections

INCIDENCE. The incidence of community-acquired varicella is approximately 1.1 case per 1000 population in a so-called endemic year. Every two or three years, the incidence doubles to approximately two cases per 1000. The majority of affected persons are between ages five and nine. Overall mortality is very low, and usually deaths occur only in newborn infants, in immunosuppressed children, or in adult patients when the disease is complicated by pneumonia or encephalitis. Reliable data on the incidence of nosocomial varicella infections are not available.

In reported series of hospitalized patients, it has been estimated that two to five cases of herpes zoster occur per 1000 discharges. The majority of infections occur in persons over 50 years of age, and fewer than 5 percent progress to disseminated infection. The incidence of zoster in hospitalized patients with neoplasms goes up to approximately eight cases per 1000. About 10 to 25 percent of patients with Hodgkin's disease develop zoster; 22 percent of these patients have zoster more than once, and 30 to 35 percent develop disseminated infection.

SOURCES. The upper respiratory tract (varicella) and skin lesions (varicella and zoster) of infected patients constitute the main sources of V-Z virus. The virus has been isolated only from patients with acute varicella or zoster infections, and asymptomatic, colonized persons probably are of little importance as a reservoir. Epidemiologic evidence suggests that most new cases follow exposure to an infected, symptomatic patient, and acute rises in antibody titers to V-Z virus rarely occur in the absence of clinical infection. The virus does not appear to infect other animals except primates; few data are available regarding its survival in the environment.

MODE OF TRANSMISSION. In varicella, V-Z virus may be transmitted by airborne and contact routes. The transmission of the virus in the incubation period prior to the onset of skin lesions and the rapidity with which new cases occur in patients with no history of direct exposure to infected patients suggest that airborne transmission occurs from the upper respiratory tract. Desquamated, infected, epithelial cells may also play a role in the airborne transmission of varicella. The presence of live V-Z virus in active skin lesions makes direct-contact transmission likely, but the relative importance of airborne and contact spread of varicella is not known.

In herpes zoster, evidence for the airborne transmission of V-Z virus is tenuous. Even though varicella may be contracted from patients with zoster, transmission has never been documented before the onset of skin lesions, and the virus has never been cultured from the pharynx of a patient with zoster. Desquamated, infected, epithelial cells may be vehicles for the airborne transmission of V-Z virus from patients with herpes zoster, but the limited (and usually covered) skin lesions in most cases make this mode of transmission infrequent.

PREVENTION. Until the skin lesions become crusted, hospitalized varicella patients should be placed in strict isolation, which requires a separately ventilated, private room. If possible, an infected patient should be on a separate ward from immunosuppressed patients.

Patients with herpes zoster require wound and skin precautions (Part I, Chapter 9) to protect other patients from direct contact spread. However, high-risk individuals—such as patients with lymphomas, leukemias, or other malignancies and children without a past history of varicella—should not be hospitalized near patients with active herpes zoster and should preferably be in areas with a different air supply. Precautions should be continued until the skin lesions are crusted.

Epidemic Infections

INCIDENCE. Nosocomial outbreaks may occur when a child who is incubating varicella is hospitalized for another reason; pediatric wards usually have susceptible children who are then exposed before the onset of symptoms in the initial case. The incidence of such outbreaks is not known.

Several small outbreaks of nosocomial herpes zoster, all in cancer hospitals, have been reported. In the largest, 13 of 26 patients in the hospital developed zoster over a three-month period. The risk of such outbreaks seems small except in these high-risk patients.

SOURCES. The reservoir of V-Z virus is the same as that for endemic infections.

MODES OF TRANSMISSION. Both contact and airborne spread probably play a role in nosocomial varicella outbreaks. Epidemics of zoster suggest exogenous acquisition of the virus rather than reactivation. All reported outbreaks of zoster have occurred when a patient with varicella or disseminated zoster has infected other high-risk patients. Transmission of the virus by direct contact can be substantiated in most cases, although the possibility of airborne spread has been raised. The role played by personnel in these outbreaks is unclear, since the importance of hand carriage of the virus is not known. CF titers to V-Z virus are not higher in employees working on cancer wards than in control employees.

CONTROL OF OUTBREAKS. A hospital varicella outbreak necessitates stringent control measures. All patients with active varicella and all exposed susceptible patients should be discharged if medically possible. Patients with active varicella who cannot be discharged should be placed in strict isolation until active vesicular skin lesions resolve (approximately seven days). Exposed susceptible patients who cannot be discharged should be placed in respiratory isolation either until discharge, until 23 days has elapsed since their last exposure, or until the resolution of varicella, whichever occurs first. New admissions without a past history of varicella or with diseases that suppress immune responses should not be placed near patients with active varicella or exposed susceptible individuals. Patients with varicella and exposed susceptible patients should not leave their rooms (e.g., to go to the x-ray department) unless absolutely necessary, and when they are out of their rooms, they should wear a mask. Visitors should be restricted to parents. Susceptible pregnant women should not be allowed on the floor. Pediatric personnel should not be rotated to other hospital areas, since susceptible staff members may be incubating the disease and could thus transmit it to hospitalized children. In order to protect susceptible staff members from acquiring varicella, temporary leave should be granted until the outbreak ends.

The control of a nosocomial zoster outbreak also requires stringent measures. Patients with localized zoster should be placed on wound and skin precautions (Part I, Chapter 9), and patients with disseminated zoster should be placed in strict isolation until their skin lesions lose infectivity (approximately

seven days). If possible, a patient with zoster should be segregated from immunosuppressed patients. Visitors should be limited to the immediate family, and pregnant women should not be allowed on the floor.

Ophthalmic *Neisseria Gonorrhoeae* Infections
General Aspects
In the past decade, the incidence of gonorrhea in this country has shown a progressive annual increase. During 1976, the reported civilian attack rate was 470 per 100,000 population. A concomitant increase in the incidence of gonococcal ophthalmic infection has accompanied this rise in community gonorrhea case rates [40]. Since this infection may have severe and permanent sequelae (i.e., visual impairment or blindness) and since it is amenable to both prevention and therapy, all hospitals should have appropriate control programs.

TRANSMISSIBILITY. Gonococci spread readily from mothers with symptomatic or asymptomatic genital infections to the conjunctivas of their vaginally delivered infants.

CLINICAL MANIFESTATIONS. Periorbital edema and erythema generally precede the development of chemosis, conjunctivitis, and a purulent ocular discharge. The onset of these signs of infection follows a one- to three-day incubation period. If untreated, corneal vascularization, ulceration, and perforation may occur.

MICROBIOLOGIC DIAGNOSIS. Microscopic demonstration of gram-negative intracellular diplococci on a Gram-stained smear of conjunctival exudate constitutes a sufficient basis for the presumptive diagnosis of gonococcal conjunctivitis. A specimen for culture should also be obtained.

CLASSIFICATION OF INFECTIONS. Most cases of gonococcal conjunctivitis occur in neonates one to three days after birth and hence are classified as nosocomial infections. Infrequent instances of neonatal gonococcal ophthalmia acquired from an infected community contact have been reported. In adults and older children, gonococcal conjunctivitis generally results either from autoinoculation or from an infected community contact.

SPECIMEN COLLECTION AND TRANSPORT. Samples of conjunctival exudate obtained with a sterile swab should be inoculated on Thayer-Martin or Transgrow medium as well as a nonselective medium.

PREDISPOSING HOST FACTORS. Infants born to mothers with vaginal *Neisseria gonorrhoeae* infection and premature rupture of membranes may acquire gonococcal conjunctivitis in utero prior to silver nitrate prophylaxis.

TREATMENT. Aqueous penicillin (50,000 to 100,000 units per kilogram of body weight per day) should be administered parenterally for two to four days to all patients with gonococcal conjunctivitis. In addition, hourly penicillin eye drops (100,000 to 200,000 units per milliliter) and saline irrigation may be of benefit. Because of the emergence of penicillinase-producing *N. gonorrhoeae,* isolates should be tested for penicillin resistance, and treated patients must be followed carefully.

Endemic Infections

INCIDENCE. Since the number of parturient women with gonorrhea in any community strongly influences the incidence of ophthalmia neonatorum, case rates of gonococcal conjunctivitis vary considerably from hospital to hospital, depending on the patient population. Annual case rates that range from zero to nearly 100 per 100,000 live births have been reported. In hospitals reporting to the NNIS, an incidence of 4.6 cases per 100,000 live births was observed in the period from 1970 to 1973. No cases were reported in adult patients.

SOURCES. In nearly all cases of ophthalmia neonatorum, an infected mother is the source of the organism. Adults with gonococcal conjunctivitis acquire the organism by autoinoculation or by contact with another infected person, but such infections are rarely nosocomial. The gonococci do not survive well in the inanimate environment, and thus nonhuman reservoirs are unimportant.

MODES OF TRANSMISSION. Gonococci spread readily via the direct contact of mucous membranes with infected tissues. Infants who develop ophthalmia neonatorum acquire the organism during passage through an infected birth canal.

PREVENTION. Measures for the prevention of this disease should be employed at every hospital; these include silver nitrate prophylaxis for all infants and prompt treatment of suspected cases with parenteral antibiotics. In hospitals that serve patient populations with a high incidence of gonococcal disease, culture screening of mothers during prenatal visits and prior to delivery may be warranted. All infants born to mothers with proved or suspected gonococcal infection, particularly when the membranes have ruptured prematurely, should have eye, pharyngeal, and rectal specimens taken for culture, and such infants should be placed under secretion precautions (Part I, Chapter 9) until effective therapy has been given for 24 hours.

Epidemic Infections

Outbreaks of gonococcal conjunctivitis attributed to infant-to-infant transmission within the nursery have not been reported.

References

1. Benenson, A. S. (Ed.). *Control of Communicable Diseases in Man* (12th ed.). New York: American Public Health Association, 1975.
2. Bennett, J. V., Shulman, J. A., Rosenstein, B. J., Trembath, B. J., Eickhoff, T. C., and Boring, J. C., III. Staphylococcal interference studies. *Am. J. Epidemiol.* 88:410, 1968.
3. Berlin, B. S., and Campbell, T. Hospital-acquired herpes zoster following exposure to chickenpox. *J.A.M.A.* 211:1831, 1970.
4. Bird, T., Ennis, J. E., Wort, A. J., and Gardner, P. S. Disseminated herpes simplex in newborn infants. *J. Clin. Pathol.* 16:423, 1963.
5. Bisno, A. L., Turpin, P., and Ledes, C. P. "Pyoderma" streptococci as a cause of nosocomial sepsis. *South. Med. J.* 66:1071, 1973.
6. Burgoon, C. F., Jr., Burgoon, J. S., and Baldridge, G. D. The natural history of herpes zoster. *J.A.M.A.* 164:265, 1957.
7. Committee on Fetus and Newborn, American Academy of Pediatrics. Skin care of newborns. *Pediatrics* 54:682, 1974.
8. Dillon, H. C. Streptococcal Infections of the Skin and Their Complications: Impetigo and Nephritis. In Wannamaker, L. W., and Matsen, J. M. (Eds.), *Streptococci and Streptococcal Diseases.* New York: Academic Press, 1972.

9. Dudding, B. A., Burnett, J. W., Chapman, S. S., and Wannamaker, L. W. The role of normal skin in the spread of streptococcal pyoderma. *J. Hyg.* (Camb.) 69:19, 1970.

10. Eichenwald, H. F., Kotsevalov, O., and Fasso, L. A. The "cloud baby": an example of bacterial-viral interactions. *Am. J. Dis. Child.* 100:161, 1960.

11. Fekety, F. R., Jr. The epidemiology and prevention of staphylococcal infection. *Medicine* (Baltimore) 43:593, 1964.

12. Francis, D. P., Herrman, K. L., MacMahon, J. R., Chavigny, K. H., and Sanderlin, K. C. Nosocomial and maternally acquired *Herpesvirus hominis* infection: a report of four fatal cases in neonates. *Am. J. Dis. Child.* 129:889, 1975.

13. Gershon, A. A., Steinberg, S., and Brunell, P. A. Zoster immune globulin: a further assessment. *N. Engl. J. Med.* 290:243, 1974.

14. Gezon, H. M., Thompson, D. J., Rogers, K. D., Hatch, T. F., Rycheck, R. R., and Yee, R. B. Control of staphylococcal infections and disease in the newborn through the use of hexachlorophene bathing. *Pediatrics* 51 (Suppl.):331, 1973.

15. Gezon, H. M., Thompson, D. J., Rogers, K. D., Hatch, T. F., and Taylor, P. M. Hexachlorophene bathing in early infancy: effect on staphylococcal disease and infection. *N. Engl. J. Med.* 270:379, 1964.

16. Goffinet, D. R., Glatstein, E. J., and Merigan, T. C. Herpes zoster-varicella infections and lymphoma. *Ann. Intern. Med.* 76:235, 1972.

17. Gordon, J. E. Chickenpox: an epidemiological review. *Am. J. Med. Sci.* 244:362, 1962.

18. Houck, P. W., Nelson, J. D., and Kay, J. L. Fatal septicemia due to *Staphylococcus aureus* 502A: report of a case and review of the infectious complications of bacterial interference programs. *Am. J. Dis. Child.* 123:45, 1972.

19. Hryniuk, W., Foerster, J., Shojania, M., and Chow, A. Cytarabine for Herpesvirus infections. *J.A.M.A.* 219:715, 1972.

20. Jack, I., and Perry, T. W. Herpes simplex infection in the newborn. *Med. J. Aust.* 46:640, 1959.

21. Kaplan, E. L., Anthony, B. F., Chapman, S. S., and Wannamaker, L. W. Epidemic acute glomerulonephritis associated with Type 49 streptococcal pyoderma. *Am. J. Med.* 48:9, 1970.

22. Klein, J. O. Family spread of staphylococcal disease following a nursery outbreak. *N.Y. State J. Med.* 60:861, 1960.

23. Levin, M. J., Gardner, P., and Waldvogel, F. A. "Tropical" pyomyositis: an unusual infection due to *Staphylococcus aureus*. *N. Engl. J. Med.* 284:196, 1971.

24. Lockhart, J. D. How toxic is hexachlorophene? *Pediatrics* 50:229, 1972.

25. Luby, J. P. Varicella-zoster virus. *J. Invest. Dermatol.* 61:212, 1973.

26. Melish, M. E., Galsgow, L. A., Turner, M. D., and Lillibridge, C. B. The staphylococcal epidermolytic toxin: its isolation, characterization, and site of action. *Ann. N.Y. Acad. Sci.* 236:317, 1974.

27. Mortimer, E. A., Jr., Wolinsky, E., Gonzaga, A. J., and Rammelkamp, C. H., Jr. Role of airborne transmission in staphylococcal infections. *Br. Med. J.* 1:319, 1966.

28. Nahmias, A. J. Infections Caused by *Herpesvirus hominis*. In Hoeprich, P. D. (Ed.), *Infecious Diseases*. Hagerstown, Md.: Harper & Row, 1972.

29. Nahmias, A. J., Alford, C. A., and Korones, S. B. Infection of the newborn with *Herpesvirus hominis*. *Adv. Pediatr.* 17:185, 1970.

30. Nahmias, A. J., and Eickhoff, T. C. Staphylococcal infections in hospitals: recent developments in epidemiologic and laboratory investigation. *N. Engl. J. Med.* 265:74, 120, 177, 1961.

31. Nahmias, A. J., and Roizman, B. Infection with herpes simplex viruses 1 and 2. *N. Engl. J. Med.* 289:667, 719, 781, 1973.

32. Payne, M. C., Wood, H. F., Karakawa, W., and Gluck, L. A prospective study of staphylococcal colonization and infections in newborns and their families. *Am. J. Epidemiol.* 82:305, 1965.

33. Powell, H., Swarner, O., Gluck, L., and Lampert, P. Hexachlorophene myelinopathy in premature infants. *J. Pediatr.* 82:976, 1973.

34. Rado, J. P., Tako, J., Geder, L., and Jeney, E. Herpes zoster house epidemic in steroid-treated patients. *Arch. Intern. Med.* 116:329, 1965.

35. Rea, W. J., and Wyrick, W. J., Jr. Necrotizing fasciitis. *Ann. Surg.* 172:957, 1970.

36. Schaffner, W., Lefkowitz, L. B., Goodman, J. S., and Koenig, M. G. Hospital outbreak of infections with group A streptococci traced to an asymptomatic anal carrier. *N. Engl. J. Med.* 280:1224, 1969.

37. Schimpff, S., Serpick, A., Stoler, B., Rumack, B., Mellin, H., Joseph, J. M., and Block, J. Varicella-zoster infection in patients with cancer. *Ann. Intern. Med.* 76:241, 1972.

38. Shinefield, H. R., Ribble, J. C., Eichenwald, H. F., Boris, M., and Sutherland, J. M. Bacterial interference: its effect on nursery-acquired infection with *Staphylococcus aureus*. V. An analysis and interpretation. *Am. J. Dis. Child.* 105:683, 1963.

39. Shuman, R. M., Leech, R. W., and Alvord, E. C.   Neurotoxicity of hexachlorophene in the human: I. A clinicopathologic study of 248 children. *Pediatrics* 54:689, 1974.

40. Snowe, R. J., and Wilfert, C. M.   Epidemic reappearance of gonococcal ophthalmia neonatorum. *Pediatrics* 51:110, 1973.

41. Srabstein, J. C., Morris, N., Larke, R. P. B., deSa, D. J., Castelino, B. B., and Sum, E.   Is there a congenital varicella syndrome? *J. Pediatr.* 84:239, 1974.

42. Stamm, W. E., Feeley, J. C., Facklorm, R. R. Wound infections due to group A streptococci traced to a vaginal carrier. *J. Infect. Dis.* 138: 287, 1978.

43. Steere, A. C., and Mallison, G. F.   Handwashing practices for the prevention of nosocomial infections. *Ann. Intern. Med.* 83:683, 1975.

44. Stern, H., Elek, S. D., Millar, D. M., and Anderson, H. F.   Herpetic whitlow—a form of cross-infection in hospitals. *Lancet* 2:871, 1959.

45. Wannamaker, L. W.   Differences between streptococcal infections of the throat and of the skin. *N. Engl. J. Med.* 282:23, 78, 1970.

21

Infectious Gastroenteritis

Herbert L. DuPont

Microorganisms that cause outbreaks of food-borne illness in the community also have the potential for causing similar events in hospitalized patients. However, certain forms of gastroenteritis—such as that caused by foodborne toxins of *Clostridium perfringens, Clostridium botulinum, Staphylococcus aureus,* and *Bacillus cereus* as well as that produced by the ingestion of food contaminated with group-A streptococci and *Vibrio parahaemolyticus*—have not been recognized to be transmissible from person to person within the hospital. The control of these diseases in the hospital depends on safe food-handling practices as discussed in Part I, Chapter 7, Section E, and such forms of gastroenteritis will therefore not be considered further in this chapter.

Infectious or communicable gastroenteritis caused by *Salmonella* other than *S. typhi, Escherichia coli, Shigella,* and rotavirus will receive primary attention within this chapter. In addition, the chapter will separately address *Yersinia enterocolitica* (an agent that has produced communicable nosocomial infections involving the gastrointestinal tract), staphylococcal enterocolitis (an important but noncommunicable form of nosocomial gastroenteritis), and necrotizing enterocolitis (a disease of uncertain, possibly infectious cause). Nosocomial transmission of *Vibrio cholera* has produced nosocomial infectious gastroenteritis in areas endemic for this disease, but it will not be discussed here, because of the rarity of endemic cases in the United States.

Infectious gastroenteritis differs from most other hospital-associated infections, which characteristically result from endogenous organisms in individuals with markedly altered resistance. Enteric infections caused by the above agents are nearly always exogenously acquired, often occur in clusters or epidemics, and are usually due to the introduction of a virulent organism by the ingestion of contaminated foods or medications, by short-term carriers among patients and hospital staff, or by patient-to-patient transmission on the hands of personnel. Although host factors such as age and debility are important, healthy patients and hospital personnel also are frequently involved in outbreaks of these infections.

Incidence

The true incidence of nosocomial infectious gastroenteritis is not known. Such enteric infections are markedly underreported in the United States because of the common occurrence of noninfectious diarrhea among hospital patients and personnel with its attendant complacency and because laboratory techniques are significantly limited in delineating some bacterial and viral pathogens. However, the number of reported infections from the National Nosocomial Infections Study (see Part II, Chapter 13) for the period of January 1970 through August 1973 can be used to indicate the relative importance of certain selected pathogens. Most reported cases of nosocomial infectious gastroenteritis in which the causative agent was established were infections with a *Salmonella* species (68 cases) or enteropathogenic *Escherichia coli* (53 cases). Nosocomial shigellosis occurred less frequently (24 cases).

Diagnostic Criteria

Clinical and Microbiologic Criteria

There is a wide variation among clinical symptoms in patients with these enteric infections. Some patients become asymptomatic excreters of a potential pathogen, while others show varying forms of diarrheal disease. Organisms that invade the intestinal epithelial lining usually elicit a febrile response in addition to causing diarrhea. In infections with pathogens that invade primarily the colonic mucosa, symptoms of colitis occur, including urgency, tenesmus, and bloody, mucoid stools (dysentery). Diarrhea or loose stools in a patient with unexplained fever should be diagnosed as infectious gastroenteritis, regardless of culture results for bacterial pathogens. When diarrhea or loose stools occur in an afebrile patient or in a febrile patient whose fever has other likely causes, the identification of a recognized infectious patho-

gen in stools or by serology is necessary for this diagnosis.

Diarrhea of noninfectious origin—such as that caused by cathartics, inflammatory diseases of the gastrointestinal tract, surgical resections and anastomoses, and the like—should be carefully differentiated from the diarrhea of infectious gastroenteritis. Alterations in the gastrointestinal flora because of antibiotic administration are commonly associated with diarrhea; such cases of diarrhea should not be reported as gastroenteritis unless enterocolitis occurs, in which event they should be reported as noninfectious gastroenteritis.

Classification of Infections

Diarrhea with onset after admission that is associated with a positive culture for organisms recognized as causative agents of infectious gastroenteritis should be regarded as a nosocomial infection. The interval between the time of admission and the onset of clinical symptoms must be greater than the known incubation periods (see subsequent sections) unless there are associated cases among other hospital patients or personnel. Alternatively, nosocomial infections may be diagnosed if a stool culture obtained shortly before or just after admission is negative for the pathogen in question and the pathogen is subsequently cultured from the patient.

Predisposing Host Factors

Defective Gastric Defenses

There is evidence to indicate that gastric acid normally plays an important role in the defense against ingested organisms. The bactericidal action of stomach acid greatly reduces or eradicates ingested organisms and thus reduces the inoculum of organisms that subsequently reach the intestine. Physiologic or pathologic achlorhydria, which is most common in premature infants and elderly patients, may underlie the increased risks of certain enteric infections seen in these groups. Although unstudied, variations in gastric acidity may also partly determine which persons become ill following the ingestion of the same contaminated common vehicle. Antacid usage has been shown to facilitate colonization of the intestine greatly with vaccine strains of *Shigella* and to increase the frequency of gastrointestinal acquisition of nosocomial strains of aerobic gram-negative rods. It is probable that anticholinergic medications act similarly. Persons with histories of gastric resection and vagotomies are known to be at higher risk of acquiring cholera than normal persons.

The time in which ingested substances are in contact with gastric acid may be important. In this regard, water without food tends to traverse the stomach more rapidly than solid food, thus reaching the neutralizing secretions of the duodenum more rapidly. The infecting inoculum of organisms is probably reduced when they are transmitted by water. Waterborne outbreaks of salmonellosis have occurred when low concentrations of the organisms were present, whereas large numbers are usually required for foodborne transmission of these organisms.

Antibiotic Therapy
The oral or systemic administration of antibiotics to which an epidemic strain is resistant greatly facilitates cross-colonization and infection. These effects presumably occur because of a reduction in the competitive interference of normal, sensitive flora against the ingested strains, which thus in effect reduces the inoculum required for establishment of the pathogen. The continued administration of the drug following acquisition of the pathogen may permit the selective outgrowth of the pathogen and result in much greater concentrations of the organism in the feces than might otherwise have occurred. Thereby, the chances of transmission and risk of disease are increased.

Crowding and Staffing Factors
An insufficient ratio of staff to patients encourages infractions in hand-washing and isolation techniques, especially in critical-care areas. Even careful hand-washing, however, is sometimes ineffective in removing gram-negative rods from the hands, and a slight but definite risk of transmitting organisms by direct contact with successive patients exists even after

hand-washing. Thus, inordinately high staff-to-patient ratios, such as may be encountered in some hospitals, may also lead to increased risks of cross-colonization and infection. Crowding of patients also increases the risks of cross-infection. While crowding of patients is often accompanied by insufficiencies in staff, it may also be independently important in that it increases the risks of indirect contact spread through environmental sources, especially in nurseries.

General Control Measures
In controlling the spread of enteric infections within the hospital environment regardless of the specific cause of such infections, a number of general measures can be taken. The most important means of cross-infection with enteric bacterial pathogens in the hospital is usually the fecal-oral route, in which indirect contact spread of organisms occurs from patient to patient on the hands of personnel. Outbreaks may also result from the ingestion of contaminated food, medication, or test materials.

Hand-washing
Since the most important means of spread of bacterial pathogens is via hand transfer, effective hand-washing is among the most important measures to prevent disease transmission. Although it is unlikely that all potentially pathogenic microorganisms can be removed by hand-washing, the level of contamination can be reduced, in most cases, below that necessary for disease transmission among healthy children and adults. Among debilitated patients or newborn infants, the required dose of enteropathogens needed to produce disease probably is substantially lower.

Surveillance
It is necessary to have an alert hospital surveillance team that continually reviews clinical patterns of infection in the hospital and evaluates bacteriologic reports from the diagnostic microbiology laboratory. Such a team is often instrumental in defining the extent of an outbreak before it has reached serious propor-

tions, and it represents the foundation of an effective infection control program.

It is necessary to maintain adequate surveillance of hospital personnel, particularly food handlers, as well as of patients. One important means of minimizing nosocomial diarrheal disease is to establish an effective personnel health service. Food handlers, nurses, and ancillary staff having direct contact with patients should be encouraged to communicate with the personnel health service when an episode of acute gastroenteritis occurs among themselves. Stool cultures should be performed, and the person removed temporarily from work until culture results and the clinical course of the disease can be evaluated.

No infant born of a mother with diarrhea should be admitted to the nursery ward, and hospital personnel with symptoms of diarrhea should be excluded from the ward. Any infant with loose, watery, or bloody diarrhea should be handled with enteric precautions until a non-infectious cause for the diarrhea has been identified.

Use of Antispasmodic Drugs

Treatment of acute gastroenteritis with drugs to decrease the motility of the gut and to produce symptomatic relief of diarrhea may have undesirable side-effects. Such drugs have been shown to prolong the time required for excretion of *Shigella,* for example, and they are also associated with an increased risk of bloodstream invasion in *Salmonella* gastroenteritis. It is probable that these effects also occur with other enteric pathogens. Thus, drugs such as Lomotil (diphenoxylate hydrochloride and atropine) should be avoided in the treatment of nosocomial gastroenteritis.

Prompt Investigation of Cases

The occurrence of two or more cases of nosocomial infectious gastroenteritis caused by the same organism within a few weeks' time should prompt a review of the exposures common to these cases. Case-control investigations are less likely to establish the source of infections conclusively when the number of cases is small, and microbiologic sampling of foods, medications, or equipment common to cases may be of special value in this circumstance. Culture surveys of other patients hospitalized in the same patient-care areas as those with cases of disease may identify asymptomatically infected persons, and such individuals should be included with symptomatic patients for purposes of epidemiologically establishing possible sources.

Hospital outbreaks of enteric disease may be caused by patients or hospital personnel who are short-term carriers of a specific pathogen. Comparison of the exposures of cases and controls to specific personnel (see Part I, Chapter 5) and culture surveys of hospital personnel and asymptomatic patients may help to identify the carriers responsible for such outbreaks. Occasionally, environmental factors—such as air, dust, bedside tables, thermometers, mattresses, and the like—are important in contact spread. If a common vehicle such as food, contaminated equipment, or contaminated oral medication or test solution can be identified, its removal or disinfection may assist in terminating the outbreak.

Secondary cases often occur following disease outbreaks caused by contaminated vehicles, and the chance of epidemiologically identifying responsible sources may be improved in such situations by focusing attention on early cases and those patients whose illnesses seem unlikely to have derived from person-to-person spread.

On occasion, epidemiologic studies may indicate that the central kitchen is responsible for the dissemination of a bacterial pathogen. Removal of food handlers with recent diarrheal disease or kitchen personnel with positive cultures on culture surveys may result in termination of the epidemic. In the vast majority of instances, however, foodborne outbreaks of nosocomial gastroenteritis derive from inadequate handling of products from food-producing animals, rather than from contamination of the food by food handlers.

Outbreak Management

During an epidemic, it is usually helpful to isolate patients with symptomatic and asymptomatic infections in separate rooms with separate lavatory facilities. Enteric isolation is necessary where glove-gown-stool precautions should be undertaken.

In nurseries where enteric isolation of individual cases is not possible, cohort systems (see Part I, Chapter 7, The Newborn Nursery) should be employed during an epidemic to minimize the risk of cross-infection. Successful control of outbreaks sometimes requires repeated culture surveys coupled with a special type of cohorting. Infants who are ill or colonized with the epidemic organism can sometimes be grouped together into a cohort that is physically separated from noninfected infants. Personnel caring for these infants must not care for noninfected infants, and no equipment should be shared between the two groups. Only milk packaged in sterile containers should be used, common equipment shared between babies should be removed, and infants should be confined to their own bassinets or isolettes. To further prevent the spread of infection, infants born outside the hospital should not enter the nursery during an epidemic of diarrhea. Unnecessary contact with the babies by hospital personnel or contact between infants should be eliminated during times of an epidemic. An adequate number of nursing and hospital staff is especially important in the management of nursery epidemics.

Not only is it important to isolate patients with active disease as long as is indicated (see Part I, Chapter 9), but infected patients should also be discharged from the hospital as soon as their condition allows them to be managed at home.

Salmonella Infections
General Aspects
CLINICAL AND MICROBIOLOGIC FEATURES. In salmonellosis, fever, nausea, and vomiting develop and are followed shortly thereafter by abdominal pain and watery diarrhea. Frequently, mucous strands can be found in stool specimens, yet rarely is there gross blood present (this provides an important means of differentiating between *Salmonella* and *Shigella* infections).

Newborns have a predisposition to disease; approximately 50 percent of exposed infants develop illness once a case is introduced into a nursery. *Salmonella* infections in infants may result in septicemia or disseminated focal disease such as meningitis, abscesses, or osteomyelitis; they may also result in asymptomatic intestinal colonization. Some neonates become persistent intestinal carriers of salmonellae, and their cultures may remain positive for over a year.

Others who are at higher risk are the aged and the debilitated. Patients with malignant disease have an unexplained predisposition to the development of salmonellosis, and the frequency of bloodstream invasion in such patients is quite high. Persons housed in nursing homes represent another segment of hospitalized patients in which explosive outbreaks may occur with high fatality rates.

In a patient with acute gastroenteritis, the isolation of *Salmonella* from a stool culture is generally sufficient to establish the cause of the disease. This suffices because of the relatively high degree of pathogenicity of these enteric bacteria, plus the fact that long-term carriers are unusual.

THERAPY. Antimicrobial therapy has been shown in numerous studies to prolong the intestinal excretion of salmonellae. Most of these studies have involved oral therapy, and recent data with ampicillin suggest that parenteral administration may be more effective. Mild, uncomplicated, *Salmonella* gastroenteritis should not be treated. However, in patients in whom bloodstream invasion occurs—most commonly newborn or extremely debilitated patients, particularly those with malignant disease—antimicrobials often are instrumental in recovery from infection and may be lifesaving. In general, ampicillin, chloramphenicol, and trimethoprim-sulfamethoxazole provide the most effective therapy.

In addition to prolonging the period of excretion of the infecting strains, the administration of antimicrobial agents may, on occasion, make the clinical infection more severe or cause clinical relapse of infection when the drug administered is one to which the infecting strain is resistant. Antimicrobial therapy also increases the chance of the infecting organism acquiring additional resistances.

Epidemiologic Considerations

CLASSIFICATION OF INFECTIONS. Incubation periods for salmonellosis vary from 6 to 72 hours. The incubation period varies inversely with the size of the infecting dose. Patients with positive cultures and an onset of gastroenteritis 72 hours or more after admission should be considered to have nosocomial infections. Persons with onsets within 6 to 72 hours of admission should be considered to have nosocomial infections only when epidemiologic evidence makes nosocomial acquisition likely. Isolation of salmonellae from a patient's stool in the absence of clinical symptoms of gastroenteritis should be reported as a nosocomial infection only if previous stool cultures during hospitalization were negative.

TRANSMISSIBILITY. While person-to-person transmission of *Salmonella* strains is unusual among healthy persons outside of the hospital environment, these organisms can be transmitted by the hands of nurses or by person-to-person spread among the aged, debilitated, or newborn patients in the hospital setting. Communicability of this organism from patients to hospital personnel or to community contacts is uncommon, because of the high dose (more than 10^7 organisms) that is usually necessary to infect healthy persons and the precautions routinely used by hospitals in managing patients with gastroenteritis.

INCIDENCE. About 50 percent of infections occur on the newborn service or on the pediatric floor. The remaining cases mainly occur among patients on the surgical or medical services.

Since 1963, the Center for Disease Control has maintained nationwide surveillance of salmonellosis. Between 1963 and 1972, 112, or 28 percent, of the total reported outbreaks occurred in institutions (hospitals, nursing homes, and custodial institutions). Approximately 3500 cases were reported in these outbreaks among institutionalized populations, which represented 13 percent of the total reported cases.

SOURCES AND MODES OF ACQUISITION. The nosocomial salmonellosis that occurs in the pediatric population, especially in newborns, is characteristically spread from person to person. The organism is typically introduced into the nursery by an infant who acquired the infection from its mother at delivery, but it can also be introduced by a carrier among the personnel or, more rarely, by foods and medications. Spread from infant to infant within the nursery then occurs on the hands of personnel. Fomites may be important in cross-infections, and persistence of the organism in dust, air, and other environmental sites is sometimes responsible for perpetuating an outbreak. Epidemics have been traced to contaminated delivery-room resuscitation equipment and the water baths used for heating infant formula [18]. A commercially distributed, special nutritional formula that contained contaminated egg albumin has caused *S. infantis* outbreaks when administered orally or by tube feeding. Outbreaks of *S. kottbus,* a serotype that has a particular tendency to be excreted from infected bovine mammary glands, have been traced to contamination of human breast milk collected to feed premature infants. Although it is unclear whether the breast milk was primarily or secondarily contaminated, inadequate storage and handling of the milk following collection allowed the organisms to proliferate to significant levels.

Outbreaks in nurseries are generally smaller than those commonly seen in nosocomial *Salmonella* infections in adults [1]. In adult infections, a common source can usually be incriminated. The common source may be previously contaminated, raw or undercooked meats or other products of food-producing animals (e.g., eggs or milk products) or food that has become contaminated after cooking because of organisms on equipment or surfaces in the kitchen [11,13]. Food contaminated by a short-term *Salmonella* carrier working in the kitchen is much less commonly responsible. On occasion, a medication contaminated by *Salmonella* serves as a vehicle, especially medications containing enzymes and hormones of animal origin (e.g., pepsin, bile salts, vitamins, and endocrine gland extracts). Sporadic cases caused by intermittent exposure to infrequently used medications can produce a puzzling epidemiologic problem that requires a careful case-control approach for its solution.

In homes for the aged, epidemics often are initiated by the ingestion of contaminated food, while the epidemic is generally perpetuated by cross-infection among debilitated patients by means of hospital nursing staff.

Less frequent sources of *Salmonella* infections include yeast, dried coconut, carmine dye, and inadequately disinfected equipment used on successive patients (e.g., Gomco suction and endoscopy equipment).

The specific serotype of *Salmonella* may sometimes provide useful clues to the source. Some serotypes commonly infecting humans, such as *S. typhimurium,* derive from a variety of sources, but some have strong associations with particular sources that may be useful in suggesting likely sources of human infection: *S. choleraesuis* is associated with porcine sources; *S. cubana,* with cochineal insects used to prepare carmine dye; *S. dublin,* with bovines; *S. pullorum,* with poultry sources; and so on. Many additional correlations between serotypes and sources exist among the 1600 or so serotypes of *Salmonella.*

CONTROL. Safe food-handling practices as outlined in Part I, Chapter 7, Section E are especially important in the prevention of nosocomial salmonellosis. In addition to the prompt epidemiologic identification and removal of common sources and the measures mentioned earlier in this chapter concerning outbreak management, thorough cleaning and disinfection of fomites and environmental surfaces in a nursery after discharge of infected infants is also important. Prophylactic antibiotics are contraindicated as a control measure.

Escherichia coli Infections

General Aspects

CLINICAL AND MICROBIOLOGIC FEATURES. *Escherichia coli* can produce gastroenteritis in children and adults by several different mechanisms. Strains that produce keratoconjunctivitis in the guinea pig eye (the Sereny test) tend to produce an invasive, *Shigella*-like illness. Disease caused by such strains appears rare in the United States, although a large common-source outbreak caused by contaminated imported French cheese has been documented. Loose, watery diarrhea, usually mild but sometimes severe and resembling that of cholera, is associated with certain strains of *E. coli* that produce enterotoxin. Both heat-labile and heat-stable toxins have been identified. Disease can be produced by either type of enterotoxin, although both are frequently produced by the same strain. Enterotoxin-producing strains appear to be major causes of travelers' diarrhea and are frequent causes of gastroenteritis in developing countries. Their importance in the United States is presently debatable; some surveys indicate them to be frequent causes but others show them to be rare causes of gastroenteritis.

E. coli belonging to the classical enteropathogenic serotypes (EPEC) appear to produce disease by mechanisms that are not yet fully understood, since disease caused by such strains cannot be explained on the basis of the above mechanisms [7]. EPEC have previously been considered common causes of nursery outbreaks, which sometimes were explosive with high attack rates and fulminating clinical courses [19]. Such outbreaks have almost disappeared in the United States in recent years. EPEC are frequently isolated from asymptomatic infants, and the diagnostic value of routinely searching for EPEC in children four years of age or less with sporadic diarrhea has recently been seriously questioned. Even during outbreaks, the isolation of EPEC from stools may not always have etiologic significance. Widespread and rapid interchange of microbial enteric flora among infants is most pronounced during outbreaks of diarrhea in nurseries. Thus, EPEC should not be considered the cause of an outbreak unless these organisms are significantly more frequently isolated from patients with disease than from matched controls without gastroenteritis, are isolated from blood cultures of affected infants, cause documented serologic conversions (i.e., increase in humoral antibody), or are demonstrated to produce enterotoxin, to invade epithelial cells, or both in tissue culture and animal studies. Tests for enterotoxin production and the invasiveness of any non-EPEC serotypes that are isolated in greater frequency from cases than controls should also be done in investigating outbreaks of gastroenteritis of otherwise unexplained cause. Most clinical laboratories, however, are not equipped to perform these tests, and strains will need to be forwarded to reference laboratories for such evaluations.

The clinical expression of EPEC infections varies considerably, probably as a result of differences in pathogenetic mechanisms, from minimal, watery diarrhea to fulminating disease with septicemia. There appears to be a great deal of unexplained variability even among strains with the same serotype, and occasional outbreaks occur in newborn nurseries in which attack rates exceed 50 percent and mortality rates are high. EPEC outbreaks are almost totally confined to newborn nurseries, and infants and young children, especially those less than two years of age, appear to be primarily at risk. The association of EPEC disease with the very young may not be totally correct, because such strains are generally only considered to occur in children less than four years of age with diarrhea.

Clinicians should be aware that the laboratory procedures used to determine the serogroup of isolates have certain deficiencies. Non-EPEC serotypes that cross-react with EPEC serotypes can agglutinate in pooled test sera to give a false-positive test result that can be identified only by complete serotyping. False-positive tests reduce both the clinical and the epidemiologic value of laboratory results.

THERAPY. Disease caused by enterotoxin-producing strains of *E. coli* has been shown to respond favorably to antibiotics to which the organisms are sensitive in studies conducted in Bangladesh, an area where such disease has a high endemic frequency. The duration and severity of diarrhea are reduced by such therapy. Although controlled trials have not been conducted, antibiotic therapy would appear to be indicated on clinical grounds for *Shigella*-like disease caused by invasive strains, and responses comparable to those seen in treatment of shigellosis (see *Shigella* Infections, below) might be anticipated.

The value of antimicrobial therapy for EPEC disease is presently controversial, and part of this controversy doubtlessly derives from the difficulty in insuring that EPEC were the cause of the gastroenteritis. In some instances, a lack of response to antibiotics may have occurred because EPEC isolated from cases were incidental findings in disease caused by other agents, especially rotaviruses. When gastroenteritis in a premature or full-term nursery occurs and a causative role can be ascribed to EPEC on the basis of the previously mentioned criteria, uncontrolled trials suggest that orally administered gentamicin, colistin, or neomycin for a one-week course of treatment may be of value. Systemic antibiotics should also be given to all such patients if sepsis occurs in one or more affected infants. Since the isolation of EPEC in a sporadic case of gastroenteritis is presently of uncertain value in establishing the cause, such laboratory findings offer little or no guidance to the clinician, and the clinical severity of the illness is the only factor useful in deciding whether to institute treatment.

Epidemiologic Considerations

CLASSIFICATION OF INFECTIONS. Incubation periods for EPEC disease are commonly 24 to 48 hours, but they may occasionally be much longer. Children with onset of gastroenteritis 48 hours or longer after admission should be considered to have nosocomial infections, as well as all infants who develop EPEC disease at any time during hospitalization following birth in the hospital. Isolation of an enteropathogenic serotype of *E. coli* from a stool culture in the absence of clinical symptoms of gastroenteritis should not be reported as an infection. For consistency in surveillance, an infection should be reported when an EPEC strain is isolated from a patient with gastroenteritis in whom no other recognized pathogen is identified, even though such isolates are of indeterminate importance in the etiology of the disease.

TRANSMISSIBILITY. The only known population at risk to develop nosocomial enteric infections due to *E. coli* strains are newborn infants and young children. When an enteropathogenic *E. coli* strain is introduced into a nursery, hospital personnel and community contacts may become asymptomatic carriers of the organism, especially during an episode of infantile diarrhea, and may serve as an important epidemiologic link in the transmission of the disease to the newborns [14]. Enteric disease caused by enterotoxigenic *E. coli* is only very rarely transmitted from person to person.

INCIDENCE. EPEC is second to *Salmonella* as a reported cause of infectious nosocomial diarrheal disease caused by bacteria in the NNIS survey. At the present time, these organisms are identified by serotype analysis, but, as noted above, serotyping of the EPEC is unreliable and may have minimal correlation with pathogenicity. Outbreaks ascribed to EPEC have become much less common over the last decade. Only five outbreaks caused by such strains were investigated by CDC in the period from 1970 to 1975 (see Part II, Chapter 13). Only a few outbreaks of nosocomial disease caused by enterotoxin-producing *E. coli* have been reported [16].

SOURCES AND MODES OF ACQUISITION. The most common source of EPEC infections usually is an infected child who is admitted to a newborn nursery or readmitted to a pediatric ward. The infant may have either acquired his or her infection at the time of delivery or acquired the organism during hospitalization and had an onset of enteric disease in the early days after discharge from the hospital. Secondary spread of the infecting strain occurs from the hospital personnel to other infants by hand transfer or from other articles in the nursery that have been contaminated with the strain during an epidemic. Pharyngeal colonization of infants is common during epidemics, and, though unproved, it may be an important intermediate step in producing disease in some cases, since proliferation of organisms at this site might produce an inoculum that is more likely to establish infection in the lower gastrointestinal tract.

Epidemics of infantile EPEC diarrhea have occurred at times when the organism can be detected in the air, dust, and fomites within the hospital environment. Asymptomatic carriers are probably important as a cause of epidemics among susceptible infants and include antepartum mothers, hospital staff, or other children without disease. During periods of infantile diarrhea outbreaks, approximately 5 percent of pediatric patients without intestinal infection

and up to one-third of antepartum females have been shown to harbor EPEC organisms in their stool. Outbreaks in the nursery usually follow the introduction of a new serotype of EPEC by a newly admitted, infected child or by colonized hospital personnel. The infecting strain is transmitted between children, generally on the hands of attendants or by articles and equipment in communal use.

A single, large, protracted, nosocomial outbreak caused by a strain of *E. coli* that produced heat-stable enterotoxin and did not belong to recognized enteropathogenic serotypes has been reported [16]. The outbreak appears to have been transmitted by means of cross-contamination of oral feedings. The epidemic strain did not colonize or produce disease in adults, despite its presence in multiple environmental sites. Illness was mild and characterized by three to five days of watery diarrhea without pus or blood in the stools. Prophylactic oral colistin, to which the multiple-drug-resistant strain was sensitive, was ineffective in preventing acquisition. Antibiotic resistances and enterotoxin production were co-linked on a transmissible plasmid of the epidemic strain [21].

CONTROL. Control measures mentioned earlier in this chapter and elsewhere [9] will be helpful in curtailing an EPEC outbreak. Such measures are not indicated, however, unless a causative role can be ascribed to an EPEC strain on the basis of the previously outlined criteria. Colonization of infants with an EPEC strain in the absence of enteric disease attributable to the strain is not an indication for control measures.

Enterotoxigenic *E. coli* strains are thought to be mainly transmitted by food and water, and prevention of disease from these sources can be accomplished by proper food handling and chlorination of water supplies.

Shigella Infections
General Aspects

CLINICAL AND MICROBIOLOGIC FEATURES. Shigellosis represents a distinct clinical entity. Fever develops in 50 percent of the patients, and mucus with or without blood can be documented in the stool within one or two days after the onset of diarrhea. Patients are usually more toxic and symptoms are more severe with this form of enteric infection than with others.

When newborns are infected by a *Shigella* strain, the mortality rate is higher and complications (e.g., intestinal perforation and septicemia) develop with a higher frequency than other common bacterial causes of gastroenteritis [8,22]. Although there is some evidence that breast-fed infants show an increased resistance to *Shigella,* nearly all hosts are extremely susceptible to these organisms.

Shigella sonnei and *S. flexneri* are the species principally responsible for disease in the United States. *S. sonnei* strains can be differentiated from each other by colicine typing, and *S. flexneri* strains by serotyping. Clinicians should be aware that *Salmonella-Shigella* agar, a popular medium for stool cultures in many clinical laboratories, is toxic to many *S. flexneri* strains. For optimal recovery of strains, specimens should not be placed in holding or transport media but should be plated directly onto blood or XLD (xylose, lysine, and deoxycholate) agar as soon as possible after collection.

THERAPY. In bacillary dysentery, appropriate antimicrobial agents are clearly beneficial in decreasing the excretion of the pathogenic shigellae and in improving clinical symptoms. In the adult, tetracycline administration may be the preferred form of therapy, and in most cases, a single oral dose of 2.5 gm. is effective when the infecting strain is sensitive. In children, because of the dental staining caused by the tetracyclines, parenteral ampicillin should be employed for six days. In vitro antimicrobial sensitivity testing should be employed to determine the most effective form of therapy, because multiple-drug-resistance, which is R-factor mediated, is common. Trimethoprim plus sulfamethoxazole, nalidixic acid, and oxolinic acid have usually shown activity against the more resistant strains. Antibiotic therapy is associated with the frequent emergence of multiple-drug-resistances in originally sensitive strains, which is presumably caused by R-factor transfer from endogenous gastrointestinal flora.

Thus, patients should remain in enteric isolation until posttreatment cultures are negative.

Epidemiologic Considerations

CLASSIFICATION OF INFECTIONS. Incubation periods for shigellosis vary from one to six days. Patients with positive cultures and an onset of gastroenteritis 24 hours or more after admission should be considered to have nosocomial infections unless epidemiologic evidence of community-acquired infection is found (e.g., occurrence of shigellosis in family contacts before the onset of the patient's illness). Isolation of shigellae from a patient's stool in the absence of clinical symptoms of gastroenteritis should be reported as a nosocomial infection only if previous stool cultures during hospitalization were negative.

TRANSMISSIBILITY. While *Shigella* strains represent the most potentially communicable of the bacterial pathogens, the striking clinical disease usually helps the physician spot the illness early and promptly institute effective therapy and control measures. Such early detection partly explains the usual, surprising lack of spread within the normal hospital environment. Other patients, hospital personnel, and community contacts appear to be at risk of developing bacillary dysentery when exposed to an infected patient, because of the very low dose of organisms (less than 10^3) necessary to produce disease.

INCIDENCE. Although any hospitalized patient is at risk of developing nosocomial shigellosis when a case is admitted, only rarely do outbreaks occur [17]. The only population at high risk are persons housed in residential institutions for the mentally retarded, where crowded living conditions, poor personal hygiene, and overworked nursing personnel all appear to be important as causes of serious outbreaks.

Shigellosis was reported to be about half as common as EPEC infections and one-third as common as nosocomial salmonellosis in NNIS data. How many of the 10,000 to 13,000 cases of shigellosis reported each year in the United States come from hospitals is unknown. Between 10 and 20 percent of the cases of shigellosis reported each year, however, come from residential institutions for the retarded.

SOURCES AND MODES OF ACQUISITION. The usual sources are short-term carriers of the disease who are either ill or in the convalescent stages of their disease. In custodial institutions, a few long-term carriers may be prevalent and may serve as an important reservoir. Long-term carriage, however, is rare. On occasion, shigellosis develops when contaminated food is ingested that was prepared by a person who was carrying the organism following an episode of disease. The vast majority of cases, however, are secondary to person-to-person spread of infection. Infections are rarely acquired by indirect-contact spread from inanimate environmental sources, since these organisms are only able to survive for short periods in the environment.

CONTROL. Antibiotics are effective in eradicating sensitive strains of *Shigella* from the gastrointestinal tract, but, as noted earlier, infecting strains have a propensity to develop multiple-drug-resistance in response to therapy. Thus, treatment of culture-positive patients should be coupled with individual enteric isolation procedures for each patient to prevent the potential emergence and continued spread of a strain that has acquired additional antibiotic resistances. Group cohorting of infected patients is not advised.

Streptomycin-dependent vaccine strains of *Shigella* have been tested as a control measure in mental institutions with high endemic rates of shigellosis. The duration of protection is short, however, as it is with the natural disease. Furthermore, multiple oral doses of vaccine must be given, vaccine strains can be transmitted to nonimmunized patients, and there is a potential risk of reversion of such strains to streptomycin-independent, virulent organisms.

Viral Gastroenteritis

Recent studies have spotlighted the major role of rotaviruses as a cause of gastroenteritis [4, 15]. Nosocomial transmission of rotavirus [2, 6,15] and adenoviruses [6] has been documented. Nosocomial adenoviral gastroenteritis appears to be much less frequent than rotaviral infections, produces milder clinical illness, and will not be further discussed in this section.

Rotavirus Infections

INCIDENCE. Rotaviruses are probably the single most frequent enteric pathogens found in persons less than five years of age in the United States, and nosocomial transmission is probably far more common than previously realized. Community-acquired rotavirus infections show a winter peak in incidence, and it is probable that nosocomial cases are also more likely at that time of year.

CLINICAL ASPECTS. Illness begins with the sudden onset of fever and vomiting and continues with moderate or severe watery diarrhea that generally lasts about five days. Dehydration severe enough to require hospitalization is frequent among patients with community-acquired illnesses. The causative agent can be identified either by the direct demonstration of virus by electron microscopy in stool or rectal swabs of patients or by serologic means. These tests, however, are generally not available in clinical laboratories. Nosocomial rotavirus gastroenteritis should be especially strongly suspected in a child one year of age or younger who develops nonbacterial gastroenteritis 72 hours or more after admission.

SOURCES AND MODES OF ACQUISITION. Rotavirus disease appears to be highly infectious, and it can be spread from patients with cases of disease to susceptible individuals by direct contact. The peak incidence in winter suggests that droplet spread from the upper respiratory tract may play a role in transmission, since respiratory spread is a common feature of most illnesses with seasonal peaks in the winter. Nosocomial transmission probably occurs indirectly from patient to patient on the hands of hospital personnel as well as by person-to-person spread from patients with disease to susceptible persons when such patients are inadequately isolated. Hospital personnel are generally immune and do not carry the virus.

PREVENTION AND CONTROL. Rotaviruses are highly immunogenic, and serologic studies indicate a high level of acquired immunity in persons over five years of age. These findings raise the possibility of ultimate control of the disease by vaccine. Children with nosocomial nonbacterial gastroenteritis should be placed in enteric isolation, and consideration should be given to the use of masks on older children to prevent droplet transmission when they are transported out of the isolation area.

Other Gastrointestinal Diseases

Staphylococcal Enterocolitis

In contrast to the preceding disease, staphylococcal enterocolitis is not transmissible as such from person to person. However, the disease may be an important source from which nosocomial strains of *Staphylococcus aureus* can be transmitted.

INCIDENCE. The true incidence of such infections is unknown. NNIS data show *S. aureus* to be the leading single cause of nosocomial bacterial diarrheal disease, and such cases are reported about one and a third times as frequently as those of salmonellosis. The proportion of such cases in which *S. aureus* was truly the causative agent of gastroenteritis is uncertain. Staphylococcal enterocolitis occurs sporadically, and epidemics have not been reported.

CLINICAL ASPECTS. In certain hosts in whom there is impaired resistance due to surgery, antimicrobial therapy, alcoholism, or diabetes mellitus, staphylococci may grow to large numbers in the intestinal tract and be responsible for morphologic damage to the intestinal mucosa that results in diarrhea and fever of varying severity. Intestinal involvement varies widely from minimal and self-limiting "enteritis" to fulminating "pseudomembranous enterocolitis" [3]. Patients with enteritis will have diarrhea of a variable nature, often mild and watery, and may have low-grade fever, but they will not be extremely toxic. Pseudomembranous enterocolitis frequently presents with fulminating and dehydrating diarrhea; bloody, mucoid stools; fever; leukocytosis; and toxemia. The entire colon may be involved with the disease, and there may be some involvement of the small intestine. Mortality rates in such patients are high and range from 10 to 50 percent.

The diagnosis is established by documenting abundant poymorphonuclear leukocytes and sheets of gram-positive cocci in stool specimens, which on subsequent cultures grow large numbers of *S. aureus*. Proctologic examination shows a white membrane that reflects areas of mucosal necrosis in those with pseudomembranous enterocolitis. It should be noted that pseudomembranous enterocolitis is not always secondary to *S. aureus* infection; it may also follow surgery or therapy with clindamycin, lincomycin, tetracycline, oral kanamycin, neomycin, etc. in cases in which *S. aureus* cannot be incriminated (see Part I, Chapter 11).

Patients should receive replacement fluid and electrolytes. Oral vancomycin [12] and fecal retention enemas from stool flora of a healthy person both appears to be of value in treating those patients with serious forms of the disease. Parenteral, semisynthetic, penicillinase-resistant penicillin treatment is advised for very toxic patients.

SOURCES AND MODES OF ACQUISITION. *S. aureus* can be cultured from stools of about 10 percent of normal adults, but it is normally present in small numbers. Intestinal carriage of these organisms is twice as common in hospitalized patients than in persons outside the hospital environment. Most strains that cause staphylococcal enterocolitis are multiple-drug-resistant, and some have been shown to produce enterotoxin in laboratory tests. Pathogenic strains are probably mainly acquired from nosocomial sources, and they proliferate to displace normal flora when antibiotics to which they are resistant are administered. Staphylococcal enterotoxin is probably not important in the pathogenesis of the disease, since otherwise identical, clinical, pseudomembranous enterocolitis occurs following infection with nonenterotoxic strains as well as other events (e.g., antimicrobial therapy) that are not associated with an overgrowth of *S. aureus*. Destruction or replacement of normal endogenous flora is probably the principal inciting factor.

PREVENTION AND CONTROL. Prompt cessation of previously administered antibiotics and administration of oral vancomycin to patients with more serious staphylococcal enteritis may prevent the disease from progressing to pseudomembranous enterocolitis. Large numbers of *S. aureus* are often disseminated from patients with these diseases, and strict, rather than enteric, isolation procedures should be considered (see Part I, Chapter 9).

Neonatal Necrotizing Enterocolitis

Neonatal necrotizing enterocolitis (NEC) is a frequently fatal disease that usually affects sick, premature infants. The disease is characterized by ischemic necrosis of the gastrointestinal tract and intramural gas (pneumatosis intestinalis), and it frequently results in intestinal perforation, peritonitis, and septicemia. NEC frequently occurs in epidemics within nurseries, which suggests an infectious cause. Three pathogenetic factors underlie the occurrence of disease: injury to the intestinal mucosa, whether due to relative ischemia from stress in newborns or other causes; the presence of intraluminal enteric bacteria; and enteral feedings that provide a metabolic substrate for the bacteria.

Most reports of NEC have not incriminated a particular bacterium as a cause of the disease, perhaps indicating that many strains of gram-negative bacteria may be involved in pathogenesis. However, a particular strain of bacteria prevalent in the nursery has occasionally been linked with an epidemic of NEC [10]. The prophylactic use of systemic antibiotics does not prevent colonization of an infant's gastrointestinal tract with gram-negative bacteria, and most studies have shown no efficacy of such drugs in preventing NEC. The prophylactic use of oral kanamycin, however, appeared effective in one study [5].

Further studies of sporadic and epidemic NEC cases, including careful aerobic and anaerobic culture studies of cases and controls, should assist in determining the role of microorganisms in this disease.

Yersinia enterocolitica Infections

Nosocomial transmission of infections caused by this agent has been rarely reported, but it probably occurs far more commonly than reports would indicate. The organism, a gram-negative rod, can easily be misidentified, and sometimes prolonged cold enrichment is required for its optimal recovery from stool specimens. Early symptoms are usually those of fever and acute enterocolitis, and the abdominal pains are frequently so similar to those of appendicitis that appendectomies are performed. Mesenteric adenitis or ileitis are generally discovered. A wide variety of other features can be seen, including arthritis and erythema nodosum. Although the reservoir of the organism is animals, person-to-person transmission also occurs, and nosocomial transmission has sometimes involved personnel [20].

A more deliberate search for this organism in otherwise unexplained, nosocomial, gastroenteritis outbreaks should be encouraged when clinical features suggest it is a possible causative agent. In addition to culture studies, serologic tests may also be helpful in establishing the diagnosis of infection with this organism.

References

1. Baine, W. B., Gangarosa, E. J., Bennett, J. V., and Barker, W. H., Jr. Institutional salmonellosis. *J. Infect. Dis.* 128:357, 1973.
2. Davidson, G. P., Bishop, R. F., Townley, R. R. W., Holmes, I. H., and Ruck, B. J. Importance of a new virus in acute sporadic enteritis in children. *Lancet* 1:242, 1975.
3. Dearing, W. H., Baggenstoss, A. H., and Weed, L. A. Studies on *Staphylococcus aureus* to pseudomembranous enterocolitis and to postantibiotic enteritis. *Gastroenterology* 38:441, 1960.
4. Echeverria, P., Blacklow, N. R., and Smith, D. H. Role of heat-labile toxigenic *Escherichia coli* and reovirus-like agent in diarrhea in Boston children. *Lancet* 2:1113, 1975.
5. Egan, E. A., Mantilla, G., Nelson, R. M., and Eitzman, D. V. A prospective controlled trial of oral kanamycin in the prevention of neonatal necrotizing enterocolitis. *J. Pediatr.* 89:467, 1976.
6. Flewett, T. H., Boyden, A. S., and Davies, H. Epidemic viral enteritis in a long-stay children's ward. *Lancet* 1:4, 1975.
7. Goldschmidt, M. C., and DuPont, H. L. Enteropathogenic *Escherichia coli*: Lack of correlation of serotype with pathogenicity. *J. Infect. Dis.* 133:153, 1976.
8. Haltalin, K. C. Neonatal shigellosis: Report of 16 cases and review of the literature. *Am. J. Dis. Child.* 114:603, 1967.
9. Harris, A. H., Yankauer, A., Greene, D. C., Coleman, M. B., and Phaneuf, M. Y. Control of epidemic diarrhea of the newborn in

hospital nurseries and pediatric wards. *Ann. N.Y. Acad. Sci.* 66:118, 1956.

10. Hill, H. R., Hunt, C. E., and Matsen, J. M. Nosocomial colonization with klebsiella, type 26, in a neonatal intensive-care unit associated with an outbreak of sepsis, meningitis, and necrotizing enterocolitis. *J. Pediatr.* 85:415, 1974.

11. Hirsch, W., Sapiro-Hirsch, R., Berger, A., Winter, S. T., Mayer, G., and Merzbach, D. *Salmonella edinburg* infection in children—A protracted hospital epidemic due to a multiple drug resistant strain. *Lancet* 2:828, 1965.

12. Khan, M. Y., and Hall, W. H. Staphylococcal enterocolitis—Treatment with oral vancomycin. *Ann. Intern. Med.* 65:1, 1966.

13. Mackerras, I. M., and Mackerras, M. J. An outbreak of infantile gastroenteritis in Queensland caused by *Salmonella bovis-morbificans* (Basenau). *J. Hyg.* (Camb). 47:166, 1949.

14. Rogers, K. B. The spread of infantile gastroenteritis in a cubicled ward. *J. Hyg.* (Lond). 49:40, 1951.

15. Ryder, R. W., McGowan, J. E., Hatch, M. H., and Palmer, E. L. Reovirus-like agent as a cause of nosocomial diarrhea in infants. *J. Pediatr.* 90:698, 1977.

16. Ryder, R. W., Wachsmuth, I. K., Buxton, A. E., Evans, D. G., DuPont, H. L., Mason, E., and Barrett, F. F. Infantile diarrhea produced by heat-stable enterotoxigenic *Escherichia coli*. *N. Engl. J. Med.* 295:849, 1976.

17. Salzman, T. C., Scher, C. D., and Moss, R. Shigellae with transferable drug resistance: Outbreak in a nursery for premature infants. *J. Pediatr.* 71:21, 1967.

18. Schroeder, S. A., Aserkoff, B., and Brachman, P. S. Epidemic salmonellosis in hospitals and institutions: A five-year review. *N. Engl. J. Med.* 279:674, 1968.

19. Taylor, J. Infectious infantile enteritis, yesterday and today. *Proc. R. Soc. Med.* 63:1297, 1970.

20. Toivanen, P., Toivanen, A., Olkkonen, L., and Aantaa, S. Hospital outbreak of *Yersinia enterocolitica* infection. *Lancet* 1:801, 1973.

21. Wachsmuth, I. K., Falkow, S., and Ryder, R. W. Plasmid-mediated properties of a heat-stable enterotoxin-producing *Escherichia coli* associated with infantile diarrhea. *Infect. Immun.* 14:403, 1976.

22. Whitfield, C., and Humphries, J. M. Meningitis and septicemia due to *Shigellae* in a newborn infant. *J. Pediatr.* 70:805, 1967.

22

Puerperal Endometritis

William J. Ledger

Nature of Infections

Incidence

There is good evidence that the incidence of puerperal endometritis reported from individual hospitals with active surveillance of these infections (1 to 4 percent) is probably unchanged from the most accurate figures available from the preantibiotic decade of the 1920s. This statement should not be construed as an apology for modern obstetrics, for the status of puerperal endometritis and sepsis has dramatically changed in that same time interval. The most severe infections—namely, those resulting in maternal death from sepsis—have virtually been eliminated from modern obstetrics.

The above incidence is higher than has been noted in the National Nosocomial Infections Study (NNIS) (see Part II, Chapter 13). In that study in the interval from January 1970 through August 1973, there were 2692 instances of endometritis among 438,228 obstetric discharges, or an incidence of 0.6 percent. Certain possible reasons for this lower incidence are noted below.

Deficiencies in Reporting Infections

Obstetricians, who are surgically oriented physicians, tend to underestimate the incidence of nosocomial infections, including postpartum endometritis. This phenomenon of individual physician inaccuracy in assessing the frequency of infections reflects commonly observed patterns of clinical practice. Most patients with the early symptoms of a postpartum endometritis, such as temperature elevation, are first discovered at night and not during the traditional early-morning rounds of physicians (Fig. 22-1). In the majority of occasions, these patients are placed on systemic antibiotics without prior culture studies. A nationwide evaluation of over 12,000 women undergoing hysterectomy who were cared for by obstetrician-gynecologists revealed that over 50 percent had received systemic antibiotics without prior culture tests [6]. A rapid response of the patient

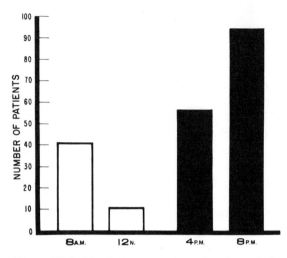

Figure 22-1. The first temperature elevation of obstetric patients with postpartum morbidity. The majority of patients had initial rises in the late afternoon or evening hours.

to the administered antibiotics with a quick return of temperature levels to normal may cause the attending physician to disregard the case as "true" morbidity. In this context, the reader must be aware that any nationwide survey will detect only a portion of all cases of endometritis during any study interval. Despite the fact that some cases are inevitably missed by surveillance systems such as that of the NNIS, pooled microbiologic data from cases that are reported do provide a good assessment of the major pathogens involved in postpartum endometritis.

Underestimates of the incidence of endometritis in modern obstetrics are also based upon continued dependence on a preantibiotic era definition of "morbidity" based on temperature elevations. This definition was established by American obstetrician-gynecologists between the first and second World Wars, and it is based on four separate oral temperature recordings each postpartum day; "morbidity" is defined as an oral temperature of 100.4°F (38°C) or greater on any two of the first 10 postpartum days, excluding the first 24 hours after delivery. This definition successfully excluded from consideration those patients with one temperature elevation shortly after delivery as well as those who had a single temperature elevation later but no evidence of a postpartum pelvic infection. On a statistical basis, nearly all the women

from the preantibiotic era who met these temperature criteria for "morbidity" had a pelvic infection, whether uterine or urinary tract. Appropriate microbiologic studies could be performed, and such patients could be isolated from other obstetric patients.

The great setback for a clear understanding of infectious disease in antibiotic era obstetrics has been the maintenance of this formerly valid standard in the face of antibiotic use. Employment of powerful systemic antibiotics in postpartum patients with the first elevation of temperature may yield an immediate clinical response with rapid and persistent defervescence of fever. If the obstetric service adheres to the old temperature-defined morbidity standards, the patient is not counted in morbidity statistics. This accounts in part for the frequent discrepancy between the low recorded morbidity figures and the high systemic antibiotic use in obstetric units.

Community-Acquired Versus Nosocomial Infections

All postpartum endometritis should be considered a nosocomial infection, unless the amiotic fluid is infected at the time of admission or the patient was admitted 48 hours or more following rupture of the membranes. Some infections in the latter group are nosocomial, however, and available microbiologic, clinical, and epidemiologic data should be carefully reviewed to determine whether the infection is community-acquired or nosocomial.

Mechanisms of Infection

The uterus has excellent local defense mechanisms to protect itself against invasion by contaminating organisms from the lower genital tract. These defenses are present in the nonpregnant state, as is demonstrated by the rapid clearance of the lower genital tract bacteria that are carried into the endometrial cavity during the insertion of an intrauterine device [13]. During pregnancy, Galask and his associates [4] have demonstrated inhibition of bacterial growth by the amniotic fluid. The stress of labor and delivery probably commonly results in uterine acquisition of organisms from the nonsterile lower genital tract, but most post-

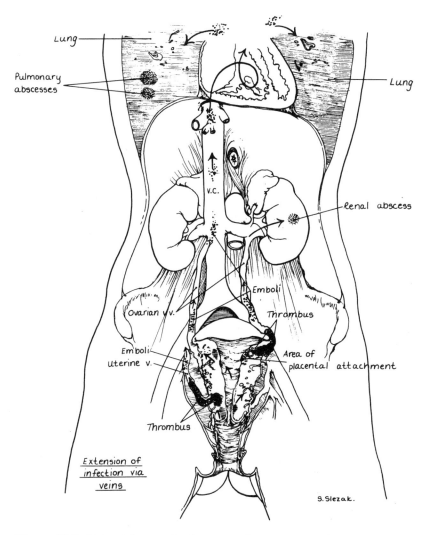

Figure 22-2. Potential spread of untreated postpartum endometritis.

partum patients remain free of symptoms as the uterus rapidly clears itself of the potentially pathogenic bacteria introduced from the vagina.

Postpartum endometritis occurs when these efficient uterine defense mechanisms are overcome by a combination of too many bacteria, the introduction of especially virulent bacterial strains, or local alterations (e.g., soft tissue damage or the incomplete removal of the placenta) that provide a nidus for the development of a postpartum infection.

Postpartum pelvic infection follows a pattern of progression (Fig. 22-2) with ascension of the organisms into the endometrial cavity, invasion of the myometrium, extension into parametrial areas beyond the uterus, and blood-

stream invasion in some instances [1]. If this progression is unchecked by the appropriate use of systemic antibiotics and anticoagulants when indicated, then myometrial, parametrial, or adnexal abscesses can occur with suppurative involvement of the pelvic veins, septic pelvic thrombophlebitis, and even distant septic metastases to the liver and lung. In addition to the appropriate use of systemic medical agents, adequate uterine drainage must be insured, and operative intervention for the drainage or removal of a pelvic abscess may be necessary for cure.

Predisposing Host Factors
Host Susceptibility
The well-nourished pregnant patient is far less likely to have infectious problems than her

poorly nourished, anemic counterpart. In addition, infection risks increase with prolonged rupture of the fetal membranes prior to delivery, with increasing length of labor, and with retention of fetal membranes or placental fragments after delivery.

Transvaginal Monitoring

In addition to reducing mortality rates, the availability of antibiotics has dramatically changed the practice philosophies of obstetrician-gynecologists. The prolonged transvaginal monitoring of maternal intraamniotic pressures and the transvaginal attachment of a fetal scalp electrode for electrocardiograph readings could not have been considered if antibiotics were not available for postpartum use by obstetricians and neonatologists. However, these advances have nonetheless been accompanied by enhanced infection risks. Although a number of studies have demonstrated no difference in endometritis rates, an increased incidence is noted when monitoring is carried out for eight hours or more [5].

Cesarean Section

Advances in the science of neonatology have increased fetal survival and have further increased the incidence of cesarean section for fetal indications in situations where the maternal risk is increased for a postpartum infection. As an example of this, the obstetric service at the Los Angeles County-University of Southern California (LAC-USC) Medical Center is now doing cesarean sections for infants estimated to weigh 1000 gm. or more, instead of 1500 gm., the limit that previously existed. The results of this philosophy have been a dramatic reduction in perinatal mortality rates [14], but these results have been achieved by judgments that increase the maternal risks for infection; my own assessment would be that the benefits of this new obstetric philosophy for the fetus outweigh the risks for the mother.

Diagnostic Criteria

Clinical

The clinical diagnosis of postpartum endometritis is based upon a number of findings, but the most significant factor is fever. Generally, these women have an oral temperature elevation to about 100.4°F (38°C) and a tachycardia consistent with this rise. Patients usually have uterine tenderness and often have tenderness beyond the uterus in the parametrial and adnexal regions. A decrease in the normal postpartum uterine lochial flow is often noted 6 to 12 hours preceding the temperature elevation, and the lochial flow may be foul smelling.

If the physician makes a clinical diagnosis of endometritis and begins administration of systemic antibiotics with or without positive culture results, the patient should be included in all infection surveillance and postpartum morbidity statistics.

Attempts to assess the presence of a postpartum endometritis through evaluation of commonly employed, indirect, hematologic measures of infection have not been successful. The phenomena of labor and delivery are accompanied by changes in the commonly employed parameters to measure the presence or absence of a bacterial infection. Thus, a normal patient in labor or postpartum who has no clinical evidence of an active bacterial infection may have an elevated white blood cell count (even above 20,000) with an increase in the percentage of immature leukocytes, an elevated sedimentation rate, and a striking increase in the percentage of white cells that have engulfed and reduced nitroblue tetrazolium during incubation. With these facts in mind, there should be no enthusiasm for dependence on such laboratory tests to determine the diagnosis of infection.

Microbiologic

Bacterial isolations in the clinical microbiology laboratory usually do not establish the diagnosis of a postpartum endometritis. The sole exception is the discovery of a group-A β-hemolytic *Streptococcus,* which should trigger specific physician responses for treatment, isolation, and investigation. The reasons for the usual lack of useful diagnostic, but not therapeutic, information from the microbiologic laboratory are manifold. Most culture techniques for sampling the postpartum endometrial cavity include a transcervical approach, which of necessity involves contamination by the abundant bacterial flora normally present in the endocervical canal of asymptomatic women. Also, the organisms recovered from the endometrial cavity of endometritis patients are usually the same as those normally inhabiting the vagina and endocervix of sexually active women.

The above considerations do not mean that the laboratory will not be helpful, for it may indirectly contribute to the diagnosis or lack of diagnosis and give therapeutic guidance for treating postpartum endometritis. Assistance in excluding the diagnosis of postpartum endometritis may be provided, for example, in the febrile postpartum patient with no localizing uterine signs of infection when a significant bacterial colony count is obtained from a properly collected urine sample, and the fever resolves successfully following therapy with an antibacterial agent (e.g., a nitrofurantoin) with limited action outside of the urinary tract.

Specimen Collection and Transport
Transvaginal Specimens
The greatest difficulty facing the clinician in his attempts to sample the postpartum endometrial cavity microbiologically is to obtain specimens that are free of vaginal and cervical contamination. To date, most techniques have stressed the transvaginal and transcervical approach to the endometrial cavity. Various techniques have been tried to decrease contamination from endocervical canal organisms, including the use of plastic or metal tubing through which specimens can be collected. There has been little physician enthusiasm for these more complicated diagnostic procedures. Also, there have been no reports of attempts to quantitate the recovery of bacteria, similar to the methods of the colony counts of urine specimens, which might separate vaginal and endocervical contaminants from the more numerous pathogens from the site of infection.

Transabdominal Specimens
An alternative microbiologic method to the transcervical technique is the transabdominal

approach. We have attempted this approach in a limited number of patients and have had no serious complications with the method. More significant has been the greater frequency of recovery of microorganisms with this approach than with a blood culture. The importance of this technique in future microbiologic sampling remains to be established by more extensive study.

Use of Blood Cultures
The most useful microbiologic technique, when it is positive, is the blood culture. A positive result usually pinpoints the most severely ill patients on the postpartum service, but more importantly, it focuses the clinician's attention on the most significant microorganisms in the infectious process. Those that invade the bloodstream are critical for the physician's therapeutic consideration. This diagnostic technique is positive in 10 percent of the febrile patients sampled.

Transport
Significant changes in microbiologic sampling and the transportation of specimens have been brought about by the growing physician awareness of the importance of anaerobic microorganisms in postpartum infections. The recovery of anaerobes is crucially dependent on the clinician's efforts to reduce exposure of the specimens to atmospheric oxygen. Time is a critical factor, because exposure of a swab of the infection site to atmospheric oxygen for a few minutes or less will reduce or eliminate certain anaerobic organisms. A number of alternative laboratory systems have been proposed to eliminate such exposure. Transport media have been used, either liquid for primary culture or semisolid for transport to the laboratory and primary plating there. Alternatively, gassed tubes, free of oxygen, have been used for transport to a laboratory where primary plating and anaerobic incubation can be performed.

There is a major weakness in all these clinical schemes for the obstetrician-gynecologist. Figure 22-1 documents the first temperature elevation of obstetric patients with postpartum morbidity, which is the logical time for initial patient evaluation [9]. It is clear that the majority of microbiologic samples will be obtained late in the afternoon or in the early evening, when laboratory coverage, particularly by technicians with familiarity in anaerobic methods, will usually be inadequate. An alternative to this scheme involves bringing the laboratory to the patient's bedside. For the clinicians at the LAC-USC Medical Center, we have made available Gas-Paks and pre-reduced blood agar plates, pre-reduced blood agar plates with vancomycin and kanamycin added, and thioglycolate broth. Inoculated medium is placed in an anaerobic chamber containing the Gas-Pak and is then placed into an ordinary incubator in the hospital. The laboratory can then work with the specimen during the daylight hours. This technique has enabled us to recover anaerobic organisms from over 70 percent of the submitted specimens.

General Control Measures

Patient-Care Practices

PRENATAL CARE. The emphasis on the preventive aspects in patient care has been heavily weighted toward patient management during pregnancy, labor, and delivery. For the patient in labor, most obstetricians believe that the results of prenatal care culminating in delivery largely determine the frequency and severity of postpartum endometritis.

RECTAL AND VAGINAL EXAMINATIONS. One of the great changes in practice patterns in obstetrics in the past several years has been the virtual abandonment of the rectal examination during labor. Rectal examination was firmly established in the preantibiotic era and was predicated on the belief that it would avoid the introduction of exogenous organisms into the vagina. Since the most feared bacterial pathogens—the group-A β-hemolytic streptococci—were often introduced into the vagina from personnel sources, prohibition of vaginal examination was undoubtedly beneficial. A number of studies have now demonstrated no differences in the postpartum endometritis rate when patients undergoing vaginal examination during labor were compared to those having rectal examination. These results probably reflect the

low frequency of involvement of exogenous organisms such as group-A β-hemolytic streptococci in postpartum endometritis. Both rectal and vaginal examinations, however, can result in the displacement of organisms from the lower genital tract to the uterus, and these manipulations, as well as other manipulations with similar risks (e.g., intrauterine placement of forceps or the physician's hand at delivery), should be limited to as few as necessary for good management of the patient.

PROPHYLACTIC ANTIBIOTICS. Recently, interest has grown in the use of prophylactic antibiotics for the patient in labor who needs a cesarean section. Although most studies to date have shown diminished postpartum morbidity, I have not been convinced that the risks of such prolonged use of antibiotics for all women undergoing cesarean section are worth the alleged maternal benefits. This subject needs continued evaluation.

HAND-WASHING AND GLOVES. In the nineteenth century, Semmelweis recognized the importance of hand transfer of organisms from the postmortem room and the autopsy in the production of endometritis, inasmuch as the physicians carried the bacterial pathogens from the autopsy room on their hands and clothing to the vagina and endocervix of the patient in labor, which led to the subsequent development of infection. Semmelweis' great achievement was to require hand-bathing by physicians in an antiseptic solution before the next patient was seen in order to break the chain of bacterial contamination and infection. Hand-washing and the use of sterile gloves for vaginal examinations remain important general control measures.

Environmental Factors

Environmental factors are infrequently involved in the development of postpartum endometritis. Indeed, the studies of the effect of ultraviolet irradiation on the rate of all postoperative wound infections [2] suggest that this would be the case in the delivery room, because they showed that there was little impact on clinical results despite reductions in the bacterial contamination of air (see Part II, Chapter 16). The lack of importance of the environment would be especially anticipated in the case of endometritis, because most of these infections derive from the patients' endogenous bacterial flora.

Therapy

The cornerstones of therapy in patients with a postpartum endometritis are adequate uterine drainage and the use of appropriate antimicrobials. Uterine drainage must be insured, and the maneuver of removing membranes provides the patient undergoing clinical examination the added benefit of an assessment of the extent of infection; a microbiologic specimen may also be obtained at this time.

Antibiotics are frequently utilized for cure. They usually are prescribed before the results of culture susceptibility tests are known, and the initial choices reflect the individual physician's philosophy of antibiotic usage, which should be based on past experiences with similar patients. At the LAC-USC Medical Center, we will frequently use a single antibiotic like ampicillin or a cephalosporin to treat the patient who is not allergic to penicillin and who has had a vaginal delivery. This course usually results in cure, even in the patient with a concomitant bacteremia, because these agents provide coverage against most of the commonly recovered organisms. In patients who have had a cesarean section, our antibiotic coverage most commonly includes a combination of penicillin and an aminoglycoside, usually kanamycin, with erythromycin substituted for penicillin in the allergic patient. We have favored kanamycin over gentamicin, because most of the gram-negative aerobes are not highly resistant in our obstetric patients. This combination of antibiotics provides coverage against most of the commonly recovered aerobes and anaerobes except *Bacteroides fragilis*. If the patient remains febrile despite such antibiotic therapy and has no clinical evidence of abscess formation that is amenable to operative drainage, we will add either clindamycin or chloramphenicol to the regimen. Tetracycline has not been utilized in postpartum patients, because of our concerns about the fatty-liver syndrome and deaths that have been reported when high doses of this agent were used in obstetric patients.

Endogenous Infections from Lower Genital Tract Flora

The microorganisms mainly responsible for postpartum endometritis are nearly always endogenous to the patient, that is, they normally reside in the gastrointestinal and lower genital tract (vagina and endocervix) of asymptomatic, sexually active, pregnant women. The stress of labor and delivery, the rupture of the membranes, the frequent vaginal examinations by the medical team caring for the patient, the use of monitoring devices, and delivery by the intrauterine placement of forceps or physicians' hands all introduce opportunities for uterine acquisition of lower genital tract flora. After introduction, they may find a suitable uterine environment where they can survive and invade.

The endogenous organisms that most frequently become pathogenic and result in an endometritis include certain aerobic streptococci ($\propto$ -hemolytic streptococci, the group-B β-hemolytic streptococci, and the enterococci); anaerobic cocci (*Peptostreptococcus* and *Peptococcus*); gram-negative enteric aerobes (*Escherichia coli, Proteus mirabilis,* and *Klebsiella* species); and finally the gram-negative anaerobic rod, *Bacteroides fragilis*. There is suggestive evidence that many patients with endometritis, particularly those with severe infections, have a mixed infection with more than one organism involved. The implications of such microbiologic findings for multiple antibiotic use have not been settled by prospective study.

Epidemics of endometritis caused by these organisms have not been recognized, and their control depends on avoiding predisposing factors, when possible, and adherence to general control measures.

Gram-Negative Aerobic Bacterial Infections

INCIDENCE. The National Nosocomial Infections Study (NNIS) data indicate that gram-negative aerobes were the most commonly recovered pathogens. From 2692 patients with endometritis, *E. coli* was recovered in 732 occasions, *Klebsiella* recovered in 179, and *P. mirabilis* in 154. This frequent recovery of *E. coli* matches our own surveillance data on endometritis and postpartum bacteria; this has consistently been the most common organism recovered. Indeed, *E. coli* is the most common pathogen isolated in modern obstetric practice.

CLINICAL FEATURES. A patient with postpartum endometritis due to a gram-negative aerobe can be seriously ill. This is particularly true in the patient with an associated bacteremia. There are no distinctive clinical signs, however, that would alert the clinician to the possibility that these organisms were involved.

THERAPY. The low frequency of antimicrobial-resistant organisms is a major advantage to the clinician treating women with endometritis due to a gram-negative aerobe. Most postpartum obstetric patients have intact host defense mechanisms and have usually neither had prolonged exposure to systemic antimicrobial therapy prior to labor and delivery nor prolonged hospitalization prior to delivery. Effective first-line drugs include the aminoglycosides, kanamycin, gentamicin, and amikacin. Since there are few resistant gram-negative aerobic organisms seen in these patients, we usually rely on kanamycin as our most frequently used aminoglycoside, with gentamicin or amikacin reserved for the patient who is suspected of having gram-negative aerobic bacterial sepsis or who had repeated exposure to antibiotics for urinary tract infections during pregnancy. The cephalosporins are highly effective against such gram-negative aerobes, and these are an acceptable alternative to aminoglycosides in patients who have been delivered vaginally. In the more serious infections seen following cesarean section, the aminoglycosides remain the drugs of choice. Ampicillin is a good second-line agent, and it is placed in this category because of the frequency of resistance to this agent seen in *Klebsiella* isolates. Chloramphenicol has shown effectiveness in the laboratory against gram-negative aerobes, but I do not prescribe it in these patients, because of my concern about bone-marrow toxicity.

Bacteroides fragilis *Infections*

INCIDENCE. The NNIS data indicate that *Bacteroides* species were the most common anaerobes isolated from patients with postpartum endometritis. Undoubtedly, the majority of these isolates were *B. fragilis*. In our own obstetric surveillance data, *B. fragilis* was one of the three most commonly recovered anaerobic organisms from the uterus and bloodstream of patients with postpartum endometritis; the others were *Peptostreptococcus* and *Peptococcus*.

CLINICAL FEATURES. Patients with postpartum endometritis due to *B. fragilis* can be seriously ill, and they frequently have lochia with a fecal odor. Prolonged rupture of the membranes, particularly for many days, has been associated with the most serious. *B. fragilis* infections that have been seen on our service. A hallmark of established postpartum pelvic infections due to this organism is their chronicity, even in the face of appropriate antibiotic coverage. This is indirectly reflected by a number of patient assessments. Such patients may require many days of antibiotic therapy and operative intervention (Fig. 22-3) before they become afebrile [7]. In addition to this clinical assessment, the urinary mucopolysaccharide/creatinine index, a measure of ground-substance turnover that is elevated in patients with a pelvic infection, remains elevated for a longer period of time in women with *B. fragilis* infection [10]. Pelvic abscess formation is not uncommon, and operative drainage or removal may be necessary for cure, despite the use of appropriate antibiotics in adequate dosages. Septic thrombophlebitis with septic emboli may also follow infections with this organism.

THERAPY. Postpartum endometritis due to *B. fragilis* requires different antibiotic strategies from those commonly employed by obstetrician-gynecologists. Frequently prescribed antibiotics—including the penicillins, cephalosporins, and aminoglycosides—are all ineffective in treating serious infections due to *B. fragilis*. Instead, the current first-line drugs of choice are clindamycin and chloramphenicol. Both seem effective, although no prospective comparative study of their effectiveness had been reported. Each has the problem of serious toxicity, which occurs very infrequently. Chloramphenicol has been associated with fatal bone-marrow aplasia in one of 10,000 to 25,000 patients treated with the drug. Clindamycin has been associated with pseudomembranous enterocolitis, a serious clinical entity that affects

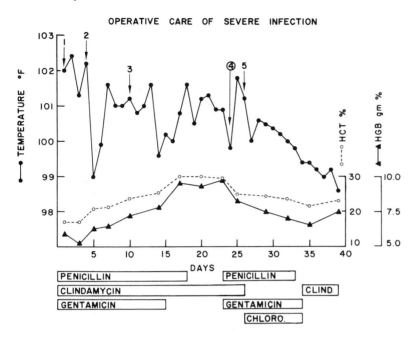

OPERATIVE CARE OF SEVERE INFECTION

Figure 22-3. The complicated postpartum course of a patient with an endometritis. This septic Jehovah's Witness was admitted to our hospital (point 1 on the graph) following a cesarean section and the development of postpartum sepsis in another hospital. Hyperalimentation was begun at point 2 and continued until point 3. At point 4, a hysterectomy and bilateral salpingooophorectomy were performed. Postoperatively (point 5), chloramphenicol was started. The *Bacteroides fragilis* organisms recovered from the excised tissue were susceptible in the laboratory to both clindamycin and chloramphenicol.

more than one in 25,000 treated patients (see Part I, Chapter 11 and Part II, Chapter 21). An alternative drug is lincomycin, but fewer strains of *B. fragilis* are susceptible to it. In addition, there is a higher incidence of diarrhea associated with its administration than with clindamycin, and an occasional patient may develop pseudomembranous enterocolitis during its administration. An exciting, newer drug is metronidazole, which is the most bactericidal of all antibiotic agents against *B. fragilis*. Only an oral preparation of metronidazole is available, however, and clinical experience has been limited. Tetracycline is less favored, because 40 to 60 percent of isolates from clinical sites of infection are not susceptible to this agent.

Operative removal and drainage of pelvic

abscesses, treatment of septic pelvic thrombophlebitis with intravenous heparin therapy, and continued use of appropriate antibiotics may result in a rapid defervescence of fever in a patient with previously persisting temperature spikes.

Peptostreptococcus and Peptococcus *Infections*

INCIDENCE. The NNIS report does not include anaerobic gram-positive cocci among the frequently recovered organisms in patients with endometritis. This undoubtedly reflects shortcomings in anaerobic microbiologic techniques in the initial culture study of patients with endometritis. Microbiologic studies of patients with postpartum endometritis in the preantibiotic era showed *Peptostreptococcus* to be the most commonly isolated organism [15]. More recent evaluations indicate that *E. coli* is now the most frequently isolated microorganism. In surveillance studies of obstetric infections with proper anaerobic culture techniques, however, *Peptostreptococcus* and *Peptococcus* are each recovered from the endometrium and bloodstream of patients with endometritis in numbers equivalent to those of *Bacteroides* species, and, if combined in the category of gram-positive anaerogenic cocci, they are numerically more common than *Bacteroides*.

CLINICAL FEATURES. A postpartum endometritis due to gram-positive anaerobic cocci can be suspected in a patient whose lochia has a putrid, fecal odor. Pelvic abscess formation can occur, and operative drainage or removal may be necessary for cure, despite the use of appropriate antibiotics as judged by in vitro antibiotic susceptibility testing. The postpartum retention of fetal membranes or placental fragments has frequently been observed with these infections.

THERAPY. The *Peptostreptococcus* and *Peptococcus* are each quite susceptible to penicillin in dosage levels that are easily exceeded in the serum by frequently administered therapeutic doses of this agent. Lincomycin and clindamycin are alternative antibiotics; both are highly effective in treating endometritis due to these organisms in patients who are allergic to penicillin. Other alternative antibiotics include the cephalosporins and erythromycin, but there is a slightly higher percentage of strains of *Peptococcus* that are resistant to these agents.

Aerobic Streptococcal Infections

INCIDENCE. The NNIS report noted that groups B and D streptococci and $\propto$-hemolytic streptococci occurred more frequently in endometritis than the group-A β-hemolytic streptococci but less frequently than any of the previously mentioned gram-negative aerobes. This frequency pattern varies from our own surveillance data on postpartum endometritis. In our patients with endometritis or an associated bacteremia, these aerobic streptococci were more frequently recovered than any organism except *E. coli*.

CLINICAL FEATURES. Postpartum endometritis due to aerobic streptococci has no characteristic clinical findings that distinguish it from endometritis due to other organisms.

THERAPY. The group-B β-hemolytic streptococci and $\propto$-hemolytic streptococci are susceptible to penicillin. An alternative antibiotic for the patient allergic to penicillin is erythromycin. The group-D β-hemolytic streptococci have unique antibiotic susceptibility patterns. In the laboratory, the organism is frequently not susceptible to penicillin or an aminoglycoside alone, but when both antibiotics are used together or when ampicillin is substituted for penicillin, there is both laboratory and clinical

evidence of a response. In the penicillin-allergic patient with enterococcal endometritis, erythromycin is the antibiotic of choice, since the cephalosporins, lincomycin, and clindamycin have little effectiveness against this group of organisms.

Group-A β-Hemolytic Streptococcal Infections
In contrast to the preceding category of infections, endometritis caused by group-A streptococci commonly derives from exogenous sources, is highly invasive and transmissible, and has produced outbreaks requiring special measures for control.

General Aspects
TRANSMISSIBILITY. The group-A β-hemolytic streptococci are highly contagious agents (see Part II, Chapter 20). For this reason, obstetricians justifiably fear the introduction of this organism into the labor-room environment lest it will be transmitted to patients in labor and result in serious cases of postpartum endometritis. A patient with an active *Streptococcus pyogenes* infection can transmit these organisms to either patients or medical personnel, resulting in colonization. Hospital personnel can be asymptomatic carriers of group-A streptococci and transmit the organism to patients in labor. Community contacts may be important in the transmission of this organism, particularly in the modern obstetric setting that so frequently allows husband and wife to be together for long periods of time during the labor and delivery. This practice can be dangerous if the husband is a carrier of group-A streptococci.

INCIDENCE. The importance of group-A β-hemolytic streptococcal infections is not based on a high frequency of infections but rather on the clinical invasiveness and epidemiologic virulence of such strains. Data from the NNIS indicate this organism was recovered in 33 of 2692 women with endometritis, an incidence of 1.2 percent of all cases of endometritis. This low frequency matches our surveillance experience with endometritis and the bacteremia associated with it.

SOURCES AND MODES OF ACQUISITION. Endogenous sources are probably mainly responsible for specific cases. The vagina of such patients is often asymptomatically colonized with group-A streptococci when the patient is admitted to the delivery room, but patients may also have an upper respiratory tract infection or skin lesion that harbors such organisms.

The most common method of spread of exogenous organisms involves direct transmission of the organism from personnel who are asymptomatic carriers to the patient. Clinically infected personnel may also be responsible (see Part II, Chapters 16, 19, and 20). Personnel may become colonized after providing care to a patient with postpartum endometritis; they may then transmit these organisms to patients in labor.

Clinical Considerations

MANIFESTATIONS. There are a number of distinctive clinical features seen in the patient with group-A β-hemolytic streptococcal endometritis. Historically, this entity has been called "puerperal fever," "puerperal sepsis," and "childbed fever." The most striking feature is the early onset of high spiking fevers (Fig. 22-4) in the postpartum patient [8]. Patients appear critically ill, but abdominal and pelvic examinations reveal diffuse tenderness with no

Figure 22-4. The early onset of a high, spiking temperature pattern in a postpartum patient with group-A β-hemolytic streptococcal endometritis. Despite the use of penicillin analogs (ampicillin and oxacillin), the patient required several days to become completely afebrile. The patient delivered at point 1 on the chart, was started on antibiotic treatment at point 2, and was discharged at point 3.

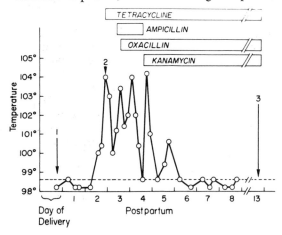

localizing signs. The cervical discharge is usually clear and watery, is not purulent, and contains many gram-positive cocci when the exudate is Gram stained. Although this organism is very susceptible to penicillin, patients with endometritis frequently do not become afebrile for 48 hours or more (see Fig. 22-4).

THERAPY. The drug of choice for treating group-A β-hemolytic streptococcal endometritis remains penicillin G. For the patient allergic to penicillin, erythromycin or the cephalosporins can be used. Although lincomycin and clindamycin are effective against this organism, we believe these antibiotics should be reserved for the patient with a suspected or proved *Bacteroides fragilis* infection. Tetracycline is not an acceptable alternative for treating patients with this infection, because of the frequency of resistant strains.

Epidemic Infections

REPORTED OUTBREAKS. In recent years, sporadic outbreaks of group-A β-hemolytic streptococcal endometritis epidemics have been reported in New York City [12] and Boston [3]. In the New York City outbreak, there were nine confirmed cases, while in Boston there were 20 women with this diagnosis.

SOURCES. In the New York City outbreak, the source of the bacteria that were disseminated around the hospital came from colonized, asymptomatic, newborn infants. In Boston, a common source was the cutaneous lesions of an anesthesiologist [3]. A preantibiotic era study of this problem found many personnel colonized with such streptococci [16]. Colonization of medical personnel and subsequent transmission to patients in labor seem to be the crucial ingredients in the maintenance of an epidemic. Another outbreak of group-A streptococcal infections affecting obstetric-gynecologic patients was ultimately traced to an anesthesiologist who was an asymptomatic rectal carrier of the organism [11]. Thus, operating-room sources of this type should be suspected in endometritis outbreaks that exclusively or primarily involve patients with cesarean sections.

Prevention and Control

PREVENTION. Infections due to this organism are so serious that the discovery of one case of puerperal sepsis should be considered an epidemic. The patient needs to be placed in wound and skin isolation, and hospital personnel should gown and glove before providing personal care (see Part I, Chapter 9). All labor and delivery room personnel on duty during this patient's labor and delivery should be screened for possible infections by history and physical examination, and cultures should be obtained on their nose, throat, and any suspected skin lesion. Lochial culture specimens should be obtained from postpartum patients who had been in the delivery room at the same time as the infected patient, and appropriate antibiotics should be given to those whose cultures are positive for group-A streptococci. Those personnel whose cultures are positive for the same strain as the one isolated from the infected patient (which is established by M and T typing) should be relieved of patient-care responsibilities until appropriate antibiotic therapy has resulted in their cultures being negative. All culture-positive personnel should be treated if the typing of strains cannot be done expeditiously.

CONTROL OF OUTBREAKS. There were a number of significant differences between the preantibiotic era epidemics and those recently reported. The preantibiotic era study reported maternal deaths, and the outbreak was controlled only by closing the maternity service of the hospital until all infected patients had been discharged [16]. The recent epidemics have been controlled by the use of appropriate antibiotics, isolation of infected patients, epidemiologic identification of disseminating carriers, and eradication of carried strains by proper treatment of colonized or infected hospital personnel. If initial nose and throat cultures of personnel epidemiologically associated with the outbreak are negative, multiple culture specimens should be obtained, including ones from rectal and vaginal sites. In Boston, all admissions to the service in the midst of the epidemic were treated with penicillin or penicillin-like antibiotics [3]. Such broad-scale prophylaxis may be especially indicated at the time an outbreak is first recognized, because it may permit a maternity unit to remain open while epide-

miologic and microbiologic investigations are undertaken. If such investigations are successful in identifying the sources and modes of spread, then attention focused on these areas should obviate the need for continued chemoprophylaxis of patients. Outbreaks should be promptly reported to local health authorities.

References

1. Eastman, N. J., and Hellman, L. M.   In Williams, L. W. (Ed.), *Obstetrics* (13th ed.). New York: Appleton-Century-Crofts, 1966.
2. Howard, J. M., Barker, W. F., Culbertson, W. R., Grotzinger, P. T., Jovine, V. M., Keehn, R. J., and Ravdin, R. G.   Postoperative wound infections: The influence of ultraviolet irradiation of the operating room and of various other factors. *Ann. Surg.* 160(Suppl.): 1, 1964.
3. Jewett, J. F., Reid, D. E., Safon, L. E., and Easterday, C. L.   Childbed fever—a continuing entity. *J.A.M.A.* 206:344, 1968.
4. Larsen, B., Snyder, I. S., and Galask, R. P. Bacterial growth inhibition by amniotic fluid. *Am. J. Obstet. Gynecol.* 119:492, 1974.
5. Larsen, J. W., Goldkrand, J. W., Hanson, T. M., and Miller, C. R.   Intrauterine infection on an obstetric service. *Obstet. Gynecol.* 43:838, 1974.
6. Ledger, W. J., and Child, M.   The hospital care of patients undergoing hysterectomy. *Am. J. Obstet. Gynecol.* 117:423, 1973.
7. Ledger, W. J., Gassner, C. B., and Gee, C. Operative care of infections in obstetrics-gynecology. *J. Reprod. Med.* 13:128, 1974.
8. Ledger, W. J., and Headington, J. T.   The Group A beta-hemolytic streptococcus. *Obstet. Gynecol.* 39:474, 1972.
9. Ledger, W. J., Reite, A. M., and Headington, J. T.   A system for infectious disease surveillance on an obstetric service. *Obstet. Gynecol.* 37:769, 1971.
10. Ledger, W. J., Thompson, G. R., and deVries, L.   The influence of infection in obstetric and gynecologic patients upon increased urinary mucopolysaccharide excretion. *Am. J. Obstet. Gynecol.* 120:407, 1974.
11. McIntyre, D. M.   An epidemic of *Streptococcus pyogenes* puerperal and post-operative sepsis with an unusual carrier site—the anus. *Am. J. Obstet. Gynecol.* 101:308, 1968.
12. Mead, P. B., Ribble, J. C., and Dillon, T. F. Group A streptococcal puerperal infection. *Obstet. Gynecol.* 32:460, 1968.
13. Mishell, D. R., Bell, J. H., Good, R. G., and

Moyer, D. L. The intrauterine device: A bacteriologic study of the endometrial cavity. *Am. J. Obstet. Gynecol.* 96:119, 1966.

14. Paul, R. H., and Hon, E. H. Clinical fetal monitoring v. Effect on perinatal outcome. *Am. J. Obstet. Gynecol.* 118:529, 1974.

15. Schwarz, O. H., and Dieckman, W. J. Puerperal infection due to anaerobic streptococci. *Am. J. Obstet. Gynecol.* 13:467, 1927.

16. Watson, B. P. An outbreak of puerperal sepsis in New York City. *Am. J. Obstet. Gynecol.* 16:157, 1928.

The Central Nervous System: Meningitis

Harry N. Beaty

Nature of Infections

Incidence

Nosocomial meningitis is extremely uncommon. A total of 298 cases, representing approximately 0.25 percent of all nosocomial infections, were reported to the Center for Disease Control during the first 44 months of the National Nosocomial Infections Study (NNIS), which began in January 1970 (see Part II, Chapter 13). About 56 percent of these infections occurred on surgical services, and 22 percent occurred in the newborn nursery. The remainder were about equally divided between medical and pediatric services.

Classification of Infections

Nosocomial bacterial meningitis can be defined as meningitis occurring in hospitalized patients who did not have evidence of the infection at the time of admission. In general, manifestations of nosocomial meningitis are not encountered within the first 48 hours of hospitalization, but meningitis secondary to infections in other sites that has a clinical onset more than 48 hours after admission should be considered nosocomial, even if the infection at the underlying site is community-acquired. Meningitis in recently discharged patients should be considered to be nosocomial only when epidemiologic evidence indicates that hospital acquisition of the organism was likely.

The onset of meningitis following potential inciting events varies with the event and the specific organisms involved. The interval between head trauma and the onset of meningitis has been reported to be from one day to eight weeks. Following spinal anesthesia or lumbar puncture, signs of meningitis may be seen as early as 12 hours or as late as 10 to 12 days. The reasons for this wide variation may be related to the inoculum or virulence of the organism involved as well as to the patient's underlying disease and the use of antibiotics for prophylaxis or treatment of other infections. The species of the infectious organism may also be important, but prolonged incubation periods have been recognized with relatively virulent strains such as *Staphylococcus* and *Pseudomonas*. In view of this, cases of meningitis with onset within a few weeks after the patient's discharge should be carefully assessed for the possibility of nosocomial acquisition during the preceding admission.

Diagnostic Criteria

Clinical

The signs and symptoms of meningitis caused by organisms that produce nosocomial infections are typical of those found in common community-acquired bacterial meningitis. These include fever, headache, nausea, vomiting, alterations in mental function, and stiff neck. None of these manifestations, however, is a sine qua non of central nervous system infection, and patients who are prone to develop nosocomial meningitis may have one or more of such findings as a consequence of head injury, recent surgery, or diagnostic procedures. For example, all the manifestations of meningitis, including nuchal rigidity, are frequently present to some degree after pneumoencephalography, and the concern about iatrogenic meningitis may be significant. Fortunately, these signs and symptoms are maximal 6 to 12 hours after the procedure and disappear by 48 to 72 hours, when the manifestations of meningitis typically would be progressively increasing in severity. For these and other reasons, the diagnosis of nosocomial meningitis depends on a high index of suspicion, knowledge of the setting in which the infection is most likely to occur, and prompt acquisition of a sample of cerebrospinal fluid for study.

Microbiologic

The diagnosis of bacterial meningitis is established definitely by demonstration of organisms in the cerebrospinal fluid. A Gram stain of the sediment of centrifuged spinal fluid should be examined routinely, because cultures are occasionally negative when the smear is positive, and the morphologic characteristics of the organisms seen on Gram stain can serve as an early guide to treatment. However, care should be taken in this circumstance to rule out nonviable organisms within the spinal fluid specimen tubes of commercial lumbar puncture traps as the source of the organisms seen on Gram smear [11]. Immunoelectrophoresis and latex agglutination may detect bacterial antigens in spinal fluid when Gram stains are negative; however, these tests are mainly of value in the diagnosis of infections that are caused by organisms that infrequently produce nosocomial meningitis. Spinal fluid for culture should be inoculated on to blood agar and chocolate agar plates that have been prewarmed in an incubator and incubated at 37°C (98.6°F) both anaerobically and in an atmosphere of 5 to 10 percent CO_2. Tests of antimicrobial sensitivity should be performed with virtually all isolates, because resistance to antibiotics is more common among isolates from cases of nosocomial meningitis than among those from infections acquired in the community.

In confirmed cases of bacterial meningitis, the cerebrospinal fluid shows an increased number of leukocytes, usually in the range of 50 to 5000 cells per cubic millimeter, and there is a preponderance of granulocytes. The concentration of protein in the spinal fluid typically is increased, being in the range of 50 to 1000 mg. per 100 ml., and the glucose concentration is low, that is, less than 40 mg. per 100 ml., or less than 40 percent of the blood glucose level determined at the same time.

A presumptive diagnosis of bacterial meningitis occasionally is made on the basis of typical spinal fluid findings when the clinical suspicion of meningitis is strong but bacteriologic confirmation is lacking. This situation frequently is due to antecedent antimicrobial therapy, which may be a particularly relevant consideration in the diagnosis of nosocomial meningitis. A cellular response with mild changes in protein and glucose concentrations in the spinal fluid may, however, be seen as a consequence of bleeding into the subarachnoid space or of a diagnostic procedure such as myelography or pneumoencephalography. This makes the diagnosis of nosocomial meningitis, in the absence of bacteriologic confirmation, especially difficult. Determination of the concentration of glucose in the spinal fluid has been particularly useful in this situation, because levels of glucose below 10 mg. per 100 ml. are unusual in the absence of bacterial infection. A physician's diagnosis of infection, with or without positive cultures of spinal fluid, should be tabulated as a "case" for surveillance purposes.

Specimens
Collection
A lumbar puncture should be performed with strict, aseptic technique to obtain spinal fluid for study. The patient should be positioned properly, and care should be taken to avoid inserting the spinal needle through or near an area of cutaneous infection. A suitable antiseptic regimen is 2% tincture of iodine in isopropyl alcohol followed by its removal with 70% isopropyl alcohol to prevent iodine burns of the skin and the possible introduction of iodine into the subarachnoid space at the time the puncture needle is inserted. A wide area around the site of the planned puncture should be treated with antiseptics, and sterile gloves should be worn to handle sterile needles, syringes, solutions, and other paraphernalia. Two to three milliliters of spinal fluid should be collected in each of three sterile tubes. The last sample collected is most suitable for cell counts and determination of protein and glucose concentrations, and bacteriologic studies should be performed with fluid in the second tube. If a routine lumbar puncture is contraindicated because of increased spinal fluid pressure or the like, a neurosurgeon should be asked to obtain fluid by cisternal puncture or some other means, because accurate bacteriologic data are essential for optimal management of the patient.

In addition to spinal fluid studies, blood cultures may be important in determining the cause of nosocomial meningitis. Blood for culture should be obtained carefully to avoid contamination, because bacteremia has great clinical significance in this setting provided technical errors can be excluded.

Transport
Spinal fluid for culture should be transported to the laboratory immediately. If a delay in processing is anticipated, the spinal fluid can be held temporarily in an incubator at 37°C (98.6°F), but a delay of more than one hour should be avoided. In most hospitals, the practice of inoculating culture media at the bedside is to be discouraged; it does not greatly increase the bacteriologic yield, and in inexperienced hands, it greatly enhances the chance of bacterial contamination.

Pathogens Typically Causing Secondary Meningitis
General Aspects
COMMON FEATURES OF INFECTIONS. Organisms frequently found among the endogenous flora of hospitalized patients—whether normal flora or flora altered by antibiotic treatment and exposure to the hospital environment—are the most common causes of nosocomial meningitis. Most nosocomial meningitis cases caused by such organisms occur secondary to trauma, neurosurgical operations, diagnostic procedures involving the central nervous system, and from infections in other sites. Meningitis is a rare or infrequent manifestation of infection caused by these agents, and colonization of other patients or personnel rarely results in meningitis.

PRINCIPAL PATHOGENS. Among the cases of nosocomial meningitis in which the cause was identified in NNIS data, 28 percent were due to *Klebsiella* species and 28 percent were due to *Escherichia coli. Staphylococcus aureus,* the next most common pathogen, was responsible for about 23 percent of cases, and this was followed by *Pseudomonas aeruginosa* at 14 percent. Reports in the literature confirm the relative importance of such pathogens, but it is clear that a wide variety of other organisms, particularly those generally accepted as opportunistic invaders, can cause meningitis in hospitalized patients. *Streptococcus pneumoniae* plays a prominent role in meningitis following skull fractures.

Clinical Features and Treatment
MANIFESTATIONS. The clinical manifestations of meningitides caused by these bacterial pathogens do not differ significantly. The pres-

ence of grossly bloody spinal fluid, however, should alert the clinician to the possibility that *E. coli* is responsible. Also, if *Pseudomonas* bacteremia is present in association with meningitis, characteristic skin lesions such as ecthyma gangrenosum may be seen.

ANTIBIOTIC TREATMENT.   Proper antibiotic treatment of patients with meningitis depends on early identification of the infecting organism. The morphologic nature of bacteria seen on a Gram smear of spinal fluid often provides the first clue to the cause and serves as a guide to initial therapy. Full identification of the organism and determination of its sensitivity to antimicrobials, however, is frequently necessary before the most effective therapeutic regimen can be employed.

When pneumococcal meningitis is suspected on the basis of morphologic characteristics seen on Gram stain, penicillin G should be given intravenously in high doses. Presumed staphylococcal meningitis should be treated with a penicillinase-resistant penicillin until sensitivity of the isolate to penicillin G is documented in the laboratory. If the organism is susceptible, penicillin G is the drug of choice. Less desirable alternatives include chloramphenicol and the cephalosporins. Lincomycin, clindamycin, or aminoglycosides should not be used despite data indicating the susceptibility of an isolate in vitro.

Intravenous gentamicin is the drug of choice for initial therapy when examination of the cerebrospinal fluid shows gram-negative bacilli.

When *E. coli* meningitis is documented but sensitivity data are not available, gentamicin administration should be continued. For sensitive organisms, ampicillin or chloramphenicol may be used. The combination of carbenicillin or ampicillin with gentamicin is perhaps the most effective form of therapy available.

Gentamicin can be used throughout the course of treatment of *Klebsiella* infections of the central nervous system, but chloramphenicol and carbenicillin penetrate the blood-brain barrier better. Therefore, the latter drugs may be preferred if sensitivity data document their potential effectiveness. Despite the fact that a high proportion of *Klebsiella* isolates are susceptible to cephalothin in vitro, this agent

should not be used alone in the treatment of meningitis. The status of other cephalosporins is less clear.

Pseudomonas meningitis should be treated with gentamicin in combination with carbenicillin. Intrathecal therapy with gentamicin is also indicated, and early consideration should be given to implantation of a reservoir to facilitate intraventricular infusion. Intrathecal therapy may also be necessary for treatment of meningitis caused by other highly resistant gram-negative organisms.

When there are no clues to the cause of suspected nosocomial meningitis, the combination of gentamicin and a penicillinase-resistant penicillin provides the greatest protection to the patient while the results of culture studies are pending.

In all instances, high doses of antibiotic should be given intravenously throughout the course of treatment. The duration of therapy should be determined by the nature of the infection, the clinical response, and the return of spinal fluid abnormalities to near normal [10].

Sources and Modes of Acquisition

Many patients who acquire meningitis in the hospital have altered resistance to infection, either because of their underlying disease and impaired cellular or humoral immunity, or because physical barriers against invasion of the central nervous system by bacteria have been compromised. Organisms may gain access to the central nervous system by hematogenous dissemination, be inoculated directly into spinal fluid, or spread from a nearby focus of infection.

LUMBAR PUNCTURE.   Organisms may be inoculated into the subarachnoid space at the time of spinal anesthesia or during diagnostic or therapeutic lumbar puncture. The frequency with which this occurs cannot be determined accurately, but meningitis as a complication of spinal anesthesia has been estimated to occur once in every 20,000 to 30,000 cases.

These organisms generally derive from the patient's skin, contaminated solutions, or unsterile instruments [4]. Contaminated needles and anesthetic solutions have been responsible for some of these cases [7]. Even small numbers of contaminating bacteria from such sources may produce infection, because host defense mechanisms in the central nervous system are inadequate to protect against a small inoculum. Indeed, sufficient organisms to produce meningitis might theoretically be inoculated into the spinal fluid of a bacteremic patient by lumbar puncture per se, since cisternal puncture in the presence of pneumococcal bacteremia in dogs may result in meningitis [8]. This hypothetical risk, however, is clearly outweighed by the potential diagnostic and therapeutic value of lumbar puncture in a septic patient with signs of meningitis.

A high proportion of cases of meningitis following lumbar puncture or spinal anesthesia are caused by *Pseudomonas*.

TRAUMA. Patients with head or spinal injuries are especially likely to develop nosocomial meningitis Penetrating wounds and extentive trauma predispose to gram-negative bacillary infection, while nonpenetrating head injury is more likely to be associated with pneumococcal meningitis [6]. Most of the cases of meningitis on surgical services occur in patients with basal skull fractures or penetrating head injuries.

NEUROSURGICAL OPERATIONS. Meningitis also may develop following craniotomy or other neurosurgical procedures, particularly if a foreign body such as a ventriculoatrial shunt has been inserted (see Part II, Chapter 28) or if a wound infection develops postoperatively (see Part II, Chapter 16). *S. aureus* and *Klebsiella* are especially important pathogens in these infections.

ADJACENT AND DISTANT INFECTIONS. Meningitis may develop in the course of bacteremia and sepsis associated with nosocomial infections at some other site, for example, infections associated with the use of intravenous catheters, bladder catheters, and the like. In the newborn nursery, meningitis frequently is part of the syndrome of neonatal sepsis. Hematogenous seeding of the meninges might also result from asymptomatic bacteremia induced by a variety of procedures (see Part II, Chapter 28). Focuses of infection in the middle ear or paranasal sinuses may be the sites from which organisms spread to the meninges. This is particularly true in adults, but it also may be a consideration in children. Organisms, especially *Pseudomonas*, occasionally infect the central nervous system through a congenital defect such as a dermal sinus or a meningomyelocele, and infection of the upper part of the face may predispose to staphylococcal meningitis.

Epidemiologic Considerations

INCIDENCE. Data from NNIS showed rates of reported nosocomial meningitis per million discharges of about 13 for *Klebsiella*, 12 to 13 for *E. coli*, 10 to 11 for *S. aureus*, and 6 to 7 for *Pseudomonas*. Although these rates doubtlessly reflect considerable underreporting, they nonetheless provide an indication of the overall relative importance of these pathogens. The relative prominence of each pathogen varies according to the service. *E. coli* is the single most frequent pathogen encountered in cases in the newborn nursery, where it is responsible for 51 percent of all cases of nosocomial meningitis in which the causative agent was identified. Overall, 46 percent of all cases of nosocomial *E. coli* meningitis occur in newborns, and 30 percent occur on surgical services. *Klebsiella* is the single most frequent pathogen seen in cases in surgical services, where it accounts for 38 percent of nosocomial meningitides in which the pathogen was identified; it also causes an unusually high proportion (73 percent) of all cases that occur on surgery, but only 13 percent of cases in newborns. *S. aureus* is the second most frequent pathogen isolated from cases with established causes on both surgical and newborn services (26.4 and 17.9 percent, respectively). The vast majority of all *Pseudomonas* cases (about two-thirds) occur on surgery.

PREDISPOSING HOST FACTORS. Factors of importance in meningitis due to gram-negative rods include very young or old age, diabetes, alcoholism, liver disease, and treatment with antibiotics, steroids, or immunosuppressive agents. Neonates are highly susceptible to infections with *E. coli* and other gram-negative bacilli, probably because of inadequate levels of circulating immunoglobulin M (IgM) in the first few weeks of life. Neonates are also particularly susceptible to *S. aureus* infections, and diabetes and antecedent antimicrobial therapy may also predispose to such infections. Of course, as noted above, infections caused by organisms in adjacent or remote sites also predispose to nosocomial meningitis.

OUTBREAKS.   Gram-negative bacillary meningitis outbreaks have followed spinal anesthesia and lumbar punctures, and contaminated needles and local anesthetic solutions have been implicated as their causes [7]. Except in these circumstances, outbreaks of nosocomial meningitis occur only as part of larger epidemics that include many more cases of infection at adjacent or distant sites. For example, an outbreak of *Pseudomonas* neurosurgical wound infections and meningitis has been reported in which a heavily contaminated shaving brush was incriminated [3]. The brush was used to assist the preoperative shaving of scalp hair of successive patients. Another outbreak, which was caused by *Klebsiella,* emphatically illustrates the adverse effects associated with widespread antibiotic use in a high proportion of patients hospitalized in a neurosurgical intensive-care unit [9]. Many patients had *Klebsiella* infections of the chest or urinary tract infections, and eight died of nosocomial meningitis. Numerous measures were instituted to control the problem, but infections continued to occur until the use of antibiotics in the unit, both prophylactically and therapeutically, was discontinued for four months. Not only was there a dramatic fall in the incidence of *Klebsiella* infections, but the rate of infection from all organisms was considerably reduced.

Clusters of cases of secondary meningitis thus follow localized outbreaks of infections at other sites. Situations posing the greatest risk for such clusters would appear to be outbreaks of neurosurgical wound infections, epidemics of staphylococcal skin disease and invasive *E. coli* gastroenteritis in newborns, and epidemics of *Pseudomonas* infections on burn units and oncology services.

Prevention

PROPHYLACTIC ANTIBIOTICS.   Antibiotics are frequently administered prophylactically in order to prevent the development of meningitis in patients with head injury. This practice is somewhat controversial, and carefully controlled, double-blind studies to document its effectiveness are lacking. Most neurosurgeons, however, provide prophylaxis to patients with basal skull fractures or penetrating wounds, because uncontrolled studies indicate that meningitis after head injury is less frequent if the patient receives antibiotics. Pneumococcal meningitis following nonpenetrating injuries is the most readily preventable infection, a fact that has made ampicillin a preferred chemoprophylactic agent in this setting, since its spectrum encompasses pneumococci and some gram-negative strains that are also associated with this type of infection.

CONTROL OF INFECTIONS AT OTHER SITES.   Many meningeal infections may be inevitable, but some can be prevented by following sound principles of patient care. If nosocomial infections of the lungs, urinary tract, skin (including burns), gastrointestinal tract, and bloodstream are prevented, for example, then hematogenous dissemination of organisms from these sites to the central nervous system is avoided. Similarly, prevention of incisional wound infections in neurosurgical operations is most important. Each of these is given extensive discussion in other chapters of this text and will not be repeated here.

Proper management and antimicrobial treatment of established infections at other sites are also of great importance in reducing the risks of bacteremic seeding of the meninges. Antibiotic use, both prophylactic and therapeutic, should be minimized. When antibiotics are necessary, the agent with the most limited spectrum that can accomplish the task should be employed.

PROPER LUMBAR PUNCTURE TECHNIQUE.   Only sterile equipment and solutions should be employed, and contamination during their use should be scrupulously avoided. Previously entered multidose vials of medications should not be used, and preparation of the skin prior to the insertion of needles should be carefully and meticulously performed (see Collection, under Specimens, above).

INVESTIGATION AND CONTROL OF OUTBREAKS.   Prompt epidemiologic investigation and control of nosocomial meningitis outbreaks as well as of infections in other sites should prevent further cases. In view of its rarity even among neurosurgical patients, clusters of two or more cases of nosocomial meningitis caused by the same organism over a short time on a particular ward or patient-care unit should prompt an investigation to unravel the common features among the cases. Suspected sources should be evaluated by microbiologic sampling and by epidemiologic comparisons with a control group of uninfected but otherwise comparable patients (see Part I, Chapter 5).

Pathogens Causing Primary Meningitis

In contrast to the preceding infections, meningitis is commonly a primary clinical manifestation of infection with group-B streptococci, *Listeria monocytogenes,* and meningococci. Also, outbreaks of meningitis due to these organisms occur without epidemic disease that involves other sites, and acquisition by healthy persons, especially newborns, poses a much higher risk of meningitis.

Group-B Streptococci

INCIDENCE. Nosocomial meningitis due to group-B streptococci is rare; only two cases were reported per 1,000,000 discharges from all services in the National Nosocomial Infections Study. There is reason to believe, however, that late-onset disease in neonates is substantially underreported, and epidemiologic studies that have focused specifically on this disease indicate that the incidence in neonates is 1 to 2 per 1000 live births. Occasional cases are also encountered on surgical and pediatric units.

SOURCES AND MODES OF ACQUISITION. The birth canal of an infant's mother is the usual source of organisms that colonize or infect infants, and infants born of mothers with positive vaginal cultures for group-B streptococci are at higher risk of colonization and disease than those born of mothers whose vaginal cultures are negative for this organism. The likelihood of maternal vaginal carriage appears to be inversely related to the socioeconomic level of the mother. Low birth weight, prematurity, and

a high degree of contamination (as is seen with premature rupture of the membranes) also increase the risk of disease in neonates.

Infants from uninfected mothers can be colonized by contact with nursery personnel who are carriers from previous exposure or who transmit strains from infant to infant by hand contact. Transmission of organisms from infants to healthy hospital personnel has been documented.

Direct acquisition from maternal sources appears to be of primary importance in disease with early onset, especially those cases with onset while the infant is hospitalized. Cross-colonization with strains while hospitalized in the nursery may be relatively more important for cases whose onsets occur later in the first month of life.

Among adults, postpartum bacteremia (see Part II, Chapter 22), diabetes, and recent neurosurgical procedures are the major underlying factors that predispose to infection.

CLINICAL ASPECTS. The bacterial meningitis due to group-B streptococci that occurs in neonates shortly after birth tends to be overwhelming, with the syndrome of neonatal sepsis predominating. Group-B streptococcal meningitis occurring later in the first month of life tends to be caused by type III strains, which are much less common in early infections, and it is clinically indistinguishable from meningitis caused by other bacterial pathogens.

Ampicillin is the treatment of choice for both adults and infants. High doses of penicillin G are also effective.

OUTBREAKS. Several nursery outbreaks of group-B streptococcal meningitis have been investigated. Most of these have typically involved a cluster of about four cases over about a month. Investigations have generally revealed about 15 percent of infants with recent nursery contact to be colonized, and carrier–case ratios average about 7 to 1. Infections with group-B streptococci are usually not seen in nursery employees, but about 20 percent of employees will be colonized. Although relatively high vaginal colonization rates in obstetric patients may be noted in association with such outbreaks, poor correlation between the culture status of the mothers and that of the infants is sometimes found [1]. This suggests that cross-colonization in the nursery may be amplifying an underlying problem that is due to a high vaginal carrier rate in the population served by the hospital.

Outbreaks appear to arise when the colonization rates in infants are high, and this may be a more important determinant than variations in the virulence of strains.

PREVENTION. Neonatal infection might be prevented by treating both pregnant women who have positive vaginal cultures and their sexual partners with penicillin early in pregnancy and again at about 32 weeks gestation. Another approach that has been proposed is to provide prophylactic treatment to infants born of infected mothers with ampicillin or penicillin G [5]. Such measures are unlikely to be cost effective unless maternal vaginal carriage rates are high, and they will not affect the nursery transmission of strains acquired by neonates from personnel.

Institution of hexachlorophene bathing of infants might help control an outbreak, but topical applications of bacitracin to umbilical areas and the circumcision site are probably safer. Topically applied triple dye is of doubtful effectiveness in preventing colonization with group-B streptococci at these sites. Neither measure has been proved effective in controlling nursery-associated group-B streptococcal infections. Emphasis on careful hand-washing is likely to be effective, and the cohorting of infants, as is practiced in the prevention of nursery-associated staphylococcal infections, should also be implemented (see Part II, Chapter 20). The possibility of controlling an outbreak through the identification and treatment of asymptomatic carriers among hospital personnel as well as the babies of infected mothers is attractive, but so far unproved.

Listeria monocytogenes

INCIDENCE. Most patients with *L. monocytogenes* meningitis, including those with predisposing factors, develop their infection outside the hospital. Neonates and people over 50 years old are predisposed to development of *L. monocytogenes* meningitis. Other contributing factors include associated diabetes, malignancy, lymphoma, leukemia, liver disease, alcoholism, collagen vascular disease, organ transplantation, and treatment with corticosteroids or cytotoxic agents.

SOURCES AND MODES OF ACQUISITION. The only identified source of *L. monocytogenes* that is important in the consideration of nosocomial infection is the birth canal of a pregnant woman. Animal contact and contaminated food have proved to be important in community-acquired infections, but not in hospitals. Spread of infection from one patient to another in the hospital has not been documented. Because infants with *L. monocytogenes* meningitis are colonized at other sites, the potential for spread by indirect contact exists, however. Patients with *L. monocytogenes* meningitis represent no recognized hazard to other patients, hospital personnel, or community contacts.

CLINICAL ASPECTS. Most cases of meningitis due to *L. monocytogenes* are indistinguishable clinically from meningitis due to the more common bacterial pathogens. In some instances, however, an indolent course with little more than headache and lethargy may be seen. Although the spinal fluid findings in most cases of *Listeria* meningitis are typical of those encountered in infections with other bacteria, a predominance of mononuclear cells rather than granulocytes is sometimes seen, and the concentration of glucose may be normal or only mildly depressed.

The treatment of choice is ampicillin. High doses of penicillin G are likely to be effective, and chloramphenicol is an acceptable but less desirable alternative.

OUTBREAKS. Reports of nosocomial epidemics of *L. monocytogenes* have not been published. Because of some similarities between the epidemiology of infections due to this pathogen and group-B streptococcal infections, the potential for similar outbreaks among neonates exists.

PREVENTION. It has been postulated that *Listeria* meningitis in neonates could be prevented by identifying infected mothers during pregnancy and treating their babies prophylactically with ampicillin at the time of birth. The sporadic cases that occur in adults probably cannot be prevented.

Should an outbreak occur in a nursery, the control measures outlined for group-B streptococcal infection (see previous section) might be instituted. Antibiotic treatment of babies born of infected mothers and of carriers among hospital personnel might be considered.

Neisseria meningitidis

INCIDENCE. Endemic nosocomial infection with *N. meningitidis* is extremely rare and has not been reported in the United States in recent years. The admission of an infected patient frequently raises important questions about the management of family and hospital contacts, however, and these are the main "nosocomial" problems associated with such infections.

SOURCES AND MODES OF ACQUISITION. The only important source of *N. meningitidis* is the nasopharynx of asymptomatic carriers or patients with clinical disease.

The meningococcus is spread only by close direct contact with patients or carriers, and it is killed rapidly on exposure to the environment. The intimate contact necessary for transmission of the organism is uncommon in the hospital setting.

Patients with meningococcal meningitis may transmit *N. meningitidis* from their nasopharynx to hospital personnel if there is close and intimate contact with nasopharyngeal secretions (e.g., in mouth-to-mouth resuscitation) before antibiotic therapy is instituted. Other patients and casual hospital or community contacts are not at risk. Indeed, studies have shown that hospital personnel who come in contact with cases are no more likely to be colonized by meningococci than hospital personnel without such exposure [2].

CLINICAL ASPECTS. The only clinical feature that is distinctive for meningococcal meningitis is a petechial or purpuric rash. Meningococcal meningitis should be treated with high doses of penicillin G. Chloramphenicol is an acceptable alternative in treating patients who are allergic to penicillin. Cephalothin should not be used.

OUTBREAKS. Epidemics of nosocomial meningococcal disease have not been reported. In the presence of a community epidemic, however, they could occur.

PREVENTION. Patients with meningococcal meningitis should be isolated during the first 24 hours of antibiotic treatment. After that, isolation is unnecessary. Hospital personnel should be considered for chemoprophylaxis if they have been involved in prolonged, intensive care of such patients without using protective masks or in mouth-to-mouth resuscitation of such a patient either before effective antibiotics are started or during the 24 hours following the start of such treatment. If the organism involved is known to be sensitive to sulfonamides, Gantrisin (sulfisoxazole) should be administered orally for four days. If the sulfa sensitivity of the isolate is in doubt, rifampin or minocycline can be used. Prophylactic doses of penicillin and ampicillin will suppress the numbers of organisms carried in the nasopharynx, but these agents will not reliably eradicate carriage, because they penetrate poorly into the nasopharyngeal area.

It is important that local health officials be notified of each case of meningococcal meningitis, so close community contacts can be identified, be given appropriate chemoprophylaxis and possibly vaccine, and then have their clinical status monitored. The risk of secondary disease among household contacts (5 percent) is substantially greater than that for less intensively exposed hospital contacts.

Polysaccharide vaccines effective against groups A and C are now available, and hospital personnel are a target group for such vaccines provided there is a protracted community epidemic due to strains of these serogroups.

References

1. Aber, R. C., Allen, N., Howell, J. T., Wilkinson, H. W., and Facklam, R. R. Nosocomial transmission of group B streptococci. *Pediatrics* 58:346, 1976.
2. Artenstein, M. S., and Ellis, R. E. The risk of exposure to a patient with meningococcal meningitis. *Milit. Med.* 133:474, 1968.
3. Ayliffe, G., Lowbury, E., Hamilton, J., Small, J., Asheshov, E., and Parker, M. Hospital infection with *Pseudomonas aeruginosa* in neurosurgery. *Lancet* 2:365, 1965.
4. Cutler, M., and Cutler, P. Iatrogenic meningitis. *J. Med. Soc. N.J.* 50:510, 1953.
5. Franciosi, R. A., Knostman, J. D., and Zim-

merman, R. A.   Group B streptococcal neonatal and infant infections. *J. Pediatr.* 82:707, 1973.

6. Jones, S. R., Luby, J. P., and Sanford, J. P. Bacterial meningitis complicating cranial-spinal trauma. *J. Trauma* 13:895, 1973.

7. Kremer, M.   Meningitis after spinal anesthesia. *Br. Med. J.* 2:309, 1945.

8. Petersdorf, R., Swarrer, D., and Garcia, M. Studies on the pathogens of meningitis.   II. Development of meningitis during pneumococcal bacteremia. *J. Clin. Invest.* 4:320, 1967.

9. Price, D. J. E., and Sleigh, J. D.   Control of infection due to *Klebsiella aerogenes* in a neurosurgical unit by withdrawal of all antibiotics. *Lancet* 2:1213, 1970.

10. Rahal, J. J.   Treatment of gram-negative bacillary meningitis in adults. *Ann. Intern. Med.* 77:295, 1972.

11. Weinstein, R. A., Bauer, F. W., Hoffman, P., Tyler, P. G., Anderson, R. L., and Stamm, W. E.   Factitious meningitis—diagnostic error due to non-viable bacteria in commercial lumbar puncture trays. *J.A.M.A.* 233:878, 1975.

24

Selected Viral Infections of Nosocomial Importance

Paul F. Wehrle

This chapter encompasses cytomegalovirus infections, measles, rubella, smallpox, and hepatitis. Certain viral infections with primary manifestations in particular sites are covered elsewhere in the text: influenza is discussed in Part II, Chapter 15; rotovirus, in Part II, Chapter 21; herpesvirus and varicella-zoster, in Part II, Chapter 20; and hemodialysis-associated hepatitis, in Part I, Chapter 7, Section A.

Cytomegalovirus Infections

Clinical syndromes associated with cytomegalovirus (CMV) infections have been termed cytomegalic inclusion disease, heterophile-negative mononucleosis, cytomegalovirus mononucleosis, and inclusion disease. CMV infection represents an important endemic infection with worldwide distribution; its prevalence, however, varies widely. Serologic evidence shows that from 20 to 90 percent of young adults in various populations have experienced infection [21]. In 1 to 2 percent of normal adults, the virus may be recovered from saliva, urine, and circulating lymphocytes; 1 to 3 percent of pregnant women excrete virus in the urine. Since approximately 1 percent of infants have been found to be infected at birth, this represents one of the most frequent perinatal infections [32]. Intermittent fecal excretion of the virus has been described [14].

Etiology

Cytomegalovirus is one of the herpesviruses and it is the sole cause of CMV infection. Since it is a prevalent infection in man, it may at least theoretically be transferred by direct or indirect contact within the hospital. Its chief importance as a nosocomial infection lies in its role as an important cause of congenital infections seen in newborn infants and in its transmission by blood transfusion or organ transplantation (see Part II, Chapter 27).

Diagnostic Considerations

CLINICAL. Clinical recognition of CMV infection is often difficult, because most infections are subclinical. When clinical manifestations are present, a single sign or several clinical signs may be present in various combinations. Congenital CMV infections may be subclinical, or the infant may have one or all of the following signs: hepatomegaly, splenomegaly, jaundice, purpura, a petechial rash, encephalopathy, microcephaly, or chorioretinitis. Intracranial calcification, particularly involving the choroid plexus, may be found after congenital CMV infection; it may also occur with toxoplasmosis and rubella infection. The onset of CMV disease may occur from before birth to shortly after birth. Intrauterine death may occur. The neonatal case fatality rate is high among severely affected infants with hemorrhagic manifestations, but the great majority of symptomatic infants survive the newborn period. Survivors may have psychomotor retardation even when no central nervous system (CNS) signs were present at birth.

Infections acquired later in life may also be subclinical, especially if the patient has preexisting antibodies. The incubation period ranges from two and one-half to seven weeks. Patients who develop clinical disease present with fever, respiratory infection (including pneumonia), hepatitis, hemolytic anemia, splenomegaly, atypical lymphocytes (seen on peripheral smear), and generalized lymphadenopathy. The latter triad, which may be observed from two to four weeks following blood transfusion, represents the usual nosocomial form of this infection [20], and it occurs with an incidence of approximately 3 percent among exposed persons without antibodies [3]. Clinical disease has also been diagnosed following transplantation procedures, especially renal transplantations [20,24]. The incidence is low if the recipient and donor are both seronegative; however, if the recipient is seronegative and the donor is seropositive, there is a 40 to 60 percent chance that the recipient will develop disease.

LABORATORY. Laboratory diagnosis of CMV infection depends on recovery of the virus from urine, pharyngeal secretions, or blood or on showing that there has been a recent antibody response to the virus. Although individual laboratory requirements may vary, samples for isolation usually should be promptly refriger-ated and then transported to the laboratory on crushed, wet ice. This method insures a temperature of 3°C to 4°C (37°F to 39°F) for the sample; freezing must be avoided. Serum samples from acute and convalescent patients are useful particularly in diagnosing acquired disease, and neutralization, complement-fixation, indirect-hemagglutination and fluorescent-antibody techniques may be employed for confirmation.

Control Measures

PATIENTS. Control measures within the hospital include precautions for respiratory secretions, urine, blood, and feces in hospitalized patients with clinically recognized infections. The use of whole-blood transfusions, particularly for those patients with illnesses or medications that reduce immunologic competence, should be considered carefully, and all risks—including the possibility of acquiring CMV infection—should be balanced against the benefits of the transfusion. At present, there is no easily applied method to exclude cytomegalovirus from blood used in transfusion. For special high-risk groups, blood donors can be screened and only seronegative donors used. In addition, one recent study has suggested that the use of frozen blood will greatly reduce the number of acquired CMV infections. Patients known to have suppressed immunologic competence should be isolated (protective isolation) from patients with CMV infection.

PERSONNEL. The risk for nurses of acquiring CMV infection on pediatric wards is 4 to 7 percent per year [42]. Because of the difficulties in making the diagnosis, it may not be possible to exclude a pregnant nurse effectively from contact with a patient with CMV infection. If there is clinical suspicion or laboratory confirmation of the diagnosis, however, then pregnant nurses should be excluded from such contact.

Therapy

Therapy of patients with CMV infection has been attempted with numerous antiviral compounds, but results are inconclusive. None can be presently recommended.

Measles

Measles is an acute, infectious, highly communicable, viral disease of susceptible children and adults. Clinical features include a two- to four-day prodromal period of cough, coryza, conjunctivitis, and fever. Koplik's spots on the buccal mucosa may be seen during the latter portion of the prodrome. Usually within 24 hours of their appearance, a typical maculopapular rash appears, beginning on the face and hairline, which spreads to the trunk and extremities within 24 hours.

Etiology

This disease results from infection by a single-stranded RNA virus of a single immunologic type. Although stable at $-70°C$ in the laboratory, it is inactivated within hours at room temperature and by drying. The virus has been propagated in cell cultures, which permitted the development of the original inactivated measles vaccine and several attenuated live-virus vaccines.

Nosocomial Infection Potential

The virus is profusely shed from the upper respiratory tract during the prodromal stages of the disease, and the cough makes transmission of measles to susceptible individuals almost a certainty, even to those with only casual contact. The coryzal symptoms may be confused with those of other respiratory illnesses unless it is known that prior exposure to measles has occurred. Accurate clinical diagnosis is made only when Koplik's spots appear or the characteristic rash is observed. Thus, children with measles may be admitted to pediatric wards and crowded outpatient clinics, thereby exposing any susceptible patients in these settings. The rash, which usually begins on the face, is easily recognized, and further exposure of susceptible individuals can be prevented by prompt isolation of the patient, although susceptible individuals may have been exposed before the diagnosis was made.

Transmission of infection from sources to susceptible persons is primarily by droplets and direct contact with respiratory secretions; indirect contact with articles freshly soiled by discharges from the nose and throat of the infected person may also serve as an avenue for spread. Airborne transmission via droplet nuclei may also occur [41].

The portal of entry may be either the respiratory tract or the conjunctiva of a susceptible individual [28,33].

Diagnostic Considerations

CLINICAL. Knowledge of whether prior exposure to recognized measles occurred, either in the community or within the hospital, is helpful in diagnosis. With prodromal or catarrhal symptoms and signs, the presence of Koplik's spots on the buccal mucosa is diagnostic. A relatively severe prodromal course that is followed within two to four days by the appearance of a typical morbilliform rash spreading downward from the face is characteristic. Many cases, however, have been mistakenly diagnosed as rubella or as a reaction to a drug prescribed for treatment of the prodromal symptoms.

Infections modified by preexisting partial immunity, either active or passive, and typical cases following vaccination with killed virus have been difficult to diagnose clinically, and laboratory confirmation may be required.

LABORATORY. Confirmation of the diagnosis can be made by hemagglutination-inhibition (HAI) or complement-fixation (CF) serologic tests; these, however, are unnecessary in most cases. Recovery of the virus is technically difficult, and it is not recommended as a diagnostic technique. Fluorescent-antibody techniques for rapid diagnosis are under study.

Control Measures

VACCINATION. Inquiry regarding recent measles exposure, particularly of children and young adults prior to hospital admission, is helpful, as is the patient's history of previous clinical measles or having been previously provided attenuated measles virus vaccine immunization at one year of age or later [11]. If immunization was attempted prior to one year of age and if inactivated vaccine was used, it may not have conferred protection. Hospital personnel who may have contact with patients infected with measles virus should be immunized if not already protected by natural or acquired immunity (see Part I, Chapter 3).

IMMUNOGLOBULIN ADMINISTRATION. If measles exposure occurs in the hospital, preventive doses (0.25 ml. per kilogram of body weight) of immune serum globulin (human) should be given to exposed susceptible individuals, since complications following measles may cause additional problems for hospitalized patients [15]. Such prophylaxis is not required if a definite history is available of prior measles or attenuated measles virus vaccine administration at more than one year of age. If doses of 0.25 ml. of immune serum globulin per kilogram of body weight are given within three days of exposure, complete protection against both infection and disease may be expected. If exposure is not recognized until the fifth or sixth day after it has occurred, a milder or modified disease is likely to ensue after immune serum globulin prophylaxis. In such exposed patients who receive prophylaxis, attenuated measles virus vaccine should be given approximately three months later to insure long-term protection (see Part I, Chapter 3).

PREVENTION OF TRANSMISSION. Exposed susceptible individuals should either be discharged from the hospital by the seventh day following known exposure, or be placed in respiratory isolation facilities to prevent transmission if hospitalization is required after the seventh day; prior to seven days after exposure, they should not be considered hazardous to others. The period of the greatest danger of transmission of infection is during the prodromal stage and early eruptive stage, that is, during the first four days of the illness. After the fever recedes and the rash has faded, the disease is no longer communicable. Since the virus is extremely fragile on exposure to light, room temperature, and drying, no special precautions other than normal cleaning procedures are required for disinfection of the room used for isolation.

Only through nearly universal immunization of all susceptible persons can this disease be prevented from posing a hazard of nosocomial infection, as well as continuing community spread [25,34].

Therapy
Since no specific antiviral therapy is available, treatment should include appropriate supportive measures and frequent observation for signs of suppurative complications, particularly otitis media and pneumonia. For the unusual occurrence of encephalitis or other infrequent complications, the reader is referred to standard textbooks for guidance. Immune serum globulin is of no value after the onset of the illness.

Rubella (German Measles)

Rubella is an endemic disease with worldwide distribution and is most prevalent during the winter and spring. At times, the disease assumes epidemic proportions. The most recent epidemic in the United States was in 1964 and 1965; this epidemic resulted in an estimated 20,000 congenital infections [13,22]. The causative agent is the rubella virus; it is a specific RNA virus and no immunologic variants of significance are known. The illness is relatively mild, and complications of serious impact are rare. Its chief importance lies in the congenital rubella syndrome, which results from intrauterine infection acquired early in pregnancy.

Nosocomial Infection Potential
Nosocomial infections occur chiefly among hospitalized children and younger members of the hospital staff. These infections are acquired from patients, usually children, who have been infected from 14 to 20 days prior to hospital admission and who develop clinical rubella disease during hospitalization. Since rubella is usually a mild or asymptomatic illness, it is seldom the primary problem initiating hospitalization. Of at least equal importance is nosocomial exposure to infants with congenital rubella. These infants are hazardous to both personnel and other infants in the nursery, during subsequent visits to clinics and physicians' offices, and during subsequent hospitalization, because they may continue to excrete rubella virus for many months [35]. Progressive panencephalitis is a

very rare disease that may occur several years later and apparently is associated with persistence of the virus [38,40]. This syndrome, however, has not yet been associated with disease transmission, and thus it is not currently considered to be related to nosocomial infections.

Diagnostic Considerations

CLINICAL. The incubation period for rubella may vary from 14 to 21 days, but it is most frequently 17 or 18 days. Clinical signs include fever from 100°F to 102°F (38°C to 39°C), mild coryza, and conjunctivitis, usually with postauricular and cervical lymphadenopathy. The rash, which initially involves the face and neck, becomes diffuse and is macular or maculopapular in character. It may resemble that of either scarlet fever or measles; rubella infection without rash may occur and is regarded as a subclinical infection. Rubella arthralgia or arthritis, if present, usually begins several days after the onset of the rash, is self-limited, and is helpful in making the diagnosis because joint symptoms do not occur with other viral exanthems. Leukopenia is characteristic early in the disease, although routine clinical laboratory tests are not very helpful in the diagnosis. Although the diagnosis may be suspected clinically, the illness is sometimes confused with syndromes associated with measles, erythema infectiosum (fifth disease), and infectious mononucleosis. The specific diagnosis for a particular patient may depend on serologic confirmation; although it is not indicated for most infections in children, laboratory investigation is essential for confirmation of suspected disease in women during early pregnancy and for determining whether pregnant women have been exposed.

LABORATORY. Confirmation of the diagnosis of congenitally acquired infection depends on the presence of rubella hemagglutination-inhibition (HAI) antibodies in the IgM fraction of the serum during the newborn period or the persistence of the HAI antibodies beyond the point (usually six months of age) when passively transferred maternal antibody would be present [18]. Recovery of virus from pharynx, urine, or spinal fluid specimens, if appropriate laboratory facilities are available, also provides proof of infection.

For infections acquired postnatally, paired serum samples obtained during the acute and convalescent stages of the illness are essential for diagnosis. Virus recovery is costly, more difficult, and seldom indicated clinically.

Control Measures

Transmission is by droplets, direct contact (nasopharyngeal secretions, blood, urine, or feces), or indirect contact (articles freshly soiled by secretions, blood, urine, or feces). Airborne spread may occur, especially from those patients with prominent respiratory symptoms (cough and coryza). Persons infected with the rubella virus may be infectious for from seven days prior to four days after developing a rash.

Appropriate measures within the hospital for the prevention of rubella include those designed to protect hospital personnel as well as those utilized for the benefit of other patients. The latter are usually young children, presumably susceptible to the infection, who may subsequently transfer the infection to both children and adults within their families upon discharge from the hospital. In some areas of the United States, the largest pool of susceptible individuals may be the older teenagers and young adults.

HOSPITAL PERSONNEL. General aspects of the protection of personnel have been discussed in Part I, Chapter 3. Preemployment procedures should include a specific inquiry regarding prior rubella immunization and, if necessary, serologic testing. Susceptible employees who will be exposed to high-risk areas, including susceptible men, should be immunized promptly with rubella vaccine. Suitable warnings should be given about temporary arthritis following vaccination. Serosusceptible women, after being advised regarding potential pregnancy, should be vaccinated and maintained on an adequate contraceptive regimen for at least three months following immunization [8]. Those who are pregnant and susceptible should not be employed in areas where they will be likely to come into contact with cases of rubella.

PATIENTS: As with other acute communicable diseases of childhood, the admitting history for all patients, and particularly pediatric patients, should include whether there has been recognized exposure to rubella during the three weeks prior to admission. For those exposed prior to hospital admission and for whom hospitalization cannot be delayed, respiratory isolation should be observed to avoid unnecessary exposure of other patients [23]. Infants with congenital rubella should be placed under strict isolation, because they may continue to excrete virus for at least several months following birth.

ENVIRONMENT. No special terminal cleaning measures are required to prepare the patient's room for subsequent occupancy by others. The virus is inactivated rapidly by sunlight, room temperature, and drying. Furniture surfaces and those areas of the walls that appear soiled should be washed with a detergent solution; routine laundering of linens is adequate for decontamination.

GENERAL. No specific antiviral therapy is available. All persons are considered susceptible until they have recovered from the natural infection, rubella HAI antibody has been demonstrated, or immunization against rubella has been provided. Immune serum globulin cannot be routinely recommended for use in those susceptible individuals exposed to the virus, because the results of such use have not been consistent.

OUTBREAKS. Nosocomial outbreaks of rubella may be prevented by the measures outlined above. Despite such precautions, a child may occasionally be admitted to the hospital with unrecognized, recent, rubella exposure who develops clinical rubella while hospitalized. Should this occur, the immune status of both hospital staff members and patients in contact with the patient must be reviewed. Previously unimmunized patients and staff, unless positive for rubella HAI antibody, should be considered susceptible and immunized promptly unless there is a contraindication to immunization (e.g., pregnancy or an immunodeficiency syndrome). Since vaccine administered after exposure may not provide protection for the current episode, the patients and their families should be notified of the possibility of disease. Because rubella cases may be infectious as long as one week prior to onset of symptoms, exposed susceptible patients should be discharged from the hospital prior to the seventh day following exposure or be placed in respiratory isolation between the seventh and the twenty-first day following contact. Furlough of susceptible hospital employees during a similar interval is recommended, although removal from patient-care duties and frequent measurement of the individual's temperature may sometimes be substituted. If the latter action is taken, the employee must remain at home if tenderness of the lymph nodes, fever, malaise, or minor respiratory complaints appear within 14 to 21 days after exposure, since these can represent the prodromal signs of rubella.

Smallpox (Variola)

Smallpox has been an important epidemic and endemic disease in virtually all countries, and numerous nosocomial outbreaks involving both patients and hospital staff have been described. Since World War II, a substantial proportion of smallpox cases in western Europe have occurred among hospital patients and personnel [39].

Rapid progress has been made toward eradication of this disease in all countries. Of the more than 30 countries with endemic disease in 1967, only five reported smallpox cases in 1975, and only two were endemic in 1977. The last case in an endemic area was reported in October 1977; worldwide eradication should be confirmed in October 1979. The possibility of infection resulting from laboratory sources and subsequent spread within hospitals will remain for an indefinite period [5,12].

Etiology

Variola virus is a poxvirus that is related both biologically and immunologically to vaccinia, cowpox, monkeypox, and other poxviruses. Man is the only source of infection; no nonhuman reservoir has been found. Two clinical forms of smallpox have been described: variola major and minor. Endemic disease of intermediate severity has also been observed, and laboratory markers indicate that there may be a family of closely related variola viruses that cause disease of varying clinical severity [5].

Nosocomial Infection Potential

Transmission of infection to others may occur during the preeruptive stage of the illness. This stage appears from 7 to 17 days after exposure, and the infectious risk is greatest from two days before to at least two weeks after the onset of rash. The correct diagnosis is usually not suspected before the distinctive clinical rash appears, unless there is a known history of exposure. Thus, extensive spread of infection within the hospital may occur prior to the initiation of isolation precautions. The incubation period varies from 7 to 17 days, but it most frequently is 10 to 12 days. Nosocomial infection is suspected if contact occurs within a hospital from 7 to 17 days prior to the onset of illness. Exposure within health-care institutions has represented a substantial portion of reported cases in nonendemic countries (e.g., England and Yugoslavia) [17,31].

While the American Hospital Association and the U.S. Public Health Service once recommended revaccination of all hospital personnel at three-year intervals, progress toward global eradication of this disease has led both groups to the belief that the risks of vaccination of health workers are greater than the benefits. Only laboratory workers who work with poxviruses require vaccination.

Diagnostic Considerations

CLINICAL. If smallpox is suspected, immediate reporting by telephone or telegraph to local or regional health authorities is mandatory.

The correct diagnosis in most cases may be made with considerable accuracy on a basis of the clinical course and physical examination. The relatively severe prodromal signs, the centrifugal distribution of vesicular rash (which is most intense on the face and distal extremities), and the relatively deep location of the individual lesions are virtually unique. Although it is not helpful in early diagnosis, the progression of the skin lesions from vesicles to pustules and crusts with relatively uniform stages of development in the same part of the body is also characteristic. Fulminant hemorrhagic disease may result in death before the typical cutaneous lesions appear, and this aspect presents a particular hazard in hospitals. Mild or atypical disease may be seen in persons vaccinated several years earlier, but such individuals are less likely to spread disease. Subclinical or inapparent infections are of no epidemiologic significance; these usually occur among individuals who are partially immune following vaccination several years earlier.

An important aid to the clinical diagnosis of smallpox is a history of possible exposure, either from being in an endemic area or from contact with travelers from endemic countries. Workers in laboratories where smallpox virus is preserved or under study should also be suspect. Furthermore, the type of illness seen in the vicinity or among contacts may be of considerable assistance.

LABORATORY. Laboratory diagnosis must be attempted in all cases. Immediate attention is required to confirm or deny each suspected case. Both laboratory consultation and experienced epidemiologic consultation are required. These are available immediately from all state health departments and, upon request, from the Center for Disease Control in Atlanta.

Appropriate specimens for laboratory diagnosis include vesicular or pustular fluid, crusts removed from drying pustules, and acute and convalescent serum samples. Consultation should be sought from the laboratory before specimens are obtained and shipped. A definite diagnosis of poxvirus infection can be made immediately by identifying the characteristic shape of the poxvirus particles in fluid or crusts by electron microscopy. The morphologic characteristics of the virus are unique and distinctly different from those of the viruses (e.g., varicella and other herpesviruses) that are most frequently mistaken clinically for smallpox. Agar-diffusion and fluorescent-antibody techniques have also been used for prompt presumptive diagnosis. Differentiation from other members of the poxvirus group is accomplished by propagating the virus in the chick embryo or in cell culture or by animal inoculation. Increases in specific antibody titers between the acute and convalescent serum samples obtained at two- to three-week intervals will also assist in confirming the diagnosis, particularly in those patients with modified or subclinical disease following earlier vaccination.

Transmission

Transmission results from contact with the nasal or pharyngeal secretions of patients or with fluid or crusts from their cutaneous lesions. Direct contact is most important, although both airborne transmission via droplet nuclei and transmission by fomites have been documented. Unlike most other diseases, subclinical infections are of no importance in transmission, and there is no carrier state or nonhuman reservoir. Susceptibility is universal; only prior vaccination within three years or a prior case of smallpox confers certain protection against disease.

Control Measures

ADMISSION REQUIREMENTS. Strict isolation is required for all patients with febrile illness when there is reason to suspect they have had contact with a smallpox case or with potentially infectious materials between 7 and 17 days prior to the onset of illness [2,23]. Since only a few hospitals are equipped to handle a patient who is suspected or proved to have smallpox, arrangements for isolating such an individual should be discussed with local, state, or federal public health authorities before admitting the patient to a hospital [23]. Isolation must be continued until a definitive diagnosis has been reached. In the event that a tentative diagnosis of smallpox is made, every effort is required to identify and vaccinate immediately every person who has had face-to-face or airborne contact with the patient. Additionally, for those persons previously unvaccinated, vaccinia immunoglobulin should be used at a dose of 0.3 mg. per kilogram of body weight. Antiviral drugs such as β-thiosemicarbazone (Marboran) are of no value for treatment and of limited value for prevention [5]. Vaccinia immunoglobulin should be used in patients in whom there is a strong contraindication to vaccination (e.g., the presence of leuke-

mia or Hodgkin's disease), and it should be used in conjunction with vaccination in those with lesser problems, such as mild eczema.

All known contacts must be kept under surveillance until 17 days have transpired following the last contact with the known case. Should contacts develop fever, prompt isolation is required until the nature of the illness has been determined.

PATIENTS. Patient-care practices must be consistent with strict isolation requirements [2,23]. The airborne route, direct contact, fomites, and indirect contact with virus in the crusts shed from patients with the disease are important mechanisms in the transfer of this infection.

ENVIRONMENT. Environmental precautions are required, because virus may persist in crusts for many months. Proper double-wrapping and disinfection of all articles leaving the patient's room is necessary. Precautions and protective garments are also required to prevent the transfer of crusts on the shoes or clothing of personnel to areas outside the isolation unit. Isolation precautions for the patient must continue until all crusts have been shed.

Terminal disinfection of the room is required after recovery or death of the patient. This involves thorough washing of all hard surfaces, including those of the walls, floors, and furniture, with a phenolic, iodophor, or chlorine-containing solution. All linens, instruments, and equipment must be wrapped carefully and autoclaved.

Therapy

Supportive measures are required in the treatment of smallpox. Attention must be given to antimicrobial treatment of secondary bacterial infections if they are recognized; such infections include pyoderma, pneumonia, and septicemia. Iododeoxyuridine (IDUR) may be used for corneal lesions [4]. Although vaccinia immunoglobulin and β-thiosemicarbazone are useful in prophylaxis, neither has been shown to be of benefit after the onset of disease. Similarly, although disseminated intravascular coagulation has been demonstrated in severe cases and heparin therapy theoretically reverses this process, no trials of heparin therapy have been reported in treating smallpox. Despite all available measures, the case fatality rate remains approximately 30 percent for variola major, although it is substantially less for infections with strains of intermediate virulence. For alastrim (variola minor), the case fatality rate is 1 percent or less.

Hepatitis

Viral hepatitis is caused by two or more viruses and is recognized by the characteristic inflammatory response of the liver. Clinical features include fever, malaise, gastrointestinal symptoms, and jaundice.

Etiology

Of the viruses presently recognized as causative agents, type A—formerly called infectious hepatitis virus—is most likely to be transmitted by the fecal-oral route. Infection with this virus follows close personal contact with infected persons (occasionally primates) or the ingestion of contaminated water or food [7,16]. A few reports have suggested transmission may occur by the airborne route [1]. Type B—formerly termed serum hepatitis virus—is more likely to be transmitted by the parenteral route via blood, blood products, blood-drawing equipment, or bodily secretions such as saliva and semen [26]. Given the proper conditions, either virus may be transmitted orally or parenterally. Recent investigations, however, provide evidence against hepatitis B being transmissible by the gastrointestinal route. Hepatitis that is not due to viruses A or B has followed transfusion and the sharing of needles for the injection of drugs, which suggests the existence of at least one other type of hepatitis virus [19, 27].

Nosocomial Infection Potential

Viral hepatitis—predominately due to type B virus but occasionally due to type A—occurs as a nosocomial infection and may follow blood transfusion or close contact with infected patients or their blood. The frequency of transfusion-associated hepatitis varies according to the blood source; more cases are reported following transfusions of blood received from commercial donors than from volunteer donors. The overall incidence varies from 4 to 20 cases of infection per 1000 transfused units; only one to seven symptomatic icteric cases occur per 1000 units transfused. Viral hepatitis is also reported frequently in hospital personnel, particularly among those working in dialysis centers (see Part I, Chapter 7, Section A), and it has long been recognized as a problem in physicians [7,9,30]. Outbreaks, probably of hepatitis A, among physicians and nurses have originated in nurseries from unsuspected nosocomial infection among the infants [7]. Cases have also been reported in laboratory workers. Currently, the great bulk of nosocomial hepatitis is due to type-B virus; evidence for this comes from studies that indicate an increased prevalence of hepatitis B surface antigen (HB$_s$Ag), antibody (anti-HB$_s$), or both among hospital workers who have close contact with blood and blood products [27].

Diagnostic Considerations

CLINICAL. Incubation periods range from two to six weeks (with an average of 25 to 30 days) in type-A infections, and from six weeks to nearly six months (average of two to three months) in type-B infections.

The onset of illness is usually more abrupt in type-A disease, and the gastrointestinal symptoms are likely to be prominent. Fever with vomiting, diarrhea, or both may be the presenting complaints. Initial symptoms in hepatitis B are more subtle and gradual in development, and they often include malaise and depression. Urticaria and arthralgias may occur and are more common in cases of hepatitis B than in hepatitis A. Jaundice is the most characteristic feature of both forms of hepatitis, especially in adult patients; dark urine and scleral icterus are often noted initially in patients with darker skin color in whom icteric skin is more difficult to recognize. In older patients, an initial symptom may be distaste for tobacco.

Similar illnesses during the preceding one or two months among family or associates provide evidence for the diagnosis of hepatitis A, while a prior blood transfusion, hospitalization, chronic renal hemodialysis, accidental inoculation involving blood-contaminated instruments, a dental procedure during the preceding two or three months, or illicit drug usage would suggest hepatitis B infection. Infected employees working in specific hospital programs, such as the dialysis center, should be suspected of having hepatitis B infection, although non-B infection may also occur. When an illness is consistent with viral hepatitis (regardless of type), greatly elevated serum glutamic-oxaloacetic or serum glutamic-pyruvic transaminase (SGOT or SGPT) levels and elevated bilirubin levels provide clinical confirmation, provided that no medications recognized to cause hepatic dysfunction (e.g., erythromycin estolate, isoniazid, or phenothiazines) were used during the several weeks prior to onset and that no exposure to potentially hepatotoxic chemicals (e.g., carbon tetrachloride) is known to have occurred. Serologic studies for HB$_s$Ag and anti-HB$_s$ should be undertaken. Similar studies for hepatitis A infection or other hepatitis viruses should be performed as indicated.

LABORATORY. The most specific tests for injury of liver cells—the SGOT and SGPT levels—are the most useful clinical determinations available in the hospital laboratory for evaluating cases of possible viral hepatitis. These, together with the documentation of an elevated direct and indirect bilirubin level, provide adequate clinical confirmation of hepatitis. Although immunologic electron-microscopic techniques have been used experimentally to identify hepatitis A virus particles in the feces of infected persons, these remain research laboratory techniques and are not generally available.

More recently, however, radioimmunoassay procedures for detection of IGM specific anti-HAV have been described [6]. Since anti-HAV appears in the IGM fraction of serum in the acute illness phase of hepatitis A and declines to undetectable levels in convalescence, it is now possible to diagnose the disease by the finding of IGM specific antibody in a single serum specimen obtained during the acute illness phase of disease. Patients with hepatitis B usually develop HB$_s$Ag during the illness, so all hepatitis patients should be tested for the presence of this antigen using the most sensitive and specific methods available (e.g., radioimmunoassay or reversed passive hemagglutination). During convalescence, most patients will become HB$_s$Ag-negative and develop anti-HB$_s$, although in a small portion (5 to 10 percent), the antigen will continue to circulate. The separation into HB$_s$Ag/ay and HB$_s$Ag/ad variants is of epidemiologic interest, but it is not essential for diagnosis.

Application of specific diagnostic tests for both hepatitis A and hepatitis B to any acute case of viral hepatitis may now also provide a diagnosis of non-A, non-B disease by exclusion, if such tests are negative for both hepatitis A and B immunologic markers. Laboratories have been screening blood for transfusion, and as a result of the elimination of HB$_s$Ag carriers among potential blood donors and the elimination of paid donors, the risk of hepatitis associated with blood transfusions has decreased during recent years.

Although some authorities advocate routine testing of hospital personnel for antigen carriage, the majority do not. A recent statement by the National Research Council and U.S. Public Health Service recommends routine surveillance among hospital personnel and patients, but not routine HB$_s$Ag screening [10]. Serologic surveillance of hospital personnel is recommended for those in high-risk occupations (e.g., in renal hemodialysis units), and it may be necessary following the occurrence of hepatitis among personnel, patients, or both in order to identify an outbreak and allow the institution of the most effective control measures.

Control Measures

IMMUNE SERUM GLOBULIN. In the past, many well-designed studies have evaluated the efficacy of standard human immune serum globulin (ISG) in preventing or modifying type-B hepatitis in hospital personnel. These studies, however, have provided conflicting evidence regarding whether ISG consistently affords protection. Most commercial lots of ISG available prior to 1971 or 1972 appeared to be ineffective in preventing or modifying type-B hepatitis acquired parenterally, and the lack of effect of such ISG preparations was presumed to be due to the absence or extremely low levels of anti-HB$_s$. However, more than 90 percent of samples of commercial ISG manufactured after 1972 that were tested by the Bureau of Biologics of the Food and Drug Administration were found to have demonstrable but low levels of anti-HB$_s$, generally in the range of 1 : 64 to 1 : 128 by passive hemagglutination (PHA). Subsequent studies on hepatitis B prophylaxis utilized standard ISG preparations manufactured after 1972 that contained low levels of anti-HB$_s$ in various doses ranging from 0.02 to 0.12 ml. per kilogram of body weight. A probable protective effect was demonstrated against the clinical manifestations and complications of hepatitis B infection when the inocula of virus were small and the exposures either percutaneous or oral. These few encouraging studies suggested that ISG with anti-HB$_s$ might be useful for prophylaxis against type-B infection and that specific hepatitis B immunoglobulins containing much larger amounts of anti-HB$_s$ should be developed and tested.

Recently, hepatitis B immunoglobulin (HB-Ig) preparations with high titers (1 : 100,000 to 1 : 500,000 by PHA) of anti-HB$_s$ have been produced and evaluated in controlled experimental trials in a variety of epidemiologic settings. These studies have included preexposure prophylaxis in hemodialysis units and postexposure prophylaxis of medical personnel following percutaneous exposure to HB$_s$Ag-containing material. When compared to placebo globulin (standard ISG with no detectable anti-HB$_s$), HB-Ig preparations afford significant value in protecting against hepatitis B when used for preexposure prophylaxis in hemodialysis units and for postexposure prophylaxis of persons who have had HB$_s$Ag-positive needle sticks. The evidence is not so clear, however, that HB-Ig preparations are of greater efficacy in such situations than standard ISG preparations with low to intermediate anti-HB$_s$ content (titers of less than 1 : 50,000 by PHA). Furthermore, some data suggest that individuals receiving low-titer ISG for prophylaxis may more often develop an active anti-HB$_s$ response (passive-active immunity) in the absence of disease.

In light of these findings, recommendations can be made for serum prophylaxis of persons exposed to hepatitis B virus. For hospital personnel who are anti-HB$_s$-negative and who have been exposed to hepatitis B through inadvertent needle puncture or other tissue inoculation with materials from patients known to be antigen-positive, HB-Ig in a dose of 0.03 ml. per pound (0.06 ml. per kilogram) of body weight should be administered intramuscularly as soon as possible, but within seven days of the exposure. The average adult dose is 3 to 5 ml. A second dose of the same amount should be given four weeks after the first dose. If HB-Ig is not available, ISG should be used (5 ml. for an adult of average weight). For exposure to hepatitis A, ISG in the dosage recommended above should be used.

VACCINE. Subunit vaccines containing highly purified and inactivated HB$_s$Ag have been prepared in several laboratories and tested in animal model systems. In general, such preparations have proved to be immunogenic in animals and have demonstrated protective efficacy in challenge studies with live virus. Studies in humans, however, are being carried out. First, small numbers of volunteers are being employed to demonstrate safety. Efficacy will then be tested by employing large numbers of persons naturally exposed to hepatitis B. Such studies are required before any preparations can be licensed for use in selected elements of the population known to be at high risk of exposure to hepatitis B.

ISOLATION REQUIREMENTS. Enteric and blood-instrument precautions are required for all patients with viral hepatitis [36]. Private rooms are necessary for children, because individual-unit isolation is more difficult to accomplish and susceptibility among contacts is likely to be greater. Gowns are recommended for all persons having direct contact with the patients in order to protect their clothing from contamination; wearing masks is not necessary. Hand-washing is an extremely effective preventive measure and should be enforced; gloves are recommended for persons having direct contact with the patient or with articles contaminated with blood, urine, or fecal material. All articles leaving the hepatitis patient's room must be disinfected or discarded. If a diagnosis of hepatitis B can be made with certainty, then enteric isolation can be omitted, since there is no firm evidence for fecal transmission of hepatitis B.

Precautions (enteric, blood, or both) should be continued during the first two weeks of the illness and for at least one week after the onset of jaundice. Blood precautions should remain in effect as long as serum specimens are HB_sAg-positive.

PATIENT CARE. Patient-care practices must be consistent with the requirements of enteric and blood precautions. Direct contact with the patient and with fomites contaminated by blood, urine, or fecal material is hazardous to hospital personnel and to others. No special environmental precautions are required, and the terminal disinfection procedure for the room should be that routinely applied to all hospital rooms within the nursing unit.

HOSPITAL PERSONNEL. Hospital personnel and others who are anti-HB_s-negative and who have been exposed to hepatitis B through inadvertent needle puncture or other tissue inoculation with materials from patients known to be antigen-positive should be considered candidates for protection with specific hepatitis B immunoglobulin (HB-Ig) when it becomes available for general use (see Part I, Chapter 3, and Chapter 7, Section A). HB-Ig has been shown to modify or prevent hepatitis with reasonable effectiveness [30]. If HB-Ig is not available, ISG should be used (5 ml. for an adult of average weight), since 90 percent of the lots of ISG tested since 1972 by the FDA Bureau of Biologics contain low levels of anti-HB_s, and clinical protection has been observed.

HOUSEHOLD CONTACTS. Household contacts may be defined as those individuals sharing the same dwelling unit and meals. Household contacts of patients with hepatitis A should receive a single intramuscular dose of 0.01 ml. per pound (0.02 ml. per kilogram) of body weight of immune serum globulin (ISG) [9]; it should be remembered that the use of ISG provides only transient (e.g., 30 to 60 days) protection. This method of prophylaxis is not currently recommended for those household contacts exposed to hepatitis B.

Therapy

Since no specific antiviral therapy is available, treatment should be directed toward the necessary supportive measures. Diet should be as tolerated, and there seems to be little evidence that any special dietary requirements or restrictions exist. For the rare development of hepatic coma or chronic progressive hepatitis, the reader is referred to standard textbooks of medicine and pediatrics for suggestions in management. Immune serum globulin therapy is of no known benefit after the onset of the disease.

Hepatitis in Newborns

HEPATITIS B. Infants born to mothers who have had hepatitis B during the last trimester of pregnancy or who are in the late incubation stages of this disease are at substantial risk of developing hepatitis B infection. The exact mode of transmission is not clear, but transplacental, perinatal, and postnatal transmission are all assumed to occur. In view of these facts, infants born to mothers who have active hepatitis B or who have had hepatitis B during the last trimester of pregnancy should be managed with blood precautions, including the use of gown and gloves for handling the infant, to reduce the risk of transmitting infection to personnel or to other infants in the nursery.

The frequency with which the cord blood of infants of asymptomatic HB_sAg-positive mothers is positive for HB_sAg is variable, although the frequency of infants in the United States who develop subsequent hepatitis or antigenemia appears to be low. Mothers whose serum is positive for e antigen (HB_eAg), however, are at increased risk of transmitting hepatitis to their infants. It is therefore unclear whether the term infant of a known, asymptomatic, HB_sAg-carrying mother needs to be managed with special precautions to protect personnel and other infants in the nursery. An infant of an HB_sAg-positive mother who remains in a nursery intensive-care unit or other area of the nursery should be tested for antigenemia at birth and periodically thereafter; an infant who develops hepatitis or antigenemia should be separated from other infants and managed with blood precautions, including the use of a gown and gloves for handling the infant and potentially antigen-contaminated equipment or supplies.

Preliminary studies have suggested that neonatal hepatitis B virus infection can be prevented in exposed infants by a prophylactic injection of specific antibody (anti-HB$_s$) during the first week of life. Although hepatitis B immune globulin (HB-Ig) may be more protective against neonatal hepatitis B infection than is standard immune serum globulin (ISG), until HB-Ig is available, ISG (0.04 ml. intramuscularly per kilogram of body weight) should be given shortly after birth to all infants of HB$_s$Ag-positive mothers.

HB$_s$Ag-positive mothers should be informed of the potential modes of transmission of their infection and of the risk of infection to the infant. The infant and mother should not be separated. Although breast milk may be antigen-positive, no studies have indicated an increased risk of transmission of hepatitis B to breast-fed infants by antigen-positive mothers.

HEPATITIS A. The risk of hepatitis A infection in newborn infants is less well described. Because fecal-oral transmission is the most frequent route, an infant born to a mother in the late incubation or early symptomatic stages of hepatitis A infection is at risk of developing disease, although the infant probably does not need to be managed with special precautions in the nursery immediately following exposure. Infants of mothers with active hepatitis A or who develop hepatitis A within a few weeks following delivery should receive ISG (0.02 ml. intramuscularly per kilogram of body weight) shortly after birth or as soon as illness develops in the mother.

References

1. Aach, R. D., Evans, J., and Losee, J. An epidemic of infectious hepatitis possibly due to airborne transmission. *Am. J. Epidemiol.* 87:99, 1968.
2. American Heart Association. *Infection Control in the Hospital* (3d ed.). Chicago: American Hospital Association, 1974.
3. Armstrong, J. A., Tarr, G. C., Youngblood, L. A., Dowling, J. N., Saslow, A. R., Lucas, J. P., and Monto, H. Cytomegalovirus infection in children undergoing open heart surgery. *Yale J. Biol. Med.* 49:83, 1976.
4. Benenson, A. S. Smallpox. In Top, F. A., and Wehrle, P. F. (Eds.), *Communicable and Infectious Diseases* (8th ed.). St. Louis: C. V. Mosby, 1976.
5. Bica, A. N., Gispen, R., Grant, F. D., Marennikova, S. S., Setiady, I. F., Singh, M., Wehrle, P. F., Foege, W. H., Henderson, D. A., Kaplin, C., and Rao, A. R. *WHO Expert Committee on Smallpox Eradication.* Second Report. Geneva: World Health Organization Technical Report Series, No. 493, 1972.
6. Bradley, D. W., and Maynard, J. E. Serodiagnosis of viral hepatitis A by radioimmunoassay. *Lab. Manage.* 16:29, 1978.
7. Capps, R. B., Bennett, A. M., and Stokes, J., Jr. Endemic infectious hepatitis in an infants' orphanage. I. Epidemiologic studies in student nurses. *Arch. Intern. Med.* 98:6, 1952.
8. Center for Disease Control. PHS Advisory Committee for immunization practices. *Morbid. Mortal. Weekly Rep.* No. 20(34):304, 1971.
9. Center for Disease Control. ISG for protection against viral hepatitis. *Morbid. Mortal. Weekly Rep.* Suppl. 21(25):1, 1972.
10. Center for Disease Control. Perspectives on the control of viral hepatitis, type B. *Morbid. Mortal. Weekly Rep. Suppl.* 25(17):3, 1976.
11. Center for Disease Control. Recommendations of PHS Advisory Committee on Immunization Practices. *Morbid. Mortal. Weekly Rep.* No. 19:359, 1976.
12. Center for Disease Control. Laboratory-associated smallpox—England. *Morbid. Mortal. Weekly Rep.* No. 27:319, 1978.
13. Cooper, L. Z., Green, R. H., Krugman, S., Giles, J. P., and Mirick, G. S. Neonatal thrombocytopenic purpura and other manifestations of rubella acquired in utero. *Am. J. Dis. Child.* 110:416, 1965.
14. Cox, F., and Hughes, W. T. Fecal excretion of cytomegalovirus in disseminated cytomegalic inclusion disease. *J. Infect. Dis.* 129:732, 1974.
15. Dover, A. S., Escobar, J. A., Duenas, A. L., and Leal, E. C. Pneumonia associated with measles. *J.A.M.A.* 234:612, 1975.
16. Eisenstein, A. B., Aach, R. D., Jacobsohn, W., and Goldman, A. An epidemic of hepatitis in a general hospital. Probable transmission by contaminated orange juice. *J.A.M.A.* 185:171, 1963.
17. Epidemic Smallpox. Symposium at University of Belgrade, Nov. 14–16, 1972. Glas Publisher, Belgrade, Yugoslavia.
18. Epstein, C. J. Current status of rubella susceptibility testing. *N. Engl. J. Med.* 286:320, 1972.
19. Feinstone, S. M., Kapikian, A. Z., Purcell, R. H., Alter, H. J., and Holland, P. V.

Transfusion-associated hepatitis not due to viral hepatitis type A or type B. *N. Engl. J. Med.* 292:767, 1975.

20. Fiala, M., Payne, J. E., Berne, T. V., Moore, T. C., Henle, W., Montgomerie, J. Z., Chatterjee, S. N., and Guza, L. B. Epidemiology of cytomegalovirus infection after transplantation and immunosuppression. *J. Infect. Dis.* 132:421, 1975.

21. Hanshaw, J. B. Cytomegalovirus Infections. In Top, F. H., and Wehrle, P. F. (Eds.), *Communicable and Infectious Diseases* (7th ed.). St. Louis: C. V. Mosby, 1972.

22. Horstmann, D. M. Rubella: the challenge of its control. *J. Infect. Dis.* 123:640, 1971.

23. *Isolation Techniques for Use in Hospitals.* U.S. Department of Health, Education, and Welfare. Washington, D.C.: U.S. Government Printing Office, Publ. No. (CDC) 76-8314, 1975.

24. Lang, D. J., and Hanshaw, J. B. Cytomegalovirus infection and the post perfusion syndrome. *N. Engl. J. Med.* 280:1145, 1969.

25. Linnemann, C. C., Jr. Measles vaccine. Immunity, reinfection and revaccination. Reviews and commentary. *Am. J. Epidemiol.* 97:365, 1973.

26. Mosley, J. W. The epidemiology of viral hepatitis: an overview. *Am. J. Med. Sci.* 270:253, 1975.

27. Mosley, J. W. Hepatitis types B and non-B: epidemiologic background. *J.A.M.A.* 233:967, 1975.

28. Papp, K., Molitor, I., and Ory, I. Experiments showing that the mode of infection of measles is by contamination of the conjunctival mucous membrane. *Rev. Immunol.* (Paris) 20:27, 1956.

29. Prince, A. M., Szmuness, W., Mann, M. K., Vyas, G. N., Grady, G. F., Shapiro, F. L., Suki, W. N., Friedman, E. A., and Stenzel, K. H. Hepatitis B "immune" globulin: effectiveness in prevention of dialysis-associated hepatitis. *N. Engl. J. Med.* 293:1063, 1975.

30. Prince, A. M., Szmuness, W., Mann, M. K., Vyas, G. N., Grady, G. F., Shapiro, F. L., Suki, W. N., Friedman, E. A., and Stenzel, K. H. Hepatitis B immune globulin—Prevention of hepatitis from accidental exposure among medical personnel. *N. Engl. J. Med.* 293:1067, 1975.

31. *Report of the Committee of Inquiry into the Smallpox Outbreak in London in March and April 1973.* London: Her Majesty's Stationery Office, 1974.

32. Reynolds, D. W., Stagno, S., Stubbs, K. G., Dahle, A. J., Livingston, M. D., Saxon, S. S., and Alford, C. A. Inapparent congenital cytomegalovirus infection with elevated cord IgM levels. *N. Engl. J. Med.* 290:291, 1974.

33. Ruti, J. Propagation of measles, chickenpox and mumps, arrested by a new method of prophylaxis in a 200-bed sanitarium for children. *Rev. Immunol.* (Paris) 21:393, 1957.

34. Schaffner, W. S., Schluederberg, A. E. S., and Byrne, E. B. Clinical epidemiology of sporadic measles in a highly immunized population. *N. Engl. J. Med.* 279:783, 1968.

35. Sever, J. L., and Monif, G. R. Limited persistence of virus in congenital rubella. *Am. J. Dis. Child.* 110:452, 1965.

36. Snydman, D. R., Bryan, J. A., and Dixon, R. E. Prevention of nosocomial viral hepatitis, type B (hepatitis B). *Ann. Intern. Med.* 83:838, 1975.

37. Surgenor, D. M., Chalmers, T. C., Conrad, M. E., Friedewald, W. T., Grady, G. F., Hamilton, M., Mosley, J. W., Prince, A. M., and Stengle, J. M. Clinical trials of hepatitis B immune globulin: development of policies and materials for the 1972–1975 studies sponsored by the National Heart and Lung Institute. *N. Engl. J. Med.* 293:1060, 1975.

38. Townsend, J. J., Baringer, J. R., Wolinsky, J. S., Malamud, N., Mednick, J. P., Panitch, H. S., Scott, R. A. T., Oshiro, L. S., and Cremer, N. E. Progressive rubella panencephalitis. *N. Engl. J. Med.* 292:990, 1975.

39. Wehrle, P. F., Posch, J., Richter, K. H., and Henderson, D. A. Airborne smallpox in a German hospital. *Bull. W.H.O.* 43:669, 1970.

40. Weil, M. L., Itabashi, H. H., Cremer, N. E., Oshiro, L. S., Lennette, E. H., and Carnay, L. Chronic progressive panencephalitis due to rubella virus simulating sclerosing panencephalitis. *N. Engl. J. Med.* 292:994, 1975.

41. Wells, W. F., and Wells, M. W. Airborne infection. *J.A.M.A.* 107:1698, 1936.

42. Yeager, A. S. Longitudinal serological study of cytomegalovirus infections in nurses and in personnel without patient contact. *J. Clin. Microbiol.* 2:448, 1975.

25

Intravenous Cannula-Associated Infections

Frank S. Rhame, Dennis G. Maki, and John V. Bennett

The terms "intravenous cannula" and "intravenous catheter" are often used interchangeably, although we prefer to restrict the use of the term "catheter" to indwelling plastic devices. Currently commercially available cannula types include a variety of catheters, straight steel needles, and "butterfly" or "scalp-vein" needles. The last are short steel needles with hub modifications for ease of insertion and taping. Catheters are made of polyethylene, polyurethane, polyvinylchloride, polypropylene fluoroethylene propylene or silicone elastomer. Barium sulfate, iodide or bismuth trioxide are often added to make catheters radiopaque.

This chapter will not consider infectious complications of the use of arteriovenous shunts, transvenous cardiac pacemakers, diagnostic vascular catheters, nonumbilical arterial catheters, or intravenous fluid. Such infection problems are discussed in Part II, Chapters 17, 26, and 28.

Intravenous (IV) cannulas may be inserted through intact skin or through a small superficial incision, or the vein may be visualized through a surgical incision (a cutdown) and cannulated directly. Normal skin defense mechanisms are bypassed with all IV cannulation, and organisms from the skin may gain access to the vein by migration along the cannula. A small fibrin-platelet aggregation rapidly develops on that portion of the cannula within the vein. This clot may become contaminated by organisms from the skin or blood or by contaminated infusions that pass through the cannula. Once contaminated, the clot may serve as a nidus for the propagation and dissemination of organisms.

Nature of Infections

The infections caused by IV cannulation include purulent thrombophlebitis, "IV site infection," and cellulitis, any one of which may be accompanied by secondary bacteremia. Cannula tips may be positive on culture tests whether or not any of these infections are present. Cellulitis will not be addressed in detail in this chapter, because its clinical features are similar to those described in Part II, Chapter 20, and the only difference is its specific relationship to IV cannulation.

Incidence

The incidence of purulent thrombophlebitis associated with IV cannulation may be estimated from data from the National Nosocomial Infections Study (NNIS). During the period from January 1970 to August 1973, there were 3,456,649 discharges from reporting hospitals. For percutaneous cannulation, the highest rates of purulent thrombophlebitis were on the medical and surgical services (Table 25-1), while for cutdowns, medical and pediatric services had the highest rates of associated purulent

Table 25-1. Incidence of Purulent Thrombophlebitis Associated with Percutaneous Intravenous Cannulation[a]

Pathogen	Service						
	Medicine	Surgery	Gynecology	Pediatrics	Obstetrics	Newborn	Overall
Staphyloloccus, coagulase-positive	10.6	5.0	0.4	7.3	0.2	2.2	5.5
Klebsiella	1.8	2.7	0.4	5.8	—[b]	1.9	2.1
Staphylococcus, coagulase-negative	2.8	2.6	0.8	2.0	—	0.5	2.0
Pseudomonas aeruginosa	1.3	1.9	—	3.4	—	—	1.3
Candida	0.5	2.6	1.3	1.0	—	—	1.3
Escherichia coli	0.8	1.2	—	2.0	0.2	0.5	0.9
Enterococcus	0.6	1.3	0.4	2.4	—	—	0.8
Enterobacter	1.5	1.1	—	—	—	0.3	0.8
Other fungi	0.3	0.9	—	1.0	—	—	0.5
Proteus mirabilis	0.5	0.5	—	—	—	0.3	0.4
β-Hemolytic *Streptococcus,* group unknown	0.5	0.5	—	1.0	0.3	0.3	0.4
Micrococcus	0.4	0.5	—	0.5	—	—	0.3
Acinetobacter	0.3	0.5	—	0.5	—	—	0.3
Proteus species	0.3	0.4	—	—	—	0.5	0.3
α-Hemolytic *Streptococcus*	0.4	0.3	—	—	0.2	—	0.3
Serratia	0.2	0.5	—	—	—	0.3	0.3
Group-A β-hemolytic *Streptococcus*	0.1	0.1	—	—	—	0.3	0.1
Other pathogens	1.2	1.3	0.4	1.5	—	—	0.9
Cultured, no pathogen identified	1.4	0.8	—	1.0	—	0.5	0.8
No culture	93.8	59.2	57.8	25.3	13.2	6.0	54.9
Overall	119.7	83.7	61.8	54.5	14.2	13.5	73.9

[a] Rate per 100,000 discharges rounded to nearest tenth.
[b] Dash indicates a rate of less than 0.1.
Data from National Nosocomial Infections Study (NNIS), January 1970 to August 1973.

thrombophlebitis (Table 25-2). The overall rate of purulent thrombophlebitis associated with percutaneous cannulation was 74 per 100,000 discharges. Since one-third to one-half of hospitalized patients receive intravenous therapy, about 0.2 percent of patients at risk will develop this complication. The fraction of patients receiving cutdowns cannot be accurately estimated, but the risk of purulent thrombophlebitis is clearly greater with cutdowns than with percutaneous cannulation. Purulent thrombophlebitis associated with percutaneous cannulation occurred about five times for each episode due to a cutdown, but the ratio of the number of percutaneous insertions to that of cutdowns is certainly more than five times greater.

Purulent thrombophlebitis occurs so infrequently in patients other than burn victims that it has been reported in only five prospective

Table 25-2. Incidence of Purulent Thrombophlebitis Associated with Cutdowns[a]

Pathogen	Service						
	Medicine	Pediatrics	Surgery	Newborn	Gynecology	Obstetrics	Overall
Staphylococcus, coagulase-positive	5.5	3.4	2.4	0.3	0.4	—[b]	2.6
Pseudomonas aeruginosa	1.3	1.0	0.7	0.3	0.4	—	0.7
Staphylococcus, coagulase-negative	0.9	0.5	0.8	0.3	—	—	0.6
Escherichia coli	0.8	2.4	0.3	0.3	—	—	0.5
Enterococcus	0.9	1.5	0.3	—	—	0.2	0.5
Klebsiella	1.1	—	0.1	0.5	—	—	0.4
Enterobacter	0.5	1.0	0.6	—	—	—	0.4
Candida	0.3	—	0.5	—	0.4	—	0.3
Proteus mirabilis	0.4	0.5	0.2	—	—	—	0.2
Other fungi	0.2	—	0.2	—	—	—	0.1
Acinetobacter	0.2	—	0.1	—	—	—	0.1
Proteus species	0.2	—	—	—	—	—	0.1
α-Hemolytic *Streptococcus*	0.1	0.5	—	0.3	—	—	0.1
Serratia	0.2	—	—	—	—	—	0.1
Group-A β-hemolytic *Streptococcus*	0.2	—	0.2	—	—	—	0.1
Micrococcus	—	—	0.1	—	—	—	<0.1
β-Hemolytic *Streptococcus,* group unknown	—	—	—	—	—	—	—
Other pathogens	0.4	—	0.5	—	—	—	0.3
Cultured, no pathogen identified	0.2	—	0.2	—	—	—	0.1
No culture	12.2	10.7	7.3	1.4	0.4	0.2	6.8
Totals	25.6	21.4	14.6	3.2	1.8	0.5	14.2

[a] Rate per 100,000 discharges rounded to nearest tenth.
[b] Dash indicates a rate of less than 0.1.
Data from National Nosocomial Infections Study (NNIS), January 1970 to August 1973.

studies of IV cannulation. In these, ten cases occurred in 4819 cannulations. This rate (0.2 percent) is in agreement with the estimate made from NNIS data.

Purulent thrombophlebitis in the burn patient represents an important special situation. Infection is the major cause of death in burn patients reaching the hospital. As techniques for controlling burn-wound sepsis have improved, several burn centers have reported that suppurative thrombophlebitis has become the most common source of infection in burn patients dying of sepsis. One burn center reported 4 percent of 1929 burn patients developed intraluminal venous suppuration between 1960 and 1968.

Rates of cannula-tip culture positivity and IV-associated septicemia may be estimated by combining data from published prospective studies of intravenous cannulation. Despite the disadvantages of grouping data from different studies from different institutions with different methods of catheter care over a span of nine years, it is probably still the best way to get estimates of complication rates. Overall, about one-fourth of catheter tips removed from cutdowns and subclavian or umbilical cannulations are culture-positive (Table 25-3). Peripheral catheters and steel needles (mainly scalp-vein needles) are culture-positive at lower frequencies (18 and 15 percent, respectively). Prospective studies of cannula tips in total parenteral nutrition (TPN) have shown similar rates of culture positivity. The significance of catheter-tip culture positivity—variously called contamination, infection, or colonization—has never been clear. Without exception, such studies have cultured catheter tips by dropping them in nutrient broth, and positive cultures may result from very few organisms. This may account for the relatively poor reported correlation between phlebitis and cannula-tip culture positivity. Recent experience with semiquantitative catheter culture (see Microbiologic Specimens, p. 439) has clarified this situation [8]. Less than one-half of catheters with positive cultures in broth show heavy growth on semiquantitative agar culture. Catheter-caused septicemia is associated only with such positive semiquantitative cultures of catheters. Catheters exposed to bacteremia from a different site do not ordinarily manifest heavy growth on semiquantitative culture.

Septicemia is far more likely to result from cutdowns than from subclavian or umbilical catheterizations (Table 25-4). Both peripheral-vein plastic catheters and steel needles (mainly scalp-vein needles in these studies) appear much less hazardous than any of the above, but their relative safety is difficult to judge, because the occurrence of just two more septicemic episodes associated with steel needles would have reversed the apparent lower frequency of septicemia with steel needles (0.2 percent) and would have made them at least as hazardous as the use of peripheral percutaneous catheters (0.5 percent).

Plastic catheters are more often inserted in emergency situations, are more frequently inserted by physicians rather than by IV team personnel, tend to be allowed to remain in

Table 25-3. Summary of Selected Literature on Cannula-Tip Contamination

	Number of of studies	Number of cannulations	Number of contaminated cannulas	Percent contaminated
Plastic cannulas:				
Percutaneous				
Peripheral	13	3031[a]	543	17.9
Subclavian	5	433	114	26.3
Umbilical	6	365	85	23.3
Cutdowns	6	248	60	24.2
Steel needles	5	677	99	14.6

[a] Includes at least 100 cutdowns.

Table 25-4. Summary of Selected Literature on IV Cannula–Associated Septicemia

	Number of studies	Number of cannulations	Septicemia episodes	Percent with septicemia
Plastic cannulas:				
Percutaneous				
Peripheral	17	7618[a]	36	0.5
Subclavian	4	393	15	3.8
Umbilical	6	374	8	2.1
Cutdowns	6	248	16	6.5
Steel needles	4	577	1	0.2
TPN[b]	15	1162[c]	139[d]	12.0

[a] Includes at least 100 cutdowns.
[b] Total parenteral nutrition (see text).
[c] Number of patients.
[d] In 10 studies that identified pathogens, 46 percent of 90 pathogens were *Candida albicans.*

place longer than steel needles, and are more likely to be inserted in sicker patients. The higher rates of contamination and sepsis with plastic cannulas seen in the composite data from these published studies no doubt reflect in part these biases. An adequate study employing random allocation of steel and plastic cannulas has not been performed.

Although almost all patients in the studies of TPN therapy presented in Table 25-4 received TPN fluid via subclavian catheters, their septicemia rates are not directly comparable with those for other subclavian catheterizations. The TPN series used the number of patients as the denominator, rather than the number of cannulations, and they tended to involve longer durations of cannulation. Patients receiving TPN are generally more debilitated than other cannulated patients. In these studies, *Candida albicans* accounted for about one-half of the septic episodes. More recently, the fraction of TPN-associated *C. albicans* sepsis has decreased but is still much higher than that occurring in the course of infusion of conventional fluids. Factors predisposing to *Candida* infection include the hyperglycemia often present during TPN therapy, the tendency of TPN patients to be receiving antibiotics, their greater debilitation, and the longer duration of cannulation.

The data presented in Tables 25-3 and 25-4 can be used to derive an estimate of the relative likelihood of a septicemic episode per culture-positive cannula. This risk is greatest for culture-positive cutdown catheters (27 per-

cent), and it is substantially less for subclavian (14 percent), umbilical (9 percent), peripheral plastic (3 percent), and steel (2 percent) cannulas.

Pathogens
The types of pathogens found in purulent phlebitis associated with percutaneous cannulation and cutdowns are given in Tables 25-1 and 25-2, respectively. For both percutaneous cannulation and cutdowns, coagulase-positive *Staphylococcus* was by far the most common pathogen identified; it represented about one-third of all pathogens that were isolated. In general, the pathogen spectrum is remarkably constant, both between the two types of cannulation and among the various services. A slightly higher rate of *Candida* infections on the surgical service may reflect a greater usage of total parenteral nutrition.

The high proportion of reported infections that were not cultured reflects the importance of purulence, regardless of the outcome of culture studies, in defining these infections. It may also reflect aggressive surveillance on the part of reporting hospitals, because uncultured infections are relatively difficult for surveillance personnel to detect. The reporting of certain pathogens, such as coagulase-negative staphylococci and α-hemolytic streptococci, however, is probably not in complete accord with our microbiologic criteria (see below).

The composite experience of published studies on pathogens isolated from cannula tips

Table 25-5. Risk of Sepsis from Contaminated IV Catheters

Organism	Number of contaminated catheter tips	Number of cases of catheter-associated sepsis	Ratio
Staphylococcus epidermidis	213	3	71 : 1
Other skin flora	70	1	70 : 1
Enterococci	30	4	8 : 1
Pseudomonas and *Citrobacter*	39	5	8 : 1
Staphylococcus aureus	78	12	7 : 1
Candida	14	2	7 : 1
Proteus	13	2	7 : 1
Klebsielleae[a]	46	8	6 : 1
Totals	503	37	14 : 1

[a] Includes *Klebsiella, Enterobacter,* and *Serratia.*
Data from eight prospective studies, each reporting at least one case of septicemia [1–4, 7, 9, 10, 12].

and from the blood of patients with IV cannula–associated sepsis indicates substantial differences in the likelihood of sepsis with different pathogens, given a contaminated catheter (Table 25-5). The most hazardous contaminants appear to be members of the tribe Klebsielleae. Perhaps this is related to their ability, in contrast to many other organisms, to proliferate in commercial, dextrose-containing, IV infusions (see Part II, Chapter 26). If so, then a certain portion of sepsis cases attributed to cannula usage probably really derive from contaminated infusion fluid.

There are no reliable data on the frequency of IV cannula-associated cellulitis.

Classification of Infections
All cannula-associated infections deriving from cannulations performed during hospitalization are nosocomial.

Clinical and Microbiologic Criteria of Infection
Purulent Thrombophlebitis
Pus draining from the point where the cannula perforates the skin, regardless of the outcome of culture studies, is considered a sign of infection. The pus may originate along the cannula tract, but whenever it extends into the cannulated vein such infections should be classed as suppurative thrombophlebitis. These infections produce greater amounts of pus, are more commonly associated with systemic symptoms and bacteremia, and pose a greater danger to the patient than IV-site infection (see below).

When an IV-associated infection is suspected and pus is not evident, it should be sought even in the apparent absence of inflammation. After careful removal of the cannula for culture, the involved vein should be compressed with a finger at a site proximal to the preceding cannula insertion site. The vein is "milked" toward the insertion site in an attempt to express pus. This process may be quite painful, but it must be done vigorously. If the clinical suspicion of purulence is high, cutdown sites should be opened prior to this milking process. Pus may sometimes be aspirated from fluctuant sites along the cannulated veins. A large-bore needle should be used, because the pus may be viscous. If the vein is to be aspirated "blindly" (e.g., in the absence of fluctuance), then at least the area just proximal to the vein-catheter junction should be aspirated. Material that is recovered from such aspirations should be cultured semiquantitatively. This method is especially helpful in interpreting cultures that yield bacteria that are not usually clinically significant (α-hemolytic streptococci, coagulase-negative staphylococci, *Bacillus* species, and diphtheroids). When sepsis persists in a patient with inflamed veins despite appropriate antibiotic therapy, it may be necessary to explore the inflamed veins surgically.

IV Site Infection
Inflamed veins that produce little or no pus are a difficult diagnostic problem, since such inflammation may be caused by infection as well as by other causes. Phlebitis (vein inflammation) and thrombosis (clot formation within a vein) may occur separately, but they usually coexist. The affected vein is warm, tender, and swollen along its course, producing a cord-like appearance. The induration may often extend from the site of insertion of the cannula to the

axilla or groin. When the inflammation is clearly separable from the vein, especially if it is distal to the insertion site, infection is usually present. Inflammation that is restricted to the course of the vein, however, may be caused by mechanical or chemical irritation from the cannula or the IV solution and its additives. In this situation, a positive semiquantitative catheter-tip culture (see below) should lead to the diagnosis of IV site infection. This diagnosis should not be made when the cannula-tip culture was performed by broth immersion only. Likewise, a diagnosis of IV site infection can be made when there is a positive semiquantitative culture from a catheter that has been removed (1) from a site where vein inspection is difficult (e.g., the subclavian vein) or (2) from a patient who has clinical septicemia consistent with an IV site origin.

Secondary Bacteremia

Any of the infections discussed above may be associated with secondary bacteremia. If clinical septicemia is present and culture of the catheter tip is positive by semiquantitative criteria, secondary bacteremia should not be reported unless it is documented by a positive blood culture.

In all such infections, it must be determined that the IV infusion fluid is not the original source of the organism(s) causing the phlebitis or sepsis. The identity of the organisms isolated from the catheter may assist in making this judgment. *Staphylococcus aureus* sepsis is not expected to derive from contaminated infusion fluid, but the presence of certain organisms that have historically been associated with infections due to contaminated infusion fluid would suggest the IV fluid, rather than the cannula, as the primary source of the problem (see Part II, Chapter 26).

Other Infections

Patients with cutdowns occasionally have an infection of the incision site that is separable from the cannula tract. Such infections should be classified as wound infections. The diagnosis of IV-associated cellulitis should comply with the criteria for cellulitis in Part II, Chapter 20, of this text.

Microbiologic Specimens

Collection

Cannula-tip culture specimen collection begins with disinfection of the skin surrounding the insertion site with 70% alcohol. The skin should be cleaned right up to the cannula, preferably with alcohol-soaked swabs. Alcohol is preferred to iodine-containing compounds because the former, after evaporation, would be less likely to kill organisms on the catheter when the catheter is removed. As the catheter is carefully withdrawn, a sterile forceps is used to avoid contact of the catheter with nonsterile surfaces. At least 5 cm. of the catheter tip and the segment beginning 1 to 2 mm. inside the point of the skin-catheter junction should be cultured. For catheters up to about 3 inches (7.6 cm.) in length, the entire catheter may be cultured. Longer catheters will require culture of two separate segments. Catheter segments are placed in sterile tubes for transport. With longer catheters, these manipulations may be performed with greater assurance of sterile technique by two people than by one.

Culture Methods

In the laboratory, the catheter segments are aseptically removed from the transport tube and placed on 100 mm. Petri plates containing a nonselective nutrient agar. Using sterile forceps, the segment is rolled several times across the agar; all surfaces of the catheter must make contact with the agar. The catheter segment may then be placed in broth; however, we do not believe that organisms that are present in the broth but not on the plate are significant. We recommend that plates with 15 or more colonies be considered as positive semiquantitative cultures. Most positive semiquantitative cultures, as defined here, show confluent growth. This technique may also be used for steel needles that can be removed from the hub by repeated bending with a sterile clamp. Confluent growth should be considered significant, and preliminary experience with the interpretation of results of steel-needle cultures indicates that 15 or more colonies on the plate should also be considered positive.

Blood cultures should be obtained at the time of catheter removal if the patient has fever of uncertain cause or if there is suspicion of IV-associated infection. Obtaining blood for culture through a catheter is a less accurate measure of the presence of bacteremia than a percutaneous aspiration, and it may lead to contamination of the IV system. Blood obtained from a catheter may provide an indication of whether or not the catheter is causing an infection, but ordinarily in such cases, the catheter should be removed.

Culturing techniques for fluid specimens are discussed in Part II, Chapter 26.

Control Measures

Patient-Care Practices

Intravenous therapy should be instituted only when it is indicated, and it should be promptly discontinued when those indications are no longer present.

Cutdowns should be avoided as much as possible, in view of the disproportionately high risk of sepsis. Scalp-vein needles rather than indwelling catheters should be used whenever the clinical situation permits. Plastic catheters will still be necessary for the provision of a secure access to the vascular system when a patient has only a few available superficial veins and a long duration of IV therapy is anticipated or when central venous pressure measurements must be made. The employment of specially trained IV therapy teams may reduce the risk of cannula-associated infections; such teams are recommended especially for large hospitals.

Cannulation of the femoral or saphenous veins should be avoided and undertaken only as an emergency measure to provide a portal for administration of large volumes of fluid rapidly. Such cannulas should be removed as soon as a satisfactory alternative portal can be established. Upper extremity, subclavian, and jugular sites of cannula insertion are vastly preferable to lower extremity sites. Some observers prefer the subclavian to the internal jugular site, because the distance between the skin-cannula junction and the vein-cannula junction is greater with the former. Subclavian catheters also pass through a fascial plain. The skin-vein distance may be lengthened by tunneling in the subcutaneous tissue after penetrating the skin, as is usually done for TPN therapy in infants; the tunneling is performed from a cutdown site.

Antisepsis should begin with thorough hand-washing. The skin at the site of insertion should be cleaned with an iodine-containing product. Two percent iodine in 70% ethanol (iodine tincture, U.S.P.) or in water (iodine solution, N.F.) is inexpensive and produces a substantial reduction in the number of organisms. An iodophor is less frequently irritating, but it requires several minutes longer to complete its action. Quaternary ammonium-containing compounds are not recommended. Sterile gloves and drapes should be utilized during cannula insertion when the cannula will be used for TPN therapy or is inserted in severely immunosuppressed patients. Cannulas inserted in emergency situations with suboptimal asepsis should be replaced as soon as possible.

An antimicrobial ointment should be applied at the skin-cannula junction at the time of insertion and every 24 hours thereafter. The composite experience of published studies suggests that antimicrobial ointments are effective in reducing the incidence of cannula-associated sepsis (Table 25-6). Antibiotic-containing ointments appear to be more effective than iodine-containing ointments in protecting against staphylococci, while iodine-containing ointments seem to be more effective in protecting against *Candida*. Accordingly, we believe the former may be recommended for conventional fluid administration and the latter for TPN therapy.

IV cannulas should be securely anchored with tape to prevent to-and-fro motion within the vein. The insertion site should be covered with a sterile dressing that is changed every 24 hours. The condition of the insertion site and vein should be carefully evaluated at the time of each dressing change.

Evidence of thrombophlebitis and cellulitis or suspicion of septic complications due to the IV cannula should lead to prompt removal of the cannula. Whenever possible, peripheral cannulas should be removed and a new cannulation performed at 48 to 72 hour intervals.

Table 25-6. Effect of Topical Antimicrobial Agents at Skin-Cannula Insertion Site on Risk of IV Cannula–Associated Sepsis[a]

Authors	Treated[b]		Placebo		Other control	
	Number of cannulations	Septic episodes	Number of cannulations	Septic episodes	Number of cannulations	Septic episodes
Zinner et al. [12]	210	1	226	1	—	—
Norden [11]	201	1	207	0	50	0
Levy et al. [7]	49	0	51	0	62	3
Moran et al. [10]	38	0	40	3	11	2
Crenshaw et al. [6]	75	0	—	—	75	0
Colvin et al. [5]	53	0	—	—	53	0
Totals	626	2	524	4	251	5
Overall percentage of sepsis	0.3%		0.8%		2.0%	

[a] Excludes TPN studies and includes only prospective studies with controls.
[b] Includes neomycin, polymyxin, bacitracin, or nitrofurazone, whether administered singly or in combinations.

Once purulent thrombophlebitis has been demonstrated, a Gram stain of the pus should be performed and appropriate antimicrobial therapy instituted. If the catheter has not yet been removed, it should be taken out. The decision regarding surgical removal of the vein depends on many factors. In a severely septic patient or in a moderately ill patient who has not responded to antimicrobial therapy, surgical removal should be undertaken. Jugular and subclavian veins are difficult to remove, and ligation is sometimes satisfactory. Purulent deep venous systems should be removed in most cases. Purulent veins in burn patients and other seriously debilitated patients are subject to emergency removal. The surgical technique for removal of such veins is to incise along the vein to a point above the suspected involvement. Free flow of blood is established by needle aspiration, and the infected segment is excised in toto.

Environmental Factors

Intrinsic contamination of IV cannulas (i.e., the presence of organisms in the cannulas prior to breaking open the package) has been reported. On at least one occasion, such contamination has led to a complete recall of a large manufacturer's cannula product line. Unfortunately, the statistics of sterility testing preclude the confident demonstration that a given lot of a product is sterile without culturing large numbers of the lot. Thus, routine culturing of cannulas and related infusion products by an individual hospital is not practical. Of course, if a hospital's surveillance program indicates the possibility of intrinsic catheter contamination, ad hoc catheter culturing is indicated. A suitable method consists of aseptically removing the catheter from its package (ideally in a horizontal laminar air-flow hood), dropping the entire cannula into a rich culture medium (such as brain-heart infusion broth enriched with 0.5% beef extract), and culturing at 35°C (95°F) for seven days.

Any environmental factor that is likely to foster contamination of the hands of hospital personnel represents a hazard of causing infection at the skin-cannula junction.

References

1. Banks, D. C., Cawdrey, H. M., Yates, D. B., Harries, M. G., and Kidner, P. H. Infection from intravenous catheters. *Lancet* 1:443, 1970.
2. Bernard, R. W., Stahl, W. M., and Chase, R. M. Subclavian vein catheterizations: a prospective study: II. Infectious complications. *Ann. Surg.* 173:191, 1971.
3. Bolansky, B. L., Shepard, G. H., and

Scott, H. W. The hazards of intravenous polyethylene catheters in surgical patients. *Surg. Gynecol. Obstet.* 130:342, 1970.

4. Collins, R. N., Braun, P. A., Zinner, S. H., and Kass, E. H. Risk of local and systemic infection with polyethylene intravenous catheters. *N. Engl. J. Med.* 279:340, 1968.

5. Colvin, M. P., Blogg, C. E., Savege, T. M., and Jarvis, J. D. A safe long-term infusion technique? *Lancet* 2:317, 1972.

6. Crenshaw, C. A., Kelly, L., Turner, R. J., and Enas, D. Bacteriologic nature and prevention of contamination to intravenous catheters. *Am. J. Surg.* 123:264, 1972.

7. Levy, R. S., Goldstein, J., and Pressman, R. S. Value of a topical antibiotic ointment in reducing bacterial colonization of percutaneous venous catheters. *J. Albert Einstein Med. Center* 18:67, 1970.

8. Maki, D. G., Weise, C. E., and Sarafin, H. W. A semiquantitative culture method for identifying intravenous-catheter-related infection. *N. Engl. J. Med.* 296:1305, 1977.

9. Mogensen, J. V., Frederiksen, W., and Jensen, J. K. Subclavian vein catheterization and infection: a bacteriologic study of 130 catheter insertions. *Scand. J. Infect. Dis.* 4:31, 1972.

10. Moran, J. M., Atwood, R. P., and Rowe, M. I. A clinical and bacteriologic study of infections associated with venous cutdowns. *N. Engl. J. Med.* 272:554, 1965.

11. Norden, C. W. Application of antibiotic ointment to the site of venous catheterization—a controlled trial. *J. Infect. Dis.* 120: 611, 1969.

12. Zinner, S. H., Denny-Brown, B. C., Braun, P., and Kass, E. H. Risk of infection with intravenous indwelling catheters: effect of application of antibiotic ointment. *J. Infect. Dis.* 120:616, 1969.

26

Intravenous Infusion-Associated Infections

Donald A. Goldmann, Dennis G. Maki, and John V. Bennett

Intravenous (IV) therapy has been an integral part of medical care for more than 50 years, but the possibility of contaminated intravenous fluid causing nosocomial septicemias has been appreciated only very recently. In 1953, Michaels and Ruebner [18] reported two cases of "coliform" septicemia that they attributed to contaminated fluid. This important observation remained unnoticed in the medical literature, however, while investigators of infusion-related infection focused their attention on the complications of the use of intravenous catheters. The study of Michaels and Ruebner was not even referenced in the American literature until 1969, when Wilmore and Dudrick [26] suggested that membrane filters might protect patients from the infusion of contaminated fluid.

Scattered reports followed of septicemia traced to intravenous fluid contaminated during use [7,22,24], but the potential magnitude of the contamination problem was not generally perceived until 1971, when contaminated infusion products of a major United States manufacturer precipitated a nationwide epidemic of septicemia [4,16]. Subsequent reports of three other outbreaks of septicemia due to contamination of intravenous solutions during the manufacturing process [5,17,21] have, one hopes, altered the complacency with which infusions were once administered. These events and subsequent studies have increased the recognition of the past inadequacies of sterility testing by manufacturers and have led to a better understanding of in-use contamination.

This chapter will mainly consider the bacterial infections acquired from infusions and will not cover bacterial or viral infections transmitted by blood or blood products (see Part II, Chapters 24 and 28). Infections from IV cannulation are covered in Part II, Chapter 25.

Incidence of Infection

In spite of increasing interest and concern, it is not yet possible to estimate accurately the incidence of septicemia caused by contaminated infusion fluid. Analysis of data compiled by the National Nosocomial Infections Study (NNIS) reveals that from January 1970 to August 1973, member hospitals reported 3541 cases of "primary" septicemia (sepsis not thought to be due to dissemination of infection from other sites, e.g., wound, respiratory tract, and urinary tract sites) among 3,456,649 discharges, an incidence of about 1 per 1000. The proportion of these septicemias that occurred while patients were receiving intravenous infusions is unknown. Furthermore, it is not known how many of the septicemias with onsets during infusion occurred coincidentally with IV administration, nor how many were actually caused by intravenous therapy. Of those caused by infusion therapy, the relative contribution of IV cannulation, in-use contamination, and intrinsic (manufacturer-derived) contamination of infusion fluid is unknown; their contributions probably occur in the order given. Attempts to interpret currently available data are complicated by the knowledge that many cases of sepsis are not recognized. Even when septicemia is documented, it is rare that appropriate cultures of blood, cannulae, and fluids are performed in an effort to determine the origin of infection.

Pathogens

Members of the tribe Klebsielleae (*Klebsiella, Enterobacter,* and *Serratia* species) have been by far the most frequent isolates from patients with sepsis caused by intravenous fluid. Of particular note has been the isolation of *Enterobacter agglomerans,* a common plant pathogen previously rarely associated with human disease, in three outbreaks caused by contaminated intravenous products of large manufacturers. The preponderance of tribe Klebsielleae septicemias is probably explained by the selective ability of these pathogens to proliferate in glucose-containing infusion fluids. *Enterobacter cloacae, E. agglomerans,* and other members of the tribe Klebsielleae have been shown to multiply rapidly at room temperature in 5% dextrose in water; concentrations of greater than 10^5 organisms per milliliter have been reached within 24 hours even when very small, washed inocula of 1 to 10 organisms are employed

[14]. The fluid remains crystal clear in spite of the high levels of bacteria.

In marked contrast to the rapid multiplication of tribe Klebsielleae organisms, other test strains—including *Staphylococcus, Proteus, Escherichia coli, Acinetobacter,* and *Pseudomonas aeruginosa*—slowly die. *Candida* grows very slowly. None of these strains proliferates appreciably in normal saline. Although some investigators have reported the multiplication of a variety of gram-negative organisms, including *P. aeruginosa,* in normal saline and other intravenous solutions, large inocula were employed and logarithmic growth was not achieved. However, *Citrobacter freundii,* an agent involved in a small outbreak of IV-associated sepsis [5], can proliferate in 5% dextrose in lactated Ringer's solution, and a high index of suspicion will undoubtedly result in the discovery of other pathogens capable of growth in various solutions. Fungal septicemia, for example, complicates total parenteral nutrition (TPN) therapy in 2 to 7 percent of patients in most series, and this may be related to the ability of organisms to grow in TPN solutions [10]. *Candida albicans* and *Torulopsis glabrata* proliferate very rapidly (more than three logarithmic factors in 24 hours at room temperature) in solutions prepared with casein hydrolysate and dextrose but more slowly in solutions prepared with synthetic amino acids and dextrose. *Serratia marcescens, Klebsiella pneumoniae,* and some strains of *Staphylococcus aureus* also proliferate rapidly in casein hydrolysate solutions, but *Escherichia coli, Enterobacter cloacae, Proteus mirabilis,* and *Pseudomonas aeruginosa* grow more slowly or die. None of the bacterial strains tested proliferates in synthetic amino-acid solutions.

Therapy

Infusion-associated septicemia usually resolves spontaneously when the infusion is terminated. Antibiotics should, however, be administered to patients who are seriously ill, are immunosuppressed, or have indwelling vascular prostheses. Therapy is also indicated when there is sufficient doubt concerning the cause of sepsis, or when clinical signs or positive cultures persist after the IV system is removed. Every possible clue to the identity of the responsible organism(s) should be diligently sought as a guide to initial antimicrobial therapy. The results of culture studies may be unrevealing, however, particularly if antibiotics were present in the infusion. A Gram stain of a drop of infusion fluid from the administration line may be helpful.

If therapy is required before culture and antibacterial sensitivity results are available, a combination of antibiotics should be used that are effective against a broad spectrum of common nosocomial pathogens, including multiple-drug-resistant gram-negative bacilli and penicillinase-producing staphylococci. An antifungal agent may, on rare occasions, be added to the initial therapeutic regimen of exceptionally ill patients who are receiving total parenteral nutrition.

Diagnostic Criteria
Clinical
Although sepsis due to the infusion of contaminated fluid may be clinically indistinguishable from sepsis of any other cause, its recognition is facilitated when septicemia occurs within a few hours after the initiation of IV infusion and presents as a catastrophic event in a stable patient, especially if the patient is without underlying diseases known to predispose to sepsis or a clinically apparent focus for secondary bacteremia. The onset of septicemia may be precipitous, with hectic fevers, rigors, diaphoresis, and hypotension or shock. Hyperventilation, nausea, vomiting, diarrhea, confusion, delirium, seizures, and obtundation occur commonly. Phlebitis at the infusion site developed in 50 percent of about 400 cases studied in a nationwide epidemic caused by intrinsically contaminated fluid [16]. Phlebitis, especially when it develops soon after cannulation, should focus the physician's attention on the infusion fluid as well as on the cannula. The infusion must be suspected even in the absence of phlebitis, especially if it has been running for more than 48 hours without change of apparatus.

Characteristically, antimicrobial therapy with agents having appropriate spectra for the in-fecting pathogens does not result in clinical improvement as long as the infusion of contaminated fluid continues. Some effect on organisms in the infusion might be expected if appropriate antibiotics are added directly to the contaminated fluid; however, antibiotic agents are more commonly given "piggy-back" and thus do not reach the reservoir of the organisms in effective concentrations. Termination of the contaminated infusion, even if antibiotics are withheld, usually produces prompt, striking, clinical improvement.

Infusion-related sepsis is considerably more difficult to recognize in patients who are already critically ill. The clinical syndrome, so distinctive in the stable patient, may be masked by previously existing hypotension, fever, or coma, and the origin of the septicemia can be particularly confusing if there are coexisting sites of infection. Unfortunately, it is these very patients who are statistically at greater risk for infusion-related sepsis, since they are more likely to receive prolonged infusions through multiple lines. Moreover, since such patients are also more disposed to IV cannula-associated sepsis, it is important to attempt to determine whether the cannula or contaminated fluid is responsible for the septicemia. Infusion fluid rather than the cannula is favored as the source when (1) the onset of sepsis occurs soon after IV infusion therapy is initiated, (2) phlebitis and other local complications of the cannulation are not present (when phlebitis is present, it is consistent with both), or (3) phlebitis is present, but steel scalp-vein needles have been employed rather than indwelling plastic cannulae.

It must also be remembered that not every patient who is given a contaminated infusion will immediately develop clinical septicemia, particularly if the concentration of contaminants in the fluid is low. Most patients probably clear small numbers of organisms from the blood without suffering ill effects. In some cases, however, particularly in the debilitated or immunosuppressed host or one with prolonged, unrecognized bacteremia, a nidus of latent infection may be established, only later to become manifest as endocarditis, endophthalmitis, or other serious infection.

Microbiologic

Although the clinical course may suggest infusion-associated sepsis, it can be very difficult—especially in the single, sporadic case—to prove that contaminated fluid is the real culprit. In one hospital, the *Limulus* assay has permitted the rapid detection of IV fluid contamination with gram-negative organisms that elaborate endotoxin [12]; however, even if this test is available and is positive, complete identification of the responsible organism must be carried out. Simultaneous recoveries of identical organisms from cultures of both blood and IV fluid is very suggestive of infusion-associated sepsis. It must be kept in mind, however, that organisms colonizing the cannula theoretically may contaminate fluid in the administration tubing in a retrograde fashion; it has been shown, for example, that motile organisms can ascend more than 5 feet against a continuous flow of fluid [25].

Several microbiologic factors may assist in judging the likely source of the organism: (1) *S. aureus* is the predominant pathogen in cases of IV cannula-associated sepsis, whereas gram-negative rods of the tribe Klebsielleae predominate in infusion-associated sepsis; (2) intrinsically contaminated fluid is favored if the identity and antibacterial susceptibility pattern of isolates from the fluid are distinctly unusual for bloodstream pathogens in the institution; and (3) cannula-derived infection is probable if cultures of fluid from the administration tubing or IV containers in use at the time of onset of sepsis are negative or contain organisms other than those cultured from the patient's blood. A positive semiquantitative culture of the catheter tip also strongly favors a cannula source (see Part 2, Chapter 25).

Failure to recover organisms from the IV container that was hanging at the onset of sepsis does not necessarily mean that a previously hanging bottle was not culpable; once introduced into the infusion system, contaminants can persist and proliferate in the administration tubing or on the cannula until reaching a level high enough to produce clinical sepsis.

It may be difficult to prove that contamination was introduced at the time of manufacture rather than during administration. Such intrinsic contamination, which may be present in low frequency, must be demonstrated by the recovery of organisms from cultures of fluid or closures from unopened bottles. This search is greatly aided by selective culturing of suspect lot numbers.

Specimen Collection

When septicemia from infusion fluid is suspected, a number of procedures should be performed in addition to careful examination of the infusion site, collection of blood culture specimens from at least two independent venipunctures, and culture of specimens from other possible sites of infection. The entire infusion system—including the bottle, administration set, and cannula—should be discontinued. The catheter and, if indicated, an aspirate from the lumen of its related vein should be cultured (see Chapter 25). After the catheter is removed and the tip of the administration set is disinfected, the clamp on the tubing should be released, and 20 ml. of fluid is collected aseptically. To estimate the level of contamination, a heat-sterilized, calibrated loop of 0.01 or 0.001 ml. capacity can be used to inoculate the surface of a blood-agar plate. Alternately, 1 ml. may be used to prepare a pour plate. The remaining fluid should be inoculated into each of two blood culture bottles. The culturing of 20 ml. of fluid aseptically withdrawn from the IV container should then be performed in an analogous fashion. Unused fluid in the bottles should be stored in a refrigerator for future tests if necessary.

In addition to culturing the fluid in use at the onset of sepsis, an attempt should be made to retrieve and culture any containers of fluid and IV additives administered to the patient in the previous 24 hours. Such products could have contaminated the infusion system but might not have contained sufficient organisms to result directly in a clinical reaction at the time they were administered. Thus, a more sensitive culture method is required. The entire volume of fluid remaining in the container may be cultured by adding to the container an equal volume of double-strength brain-heart infusion broth enriched with 0.5% beef extract (or a proportionately smaller quantity of concentrated broth) and incubating at 37°C. Alternative but less sensitive culture methods include (1) substitution of trypticase soy broth for enriched brain-heart infusion broth and (2) passage of the remaining contents of the container through a 0.22 μ filter, followed by culture of one-half of the filter on blood agar and one-half in broth. Empty containers may be cultured by adding a small amount of enriched broth and swirling the medium in the bottle.

All culturing should be performed in a clean, sheltered part of the laboratory and, if possible, under a horizontal laminar-flow hood. The working area should be monitored with settling plates. All cultures should be incubated for at least one week before being discarded as negative. All isolates should be speciated and tested for antimicrobial susceptibility. Isolates should be saved until the scope and cause of the problem have been elucidated.

It is important to record the nature and lot numbers of all fluids suspected of causing sepsis. If epidemiologic investigation suggests contamination during manufacture, all fluids with implicated lot numbers should be reserved for a Food and Drug Administration (FDA) representative, and the FDA and local authorities should be notified immediately. Final resolution of the problem may require the culturing of large numbers of unopened fluids or other products; such culturing is best performed by state and federal agencies equipped to examine large numbers of samples using sensitive techniques and laminar-flow facilities.

Contamination of Intravenous Fluids During Manufacture

Epidemics

Four recent outbreaks of nosocomial septicemia have dramatized the possibility of IV product contamination during the manufacturing process. The first, largest, and most extensively studied outbreak began in the summer of 1970 and persisted for approximately eight months [16]. About 400 cases of septicemia due to *Enterobacter agglomerans* (formerly *Erwinia,* herbicola-lathyri group) and *Enterobacter cloacae* were documented in 25 hospitals that

were selected for study; it may be estimated that several thousand cases occurred nationwide. Septicemia contributed to the death of approximately 13 percent of patients developing sepsis from these organisms. Epidemiologic investigation traced the epidemic to contaminated infusion products of an American manufacturer. Specifically, the epidemic was triggered by the distribution of IV fluids with a newly introduced, elastomer-lined, screw-cap closure. Over 30 microbial species, including *E. cloacae* and *E. agglomerans,* were isolated from elastomer liners from previously unopened bottles. The epidemic strains were also found in fluid from about six per 1000 unused bottles from stock supplies, and organisms were demonstrated to gain access regularly to the infusion fluid when bottles were manipulated under conditions duplicating those of normal, in-hospital use. Moreover, the epidemic organisms were simultaneously isolated from blood and from solutions being administered to patients, and they were also found throughout the environment of the manufacturing plant. The epidemic was abruptly terminated by an FDA recall of the contaminated products in March 1971.

The second outbreak [21] occurred when softened, deionized, distilled water prepared by a London hospital for its own use became contaminated with *Pseudomonas thomasii,* a cepacia-like organism. Forty cases of nosocomial infection, including eight cases of sepsis, were linked to the contamination. Contaminated water, which was used as a coolant in a rapid-cooling autoclave, was found to remain beneath the foil seal of rubber-stoppered, IV fluid bottles and to enter the bottles when administration sets were attached. The outbreak demonstrated that rubber-stoppered bottles as well as screw-top bottles could become contaminated under the appropriate conditions.

In the third outbreak [17], five patients who had undergone uncomplicated surgical procedures at a hospital in Plymouth, England, suddenly experienced fatal septicemia after receiving 5% dextrose in water solution that was manufactured by a British company. Blood cultures were apparently not obtained, but unopened bottles were found to be contaminated with high concentrations of a number of organisms, including *E. agglomerans, E. aerogenes,* and *P. thomasii.* Faulty maintenance of autoclaving equipment at the manufacturing plant was incriminated.

The fourth outbreak [5] was caused by intrinsically contaminated 5% dextrose in lactated Ringer's solution manufactured by an American company. Five patients developed septicemia; *Citrobacter freundii* was recovered from the blood of three patients, *E. cloacae* from one patient, and *E. cloacae* and *E. agglomerans* from one patient. The precise mechanisms of contamination are uncertain, but they probably involved contaminated autoclave cooling water and the adoption of a different autoclave cycle that resulted in greater stress on the containers and their closures during the autoclave cooling phase.

Prevention

Control of contamination during the manufacturing process is the responsibility of industry and regulatory agencies. The statistics of sterility testing preclude the confident demonstration that any given autoclave load or lot is sterile without excessive sampling for culture tests. Present requirements for sterility testing will permit nearly all autoclave loads contaminated at low frequencies to be released for consumer use. Revisions of sterility testing procedures at the manufacturing level and methods of their analysis are needed and are being considered. Reasonable, practical, sampling procedures can be devised to detect ongoing production problems that may result in low-level contamination. Sequential sampling schemes to monitor the production process seem well suited for this purpose, because they are designed to reject products efficiently that are contaminated at unacceptable frequencies and to take into account automatically the results of previous sterility testing in interpreting the acceptability of present tests.

All the fluid in test bottles should be cultured, since low-level contamination may be missed by less thorough techniques. The value of microbiologic sampling can be further enhanced by identifying gram-negative contaminants to the species level. Isolation of the same organism from a few bottles or a tribe Klebsielleae strain from only one bottle should certainly prompt a complete review of manufacturing methods. Of course, microbiologic sampling is not a substitute for actual monitoring of the sterilization process; the adequacy of autoclave temperatures must be verified by accurate recording thermocouples and properly placed biologic indicators. Even though autoclave function is of critical importance, it should be emphasized that three of the four epidemics that have been mentioned did not appear to derive from faulty autoclave function.

Outbreaks of nosocomial septicemia associated with intrinsic contamination of IV fluid may be extremely difficult to recognize, particularly if the events are of low frequency and occur in scattered hospitals. Recognition of such problems can be greatly facilitated by awareness at the local hospital level and by nosocomial infection surveillance at the national level.

Infusion products should be carefully inspected prior to use for turbidity, particulate matter, and the presence of cracks or leaks. Loss of vacuum or damage to the closure of the bottles should also be noted. Any such observation should be reported promptly to the hospital pharmacist, who should then contact the FDA and the manufacturer. It should be kept in mind that fluids containing more than 10^5 organisms per milliliter may give no visual evidence of abnormality. Regular changes of bottles, administration lines, and cannulae are recommended (see below) and should be of benefit in preventing sepsis from the infusion of small numbers of intrinsically contaminating microorganisms. Such periodic changes, however, will be of no value in preventing adverse consequences from the infusion of fluid containing large numbers of organisms at the time the bottle is used.

It is not practical, nor should it be necessary, for hospitals to perform ongoing microbiologic quality control checks on infusion products in sufficient numbers to detect low-level contamination reliably.

In-Use Contamination

Incidence

Even if infusion fluid is sterile when it arrives from the manufacturer, it frequently becomes contaminated during use. When fluids have been cultured after the introduction of additives but before delivery to patients, 2.5 to 18 percent of bottles have been found to be contaminated [1,11,20]. Microbiologic studies of fluid collected during administration have revealed contamination rates between 3 and 35 percent [6,7,15,26]. In view of the rather high incidence of sepsis complicating total parental nutrition therapy, it is particularly disturbing to note reported rates of TPN fluid contamination as high as 29 percent [19] and 38 percent [6]. In one study [11], 2.5 percent of bottles of TPN solution were found to be contaminated even before leaving the pharmacy where they were prepared. IV systems in use continuously for more than 48 hours are more frequently contaminated (15 percent) than are systems in use for less than 48 hours (3 percent) [13]. Contamination usually is low level and due to relatively avirulent organisms, but tribe Klebsielleae organisms are occasionally found in very high concentrations [15].

The incidence of nosocomial septicemia from in-use contamination of infusion fluid is unknown, but it doubtlessly occurs more frequently than is suggested by the number of reports in the literature in which a direct, causal relationship has been documented [7,18,22,24]. In most cases, septicemia has been caused by organisms of the tribe Klebsielleae (*Enterobacter, Klebsiella,* and *Serratia*).

Sources

Contamination can occur at virtually every point in the IV system (Fig. 26-1). Addition of medications to the IV container; injections into the tubing; administration of "piggy-back" infusions; introduction of stopcocks, manometers, and other devices into the lines; changes of bottles and administration sets; irrigation of clogged catheters; and the use of the IV system to obtain blood samples all increase the risk of contamination.

IV fluid may also be contaminated by the influx of unfiltered air, which occurs when the vacuum of the IV bottle is broken during attachment of the administration set and as air enters the bottle during infusion [1]. Most manufacturers have attempted to combat this danger by placing a filter in the air vent. Flexible plastic containers avoid the influx of air altogether, but accidental punctures, which may not be evident unless the plastic bag is squeezed, may provide points of entry for organisms.

The natural rubber bungs used as closures for some bottles have been responsible for fluid contamination in the past. Fungal elements were found in almost one-half the bottles sampled in an Australian study [8]. Fungi reached the fluid from blisters on the bung and by coring when the bung was pierced by the administration set. All American manufacturers now use coated bungs, and this source of contamination is presumably no longer a significant problem.

Hairline cracks in IV bottles may provide a portal of entry for contamination [22]; organisms can apparently gain entry to the bottle through cracks so small that fluid does not leak.

As mentioned previously, infusion fluid theoretically can become contaminated by the retrograde spread of organisms that colonize the IV catheter.

Prevention

Control of in-use contamination of IV fluids requires extraordinary vigilance by pharmacists, nurses, and physicians at every stage of the administration process. Rigorous aseptic techniques and the avoidance of unnecessary manipulations of the infusion system are the cornerstones of infection control.

Mixing all solutions in a centralized pharmacy additive service—in addition to reducing medication errors, avoiding drug incompatibilities, and increasing awareness of rational therapeutics—should theoretically decrease the incidence of IV fluid contamination. Adherence to strict aseptic procedures is probably greater in a pharmacy than on a hectic ward where nurses have a variety of tasks. Moreover, contamination by airborne organisms should be reduced by mixing fluids in a laminar-flow

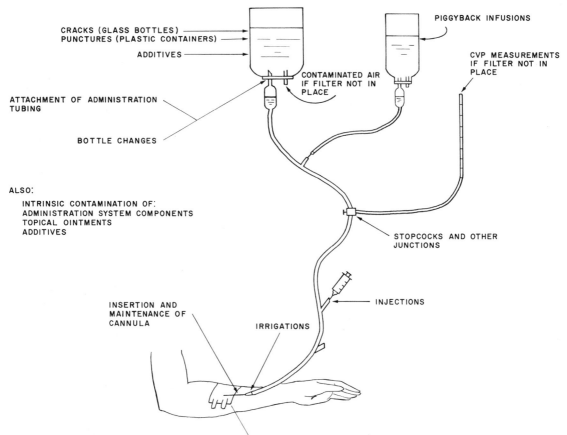

CRACKS (GLASS BOTTLES)
PUNCTURES (PLASTIC CONTAINERS)
ADDITIVES

PIGGYBACK INFUSIONS

CVP MEASUREMENTS
IF FILTER NOT IN
PLACE

CONTAMINATED AIR
IF FILTER NOT IN
PLACE

ATTACHMENT OF ADMINISTRATION
TUBING

BOTTLE CHANGES

ALSO:

INTRINSIC CONTAMINATION OF:
ADMINISTRATION SYSTEM COMPONENTS
TOPICAL OINTMENTS
ADDITIVES

STOPCOCKS AND OTHER
JUNCTIONS

INJECTIONS

INSERTION AND
MAINTENANCE OF
CANNULA

IRRIGATIONS

SEPTICEMIA (RETROGRADE CONTAMINATION OF INFUSION SYSTEM)

Figure 26-1. Potential portals for contamination of intravenous infusion systems.

hood. However, no difference in contamination rates of fluid prepared on nursing units and in the hospital pharmacy was noted in one study [20]. Also, a break in aseptic technique in the pharmacy could expose a large number of patients to contaminated fluid. Moreover, preparation of solutions in a laminar-flow hood cannot be expected to eliminate contamination completely. Even if solutions prepared in the pharmacy are initially contaminated less frequently than solutions prepared on the ward, the probable lengthening of the interval between preparation in the pharmacy and administration would allow more time for the proliferation of contaminants. Further studies should be done to determine the usefulness of additive services in reducing the risk of clinical disease. The time between preparation and use of the fluid, we believe, is a major determinant of this risk.

Regardless of the care with which IV fluids are administered, it seems inevitable that contamination will occasionally occur. The chance that a single infusion system will become contaminated increases the longer it remains in use. Moreover, common hospital pathogens, particularly members of the tribe Klebsielleae, can persist and even proliferate in IV administration lines despite repeated replacements of the bottle, thus exposing the patient to an increasing inoculum of organisms with the passage of time. This dangerous situation can be combated by several infection control measures. IV fluid should be used as soon as possible after opening, and no IV bottle or plastic bag should be left in use for more than 24 hours. It may be of benefit to change the infusion apparatus (container and administration set) every 24 to 48 hours, particularly in high-risk patients; however, this procedure may not be cost-effective in institutions with low rates of in-use contamination. Whenever clinically possible, cannulae should be changed at 48-hour intervals. An entirely new system should be started after each cannula change. The infusion apparatus should also be replaced after the administration of blood products, because minute amounts of blood increase the spectrum of pathogens capable of growing in dextrose-containing IV fluids [14], presumably by buffering the solutions and providing organic nutrients for fastidious organisms.

In-line membrane filters have been employed by some IV programs, particularly for TPN therapy, in the hope of preventing fluid contaminants from reaching the patient. A 0.45 μ filter will block the passage of fungi and most bacteria, except for L forms and some types of *Pseudomonas*. A 0.22 μ filter will block virtually all bacteria, but it is seldom used, because a pump is necessary to deliver viscid solutions such as TPN fluid. Such filters prevent air emboli and the passage of inanimate particles often found in IV fluid, although larger pore (1 μ or 2 μ) filters that are less subject to clogging would accomplish the same task [2]. Membrane filters cannot prevent the passage of endotoxin.

Although one controlled study has suggested that in-line filters reduce the risk of phlebitis [23], studies have not yet determined the utility of filters in reducing the incidence of infection. Theoretically, filters should reduce the infection hazard from intrinsically contaminated solutions and from in-use contamination occurring above the filter, but they have no effect on organisms entering the system below the filter. Moreover, the insertion of any device into the IV system increases the likelihood of contaminating the system, although incorporation of filters into the tubing during manufacture would eliminate this problem.

Because TPN solutions support the proliferation of fungi and have been associated with a significant risk of *Candida* septicemia, some investigators have advocated flushing the TPN administration system every few days with small quantities of amphotericin B [3]. The safety and efficacy of this procedure, however, have not been evaluated in controlled clinical trials.

Uniform adherence to infection control standards can be promoted by the formation of IV therapy teams composed of specially trained nurses and technicians. Such teams may be especially useful in the care of TPN delivery systems, which must be maintained with military precision if infection is to be minimized. In addition, IV teams facilitate the surveillance of infusion-related infections.

References

1. Arnold, T. R., and Hepler, C. D.   Bacterial contamination of intravenous fluids opened in unsterile air. *Am. J. Hosp. Pharm.* 28:614, 1971.
2. Avis, K. E.   Chemicals and Particulate Matter. In *Symposium on Total Parenteral Nutrition.* American Medical Association, 1972, p. 147.
3. Brennan, M. F., Goldman, M. H., O'Connell, R. C., Kundsin, R. B., and Moore, F. D. Prolonged parenteral alimentation: *Candida* growth and the prevention of candidemia by amphotericin instillation. *Ann. Surg.* 176:265, 1972.
4. Center for Disease Control.   Nosocomial bacteremias associated with intravenous fluid therapy—U.S.A. *Morbid. Mortal. Weekly Rep.* 20(Suppl. 9), 1971.
5. Center for Disease Control.   Septicemias associated with contaminated intravenous fluids. *Morbid. Mortal. Weekly Rep.* 22(11):99, 1973.
6. Deeb, E. N., and Natsios, C. A.   Contamination of intravenous fluids by bacteria and fungi during preparation and administration. *Am. J. Hosp. Pharm.* 28:764, 1971.
7. Duma, R. J., Warner, J. F., and Dalton, H. P. Septicemia from intravenous infusions. *N. Engl. J. Med.* 284:257, 1971.
8. Garvan, J. M., and Gunner, B. W.   The harmful effects of particles in intravenous fluids. *Med. J. Aust.* 2:1, 1964.
9. Goldmann, D. A., Maki, D. G., Rhame, F. S., Kaiser, A. B., Tenney, J. H., and Bennett, J. V.   Guidelines for infection control in intravenous therapy. *Ann. Intern. Med.* 79:848, 1973.
10. Goldmann, D. A., Martin, W. T., and Worthington, J. W.   Growth of bacteria and fungi in total parenteral nutrition solutions. *Am. J. Surg.* 126:314, 1973.
11. Hak, L. J., Long, J. M., and Ruberg, R. L.

Contamination incidence in IV solutions with additives. Presented to the Annual Meeting of the American Society of Hospital Pharmacists, March 31, 1971.

12. Jorgensen, J. H., and Smith, R. F. Rapid detection of contaminated intravenous fluids using the *Limulus in vitro* endotoxin assay. *Appl. Microbiol.* 26:521, 1973.

13. Maki, D. G., Anderson, R. L., and Shulman, J. A. In-use contamination of intravenous infusion fluid. *Appl. Microbiol.* 28:778, 1974.

14. Maki, D. G., Goldmann, D. A., and Rhame, F. S. Infection control in intravenous therapy. *Ann. Intern. Med.* 79:867, 1973.

15. Maki, D. G., and Martin, W. T. Nationwide epidemic of septicemia caused by contaminated infusion products: IV. Growth of microbial pathogens in fluids for intravenous infusion. *J. Infect. Dis.* 131:267, 1975.

16. Maki, D. G., Rhame, F. S., Mackel, D. C., and Bennett, J. V. Nationwide epidemic of septicemia caused by contaminated intravenous products. I. Epidemiologic and clinical features. *Am. J. Med.* 60:471, 1976.

17. Meers, P. D., Calder, M. W., Mazhar, M. M., and Laurie, G. M. Intravenous infusion of contaminated dextrose solution: The Davenport incident. *Lancet* 2:1189, 1973.

18. Michaels, L., and Ruebner, B. Growth of bacteria in intravenous infusion fluids. *Lancet* 1:772, 1953.

19. Miller, R. C., and Grogan, J. B. Incidence and source of contamination of intravenous nutritional systems. *J. Pediatr. Surg.* 8:185, 1973.

20. Miller, W. A., Smith, G. L., and Latiolais, C. J. A comparative evaluation of compounding costs and contamination rates of intravenous admixture systems. *Drug Intelligence Clin. Pharmacol.* 5:51, 1971.

21. Phillips, I., Eykyn, S., and Laker, M. Outbreak of hospital infection caused by contaminated autoclaved fluids. *Lancet* 1:1258, 1972.

22. Robertson, M. H. Fungi in fluids—a hazard of intravenous therapy. *J. Med. Microbiol.* 3:99, 1970.

23. Ryan, P. B., Rapp, R. P., and DeLuca, P. P. In-line final filtration—a method of minimizing contamination in intravenous therapy. *Bull. Parenter. Drug Assoc.* 27:1, 1973.

24. Sack, R. A. Epidemic of gram-negative organism septicemia subsequent to elective operation. *Am. J. Obstet. Gynecol.* 107:394, 1970.

25. Weyrauch, H. M., and Bassett, J. B. Ascending infection in an artificial urinary tract: An experimental study. *Stanford Med. Bull.* 9:25, 1951.

26. Wilmore, D. W., and Dudrick, S. J. An inline filter for intravenous solutions. *Arch. Surg.* 99:462, 1969.

27

Transplant-Associated Infections

John E. Swartzberg and
Jack S. Remington

In recent years, the transplant recipient has been added to the growing legion of patients who are seriously predisposed to nosocomial infections. At the close of 1962, there had been only 200 organ transplants reported to the National Institutes of Health (NIH) Organ Transplant Registry; all were renal allografts. By July 1977, this number had increased more than 100 times, and, although most were renal transplants, heart, liver, lung, pancreas, and bone-marrow transplants have been added to the Registry (Table 27-1). Because infection is the leading cause of morbidity and mortality in most series of transplant recipients, it has become incumbent upon physicians caring for this growing number of transplant patients to acquire new knowledge related to the special circumstances of infection in this unique population. They must be aware of the variety of infections that may develop and their manifestations. They must have an understanding of the ever-enlarging group of opportunistic pathogens and the conditions that favor their opportunism, and they must be cognizant of the most efficient and effective means for diagnosis, management, and prevention of the infections caused by such pathogens.

Among the factors that account for infections in transplant patients are the underlying disease and the severe debility that results from it, the major surgical procedure, the foreign body transplant, the immunosuppressive therapy given to prevent organ graft rejection, and finally, the prolonged period of hospitalization and the resulting exposure to an environment of pathogenic organisms.

Major Determinants of Infection

The type, frequency, and severity of an infection depend on at least two major determinants: the local factors associated with the specific type of transplant and the immunosup-

This work was supported by a grant from the National Institutes of Health (AI 04717).

Table 27-1. Organ Transplants

| | Number of transplants | | | | |
	Heart	Liver	Lung	Pan-creas	Kidney
Transplant teams	66	43	22	16	301
Transplants	346	318	37	57	25,108
Recipients	338	302	37	55	22,261

Adapted from the American College of Surgeons-National Institutes of Health Organ Transplant Registry. Cases reported to the Registry as of July 1, 1977 are included, except for kidney cases, which were reported to May 1, 1976.

pressive state induced to prevent rejection of the graft.

Local Factors

Certain types of infectious problems appear to be related to the specific type of allograft. The lung, for example, is the most common site of infection in heart and lung transplant recipients, septicemia occurs more frequently in liver transplant patients, and the urinary tract is the site of infection most often observed in renal transplant patients. Because of these differences, the types of infections observed in each organ transplant group will be reviewed separately.

KIDNEY. Of 224 renal transplant procedures at the University of Colorado performed between 1962 and 1968, 35 percent of the patients had infections of the urinary tract [3]. Bacteriuria was present following transplantation in 44 of 56 renal transplants performed from 1965 to 1969 at the Massachusetts General Hospital in Boston [14]. This high incidence of urinary tract infections was also noted by other groups [88,122,151], and it is unique to renal transplant patients. In an attempt to assess the factors responsible for this, Bennett and co-workers [14] compared the 44 bacteriuric and 12 nonbacteriuric patients at the Massachusetts General Hospital and noted that only preoperative bacteriuria and postoperative urologic complications were significantly related to postoperative bacteriuria.

The natural history of chronic bacteriuria in renal transplant patients is not known, but there is evidence that urinary tract infections in such patients are a frequent cause of bacteremia. Myerowitz and associates [134] from the Peter Bent Brigham Hospital in Boston reviewed the 53 bacteremic episodes that occurred in 37 of their 140 renal transplant patients between 1964 and 1969. Thirty-two (60 percent) of these episodes were due to focuses of infection in and around the revised urinary tract. Certain groups have stated that it would seem advantageous to insure sterility of the urine prior to transplantation, to remove the kidneys at an earlier operation if they are known or suspected of being infected [14,181], to limit urinary tract manipulations to the minimum essential for patient care, and to look actively for and treat vigorously posttransplant urinary tract infections [14,134,181]. Hamshere and associates at the Hammersmith Hospital [83] evaluated the significance of urinary tract infections three months after renal transplantation. The incidence of infection was 83 percent in females and 43 percent in males. There was no evidence that these infections affected the function of the transplanted kidney.

Moore and Hume [130] have noted another urinary-tract infectious problem peculiar to the renal transplant recipient, "transplant nephrectomy site sepsis." This was a particularly hazardous occurrence in their patients. Between 1962 and 1968, there were 119 patients who underwent renal transplantation at the Medical College of Virginia. Operations were carried out for removal of nonfunctioning renal transplants in 17 patients. Eight of these patients developed an abscess at the site of the nephrectomy; six patients died and sepsis was the major cause of death in four of these six. The authors emphasized that more extensive removal of host tissue adjacent to the transplant, greater care in wound closure, irrigation of dead space, and meticulous removal of all transplant tissue at the time of transplant nephrectomy may help diminish the incidence of this very serious complication.

HEART. The largest series of heart transplants is from Stanford University Hospital, where 121 transplants had been performed by March 1977. Complete analysis of the first 70 cases (to March 1974) revealed that 60 of

Table 27-2. Organisms Producing Infections in Heart Transplant Patients at Stanford University Hospital[a]

Site of infection	No. of episodes/ No. of patients	Bacteria				Funguses and nocardia						Virus					Parasites			
		Gram-negative	Gram-positive	Anaerobic	Total	Aspergillus	Nocardia	Candida	Phycomycetes	Other	Total	Cytomegalovirus	Herpes simplex	Varicella-zoster	Other	Total	Pneumocystis	Toxoplasma	Other	Total
Lung	99/51	47	10	15	72	19	7	1	0	3	30	8	0	0	0	8	6	1	0	7
Blood	25/19	17	8	1	26	0	0	1	0	0	1	0	0	0	0	0	0	0	0	0
Urinary tract	14/19	14	0	0	14	0	0	1	0	0	1	0	0	0	0	0	0	0	0	0
Nervous system	6/6	0	1	0	1	1	0	0	2	1	4	0	0	0	1	1	0	0	0	0
Other	31/23	7	6	1	14	0	1	1	2	0	4	6	3	6	11	26	0	1	1[b]	2
Totals		85	25	17	127	20	8	4	4	4	40	14	3	6	12	35	6	2	1	9

[a] Experience summarized for time period ending March 1974 in 70 heart transplant recipients.
[b] Sporozoan, classification unknown.

these patients experienced one or more infections, of which 99 cases of infection involved the lungs (Table 27-2). The reasons for this high incidence of pulmonary infection probably involve several factors. Prior to the transplant, all patients were in severe congestive heart failure. La Force and associates [108] have shown that chronic pulmonary edema adversely affects the clearing mechanisms of the lungs, and this may be the major reason that patients with excessive lung parenchymal fluid are more susceptible to pulmonary infection. Following the surgical procedure, patients have atelectasis, pleural fluid, and chest tubes, which predispose to pleuropulmonary infection. Furthermore, the difficulty encountered in deep coughing after thoracotomy precludes the natural use of this defense mechanism. To this already compromised pulmonary situation is added the exposure to the hospital environment and assisted-inhalation equipment. Such inhalation equipment may be contaminated with a variety of pathogens [154] and may drive into the lungs organisms such as *Aspergillus* that may be present as contaminants of the upper respiratory tract [80].

Cardiopulmonary bypass may also contribute to the risk of postoperative infection, because leukopenia [69], decreases in serum bactericidal activity [81], defective clearance of bacteria by the reticuloendothelial system [199], and decreased phagocytic function by polymorphonuclear leukocytes [180] have all been associated with such bypass procedures.

LIVER. Approximately 300 liver transplants had been performed by July 1977. The largest number of cases (124 patients as of March 1977) are those of Starzl and his colleagues at the University of Colorado, and the most frequent infectious complication they observed was septicemia [190]. In their first 93 recipients of 102 orthotopic liver homografts, the incidence of bacteremia or fungemia exceeded 70 percent [174].

There are several factors that may account for this high incidence of septicemia. First, the graft is exposed to the endogenous flora of the gastrointestinal tract via the biliary system. Starzl [192] feels that this exposed relation of the duct system of the orthotopic liver is "the first step in bacterial leak through the homograft which may well be bacteriologically porous without the presence of histopathologically significant cholangitis." Second, since the liver receives its portal inflow from the nonhepatic splanchnic bed, it may be directly inoculated with bacteria. Finally, because of the transplant procedure, immunosuppressive agents, and graft rejection, the reticuloendothelial system of the homograft likely does not function optimally [190]. The impairment of function of the reticuloendothelial system may influence the efficiency of host defense against infection [190].

A syndrome of septic infarction of the homograft was seen in five consecutive patients by Starzl [190]. The syndrome consisted of gram-negative sepsis, evidence of massive liver necrosis as shown by transaminase determinations, and evidence from serial liver scans of large areas of persistently absent isotope concentration in the homograft. At autopsy or surgery, four of these patients were found to have a thrombosed right hepatic artery. Subsequently, studies from fresh human cadavers demonstrated that an anatomic distortion of the course of the right hepatic artery could accidentally be produced during transplantation in man, partly because of the erect position assumed by higher primates [191]. Another factor that may have been important was incomplete control of rejection during the early postoperative period. Attention to such factors has apparently been the solution to this problem, because none of their subsequent homograft recipients has experienced this syndrome.

Problems associated with the biliary duct have been the major postoperative cause of morbidity and mortality among liver transplant recipients. Waldram and colleagues [206], in looking for the cause of bile duct obstruction, studied the bile drainage in two liver transplant recipients with T-tubes in the bile ducts. They concluded that while bile may become more lithogenic during rejection, the effect of infection on bile composition might be more important in inducing stones after transplantation. *Escherichia coli* can lead to deconjugation of bilirubin and the precipitation of insoluble free bilirubin, which was the main component of a bile cast found in one liver transplant patient at necroscopy [115]. Another cause of biliary tree obstruction might be viral infection. Among the first 44 liver transplant patients at the University of Colorado, there were four cases of cystic duct obstruction. All patients died, and in three, cytomegalovirus (CMV) infection was found in the biliary tree.

Papopavirus infection of the epithelial cells lining a homograft ureter has been responsible for urethral obstruction, and it seems reasonable that CMV infection could do the same in the biliary tree [72].

BONE MARROW. Recipients of allogeneic bone-marrow transplants may be more susceptible to infection than recipients of other types of homografts. Winston and co-workers [216] from the University of California at Los Angeles documented 262 individual infections in 73 patients receiving transplants of allogeneic bone marrow. There are several reasons for this high incidence of infection. Candidates for marrow transplantation have serious underlying diseases, such as acute lymphocytic leukemia, acute myelogenous leukemia, aplastic anemia, and immunodeficiency syndromes, all of which are associated with significant impairment of host defense mechanisms. Clift and associates [36] noted that 21 of 52 allogeneic bone-marrow transplant patients at the University of Washington had clearly defined infection when the marrow transplant was initiated. Because of the severity of their underlying disease, marrow transplant patients usually have been in a hospital environment for extended periods of time prior to the transplantation and therefore have significant exposure to nosocomial pathogenic organisms. Bone-marrow transplant patients also frequently require significantly more immunosuppression than other transplant patients. Bone marrow differs markedly from a graft such as a kidney, which cannot originate significant immunologic reactions against the recipient. Also, suspensions of allogeneic cells are more accessible to the immune system of the recipient and are more easily inactivated than solid tissue grafts. Finally, graft-versus-host disease (GVHD) is associated with a pronounced degree of immunologic incompetence because of the production of lymphoid atrophy, bone marrow depression [18], and impaired neutrophil chemotaxis, and it may cause severe damage to the intestinal mucosa, resulting in continuous seeding of enteric organisms into the blood [46]. In 61 marrow transplant patients from the University of Washington, fatal infections were observed in 26 of 36 with severe GVHD but in only 4 of 25 with minimal or no GVHD [35]. Six of the nine patients reported by Solberg and associates [186] from the University of Minnesota had GVHD. They experienced 18 separate infectious episodes. Two of the three patients who died did so from septicemia; both had multiple intestinal ulcerations, and identical organisms were isolated from blood and stool cultures.

Because there are no specific local factors associated with the primary underlying diseases exhibited by marrow transplant patients, no predominant type of infection has been seen in them. Solberg and associates [186] noted eight episodes of septicemia in six patients, eleven episodes of pneumonia in six patients, and eleven episodes of urinary tract infection in seven patients. Clift and associates [36] found pneumonia (28 patients) and septicemia (34 patients) to be the most frequent infections in their 52 patients. Winston and associates [216] found an equal number of episodes of septicemia and pneumonia (56 episodes) in their 78 patients. Most of the episodes of pneumonia were interstitial; posttransplant pneumonia is discussed below (see Cytomegalovirus, under Organisms Causing Infections in Transplant Patients; Viruses).

The types of organisms causing infection in bone-marrow transplant patients are similar to those seen in other organ transplant patients. Gram-negative organisms cause infection predominantly in the first 30 days after transplantation [36], whereas infections with opportunistic organisms occur later [125]. Clift and coworkers [36], for example, noted six patients with "mildly generalized" herpes-zoster infection. One patient developed this disease 28 days after the transplant; the others developed it more than 100 days after transplantation. Winston and colleagues [216] found that infections during the severely leukopenic period between the day of transplant and 30 days post transplant are primarily localized processes or gram-negative bacteremias or pneumonias. After 30 days post transplant, GVHD and/or steroid therapy are associated with gram-negative bacteremias, fungemias, and interstitial pneumonia. The greater use of empirical amphotericin B and the routine use of trimethoprim-sulfamethoxazole markedly reduced the

incidence of fungal and pneumocystic infections respectively.

LUNG. Infection has been the major cause of death in lung transplant patients [45], and the most frequent infection in such patients is pneumonia. Wildevuur and Benfield [214] reviewed the first 20 lung transplant patients throughout the world and found pneumonia to be the direct cause of death in eight of them.

There are several reasons why pulmonary infection occurs so frequently in these patients. First, most donors have been unconscious without a cough reflex and have required assisted ventilation for significant periods of time before the lung could be available for transplantation [11]. Invariably, this results in atelectasis and infection; Blumenstock [19] has stated that infection can be expected to be present in all cadaver lungs used in transplantation. Second, although the transplanted lung is protected within the thoracic cavity, its internal surface is in constant contact with the outside environment. Third, the remaining lung of the recipient may be infected, and this is in direct contact with the bronchial system of the allograft [45].

There are subtle changes associated with lung transplantation that may predispose the recipient to pulmonary infection. Edmunds [53] has shown that transplanted lungs of canines are less able to clear foreign matter from their bronchi. He concluded that lung denervation adversely affected the bronchial mucous glands, and this was probably the cause of the delayed clearance. Drews and associates [51] demonstrated that immunosuppressive therapy, especially in "toxic" doses, severely depresses the number of recoverable alveolar macrophages obtained by bronchopulmonary lavage in canines. This could be a factor that contributes to the pathogenesis of pneumonia in all types of transplant recipients, including the lung transplant patient.

Immunosuppression
Suppression of cell-mediated immunity is necessary to circumvent rejection of grafts. However, the severe and generalized deficits caused by immunosuppressive drugs, whether used for this or other purposes, have been associated

with an increase in clinical infection with a variety of infectious agents. Lopez and co-workers [118] analyzed the effect of immunosuppression on both humoral and cell-mediated immunity in 61 renal transplant patients in an attempt to correlate these findings with the clinical courses of the patients. For most of them, the immunosuppressive agents (antilymphocyte globulin, azathioprine, or corticosteroids) did not adversely affect circulating immunoglobulins or the antibody response to CMV infection. A notable exception was a group of four patients who were so severely immunosuppressed that their lymphocytes did not respond to phytohemagglutinin in autologous plasma and whose antibody response to CMV infection was impaired. Immunoglobulin levels determined in two of these patients were found to be more than two standard deviations below the normal mean. All four patients died from infection, whereas almost all patients who did not have these defects survived. Their data indicated that the degree of immunosuppression was dependent on the concentration of immunosuppressive agents in the peripheral blood. The authors suggested that some patients may not be able to clear such drugs from their blood as quickly as others, and the accumulation may cause excessive immunosuppression [118].

The effects of various classes of immunosuppressive drugs used by transplant teams have been discussed extensively in the literature and therefore will be covered only briefly here.

CORTICOSTEROIDS. The immunosuppressive effect of corticosteroids appears to be related to their suppression of the inflammatory response. These agents can reduce the number of leukocytes migrating into inflammatory exudates by a factor of four to ten [21]. Yu and co-workers [222] have demonstrated that 60 mg. of prednisone given to normal subjects causes a transient decrease in circulating thymus-derived (T) and bone marrow-derived (B) lymphocytes, the former being suppressed more than the latter. Butler and associates [26] have shown that a short course of methylprednisolone treatment in normal individuals causes a pronounced and sustained decrease in serum immunoglobulin G (IgG) levels because of in-

creased catabolism during drug administration and decreased synthesis during and for a variable time after drug administration. Rytel and Balay [168] have studied interferon production induced by Newcastle disease virus in 15 renal transplant patients receiving corticosteroids and azathioprine and found that its production by peripheral lymphocytes was impaired. Whereas azathioprine has no apparent effect on interferon production [218], corticosteroids in experimental animals have been shown to have a significant effect, and they may be the major cause of impaired interferon production observed in transplant recipients [169]. How these findings may be related to the transplant patient's increased susceptibility to viral infections is unclear, because most viral infections in these patients are secondary to DNA viruses that are thought to be relatively insensitive to interferon. Other immunosuppressive effects of corticosteroids include stabilization of lysosomal membranes [212] (which would tend to reduce the release of lysosomal enzymes necessary for destruction of phagocytized pathogens), interference with wound healing [114], inhibition of the action of migratory-inhibition factor on macrophages [10], and hyperglycemia [75]. Anderson and associates [3] have correlated the latter effect with infection in renal transplant recipients at the University of Colorado.

CYTOTOXIC DRUGS. The two most commonly used cytotoxic drugs in transplant patients are cyclophosphamide and azathioprine. Table 27-3 summarizes the features of these drugs that may contribute to the host's increased susceptibility to infection.

ANTILYMPHOCYTE GLOBULIN. Because the bulk of data on antilymphocyte globulin (ALG) in humans has been obtained from transplant patients who are under severe surgical stress and who are receiving multiple additional forms of immunosuppressive therapy, the immunologic effects attributable to ALG in man have not been extensively studied. Pirofsky and associates [146] studied a group of nonsurgical patients who were receiving ALG as their sole immunosuppressive therapy. In this population, ALG was shown to depress significantly cellular immune reactivity, increase the survival

*Table 27-3. Summary of Effects of Cyclophospha-
mide and Azathioprine*

Effect	Cyclo-phospha-mide	Azathio-prine
Decreased primary immune response	++	++
Decreased secondary immune response	++	±
Decreased immune complexes in NZB mice	++	0
Antiinflammatory effect	±	++
Mitostatic effect	+	++
Decreased delayed hypersensitivity	++	? antiin-flammatory
Suppression of passive transfer of cellular immunity	++	±
Lymphopenia	++	±
Tolerance induction	++	+

Adapted from Hurd, E. R. *Arthritis Rheum.* 16:84,
1973.

time of allogeneic skin grafts, and depress primary IgG and IgM response following typhoid
vaccination.

In association with the significant impairment of host defenses by these classes of drugs,
many commensal microorganisms have been
elevated to the status of significant pathogens.
Such "opportunistic" organisms can now be
found in all the major taxonomic classifications: bacteria, viruses, funguses, protozoa, and
helminths. The following section will focus on
the organisms that cause disease in the transplant population.

Organisms Causing Infections in Transplant Patients

Bacteria

Bacteria are the most common infectious cause
of morbidity and mortality in transplant patients. Myerowitz and co-workers [134] reported that bacteremia occurred at least once
in every four patients in a series of 140 patients who received a kidney homograft between 1964 and 1968. One-third of those patients with bacteremia were considered to have
died as a result of the bacteremia. Of the total

number of bacteremic episodes in this study,
25 percent were fatal. In those patients who
survived their bacteremia, nearly one-half required nephrectomy or died of renal failure
shortly thereafter. In the review of the first 17
liver transplant patients at the University of
Colorado by Fulginiti and associates [67], there
were more than 50 serious bacterial infections.
Of the 32 heart transplant patients reported by
Montgomerie and associates [127] from Houston, 30 had intercurrent infections, of which
14 were caused by bacteria. Six of the nine
deaths in this series were caused by bacteria.

Bacterial infection in transplant patients is
frequently associated with infection with other
classes of opportunistic pathogens. Eickhoff
[55] found that bacteria associated with fungus,
Pneumocystis carinii, or both caused death in
14 of the 50 renal transplant patients who died
of infections. We have had a similar experience
with the heart transplant patients at Stanford.
Bacteria in conjunction with fungus, *P. carinii,*
or both were found at autopsy in 10 of 70 patients.

AEROBIC GRAM-NEGATIVE RODS. The relatively recent emergence of gram-negative organisms as a significant cause of infection in
hospitalized patients has been amplified by the
report of Finland and co-workers [62]. More
recently, such findings have been confirmed in
the transplant patient population as well. Table
27-4 summarizes the distribution of bacterial
organisms causing bacteremia in some of the
larger transplant series. The types of bacteria
seen were similar for urinary tract infections,
pneumonia, and wound infections; gram-negative bacterial infections significantly outnum-
bered those due to gram-positive bacteria. Of
the gram-negative organisms, *Klebsiella, Escherichia coli,* and *Pseudomonas* were the most
frequent offenders. Montgomerie and associates
[129] found *Klebsiella* to be a frequent cause
of infection in renal transplant patients at
Auckland Hospital, New Zealand. In a prospective evaluation of possible sources of the
infection in ten of these patients, large numbers
of *Klebsiella* were found in milkshakes served
at the hospital. The mixer was contaminated
with this organism as well. Infection by *Klebsiella* (singly or with other bacteria) occurred

Table 27-4. Bacteria Causing Bacteremia in Selected Series of Transplant Patients

Organism	Boston,[a] renal[b] [14][c]	Minnesota, renal [181]	Colorado, renal [55]	London, renal [111]	Paris, renal[d]	Stanford, heart[d]	Colorado, liver [190]
Gram-positive cocci	19	6	10	5	9	8	5
Staphylococcus[e]	15	6	7	4	4	5	1
Enterococcus	3	0	0	0	0	2	1
Other	1	0	3	1	5	1	3
Gram-negative bacilli	39	45	35	12	11	14	36
Klebsiella	7	22	4	1	3	8	12
E. coli	10	5	10	4	3	3	18
Pseudomonas	5	10	18	7	0	2	5
Proteus	4	8	0	0	0	0	0
Other	1	0	3	0	3	0	1
Serratia	9	0	0	0	2	1	0
Enterobacter	3	0	0	0	0	0	0
Anaerobic organisms (gram-positive and gram-negative)	2	1	0	1	0	1	0

[a] Location of transplant center.
[b] Type of organ transplant.
[c] Reference number (see References).
[d] Unpublished data.
[e] Coagulase positive and negative.

in six patients on nine occasions. Serotyping of the organism, from both the infection and the bowel, revealed that the strains of *Klebsiella* were identical in three of five patients. In these three patients, the organism appeared in the fecal flora before it was isolated from the site of the infection, which strongly suggested that the bowel was the source.

Recently, Legionnaires' bacillus has emerged as a pathogen in renal transplant recipients. Legionnaires' disease in these patients has caused significant morbidity and mortality [12, 102]. Six of twelve renal homograft recipients at the Wadsworth Veterans Administration Hospital in Los Angeles developed pneumonia due to Legionnaires' disease bacillus in 1977. The renal transplant program at that institute was suspended until the risk of Legionnaires' disease could be reduced [102].

INTRACELLULAR BACTERIA. Facultative intracellular bacteria uncommonly cause disease in the transplant patient. In over 200 transplants (including both heart and kidney) at Stanford, there has been only one documented infection with *Listeria monocytogenes* and none with *Salmonella*. Listeriosis has been reported by a number of renal transplant teams [58,96,120,124,141]. Unpublished data of Acar and his colleagues in Paris (personal written communication, 1974) include three cases of bacteremia (one had meningitis also) due to *L. monocytogenes* among 87 renal transplant patients. In over 700 renal transplants at the University of Colorado, *L. monocytogenes* infection was observed in 13 patients. The central nervous system was involved in seven of these patients [175]. Gantz and associates [70] reported a cluster of eight cases of listeriosis in a single hospital during 15 months. Five of the eight patients were renal transplant recipients. The possibility of a common source of exposure was considered although the source and mode of acquisition were not determined. Watson and colleagues [209] reviewed 20 cases of listeriosis in renal transplant patients and added three additional cases.

In those patients who received three weeks or less of antibiotic therapy, there was a 35 percent rate of relapse.

Tuberculosis is an uncommon cause of infection in transplant patients. At the University of Colorado between 1962 and 1972, only 3 of approximately 400 patients who received a renal transplant developed infection with *Mycobacterium tuberculosis*. (Of these three patients, one developed miliary tuberculosis, the pulmonary lesions of which resolved almost completely during the first three weeks of antituberculosis therapy. When this patient was given his second renal transplant, tuberculosis relapsed in spite of 20 months of isoniazid and ethambutol therapy [138]). In Australia, Oliver [142] reported two infections, one fatal, in a transplant unit which performs between 18 and 22 transplants per year. Bell and Williams [13] from England reported four cases in 82 renal transplants over seven years. All were treated successfully with no fatalities or deterioration in renal function. In spite of the infrequency of infection with *M. tuberculosis,* some authors suggest that all potential transplant recipients be tuberculin tested before transplant and their chest roentgenogram be carefully reviewed. If there is radiologic evidence of old infection or if the skin test is positive, isoniazid prophylaxis should be instituted. Atypical mycobacterial infections are even less common than tuberculosis. Graybill and associates [77] documented disseminated *Mycobacterium abscessus* in two renal homograft recipients. Fraser and colleagues [64] have reported a case of disseminated *M. kansasii* infection in a renal homograft recipient. In all these cases, the infections presented as skin lesions. This was true also in two of our seven transplant patients at Stanford who acquired atypical mycobacterium abscesses post transplant. Hamburger and associates [82], in reviewing 45 kidney transplants in 1965 in Paris, noted one case of miliary tuberculosis, which was readily cured by chemotherapy without interruption of the immunosuppressive drugs. Hamburger and associates, in the series mentioned above, also reported one case of "benign salmonella" due to *Salmonella paratyphi* B. Two cases of *Salmonella* septicemia were noted among the first 50 liver transplant patients at the University of Colorado [190].

ANAEROBES. Anaerobic bacteria constitute a small percentage of the bacteria causing infections in the transplant population. At Stanford, among the 70 heart transplant patients, there were 17 anaerobic bacterial infections. The organisms were *Bacteroides* species (six patients), *Clostridium* species (one patient), anaerobic diphtheroids (two patients), and unspecified (eight patients). Of the 64 clinical infections in Starzl's first 17 liver transplant patients, five were caused by anaerobic bacteria; all were due to *Bacteroides fragilis* [67]. The occurrence of anaerobic bacterial infections may be greater than that indicated in these two series, because the techniques for obtaining and handling anaerobic cultures have improved considerably in recent years.

Viruses

SOURCES OF INFECTION. Those viruses that cause the most significant morbidity and mortality in transplant recipients are the DNA viruses, which produce latent infection in a significant segment of the normal population. The question arises as to how often clinical disease in the transplant population is due to initial infection from exogenous sources and how often it is due to reinfection (including transplanted tissue) or reactivation of an endogenous virus. Each of these mechanisms probably occurs, but the relative importance of each has not been clearly established. Information has accumulated from studies with the herpes group of viruses in transplant patients that shed considerable light on this subject.

Strauch and associates [198] measured Epstein-Barr virus (EBV) shedding in renal transplant patients and compared the results with those obtained in other patients treated with immunosuppressive drugs, patients with chronic uremia, and healthy hospital staff associated with a dialysis unit. EBV was recovered from 47 percent of the first group, 35 percent of the second, 14 percent of the third, and 17 percent of the fourth. Only individuals with EBV capsid antigen in their blood shed virus in their urine. These results are compatible with the hypothesis that in immunosuppressed patients, EBV shedding results from reactivation of a latent infection.

Craighead and co-workers [41] have shown that disease due to cytomegalovirus (CMV) occurs more frequently in patients with antibody to CMV present before transplantation, which also suggests reactivation of latent infection. Fiala and colleagues [60] demonstrated that 12 of 13 renal transplant patients whose complement-fixation (CF) antibody titers were less than 1 : 8 before transplantation and all 13 patients who developed antibody at a titer equal to or greater than 1 : 8 before transplantation developed a positive virus culture or antibody response after the transplantation. Active CMV infection was not detected in the hemodialysis or transplant unit staff, and only three patients had evidence of CMV infection during the hemodialysis phase of their treatment. Reactivation of infection with herpes simplex virus (HSV), varicella-zoster virus (V-Z), adenovirus, or measles virus was detected at about the same time as CMV reactivation in those patients with dual or triple infections. Such findings are more consistent with endogenous than with exogenous sources of these viruses.

Nagington [136] from Cambridge, England, reviewed the sera from 50 renal transplant recipients for antibody against CMV and reported that the incidence of pretransplant CMV infection was at least 84 percent and possibly as high as 92 percent. Both he and Weller [213] have emphasized that the complement-fixation (CF) technique is not highly sensitive and that the absence of CF antibody is inadequate evidence that previous CMV infection has not occurred. Furthermore, several investigators have shown that the CF antibody titer to CMV can fall to undetectable levels in some children two or three years after infection [1, 109,188]. Therefore, a diagnosis of primary CMV infection in a transplant patient cannot be made if a positive CF titer appears following transplantation. Detailed comparison is required between the primary infecting viral strain and the virus recovered subsequently before the question of primary infection versus reactivation or reinfection can be adequately resolved.

Several authors have implicated the donor kidney as a source of virus infection. Ho and colleagues [89] and Betts and associates [15] showed that seronegative recipients from seropositive donors had a higher incidence of CMV infection than those whose donors were seronegative. The data by Howard and colleagues [91] supported these findings by showing that the lowest incidence of CMV infection occurred among the recipients who lacked CMV-CF antibodies and whose donors were seronegative. But these latter authors acknowledged the imprecision of CF testing and concluded that the number of recipients who never had CMV infection was probably overestimated. They therefore concluded that the donor organ is a source of virus in pre-renal transplant recipients. In support of this conclusion, Pien and co-workers [145] studied CMV titers in 16 donor-recipient pairs and found no correlation between the presence of CMV titers in the donor and subsequent viral isolation in the recipient.

Nagington and colleagues [137] have reexamined the sera of transplant patients, using a test for antibody against the core of the 42-nm (Dane) particle. When the first serum of each patient admitted to the Cambridge Transplant and Dialysis Unit was examined for anti-HBcAb, 23 of 380 (6.1 percent) patients were found positive. Since the presence of anti-HBc is evidence of previous infection, the occurrence of antigenemia in three of the positive patients when they were immunosuppressed after transplant was interpreted to be due to reactivation of latent infection.

The individual viruses that cause disease in the transplant patient population are discussed separately below.

CYTOMEGALOVIRUS. Cytomegalovirus (CMV) was initially incriminated as a potential cause of disease in organ transplant recipients by Hill and co-workers [87]. Subsequently, prospective studies with virus isolation procedures and serial serologic determinations have indicated the incidence of CMV infection in renal allograft recipients to be 22 to 96 percent [60,136]. The clinical importance of CMV in such patients, however, has been difficult to evaluate, because this virus is often found incidentally at autopsy in various organs.

In most organ transplant series, cases of CMV pneumonitis have been observed that appear related to the compromised state of the posttransplant patient. A case of fatal CMV pneumonia in a renal transplant recipient was reported in 1965 by Hedley-Whyte and Craighead [85]. Rifkind and associates [161] in 1967 found evidence of CMV in the lungs of 27 of 51 (52 percent) autopsied renal transplant patients. In several of these patients, multiple small (2 to 4 mm.) nodular densities were seen scattered throughout both lung fields on chest radiographs; at autopsy, cytomegalic cells were found in the nodules in all but one patient. In all patients who demonstrated pulmonary cytomegalic cells in association with pneumonia, another infectious agent was also found in the lungs. They concluded that CMV may be of importance in such patients in two regards: first, in the production of clinical disease and, second, in predisposing to pulmonary involvement with additional infectious agents. Neiman and associates [139,140] in reviewing the experience at the University of Washington with 80 consecutive bone-marrow transplant recipients, found interstitial pneumonia to be a serious complication in 43 patients; in 28 of these cases, the outcome was fatal. It occurred principally in the first three months following transplantation. In 20 of these 43 patients, there was histologic, culture, or serologic evidence of infection with CMV. *Pneumocystis carinii* alone (four cases) or with CMV (five cases), and HSV alone (two cases) or with CMV (one case), accounted for the remaining cases in which an etiology was determined. The data also suggested that patients with poor or absent serologic responses to CMV tended to develop disseminated infection with fatal pneumonia, whereas those with rises in antibody titers to CMV either showed no clinical symptoms attributable to CMV or developed only transient pneumonia.

A causal role of CMV has been suggested in the production of cryptogenic fever and atypical lymphocytosis (CMV mononucleosis) occurring within three months following transplantation. In 1969, Balakrishnan and associates [9] reported a case of a renal allograft recipient who developed fever and atypical lymphocytosis one month after transplantation. The findings lasted one week and subsided. CMV was isolated during and after this illness from blood and urine, and serial CF antibody tests demonstrated a rise in titer. Anderson and Spencer [2] described three similar patients the same year. All had a rise in CF antibody titers and self-limited clinical illness between the forty-third and eighty-third posttransplant day. Fine and co-workers [61] cited nine renal allograft recipients who developed prolonged fever and hematologic abnormalities (leukopenia, lymphocytosis, thrombocytopenia, and anemia) during the first three months following transplantation. CMV was incriminated as the causative agent by the findings of viremia, viuria, a rise in CF antibody titer, or a combination in each patient. The difficulty in interpreting the data in some of these cases is that CMV has been isolated and a rise in the CF antibody titer has been documented in asymptomatic allograft recipients. If such clinical episodes were due to CMV, there is no way of knowing whether they were due to a recently acquired infection or to reactivation of a latent infection.

Between April 1970 and October 1971, 13 (38 percent) of 34 renal transplants at Stanford University Hospital developed a clinical syndrome that may represent another manifestation of CMV disease in the organ transplant recipient [40]. About 40 days following transplantation, daily fevers began and recurred for periods of four to six weeks; the fever frequently occurred in conjunction with a diffuse interstitial pneumonitis and impaired hepatic and renal function. In three of the four patients in whom liver biopsy was performed, inclusion bodies characteristic of CMV were seen, and CMV was cultured from the liver biopsy specimen of one patient. Two of the patients with pneumonitis had inclusion bodies in sections of lung biopsy material, and in one of these, inclusion bodies were seen in the kidney as well. Armstrong and associates [5] reported a case of hepatitis that was presumably secondary to CMV infection, and in the previously mentioned nine cases reported by Fine and co-workers [61], there was evidence of hepatitis in two and of pneumonitis in three. In two of their three patients with pulmonary involvement, CMV was recovered from the lung at autopsy.

The diffuse interstitial pneumonitis described in renal transplant patients at Stanford University Hospital [40] and by Fine and colleagues [61] is consistent with what Rifkind called "transplantation pneumonia" [163]. Subsequent reports have adopted the term "transplant lung," since this term does not necessarily suggest an infectious cause. Episodes of transplant lung frequently follow a rejection crisis or a reduction in the dosage of corticosteroids. The clinical picture is characterized by fever, pulmonary infiltrates, and arterial hypoxemia. The episodes have occurred both early and late following transplantation, and various causes have been considered for this entity. Slapak and associates [183] and Jeannet and associates [98] have suggested that immunologic cross-reactivity between the kidney and lung might explain the association of transplant rejection and pulmonary infiltrates. The presence at autopsy of CMV and *P. carinii* in the lungs of some of these patients has suggested an infectious cause [163]. Uranga and co-workers [204] have presented cases that are typical of transplant lung that responded to vigorous diuretic therapy. They suggested that with renal graft rejection, there often are fever, subsequent water retention, and pulmonary congestion. Instead of the blanket term "transplant lung," which suggests numerous diagnoses and possible therapeutic modalities, it is wisest to approach each case from the differential diagnosis of pulmonary infiltrative disease.

Luby and associates [119] from the University of Texas Southwestern Medical School, in an attempt to define the occurrence of hepatitis after renal transplantation and to delineate its relation to CMV, screened 44 consecutive recipients of renal transplants both before and after transplantation for titers to CMV, herpes simplex virus, type 1 (HSV$_1$), and hepatitis B antigen (HBAg). Twenty of these patients developed evidence of hepatitis following transplantation. Eleven did not have HBAg, and nine of these had hepatitis while undergoing seroconversion to CMV. The attack rate of HBAg-negative hepatitis was higher in persons who had greater maximal rises in antibody titer to CMV. Based on these data, the authors felt that CMV may be an important cause of hepatic functional abnormality in the transplant recipient.

Involvement of the central nervous system by CMV in the transplant population was first described by Schneck [171] in 1965, who noted a glial-nodule encephalitis in renal transplant recipients who had histologic evidence of CMV infection in other organs. In 1973, Dorfman [49] described three renal transplant patients at Stanford University Hospital who developed encephalitis as a late complication of CMV infection. The cerebral involvement was difficult to diagnose with certainty ante mortem, because the clinical findings were nonspecific, and the cerebrospinal fluid was normal in the two patients in whom this test was done. At autopsy, each of the patients had widespread glial-nodule encephalitis without meningitis or perivascular inflammatory-cell infiltration. Cytomegalic cells were found in one patient, and the virus was cultured from body fluids in each case, but not from brain or cerebrospinal fluid.

CMV may also be associated with transplant rejection. In 1970, Simmons and co-workers [181] suggested that mild febrile illnesses appeared to precede and accompany renal graft functional deterioration; this deterioration was consistent with allograft rejection. Others noted this same association, and in 1974, Lopez and associates [117] strengthened this hypothesis. Screening 61 immunosuppressed renal transplant patients for viral infection, they found that patients without viral infections were usually asymptomatic, whereas those with viral infections had a characteristic syndrome of fever, leukopenia, and renal allograft rejection. These viruses were all herpesviruses, and more than 75 percent were CMV, which suggested a pathogenic relationship between virus infections and graft rejection episodes. The two mechanisms postulated to explain this relationship were (1) the virus acts as an adjuvant and triggers the rejection of the allograft, or (2) the allograft rejection activates a latent viral infection. Betts and associates [16] have evaluated the influence of CMV infection on the outcome of renal allografts in 91 consecutive patients. Reactivation of latent infection occurred in half (45 patients). Primary infection, which occurred when a seronegative recipient received an allograft from a seropositive donor, was significantly associated with clinical illness in the second and third months following transplant and with allograft rejection [16]. Rand and associates [153] demonstrated that cardiac transplant patients who were seronegative for CMV before transplantation had both a significantly greater overall mortality and a higher bacterial pulmonary infection rate than those who were seropositive. Also, those who survived long enough to demonstrate CMV seroconversion had a significantly increased incidence of bacterial pneumonia and abscess in the first 90 days after transplantation.

At postmortem examination, CMV has also been cultured or seen in many other organs of transplant recipients, including the submandibular glands, adrenals, ureters, parathyroid glands, and lymph nodes [213], as well as retina and pancreas. The role of CMV as a cause of disease is less clear in such circumstances, except for retinal and pancreas involvement. Wyhinny and co-workers [219] described a case of CMV retinitis in a 27-year-old patient with a renal transplant. The diagnosis was made by what the authors felt to be distinctive fundal findings of CMV retinitis: broad yellow-white, granular, necrotic lesions admixed with patches of flame-shaped intraretinal hemorrhage. These findings were confirmed to be due to CMV on postmortem examination. Acute hemorrhagic pancreatitis caused death in two renal transplant patients reported by Tilney and associates [202] from the Peter Bent Brigham Hospital. Virus particles consistent with CMV were cultured from the pancreas in one patient, and, although no virus was cultured from the pancreas of the other, CMV was cultured in the lungs post mortem.

HERPES SIMPLEX VIRUS. Herpes simplex virus (HSV) may cause fulminant and lethal disease in the transplant recipient, or the infection may be benign. Of the first 70 heart transplant patients at Stanford University Hospital, two patients died of disseminated HSV infec-

tion, and one other had cutaneous and pulmonary lesions. Montgomerie and associates [129] reported four cases of severe HSV infection in renal transplant recipients. The infection produced extensive lesions on the face, mouth, and neck. One patient died as a result of herpetic lesions involving the face, mouth, esophagus, ileum, and anogenital areas; in the other three, the infection was considered an important factor in causing death. In reporting on intercurrent infections in 32 heart transplant patients from Houston, Texas, Montgomerie and co-workers [127] noted that 25 percent had apparent cutaneous infection with HSV. HSV may also involve the lungs in the transplant patient population. Douglas and associates [50] reported a case of a patient with a lung transplant who developed oral ulcerations secondary to HSV postoperatively. The allograft developed an infiltrate, and the patient died. At autopsy, HSV was cultured from both tracheal aspirates and lung biopsy material; electron microscopy revealed intracellular, HSV-like particles. A renal transplant patient was reported who died with HSV laryngotracheitis, bronchopneumonia, and esophagitis; CMV was also present in his lungs and pancreas [112].

Contrary to the preceding reports, Spencer and Anderson [187] noted that of the 55 living renal transplant patients in their study, 16 had suffered from HSV lesions about the mouth before transplantation. In only one of these was there an increased occurrence after transplantation; six of these patients thought they had fewer outbreaks. There were four cases of labial herpes following the transplant, two of which persisted for a prolonged period of time (two to three months).

VARICELLA-ZOSTER. The frequency of disease due to varicella-zoster (V-Z) infection in the transplant population may be no greater than the 9 percent reported in the noncompromised host over 50 years of age [90]. From Denmark, Spencer and Anderson [187] reported that 7 of 74 patients with renal transplants developed typical zoster lesions between 84 and 686 days following the surgical procedure; none was disseminated. Turcotte [203] noted three cases in 101 consecutive renal transplant patients. There have been four cases of localized herpes zoster in the first 70 heart transplant patients at Stanford University Hospital. Rifkind [159] reported herpes zoster in six (8.2 percent) of the first 73 patients with renal transplants at the University of Colorado. None was accompanied by complications. In five of the six patients, V-Z appeared 5 to 23 days following the use of local radiation therapy, either for "therapeutic antirejection" or for diagnostic purposes. All six cases were accompanied by a prompt rise in antibody titer to V-Z. Rifkind postulated that the figure of 9 percent incidence in individuals over 50 years old may represent the percentage of persons in whom V-Z virus persists in a state of latency following initial varicella infection.

Death due to V-Z has been described in transplant patients. Calne and co-workers [27] reported a case of hemorrhagic varicella in a patient four weeks after a renal transplant, and of the four renal transplant patients who died of viral infection that were reported by Eickhoff [55], one had disseminated V-Z infection.

HEPATITIS. The significance of the presence of hepatitis B antigenemia or hepatitis in a transplant recipient candidate is unclear. In reviewing 140 renal transplants at the Medical College of Virginia from 1962 to 1968, Moore and Hume [130] found hepatitis to be one of the more hazardous complications. Fifteen of their patients were afflicted with hepatitis from 60 days to 54 months after the procedure, with most cases occurring between 60 and 108 days. Six of these 15 patients died due to hepatic failure. Also, the hepatitis was four times as frequent and three times as lethal in the cadaver-donor recipient. Although no virologic or serologic studies were done, the authors felt that an agonal viremia resulting from hepatic cell lysis and the release of intracellular virus may occur in cadaver-donor recipients and account for the greater incidence of hepatitis in such patients. Pattison and co-workers [144] from Stockholm reported 23 cases of hepatitis in 88 renal transplant patients; 14 were tested for hepatitis B surface antigen (HB$_s$Ag), and 11 were positive. Hepatic insufficiency was considered an important complication in five of the nine who

died. Pirson and associates [147] studied 121 renal graft recipients to determine the effects of HB$_s$Ag antigenemia on patient and graft survival. Although HB$_s$Ag antigenemia appeared to have no effect on graft or patient survival in the first 24 months following transplantation, from 36 months onward there was an increased number of patients with severe liver disease and decreased patient survival in the carriers of this antigen [147]. Arnoff and associates [6] reported 13 patients with hepatitis among 125 renal transplant patients over a seven-year period; five died, two from acute hepatic failure, and in three, the hepatic dysfunction appeared to be a major factor in causing death. Fifteen patients with hepatitis were tested for HB$_s$Ag and 12 were positive. On the basis of these findings, the authors concluded that HB$_s$Ag antigenemia persisting beyond three months prior to transplantation should be considered a contraindication to the transplantation procedure.

In contrast to the above experiences, the results of other workers suggest that hepatitis B antigenemia should not exclude patients from transplantation. Briggs and co-workers [23] from the Peter Bent Brigham Hospital reported a major outbreak (38 patients) of hepatitis that affected dialysis and transplant patients, medical personnel, and one patient's spouse between March 1969 and July 1970. The immunosuppressed posttransplant patients had a benign clinical course compared with the dialysis patients and the contact cases. Azathioprine therapy adversely influenced the course of hepatitis in some posttransplant patients, and its temporary discontinuation was associated with rapid clinical and biochemical recovery and with a change from positive to negative test results for HBAg in two of four patients. Starzl and Putnam [193] reported that about 12 percent of renal transplant recipients were HBAg-positive before transplantation; hepatic dysfunction correlated poorly with antigenemia and occurred with almost equal frequency in HBAg-negative recipients. Steiness and Shinhoj [195] described 12 patients who were HB$_s$Ag-positive after renal transplantation. Retrospectively, pretransplant serum specimens were tested in four, and HB$_s$Ag was present in three. These patients were all well, and only one became jaundiced. Chatterjee and colleagues [34] from the University of Southern California examined 16 renal transplant patients who were HB$_s$Ag-positive before transplantation and 7 patients who developed HB$_s$Ag antigenemia after the procedure. They did not find serious hepatic disease in any patients given transplants, either in the presence of chronic HB$_s$Ag antigenemia before transplantation or when persistent antigenemia was acquired after transplantation. Similar results have been obtained by Shons and co-workers [179] in a case-control study of 35 HB$_s$Ag-positive patients. Both in this study and in the study by Chatterjee and colleagues, the follow-up period was less than 24 months. Recent work has suggested that HB$_s$Ag antigenemia may be associated with an improved early graft survival. London and associates [116] studied the relation between host response to hepatitis B infection before transplantation and the survival of renal homografts in 79 patients receiving 87 transplants. Homograft recipients with antibody to HB$_s$Ag prior to transplant had early graft rejection, whereas recipients with prior HB$_s$ antigenemia had delayed graft rejection. Cuthbert and associates [42] were unable to confirm these associations in a retrospective study of 158 patients receiving 160 renal transplants at Parkland Memorial Hospital.

From the above information, it is obvious that the risks of renal transplantation in patients with HB$_s$Ag antigenemia remain controversial, whereas the risks involved in chronic dialysis are well defined (e.g., shunt infections, surgical procedures for new shunts, and the like). Therefore, HB$_s$Ag antigenemia alone does not necessarily appear to be a contraindication to organ transplantation. Further information on the natural history of the carrier state of HB$_s$Ag, including determination of the presence of Dane particles, DNA polymerase, e antigen, and anti-e, is needed. Until then, however, it appears that the prevention of hepatitis B may be an important factor in improving the long-term survival of renal transplant patients.

EPSTEIN-BARR VIRUS. Although it is known that immunosuppressive drugs are associated with the reactivation of latent Epstein-Barr virus (EBV) infections in transplant patients, there is little information on how these patients respond clinically to primary EBV infections [31,198]. Grose and colleagues [79] have reported a case of a child with a renal homograft and a primary EBV infection. He developed a clinical picture of fever and pneumonitis which closely resembled a posttransplant syndrome associated with CMV infection.

POLYOMAVIRUS. Coleman and co-workers [39] from St. Mary's Hospital in London studied 74 renal transplant recipients with functioning allografts to detect polyomavirus infection of the urinary tract. Over a period of two years, ten patients were found to excrete this virus, and in four of them, a type of polyomavirus, BK, was isolated. Serologic studies in this same population revealed that 26 of 69 patients had a significant rise in antibody titers to BK antigen, suggesting the presence of an active infection. Gardner [71] had previously found that primary infection with BK occurs in childhood, and antibody is common in the adult population. Thus, reactivation of latent virus during immunosuppressive therapy may have been responsible for the changes in antibody titers. The only human disease with which polyomaviruses have thus far been associated is progressive multifocal leukoencephalopathy, a disease usually found in patients with immunologic defects [121]. Four renal transplant patients have developed this disease, and McCormick and colleagues [123] have suggested that progressive multifocal leukoencephalopathy may be emerging as a "serious problem in renal transplant recipients."

PAPOVAVIRUS. In 1970, Spencer and Anderson [187] in Denmark reported that 42 percent of 74 renal transplant recipients developed verrucae, the incidence increasing with the length of time from transplantation. Koranda and associates [105] studied dermatologic complications in a consecutive series of 200 renal transplant patients. Verrucae developed in 43 percent. These observations are in contrast to the 11 to 16 percent incidence of verrucae expected in the general population, and they suggest that either transplant patients are more frequently exposed to papovaviruses or immunosuppression reactivates latent papovavirus infection.

ADENOVIRUS. Myerowitz and associates [135] have described a 61-year-old woman who died of disseminated adenovirus infection 55 days after receiving a cadaveric renal allograft. The virus was serologically distinct from all known human adenoviral serotypes. Although the source of infection was not clear, the authors speculated that the source was a latent infection in the donor kidney.

Protozoa and Helminths

TOXOPLASMOSIS. *Toxoplasma gondii* is a ubiquitous latent parasite of man; for instance, it infects approximately 50 to 60 percent of the adult population of the United States, 80 to 90 percent of the adult population of much of France, and greater than 90 percent of the adult population of Central America. In recent years, it has become increasingly evident that

this organism can cause severe, often fatal, infections in patients with altered defense mechanisms [166]. In experimental animals, corticosteroids in combination with radiation therapy have been shown to activate latent *Toxoplasma* infection [66].

At least ten transplant patients have had significant *Toxoplasma* infection, and three died of this disease (Table 27-5). From the available data, it was not always possible to determine whether the patients developed disease by reactivation of latent infection or from primary infection. In two of them, it is considered likely that the organism was transmitted with the transplant [167]. Four patients had *Toxoplasma* serologic tests performed before transplantation, and the results were negative. Low or even negative *Toxoplasma* antibody titers, however, may be observed in patients with acute toxoplasmosis who are receiving immunosuppressive drugs [166].

Autopsy findings were reported in nine of the patients, and in seven of them, the central nervous system was involved (Table 27-5).

Table 27-5. Toxoplasma gondii *Infection in Transplant Patients*

Transplant center	Transplant	*Toxoplasma* serology	Tissue involvement at autopsy
Peter Bent Brigham Hospital [158][a]	Renal	Negative prior to transplant; rising after transplant	Brain, lungs, heart, skeletal muscle, liver, testis, parathyroid, kidney
University of California, San Francisco [38]	Renal	Negative prior to transplant	Brain, heart
Hospital Universitaire Brugmann, Brussels [63]	Renal	NR[b]	Brain
Stanford University Hospital [197]	Heart	NR	Lungs
Stanford University Hospital	Heart	NR	Disseminated
Stanford University Hospital [167]	Heart	Negative prior to transplant	Brain
Stanford University Hospital [167]	Heart	Negative prior to transplant	Brain, lungs, heart
Institut Pasteur[c]	Renal	NR	Lungs
University of Colorado [4]	Liver	NR	Brain, heart, lungs, bone marrow, urinary bladder
Albert Einstein College of Medicine [74]	Renal	NR	Brain

[a] Reference number (see References).
[b] Not reported.
[c] Unpublished data.

Two of these patients had symptoms of a diffuse encephalopathy and two of a space-occupying lesion. The rest of the patients had no symptoms referable to the central nervous system. Although all organs of the body may be infected with *Toxoplasma* during the acute and latent infection, the central nervous system appears to be remarkably vulnerable in adults with advanced malignancy and in those receiving immunosuppressive therapy [155,205].

STRONGYLOIDES STERCORALIS. Rogers and Nelson [164], in commenting on the opportunistic nature of helminths in general and on *Strongyloides stercoralis* in particular, have stated that "if a lowly fungus can be called 'opportunistic,' surely the opprobrium can be applied to a parasitic worm invading a weakened host."

S. stercoralis usually infects only the mucosa of the small intestine. Hyperinfection, or invasion of other organs by filariform larvae,

usually occurs only in the compromised host; it is a life-threatening condition. Puritilo and co-workers [152] cited 32 patients with strongyloidiasis who were studied at autopsy. All had underlying disease characterized by depressed cell-mediated immunity. Although none of these patients had received transplants, they warned that the transplant group also might be threatened by fatal strongyloidiasis. To our knowledge, this had been reported only once. Fagundes and associates [59] from Brazil mentioned a renal transplant recipient who died as a result of massive infection due to *S. stercoralis*.

PNEUMOCYSTIS CARINII. *P. carinii* pneumonia may be the most common cause of interstitial pneumonitis in the transplant patient population. Table 27-6 gives details on six of the first 70 heart transplant patients at Stanford University Hospital, in whom a diagnosis of this disease was made between January 1968

Table 27-6. Stanford Heart Transplant Patients with Pneumocystic carinii Infection *

Transplant series number	Organ involved	Onset of *P. carinii* infection (days post transplant)	Treatment of *P. carinii*	Other infections	Outcome
2	Lung	46	Pentamidine	Bacteremia, urinary tract infection	Death due to *P. carinii* infection
6	Lung	65 (diagnosis made at autopsy)	None	Pneumonia (*E. coli,* bacteroides, *Aspergillus, Toxoplasma,* [CMV], urinary tract infection)	Death due to pneumonia
43	Lung	215	Pentamidine	Pulmonary abscess (*Nocardia*)	*P. carinii* infection eradicated
47	Lung	80	Pentamidine	Pulmonary abscess (*Aspergillus*), pneumonia (*E. coli*)	*P. carinii* infection eradicated
31	Lung	253 (diagnosis made at autopsy)	None	Peritonitis, pulmonary abscess (*Aspergillus*), bacteremia, pneumonia (*S. aureus*), herpes zoster	Death due to *P. carinii* infection
52	Lung	100	Pentamidine	Bronchitis	*P. carinii* infection eradicated

* Among the first 70 heart transplant recipients.

and May 1974. This represents an incidence of 8.6 percent. Since that time, seven additional patients among the 121 heart transplants performed to March 1977 have had *P. carinii* pneumonia. In reviewing the 264 renal transplant patients at risk between 1968 and 1972 at the University of Colorado, Eickhoff [55] cited 25 episodes of pneumocystosis in 24 patients, an incidence of 9.5 percent. Fourteen of these patients died, eleven secondary to respiratory failure. Eickhoff considered that these figures seriously underestimated the overall risk of infection by this organism, since most of these diagnoses were made at autopsy. The experience at Auckland Hospital, New Zealand, with 81 cadaveric renal transplant patients was reviewed in 1973 by Doak and associates [47]. Eleven patients developed dyspnea, hypoxia, and pulmonary infiltrates ("transplant lung") 38 to 390 days after transplantation. Seven patients died of respiratory failure, and at necropsy, *P. carinii* was found in five of the six patients examined. One other patient was shown to have pneumocystosis by lung biopsy.

The characteristic clinical picture of this disease in the transplant population is that of the insidious onset of nonproductive cough, dyspnea, and tachypnea, with or without fever, several months after the transplantation. The typical chest roentgenogram appearance is that of bilateral perihilar interstitial infiltrates that progress to an alveolar confluence, with sparing of the apices and peripheral lung fields. This "typical" clinical and roentgenographic appearance is often not present. One reason for this is that the patient with pneumocystosis frequently has other organisms infecting his lungs as well.

Table 27-7 is adapted from a review of the first ten renal transplant patients at the University of Colorado who died with *P. carinii* pneumonia [160]. The group is biased by the fact that it is an autopsy series, but it does illustrate something of the spectrum of organisms with which *Pneumocystis* may be associated. The association with CMV has been noted in other transplant series as well. Wang and co-workers [207] reported a case of combined *P. carinii* and CMV infection in a renal transplant recipient. Based upon light and electron microscopic data, the authors suggested that *P. carinii* may contain CMV and act as an intermediate host for this DNA virus. Rifkind and associates

Table 27-7. Concomitant Infections Seen with Pneumocystis carinii *Pneumonia at the University of Colorado in Renal Transplant Cases*

Patient no. in transplant series	Age	Sex	Infections	
			Pulmonary	Extrapulmonary
LD 19	17	M	CMV	CMV (generalized)
LD 36	43	M	CMV	*Staphylococcus* (septicemia)
LD 47	40	M	CMV, *Aspergillus*	CMV (stomach), sporozoan (liver, heart)
LD 56	26	F	None	None
LD 66	38	M	CMV, *Nocardia*	None
LD 76	27	M	*Aspergillus, Pseudomonas*	None
LD 82	36	M	CMV	CMV (brain)
LD 83	21	F	CMV, *Staphylococcus, Pseudomonas*	CMV (kidney)
LD 97	17	M	CMV, *Nocardia*	None
SD 3	17	M	*Aspergillus, Histoplasma*	*Aspergillus* (brain)

Adapted from Rifkind, D., et al. *Ann. Intern. Med.* 65:943, 1966.

[160] suggested that the association of these two organisms may be coincidental. Of 51 autopsies in renal transplant patients, there were 10 patients with pneumocystosis, and CMV was found in the lungs of 27 patients (53 percent) [160].

Although *P. carinii* is thought of as a pulmonary pathogen, cases of extrapulmonary pneumocystosis have been reported. A renal transplant patient reported by Awen and Baltzan [7], for example, who died of *P. carinii* pneumonitis was found at autopsy to have this organism in hilar lymph nodes, pericardium, thymic capsule, ascending colon, liver, pancreas, homograft kidney, periureteral retroperitoneal tissue, hard palate of the mouth, and bone marrow, in addition to the lungs.

The pathogenesis and epidemiology of *P. carinii* infection in the transplant population requires further elucidation. Attempts to assess accurately the prevalence and infectivity of the organism have been hampered by an inability to propagate the agent on artificial media or tissue culture. Most available evidence favors the hypothesis that overt *P. carinii* infection represents activation of prior latent infection.

This has been demonstrated in animal models [65,86], and subclinical or latent infection with the parasite has been documented in man [177, 211]. That an exogenous source may be important for the development of clinical disease by *P. carinii* is suggested by data such as those of Rifkind and associates who noted that all ten of their cases of pneumocystis in renal transplant patients occurred at Colorado General Hospital; none occurred in the patients at the Denver Veterans Administration Hospital [160]. Because the two hospitals are located within a block of each other and because all patients were treated by the same surgical and medical teams, an environmental source of infection is suggested.

Fungi and Nocardia
The major fungi that cause infection in transplant patients are shown in Table 27-8. Relatively little is known about normal host resistance against such agents, and the specific defects predisposing to fungal infection in transplant recipients are unknown. Rifkind and associates [162], in evaluating 23 renal transplant patients with fungal infections who came to au-

Table 27-8. Fungal Infections in Transplant Patients

Transplant center	No. of patients in series	Time of diagnosis	Type of transplant	Organism				Total fungal infections
				Aspergillus	*Candida*	Phycomycetes	Other[a]	
Stanford University Hospital	70	Premortem, autopsy	Heart	20	4	2	4	30
University of Colorado [67][b]	23	Premortem, autopsy	Liver	0	20	0	2	22
Baylor Medical Center [128]	32	Premortem, autopsy	Heart	0	4	1	0	5
University of Michigan [203]	22	Autopsy	Renal	2	0	0	0	2
University of Minnesota [181]	46	Autopsy	Renal	3	6	0	1	10
University of Colorado [162]	51	Autopsy	Renal	7	14	0	2	23
Massachusetts General Hospital [8]	54	Premortem, autopsy	Renal	11	2	1	2	16
St. Mary's Hospital, London [149]	65	Premortem, autopsy	Renal	6	2	0	0	8

a Infections caused by *Penicillium, Histoplasma, Cryptococcus,* and unspecified organisms.
b Reference number (see References).

topsy, found no correlation between the occurrence of these fungal infections and the duration of high-dose (40 mg. or more of prednisone daily) corticosteroid therapy. The patients did not receive antibiotics for significantly longer periods than patients who escaped fungal infection. Bach and co-workers [8] reviewed 20 fungal and nocardial infections that occurred in 51 renal transplant patients and found a statistically significant correlation between infections with such agents and the treatment of rejection episodes. This relationship was magnified if the rejection episodes were multiple or occurred 30 days or more after transplantation. Gurwith and colleagues [80] suggested that the high incidence of *Aspergillus* infections in heart transplant patients at Stanford University Hospital might be related to the use of antilymphocyte globulin (ALG). In most series in which antilymphocyte globulin has been used in conjunction with azathioprine and prednisone, however, an increased incidence of fungal or nocardial infection that can be correlated with this treatment (ALG) has not been observed [126].

The role of sex hormones in predisposing the transplant patient to fungal infection has been suggested by Rifkind and co-workers [162]. They noted that 22 of 23 patients with fungal infection who came to autopsy were males. In contrast, the male-to-female ratio in their entire series of 107 cases was 3 : 1, and in all 51 autopsy cases, it was 5.4 : 1. This greater male-to-female ratio in all autopsy cases as compared to the total series was entirely accounted for by the excess of male patients in the group with systemic fungal infections.

ASPERGILLUS. *Aspergillus,* like *Candida,* is an uncommon cause of serious disease in the noncompromised host. In the transplant patient population, however, these two organisms have accounted for more than 90 percent of serious fungal infections. Of interest is the observation that transplant teams that report frequent systemic fungal infections uncommonly see a high incidence of both of these organisms among such patients; it is usually one or the other that is the major cause of systemic disease at a particular institution (see Table 27-8). The reasons for this are not immediately apparent, and the role of the hospital environment in each series of patients has been implicated but not proved.

Burton and associates [24] cited four cases of aspergillosis in renal transplant patients in which the hospital environment may have been important in the spread of the infection. Over the same six-month period in which these infections occurred, *Aspergillus fumigatus* was isolated from the air ducts in the patient's isolation room, and pigeon excretions were found at the external air inlets. There were no cases of aspergillosis in 20 subsequent renal transplants in the year following the revision of this ventilation system to prevent pigeons from reaching the inlets.

There is considerable experimental work to suggest that corticosteroids, as well as environmental factors, are significant in predisposing the transplant patient to infection with *Aspergillus.* Iwata and co-workers [97] have demonstrated germination of phagocytized *Aspergillus* spores in isolated peritoneal leukocytes from cortisone-treated animals but not in cells from control animals. Of interest, in relation to pulmonary infection with this fungus, Epstein and associates [57] found a significant decrease in the release of lysosomal factors from alveolar macrophages of corticosteroid-treated animals following in vivo phagocytosis of *Aspergillus* spores.

Pulmonary involvement is the most common presentation of aspergillosis in the transplant patient. Each of the 20 heart transplant patients at Stanford University Hospital with aspergillosis cited in Table 27-2 and the five subsequent patients with this infection presented with a pulmonary infiltrate, pulmonary cavitation, or both. The most common pattern in the renal transplant patients studied by Bach and co-workers [8] was sudden onset of pleuritic chest pain, a pleural friction rub, tachypnea, and fever followed by progressive hypoxemia, production of pulmonary infiltrates, and a rapidly fatal outcome. Infection with *Aspergillus* in the transplant population may less commonly present as acute bacterial sepsis or as gastrointestinal bleeding secondary to *Aspergillus* invasion of the bowel.

Regardless of the type of presentation, when

a transplant patient develops infection with *Aspergillus,* the data suggest that the prognosis for survival is poor. All 11 of the 51 renal transplant patients at Boston City Hospital between 1969 and 1971 (premortem and postmortem data) who became infected with *Aspergillus* died [8]. Of these 11, *Aspergillus* was judged to be the principal cause of death in eight. Of the 20 cited heart transplant patients at Stanford University Hospital with aspergillosis, only five survived. *Aspergillus* infection was the direct cause of death in seven of these patients and was a major contributing factor of death in three of them.

Although early clinical manifestations of infection with *Aspergillus* are usually referable to the lungs, the fungus is often found in other organs at autopsy. Rifkind and associates [162], for instance, noted that of the six renal transplant patients with aspergillosis at autopsy, only one had this fungus limited to the lungs. Three had involvement of the central nervous system, four of the heart, two of the kidney, and one each of the liver and thyroid. The experience with heart transplant patients at Stanford University Hospital has been similar.

Aspergillosis in transplant patients is frequently associated with other organisms. Simmons and associates [181] noted that in the three patients in whom death was caused by aspergillosis, each was also infected with *Candida.* Of the seven cases of aspergillosis in liver transplant patients at the University of Colorado, one also had *Candida* infection of the heart [173]. Only one of the six renal transplant patients with aspergillosis mentioned by Rifkind and associates [162] had infection solely with this fungus; cytomegalovirus was found in the lungs of three patients, gram-negative bacillary pneumonia in three patients, *P. carinii* pneumonia in two patients, and a sporozoan in the lungs of one patient. Each of our 20 heart transplant patients with aspergillosis had a concomitant viral, fungal, protozoal, or mixed infection.

The diagnosis of pulmonary aspergillosis in patients with acute nonlymphocytic leukemia may be facilitated by nasal cultures [194]. Furthermore, the risk of pulmonary disease in such patients is substantially higher among those who have had prior positive nasal cultures. At present, there have been no reported studies evaluating whether these observations also apply to transplant patients.

CANDIDA. In contrast to *Aspergillus, Candida* is frequently found in fecal specimens and the oropharynx in normal persons, which suggests an endogenous source for infection by this fungus [176]. Although the respiratory tract acts as a portal of entry for *Candida* in certain cases, of 14 patients with systemic candidiasis in one series, four had no pulmonary involvement; instead, invasion of the gastrointestinal tract was found [162]. In all 18 liver transplant patients with *Candida* infection at the University of Colorado, some sort of damage to the gastrointestinal tract or else a surgical complication was obvious clinically or at autopsy [173].

Table 27-9 depicts the types of infections caused by *Candida* in such patients. In contrast to *Aspergillus* infections, there is no typical clinical presentation for patients with deep-seated *Candida* infection. Pulmonary involvement may be asymptomatic with roentgenographic evidence of an abscess, infiltrate, or both; gastrointestinal involvement may be in the form of thrush, esophagitis, or upper or lower gastrointestinal bleeding with or without diarrhea. The patient with fungemia may be asymptomatic or may appear to have gram-negative sepsis.

Involvement of the urinary tract by *Candida* deserves special mention. *Candida* is the most common fungal organism cultured from urine. Unfortunately, the meaning of candiduria is unclear. This fungus has disappeared spontaneously in some renal transplant patients, while in others, the candiduria represented significant upper urinary tract disease. Shelp and coworkers [178] reported a case of *Candida* pyelitis with ureteral obstruction, and Knepshield and associates [104] cited a case of renal papillary necrosis due to *Candida* in renal allograft patients. In both humans and experimental animals with systemic candidiasis, the kidney is frequently the most extensively damaged organ [56]. Thus, candiduria may reflect not only severe local infection, but disseminated disease as well.

As with *Aspergillus* infection, the transplant

Table 27-9. Organ Involvement by Candida *in Transplant Patients*

Transplant center	Number of patients in series	Number of patients with candidiasis	Time of diagnosis	Type of transplant	Site					
					Lung	Urinary tract	Gastro-intestinal tract	Central nervous system	Blood	Other
Stanford University Hospital	70	4	Premortem, autopsy	Heart	1	1	0	0	1	1[b]
University of Colorado [162][a]	51	23	Autopsy	Renal	10	2	8	2	0	3
University of Colorado [167]	23	22	Premortem, autopsy	Liver	4	6	6	0	4	3

[a] Reference number (see References).
[b] Disseminated.

patient infected with *Candida* is usually infected with other organisms. Rifkind and associates [162] found, for example, that all 14 of their autopsy patients with systemic candidiasis were infected with a gram-negative bacillus or *Staphylococcus* as well. In addition, one patient was infected with *Aspergillus* and another with *Nocardia*.

CRYPTOCOCCUS. Cryptococcosis is an infection whose incidence in man is unknown, because of the difficulty in determining inapparent infection. As an increasing proportion of infections by these organisms is being observed in immunologically compromised patients, infection with this fungus can be considered opportunistic [25,84].

The first report of cryptococcosis in a renal allograft recipient was by Slapak and co-workers [183] in 1968; the outcome was fatal. Subsequently, Bach and associates [8] cited two renal transplant patients with cryptococcosis. One, with cryptococcal meningitis, recovered after receiving 2 gm. of amphotericin B. The other, with pulmonary cryptococcosis, received 1.25 gm. of amphotericin B, which was followed by resolution of a lung nodule and elimination of the fungus from his sputum. Simmons and co-workers [181] noted cryptococcosis to be the cause of death in one of 46 septic deaths following renal transplantation. Swenson and colleagues [200] reported a case

of a 40-year-old woman with primary pulmonary cryptococcosis and renal failure. She was treated with amphotericin B, and slight objective improvement of her pulmonary lesions was noted. She then received a renal allograft and, during the postoperative period, received immunosuppressive agents. Twenty-five days following transplantation, her chest roentgenogram demonstrated an exacerbation of the pulmonary disease. This was successfully treated by decreasing the immunosuppressive therapy and by another course of amphotericin B. Woodruff and co-workers [217] from Edinburgh described a patient who developed backache and fever 14 months after her renal transplant. She was found to have *Cryptococcus neoformans* in her cerebrospinal fluid and urine. After 45 days of treatment with amphotericin B, her only evidence of central nervous system dysfunction was mild euphoria.

Schröter and associates [173] from the University of Colorado noted one case of disseminated cryptococcosis among their first 100 liver transplants. The infection was associated with disseminated candidiasis and, in spite of amphotericin therapy, the patient died. Acar and colleagues (personal communication) observed one case of cryptococcal meningitis among 87 renal transplant patients. The patient survived with antimicrobial therapy. The largest series of cryptococcal infections in transplant patients are those reported by Platt and co-workers [148] from the University of California at Los Angeles and by Murphy and co-workers [131] from the University of Michigan. In the former series, six cases of disseminated cryptococcosis in 188 renal transplants were described.

Although the onset was heralded by transient pulmonary infiltrates in four patients, central nervous system involvement occurred in all cases. Cutaneous lesions were noted in three patients, and biopsy specimens from two of these revealed *C. neoformans. Candida albicans* was isolated in four of the six cases, and this organism persisted in one case after *Cryptococcus* was isolated. All patients were treated with amphotericin B, and three were alive at five months after the diagnosis of their disease.

In the series of Murphy and co-workers [131], *C. neoformans* caused seven cases of meningitis in 149 renal transplant recipients. The authors speculated that this high rate of infection might be related to the ability of this organism to use creatinine as a nitrogen source and a consequent preference for patients with renal failure. Although most cases of cryptococcosis in transplant patients are thought to be due to reactivation of latent infection, on at least one occasion transmission of *C. neoformans* probably occurred by way of the corneal transplant tissue [17].

COCCIDIOIDES. Immunosuppressive drug therapy has been associated with primary and relapse coccidioidomycosis, but there is no evidence as yet that *Coccidioides* is a common opportunistic invader [44]. Of the 41 cases of coccidioidomycosis seen between 1961 and 1969 at Stanford University Hospital, only two occurred in compromised hosts [84]. One of these cases was a patient who had been diagnosed four years prior to renal transplantation as having coccidioidal pulmonary nodules. The administration of immunosuppressive drugs following transplantation led to disseminated coccidioidomycosis that caused the patient's death. The diagnosis was not made ante mortem. Schröter and colleagues [172] have reported two cases of coccidioidomycosis in a group of more than 750 renal transplant recipients. The first patient died of unsuspected disseminated coccidioidomycosis six days after his second transplantation. The second patient had pulmonary coccidioidomycosis treated by lobectomy and amphotericin B before transplant. At a five-year posttransplant follow-up, there was no evidence of recurrence. Table 27-10 displays other cases of coccidioidomycosis that have been reported in transplant patients.

PHYCOMYCETES. Fungi of the order Phycomycetes are usually encountered as innocuous human saprophytes. In the United States,

Table 27-10. Cases of Coccidioidomycosis in Transplant Patients

Transplant center	Type of transplant	Site(s) of involvement	Treatment	Outcome
Peter Bent Brigham Hospital [215][a]	Renal	Meninges	Amphotericin B	Fatal
Wadsworth VA Hospital [43, 143]	Renal	Disseminated	No data	Fatal
Wadsworth VA Hospital [43, 143]	Renal	Disseminated	Amphotericin B	Survived
Children's Hospital of Pittsburgh [132]	Renal	Lungs, spleen, lymph nodes	No data	Fatal
University of Washington [30]	Renal	Disseminated	Amphotericin B	Fatal
University of Colorado [133]	Renal	Disseminated	None	Fatal
University of Colorado [133]	Renal	Pulmonary	Amphotericin B Lobectomy	Survived
Stanford University Hospital [84]	Renal	Lungs, liver, lymph nodes	None	Fatal

[a] Reference number (see References).

Table 27-11. Cases of Phycomycosis in Transplant Patients

Transplant center	Type of transplant	Site(s) of involvement	Treatment	Outcome	Other infections
University of Colorado [196][a]	Renal	Nasal	Amphotericin B, surgical	Cure	None
Baylor Medical Center [127]	Heart	Disseminated	None	Died	Herpes simplex, bacterial peritonitis
Stanford University Hospital	Heart	Rhino-cerebral	Amphotericin B	Cure with residual CNS damage	Bacterial septicemia, CMV (serology)
Massachusetts General Hospital [8]	Renal	Liver	None	Died	*Aspergillus, Candida* (both disseminated)
St. Mary's Hospital, London [95]	Renal	Lung	None	Died	Pneumocystosis
Chaim Sheba Medical Center, Tel Aviv [22]	Renal	Rhino-cerebral	Amphotericin B	Cure	None
Chaim Sheba Medical Center, Tel Aviv [22]	Renal	Rhino-cerebral	Amphotericin B	Cure	*Pseudomonas aeruginosa* osteomyelitis

[a] Reference number (see References).

infection with these fungi almost always develops under conditions of impaired host resistance. The rhinocerebral form has been classically associated with uncontrolled diabetes mellitus, while the pulmonary or disseminated form is characteristic of the immunosuppressed patient. This has not been the case, however, with transplant patients (Table 27-11). Although mucormycosis is an opportunistic infection, it accounts for only a small proportion of the fungal infections reported in transplant patients.

NOCARDIA. Opportunistic infection due to *Nocardia* has caused serious morbidity and death in transplant patients. At Stanford University Hospital, seven of the first 70 heart transplant patients have been infected with this organism. Data on these patients, including the sites of involvement, are shown in Table 27-12. In one patient, extensive destruction of the muscles of the leg due to spread of nocardial infection from an adjacent subcutaneous abscess necessitated amputation of the leg. Interestingly, all these cases appeared in a 22-month period from March 1971 to January 1973 [106]. In only one of the patients who definitely developed the infection in the hospital could a nosocomial source be implicated. Following the report of these seven cases, we have

observed an additional nine heart transplant patients with *Nocardia* infection among the total of 121 heart transplant patients (data as of March 1977). Bach and associates [8] diagnosed five cases of *Nocardia* infection in 51 renal transplant patients. In four patients, the infection presented with fever, dry cough, and pulmonary infiltrates or nodules, and *Nocardia* organisms were detected by Gram stain and culture of the sputum. The sudden appearance of skin nodules heralded the onset of disease in the remaining patient. All patients were treated, and they experienced clearing of their lesions. Rifkind and co-workers [162] cited two autopsy cases of *Nocardia* infection. Both presented with pulmonary symptoms. One had disease localized (along with CMV and *P. carinii*) to the lungs; the other had disseminated infection. Neither had been treated for their *Nocardia* infection. One case of *Nocardia* pulmonary infection in 87 renal transplant patients was personally reported to us by Acar and his colleagues in Paris.

OTHER FUNGI. Rifkind and associates [162] noted two cases of histoplasmosis in 51 renal transplant autopsy cases; one of them also had aspergillosis. King and Kraikitpanitch [101] observed two renal transplant patients who developed granulomatous subcutaneous

Table 27-12. Nocardia *Infections in Heart Transplant Patients at Stanford University Hospital**

Patient number in transplant series	Onset of infection (months posttransplant)	Site of involvement	Treatment	Outcome
54	29½	Lung	Sulfisoxazole, kanamycin	Died (no evidence of lung infection at autopsy)
44	18	Lung, skin	Sulfisoxazole, kanamycin	Died (no evidence of lung infection at autopsy)
48	28	Lung, skin, muscle	Sulfisoxazole, tetracycline, gentamicin, clindamycin, erythromycin, minocycline	Infection suppressed
36	2	Lung	Sulfisoxazole, kanamycin	Infection suppressed
47	3½	Lung	Sulfisoxazole, kanamycin	Died of pulmonary aspergillosis
32	8	Lung	Sulfisoxazole	Infection suppressed
19	7½	Lung	Sulfisoxazole	Death due to other causes; *Nocardia* pulmonary abscess found at autopsy

* Among the first 70 heart transplants.

nodules caused by *Histoplasma capsulatum* with other evidence of disseminated disease. To our knowledge, only one case of blastomycosis (causing pneumonia only) has been reported in transplant patients. Young and co-workers [221] described an infection due to *Phoma* species occurring in a patient with a transplanted kidney who had been maintained on prolonged immunosuppressive therapy prior to the clinical appearance of the infection. *Penicillium* species caused pulmonary lesions in one heart transplant patient at Stanford University Hospital.

Classification of Infections

Clinical disease caused by these agents and having onset during hospitalization should be considered a nosocomial infection, even though the source of the organism may have been endogenous. This approach is consistent with that employed in classifying other infections. Urinary tract infections, for example, which are commonly caused by endogenous bacteria, are classified as nosocomial if their onsets occur during hospitalization. Clinically significant infections with onset within the first few months after discharge are more difficult to classify. Such episodes should probably be considered community-acquired unless (1) subclinical ac-

tivity of the infection was detected during hospitalization (e.g., shedding of or colonization with the organism, serologic or skin test responses, and so on) or (2) nosocomial acquisition of the organism is probable based on incubation periods, when applicable, or on known exposures of the patient during hospitalization.

Except for their effect on surveillance data, such distinctions are of limited importance at present. Nosocomial infections in these compromised hosts may, however, ultimately become more amenable to control. All nosocomial infections caused by exogenous organisms in these patients are theoretically preventable, but effective methods do not currently exist to prevent all of them. Even those infections caused by endogenous organisms may eventually become controllable, as advances are made in chemotherapeutic agents and methods of immunosuppression.

Diagnosis, Treatment, and Prevention
Diagnosis
The increased potential for rapid progression of infections in patients on immunosuppressive therapy necessitates early instigation of appropriate therapy and, therefore, an aggressive approach to diagnosis [156]. The clinical diagno-

sis of infection in such patients is complicated by the fact that immunosuppressive therapy may mask many typical clinical and laboratory signs of the infection. The roentgenographic changes associated with bacterial pneumonias in the otherwise normal host, for example, may not appear in patients on high-dose corticosteroid or cytotoxic drug therapy, because of the depressed inflammatory response that occurs as a result of such therapy.

Since a number of opportunistic pathogens remain dormant in tissues of normal individuals and become activated in a setting of impaired immunity, diseases caused by such agents should be considered early in the differential diagnosis of infection in the transplant patient (Table 27-13). Latent infection must also be considered in the tissues of the donor. This rate of infection has been highlighted by the case of a 53-year-old male who died from Creutzfeldt-Jakob disease, a slow-virus disease of the central nervous system [52]. A corneal transplant was performed from this patient to a 55-year-old female, and approximately 18 months later, she developed signs and symptoms of central nervous system dysfunction and died eight months later. At autopsy, her brain had the characteristic changes of Creutzfeldt-Jakob disease.

Historical data from the transplant patient that may yield useful diagnostic information before clinical infection occurs include a history of tuberculosis or positive tuberculin skin test, areas of habitation and travel, type of work, and animal exposure. Also, physicians must gain a perspective of the types of infections seen in the transplant patients at their institu-

tion through ongoing surveillance of infections. Such prior knowledge will assist in the approach to the patient in whom infection is being considered. The unusually high incidence of infections by *Nocardia* and *Aspergillus* in heart transplant patients at Stanford University Hospital, for example, has made such organisms prime suspects in those patients who develop pulmonary lesions.

In addition to screening tests on patients (Table 27-14) that may provide information of diagnostic value if the patient subsequently develops infection and the causative agent is unclear at the time infection is suspected, there are certain procedures that maximize the opportunity for detecting the pathogen early enough to institute therapy. Cultures of sputum, urine, and blood should be ordered routinely. It is important to emphasize the collection of sputum, which may have to be induced, rather than that of saliva, which frequently does not reveal or allow recognition of the actual pathogen. In addition, cultures of both stool and cerebrospinal fluid should be obtained if there is any indication that infection exists in the gastrointestinal tract or beyond the blood-cerebrospinal fluid barrier. A lumbar puncture should be performed if a patient has an unexplained fever or if there is suspicion of cryptococcal or coccidioidal infection. When appropriate, cultures should be set up anaerobically as well as aerobically, and they should include media for fungi, bacteria, and mycobacteria.

In addition to culturing procedures, spinal fluid should be examined for cryptococci by India ink preparations and for cryptococcal antigens [76]. If a patient comes from or has been in areas known to be endemic for certain diseases (e.g., coccidioidomycosis in the San Joaquin Valley), appropriate serologic and skin testing [112] should also be performed. Smears—whether obtained from sputum, pus, cerebrospinal fluid, or any other body fluid—should be stained with acid-fast, Gram, and silver (for fungi and *P. carinii*) stains, and potassium hydroxide (KOH) and India ink preparations should be made.

The presence or even suspicion of pulmonary infection necessitates studies that go beyond the routine outlined above. A transtra-

Table 27-13. Organisms Causing Latent Infections in Man that May Be Reactivated in Transplant Recipients

Bacterial:	Fungal:
Mycobacterium	*Cryptococcus*
tuberculosis	*Coccidioides*
Viral:	Helminths:
Cytomegalovirus	*Strongyloides*
Herpes simplex	Other:
Varicella-zoster	*Pneumocystis*
Protozoal:	
Toxoplasma	

Table 27-14. Screening Tests for Transplant Patients

Cultures:	Serologic tests:
Oropharynx or tracheostomy	Cytomegalovirus
	Herpes simplex virus
Urine, stool	*Cryptococcus neoformans*
Intravenous sites	*Coccidioides immitis*
Wounds	*Toxoplasma gondii*
Skin tests:	*Aspergillus* species
Tuberculin	Other:
Coccidioides	Stool examination for ova
Streptokinase-	and parasites
streptodornase	Urine culture and
Mumps	cytology for cyto-
Trichophyton	megalovirus

cheal aspirate should be considered in all patients whose chest roentgenograms are consistent with the diagnosis of pneumonia. An example of the usefulness of this procedure is the experience in the first 20 heart transplant patients at Stanford University Hospital. Sixteen clinically apparent pneumonias among nine individuals were studied with the aid of transtracheal aspiration. Ten of the 12 infections that yielded specific causative diagnoses were bacterial, and in every one of these, multiple bacteria were present in the sputum. In all, transtracheal aspiration was performed 40 times, with only three false-negative results. Lau and co-workers [110] have documented the value of a transtracheal aspirate in the diagnosis of pneumonia due to *Pneumocystis carinii*. The transtracheal aspirate is also useful in monitoring patient response to therapy. This use of the method is particularly appropriate when sputum cultures are negative; the continued presence of organisms can be determined by culturing the aspirate.

If a transtracheal aspirate is negative and there is roentgenographic evidence of increasing pulmonary lesions, direct sampling of lung to obtain tissue for culture and histologic examination is necessary. Bronchial washings with bronchoscopy, transbronchial biopsy, brush biopsy, lung aspiration, and open lung biopsy have all been used with success to achieve this end [73]. At Stanford University Hospital, we usually proceed with direct needle aspiration, and surgery is scheduled the same or following day for open biopsy if the former procedure is

not diagnostic. When open lung biopsy is resorted to, it is advisable to do an impression smear with immediate silver staining or other rapid stain methods (e.g., Giemsa or polychrome methylene blue), rather than wait for the results of permanent sections [100].

The study of material from skin lesions may be of value in identifying an infectious agent. The hallmark of HSV or V-Z, for example, is the presence of multinucleated giant cells; a diagnosis of disseminated *Nocardia* [182] and cryptococcal infection may be made by biopsy of skin nodules; and the lesions seen in *Pseudomonas* sepsis are characteristic enough to suggest the diagnosis [48].

Infection with *Candida* has been particularly difficult to identify ante mortem. In only 2 of 14 renal transplant patients with systemic candidiasis studied by Rifkind and colleagues [162], for example, was the condition diagnosed pre mortem. There are several reasons for this. First, the majority of patients with disseminated candidiasis that is proved by demonstration of the fungus in tissue do not have positive blood cultures ante mortem [92,201]. Second, with regard to the significance of candidemia in a patient who does not have clear evidence of disseminated disease, the data are not adequate to permit reliable differentiation between the patient who needs antifungal therapy because disseminated candidiasis is developing, or is already present, and the patient who does not need treatment because the fungemia is benign and transient. There are clinical and laboratory techniques that may be helpful in making this differentiation. The occurrence of *Candida* endophthalmitis or retinitis indicates disseminated disease [54]. A careful urinalysis may reveal clumps of hyphae and pseudohyphae in patients with candidal renal involvement. Several serologic methods have been analyzed for diagnostic potential. The two that seem to hold the most promise for the early diagnosis of systemic *Candida* infections are the determination of agglutinin and precipitin titers [68,157,201].

Treatment
Table 27-15 lists the preferred agents for treatment of infections caused by certain of the less

Table 27-15. Antimicrobial Agents for Less Familiar Opportunistic Pathogens

Organism	Preferred agent(s)
Nocardia	Sulfonamides
Herpes simplex virus	Adenine arabinoside (?), interferon (?)
Cytomegalovirus	Adenine arabinoside (?)
Varicella-zoster virus	Adenine arabinoside (?), interferon (?)
Toxoplasma gondii	Pyrimethamine plus sulfadiazine or triple sulfonamides
Candida	Amphotericin B, 5-fluorocytosine,[a] miconazole (?)
Cryptococcus neoformans	Amphotericin B, 5-fluorocytosine,[a] miconazole (?)
Aspergillus	Amphotericin B
Phycomycetes	Amphotericin B
Pneumocystic carinii	Pentamidine isethionate, pyrimethamine plus sulfadiazine or triple sulfonamides, and trimethoprim plus sulfamethoxazole

(?) = Efficacy as yet unproved; evaluation of drug is presently in progress.
[a] We do not recommend the use of 5-fluorocystosine alone but in combination with amphotericin B.

familiar opportunistic pathogens. Many of these antimicrobial agents carry with them the hazard of toxicity, and their use is rarely justified unless a specific causal indication has been established.

Whether or not to discontinue or at least to decrease the immunosuppressive therapy that has facilitated the emergence of the infection is a dilemma often faced by the transplant team. In renal transplant patients, where there often is an alternative to transplantation (i.e., dialysis, retransplantation, or both), life-threatening infection usually necessitates discontinuation of immunosuppressive therapy. In other transplant patients, it would only complicate matters to superimpose upon a patient with an already serious infection the problems associated with acute graft rejection.

Appropriate antimicrobial sensitivity testing should be performed on all suspect isolates. It is frequently useful to determine the minimum inhibitory concentration of various antimicrobial agents against the offending organism as well as the serum levels of the antibiotics being used (e.g., aminoglycosides) to make certain an efficacious agent has been chosen and to insure that the frequency and route of administration and dosage are optimal. If such tests are not readily available, the determination of serum killing levels against the patient's own organism may prove helpful [103]. We consider it of utmost importance for there to be close cooperation and open communication between the members of the transplant team, the infectious disease consultant, and the infectious disease diagnostic laboratory. This is well illustrated by the experience at Johns Hopkins Hospital [33].

Prevention

As has previously been pointed out, once infection is established in a transplant patient, appropriate therapy may not necessarily be successful. Certainly, prevention of infection is preferable, and, where applicable, it has been discussed above under the headings of the organ transplant. There are several instances where antimocrobial agents are or may be of prophylactic value. Kemeny and associates [99] from Budapest found that pentamidine isethionate given every other day for 14 days to premature infants prior to the second week of life was efficacious in preventing disease from *P. carinii*. Post and co-workers [150] found that the biweekly administration of the combination of pyrimethamine and sulfadiazine to infants in an Iranian orphanage where *P. carinii* is endemic prior to the second month of life entirely erased pneumocystosis from the institution. Hughes and co-workers [94] demonstrated the efficacy of a combination of trimethoprim and sulfamethoxazole in the prevention of pneumocystosis in cortisone-treated rats and, more recently, in children with leukemia [93].

Other chemotherapeutic modalities that may be effective in preventing disease in the transplant patient include isoniazid for the patient with a positive tuberculin skin test, thiabendazole if the patient is shedding *S. stercoralis* in the stool, and influenza vaccine [28,107] and amantadine hydrochloride [210] to prevent or modify influenza infection.

Studies in nontransplant patients suggest that granulocyte transfusions complement appropriate antibiotic treatment of gram-negative septicemia associated with granulocytopenic patients. Clift and colleagues [37] at the University of Washington used granulocytes prophylactically with bone-marrow transplant patients in a randomized trial. Although there was no substantial difference in survival between the two groups, the transfused group had significantly fewer local and systemic infections than did the control group.

Several groups have demonstrated that life island units and laminar airflow rooms effectively provide a patient environment with a minimal amount of microbial contamination and a substantial reduction in exposure to potential pathogenic organisms [20,113,170,220]. Although no controlled studies have been done in transplant recipients, this environmental protection might be beneficial to transplant patients, because pneumonias due to organisms from an exogenous source are frequent in such groups, especially in the case of heart and lung transplants. Effective suppression of gut flora can be obtained by using nonabsorbable antibiotic regimens [113], and it is possible that this might minimize infection in the hepatic and bone-marrow transplant patients, in whom sepsis from the gastrointestinal flora is common [185]. Although the methods utilized to reduce patient exposure to environmental and gut organisms are expensive, the benefits may be considerable in the prevention of infectious complications in this population. Unfortunately, such methods do not interfere with the infective potential of latent endogenous pathogens. Until controlled studies are completed with transplant patients, no statement can be made regarding the efficacy of these techniques.

References

1. Andersen, H. Complement-fixing and neutralizing antibodies against cytomegalovirus strain AD 169 in sera from infants with cytomegalovirus infection. *Scand. J. Infect. Dis.* 1:141, 1969.
2. Andersen, H., and Spencer, E. Cytomegalovirus infection among renal allograft recipients. *Acta Med. Scand.* 186:7, 1969.
3. Anderson, R., Schafer, L., Olin, D., and Eickhoff, T. Septicemia in renal transplant recipients. *Arch. Surg.* 106:692, 1973.
4. Anthony, C. Disseminated toxoplasmosis in a liver transplant patient. *J. Am. Med. Wom. Assoc.* 27:601, 1972.
5. Armstrong, D., Balakrishnan, S., Steger, L., Yu, B., and Stenzel, K. Cytomegalovirus infections with viremia following renal transplantation. *Arch. Intern. Med.* 127:111, 1971.
6. Arnoff, A., Gualt, M., Huang, S., Lal, S., Wu, K., Moinuddin, M., Spence, L., and MacLean, L. Hepatitis with Australia antigenemia following renal transplantation. *Can. Med. Assoc. J.* 108:43, 1973.
7. Awen, C., and Baltzan, M. Systemic dissemination of *Pneumocystis carinii* pneumonia. *Can. Med. Assoc. J.* 104:809, 1971.
8. Bach, M., Sahyoun, A., Adler, J., Schlesinger, R., Berman, J., Madras, P., P'eng, F., and Monaco, A. High incidence of fungus infection in renal transplant patients treated with antilymphocyte and conventional immunosuppression. *Transplant. Proc.* 5:549, 1973.
9. Balakrishnan, S., Armstrong, D., Rubin, A., and Stenzel, K. Cytomegalovirus infection after renal transplantation. *J.A.M.A.* 207:1712, 1969.
10. Balow, J., and Rosenthal, A. Glucocorticoid suppression of macrophage migration inhibitory factor. *J. Exp. Med.* 137:1031, 1973.
11. Beall, A., Jenkins, D., Weg, J., Stevens, P., Noon, G., Johnson, P., Bell, R., Knight, J., Rossen, R., Butler, W., Douglas, R., Williams, T., Lewis, J., Morgan, R., MacIntyre, R., Anderson, M., Balsaver, A., and DeBakey, M. Human lung allotransplantation. *Am. J. Surg.* 119:300, 1970.
12. Beaty, H. N., Miller, A. A., Broome, C. V., Goings, S., and Phillips, C. A. Legionnaires' disease in Vermont, May to October 1977. *J.A.M.A.* 240:127, 1978.
13. Bell, T. J., and Williams, G. B. Successful treatment of tuberculosis in renal transplant recipients. *J. R. Soc. Med.* 71:265, 1978.
14. Bennett, W., Beck, C., Young, H., and Russell, P. Bacteremia in the first month following renal transplantation. *Arch. Surg.* 101:453, 1970.
15. Betts, R. F., Freeman, R. B., Douglas, R. G., Jr., Talley, T. E., and Rundell, B. Transmission of cytomegalovirus infection with renal allograft. *Kidney Int.* 8:385, 1975.
16. Betts, R. F., May, A. G., and Freeman, R. B. Influence of Cytomegalovirus Infection on Outcome of Renal Allograft (Abstract No. 132). In Program and Abstracts of the 16th Interscience Conference on Antimicrobial Agents and Chemotherapy, October 1976,

Chicago, Ill. Washington, D.C.: American Society for Microbiology, 1976.

17. Beyt, B. E., and Waltman, S. R. Cryptococcal endophthalmitis after corneal transplantation. *N. Engl. J. Med.* 298:825, 1978.

18. Blaese, R., Martinez, C., and Good, R. Immunologic incompetence of immunologically runted animals. *J. Exp. Med.* 119:211, 1964.

19. Blumenstock, D. Transplantation of the lung. *Transplantation* 5(Suppl.):917, 1967.

20. Bodey, G., and Johnston, D. Microbiological evaluation of protected environments during patient occupancy. *Appl. Microbiol.* 22:828, 1971.

21. Boggs, D., Athens, J., Cartwright, G., and Wintrobe, M. The effect of adrenal glucocorticosteroids upon the cellular composition of inflammatory exudates. *Am. J. Pathol.* 44:763, 1964.

22. Braj, Z. F., Altman, G., and Ostfeld, E. Fungal infections after renal transplantation. *Isr. J. Med. Sci.* 12:674, 1976.

23. Briggs, W., Lazarus, J., Birtch, A., Hampers, C., Hager, E., and Merrill, J. Hepatitis affecting hemodialysis and transplant patients. *Arch. Intern. Med.* 132:21, 1973.

24. Burton, J., Zachery, J., Bessin, R., Rathbun, H., Greenough, W., Sterioff, S., Wright, J., Slavin, R., and Williams, G. Aspergillosis in four renal transplant recipients. *Ann. Intern. Med.* 77:383, 1972.

25. Butler, W., Alling, D., Spickard, A., and Utz, J. Diagnostic and prognostic value of clinical and laboratory findings in cryptococcal meningitis. *N. Engl. J. Med.* 270:59, 1964.

26. Butler, W. T., and Rossen, R. D. Effects of corticosteroids on immunity in man. *J. Clin. Invest.* 52:2629, 1973.

27. Calne, R., Evans, D., Herbertson, B., Joysey, V., McMillan, R., Maginn, R., Mellard, P., Pena, J., Salaman, J., White, H., Withycombe, J., and Yoffa, D. Survival after renal transplantation in man: An interim report on 54 consecutive transplants. *Br. Med. J.* 2:404, 1968.

28. Carroll, R., Marsh, J., O'Donoghue, E., Breeze, D., and Shackman, R. Response to influenza vaccine by renal transplant patients. *Br. Med. J.* 2:701, 1972.

29. Castleman, B., Scully, R., and McNeely, B. Clinico-pathological exercise at Massachusetts General Hospital. *N. Engl. J. Med.* 288:780, 1973.

30. Chandler, J., Kalina, R., and Milan, D. Coccidioidal choroiditis following renal transplantation. *Am. J. Ophthalmol.* 74:1080, 1972.

31. Chang, R. S., Lewis, J. P., Reynolds, R. D., Sullivan, M. J., and Neuman, J. Oropharyngeal excretion of Epstein-Barr virus by patients with lymphoproliferative disorders and by recipients of renal homografts. *Ann. Intern. Med.* 88:34, 1978.

32. Charache, P. Unpublished data, 1974.

33. Charache, P., Walker, W., and Williams, G. Management of infectious disease in renal homotransplant patients. *Clin. Res.* 21:731, 1973.

34. Chatterjee, S., Payne, J., Bischel, M., Redeker, A., and Berne, T. Successful renal transplantation in patients positive for hepatitis B antigen. *N. Engl. J. Med.* 291:62, 1974.

35. Clark, R. A., Johnson, F. L., Klebanoff, S. J., and Thomas, E. D. Defective neutrophil chemotaxis in bone marrow transplant patients. *J. Clin. Invest.* 58:22, 1976.

36. Clift, R. A., Buchner, C. D., Fefer, A., Lerner, K. G., Neiman, P. E., Storb, R., Murphy, M., and Thomas, E. D. Infectious complications of marrow transplantation. *Transplant. Proc.* 6:389, 1974.

37. Clift, R. A., Sanders, J. E., Thomas, E. D., Williams, B., and Buckner, C. D. Granulocyte transfusions for the prevention of infection in patients receiving bone-marrow transplants. *N. Engl. J. Med.* 298:1052, 1978.

38. Cohen, S. Toxoplasmosis in patients receiving immunosuppressive therapy. *J.A.M.A.* 211:657, 1970.

39. Coleman, D., Gardner, S., and Field, A. Human polyomavirus infection in renal allograft recipients. *Br. Med. J.* 3:371, 1973.

40. Coulson, A., Lucas, Z., Condy, M., and Cohn, R. An epidemic of cytomegalovirus disease in a renal transplant population. *West. J. Med.* 120:1, 1974.

41. Craighead, J., Hanshaw, J., and Carpenter, C. Cytomegalovirus infection after renal allotransplantation. *J.A.M.A.* 201:99, 1967.

42. Cuthbert, J., Ware, A., Combes, B., Mauk, R., and Hull, A. Transplant survival and antibody to hepatitis virus. *N. Engl. J. Med.* 297:1068, 1977.

43. Davis, A., Klasky, I., and Koppel, M. Disseminated Coccidioidomycosis in Renal Transplant Patients Receiving Immunosuppressive Therapy. In *Report of the Veterans Administration Armed Forces Coccidioidomycosis Study Group*, 1968.

44. Deresinski, S. C., and Stevens, D. A. Coccidioidomycosis in the compromised host. *Medicine* (Baltimore) 54:377, 1974.

45. Derom, F., Barbier, F., Ringoir, S., Versieck, J., Rolly, G., Berzsenyi, G., Vermeire, P., and Vrints, D. Ten month survival after lung homotransplantation in man. *J. Thorac. Cardiovasc. Surg.* 61:835, 1971.

46. DeVries, M., Crouch, B., VanPutten, L., and

VanBekkum, D. Pathologic changes in irradiated monkeys treated with bone marrow. *J. Natl. Canc. Inst.* 27:67, 1961.

47. Doak, P., Becroft, D., Harris, E., Hitchcock, G., Leeming, B., North, J., Montgomerie, J., and Whitlock, R. *Pneumocystis carinii* pneumonia—transplant lung. *Q. J. Med.* 42:59, 1973.

48. Dorf, G., Geimer, N., Rosenthal, D., and Rytel, M. Pseudomonas septicemia: Illustrated evolution of its skin lesion. *Arch. Intern. Med.* 128:591, 1971.

49. Dorfman, L. Cytomegalovirus encephalitis in adults. *Neurology* (Minneap.) 23:136, 1973.

50. Douglas, R., Anderson, M., Weg, J., Williams, T., Jenkins, D., Knight, V., and Beall, A. Herpes-simplex virus pneumonia. *J.A.M.A.* 210:902, 1969.

51. Drews, J., Shimada, K., White, P., and Benfield, J. The pulmonary alveolar macrophage in lung transplantation. *Transplantation* 17:319, 1974.

52. Dufly, P., Wolf, J., Collins, G., DeVoe, A., Streeten, B., and Cowen, D. Possible person-to-person transmission of Creutzfeldt-Jakob disease. *N. Engl. J. Med.* 290:692, 1974.

53. Edmunds, H. A case of clinical lung allotransplantation. In discussion, Hardy, J., Alican, F., Moynihan, P., Timmis, H., Chavez, C., and Davis, J. *J. Thorac. Cardiovasc. Surg.* 60:411, 1970.

54. Edwards, J., Foos, R., Montgomerie, J., and Guze, L. Ocular manifestations of candida septicemia: Review of 76 cases of hematogenous candida endophthalmitis. *Medicine* (Baltimore) 53:47, 1974.

55. Eickhoff, T. Infectious complications in renal transplant recipients. *Transplant. Proc.* 5:1233, 1973.

56. Ellis, C., and Spivack, M. The significance of candidemia. *Ann. Intern. Med.* 67:511, 1967.

57. Epstein, S., Verney, E., Miale, T., and Sidransky, H. Studies on the pathogenesis of experimental pulmonary aspergillosis. *Am. J. Pathol.* 51:769, 1967.

58. Etheredge, E. E., Light, J. A., Perloff, L. J., and Spees, E. K. *Listeria monocytogenes* meningitis in a transplant recipient. *J.A.M.A.* 234:78, 1975.

59. Fagundes, L., Bausto, O., and Brentano, L. Strongyloidiasis: Fatal complication of renal transplantation. *Lancet* 2:439, 1971.

60. Fiala, M., Payne, J. E., Berne, T. V., Moore, T. C., Henle, W., Montgomerie, J. Z., Chatterjee, S. N., and Guze, L. B. Epidemiology of cytomegalovirus infection after transplantation and immunosuppression. *J. Infect. Dis.* 132:421, 1975.

61. Fine, R., Malekzadeh, M., Grushkin, C., and Wright, H. Cytomegalovirus syndrome post-renal transplantation. *Calif. Med.* 118:46, 1973.

62. Finland, M., Jones, W., and Barnes, M. Occurrence of serious bacterial infections since introduction of antibacterial agents. *J.A.M.A.* 170:2188, 1959.

63. Flament-Durand, J., Coers, C., Waelbroeck, C., VanGeertruyden, J., and Toussaint, C. Encephalité et myosité à Toxoplasmes au cours d'un traitement immuno-dépresseur. *Acta Clin. Belg.* 22:44, 1967.

64. Fraser, D. W., Buxton, A. E., Naji, A., Barker, C. F., Rudnick, M., and Weinstein, A. J. Disseminated *Mycobacterium kansasii* infection presenting as cellulitis in a recipient of a renal homograft. *Am. Rev. Resp. Dis.* 112:125, 1975.

65. Frenkel, J. Effects of cortisone, total body irradiation and nitrogen mustard on chronic latent toxoplasmosis. *Am. J. Pathol.* 33:618, 1957.

66. Frenkel, J., Good, R., Jr., and Schultz, J. Latent *Pneumocystis* infection of rats, relapse, and chemotherapy. *Lab. Invest.* 15:1559, 1966.

67. Fulginiti, V., Scribner, R., Groth, C., Putnam, C., Brettschneider, L., Gilbert, S., Porter, K., and Starzl, T. Infections in recipients of liver homografts. *N. Engl. J. Med.* 279:619, 1968.

68. Gaines, J., and Remington, J. Diagnosis of deep infection with Candida. *Arch. Intern. Med.* 132:699, 1973.

69. Galletti, P. Laboratory experience with 24 hour partial heart-lung bypass. *J. Surg. Res.* 5:97, 1965.

70. Gantz, N. M., Myerowitz, R. L., and Medeiros, A. A. Listeriosis in immunosuppressed patients. *Am. J. Med.* 58:637, 1975.

71. Gardner, S. Prevalence in England of antibody to human polyomavirus (B.K.). *Br. Med. J.* 1:77, 1973.

72. Gardner, S., Field, A., Coleman, D., and Hulme, B. New human papovavirus (B.K.) isolated from urine after renal transplantation. *Lancet* 1:1253, 1971.

73. Gentry, L., Ruskin, J., and Remington, J. *Pneumocystis carinii* pneumonia. *Calif. Med.* 116:6, 1972.

74. Ghatak, N., Bon, T., and Zimmerman, H. Toxoplasmosis of the central nervous system in the adult. *Arch. Pathol.* 89:337, 1970.

75. Goodman, L., and Gilman, A. *Pharmacological Basis of Therapeutics* (4th ed.). New York: MacMillan, 1970, p. 1615.

76. Gordon, M., and Vedder, D. Serologic tests

in diagnosis and prognosis of cryptococcosis. *J.A.M.A.* 197:961, 1966.

77. Graybill, J. R., Silva, J., Fraser, D. W., Lordon, R., and Rogers, E. Disseminated mycobacteriosis due to *Mycobacterium abcessus* in two recipients of renal homografts. *Am. Rev. Resp. Dis.* 109:4, 1974.

78. Greenman, R. L., Goodall, P. T., and King, D. Lung biopsy in immunocompromised hosts. *Am. J. Med.* 59:488, 1975.

79. Grose, C., Henle, W., and Horwitz, M. S. Primary Epstein-Barr virus infection in a renal transplant recipient. *South. Med. J.* 70:1276, 1977.

80. Gurwith, M., Stinson, E., and Remington, J. *Aspergillus* infection complicating cardiac transplantation. *Arch. Intern. Med.* 128:541, 1971.

81. Hairston, P., Manos, J., Graber, C., and Lee, W. H. Depression of immunological surveillance by pump-oxygenation perfusion. *J. Surg. Res.* 9:587, 1969.

82. Hamburger, J., Crosnier, J., and Dormont, J. Experience with 45 renal homotransplantations in man. *Lancet* 1:985, 1965.

83. Hamshere, R. J., Chisham, G. D., and Shackman, R. Late urinary-tract infection after renal transplantation. *Lancet* 2:793, 1974.

84. Hart, P., Russell, E., and Remington, J. The compromised host and infection. II. Deep fungal infection. *J. Infect. Dis.* 120:169, 1969.

85. Hedley-Whyte, E., and Craighead, J. Generalized cytomegalic inclusion disease after renal homotransplantation. *N. Engl. J. Med.* 272:473, 1965.

86. Hendly, J., and Weller, T. Activation and transmission in rats of infection with *Pneumocystis carinii*. *Proc. Soc. Exp. Biol. Med.* 137:1401, 1971.

87. Hill, R., Rowlands, D., and Rifkind, D. Infectious pulmonary disease in patients receiving immunosuppressive therapy for organ transplantation. *N. Engl. J. Med.* 271:1021, 1964.

88. Hinman, F., Schaelzie, J., and Belzer, F. Urinary tract infection and renal homotransplantation. II: Post-transplantation bacterial invasion. *J. Urol.* 101:673, 1969.

89. Ho, M., Suwansirikul, S., Dowling, J. M., Youngblood, L. A., and Armstrong, J. A. The transplanted kidney as a source of cytomegalovirus infection. *N. Engl. J. Med.* 293:1109, 1975.

90. Hope-Simpson, R. The nature of herpes zoster. *Proc. R. Soc. Med.* 58:9, 1965.

91. Howard, R. J., Kalis, J. M., Balfour, N. H., Marker, S. M., Simmons, R. L., and Najarian, J. S. Viral infections in kidney donors and

recipients: A prospective study. *Transplant. Proc.* 9:113, 1977.

92. Hughes, J., and Remington, J. Systemic candidiasis, a diagnostic challenge. *Calif. Med.* 116:8, 1972.

93. Hughes, W. T., Kuhn, S., Chaudhary, S., Feldman, S., Verzosa, M., Aur, R. J. A., Pratt, C., and George S. L. Successful chemoprophylaxis for *Pneumocystis carinii* pneumonitis. *N. Engl. J. Med.* 297:1419, 1977.

94. Hughes, W. T., McNabb, P. C., Makres, T. D., and Feldman, S. Efficacy of trimethoprim and sulfamethoxazole in the prevention and treatment of *Pneumocystis carinii* pneumonia. *Anticimrob. Agents Chemother.* 5:289, 1974.

95. Hulme, B., Kenyon, J., Owen, K., Snell, M., Mowbray, J., Porter, K., Starkie, S., Muras, H., and Peart, W. Renal transplants in children. *Arch. Dis. Child.* 47:486, 1972.

96. Isiadinso, O. A. *Listeria* sepsis and meningitis. *J.A.M.A.* 234:842, 1975.

97. Iwata, K., Awadaguci, S., and Yonekura, Y. Influence of adrenal cortex hormones on phagocytosis. I. Studies on phagocytosis of *Aspergillus* spores by leukocytes in vitro. *Jap. J. Bacteriol.* 16:21, 1961; Influence of adrenal cortex hormones on phagocytoses. II. Studies on effects of cortisone on phagocytoses of *Aspergillus* spores by leukocytes. *Jap. J. Bacteriol.* 16:210, 1961.

98. Jeannet, M., Pinn, V., Flax, M., Winn, H., and Russell, P. Humoral antibodies in renal allotransplantation in man. *N. Engl. J. Med.* 282:111, 1970.

99. Kemeny, P., Adler, T., Szokolai, V., and Szirmai, S. Prevention of interstitial plasma-cell pneumonia in premature infants. *Lancet* 1:1322, 1973.

100. Kim, H., and Hughes, W. Comparison of methods for identification of *Pneumocystis carinii* in pulmonary aspirates. *Am. J. Clin. Pathol.* 60:462, 1973.

101. King, R. W., and Kraikitpanitch, S. Subcutaneous nodules caused by *Histoplasma capsulatum*. *Ann. Intern. Med.* 86:586, 1977.

102. Kirby, B. D., Snyder, K. M., Meyer, R. D., and Finegold, S. M. Legionnaires' disease: Clinical features of 24 cases. *Ann. Intern. Med.* 89:297, 1978.

103. Klastersky, J., Daneau, D., Swings, G., and Weerts, D. Antibacterial activity in serum and urine as a therapeutic guide in bacterial infections. *J. Infect. Dis.* 129:187, 1974.

104. Knepshield, J., Feller, H., and Leb, D. Papillary necrosis due to *Candida albicans* in a renal allograft. *Arch. Intern. Med.* 122:441, 1968.

105. Koranda, F. C., Dehmel, E. M., Kahn, G.,

and Penn, I. Cutaneous complications in immunosuppressed renal homograft recipients. *J.A.M.A.* 229:419, 1974.

106. Krick, J., Stinson, E., and Remington, J. Infection due to Nocardia in heart transplant patients. *Ann. Intern. Med.* 82:18, 1975.

107. Kumar, S. S., Ventura, A. K., and Vander-Werf, B. Influenza vaccination in renal transplant patients. *J.A.M.A.* 239:840, 1978.

108. LaForce, F., Mullane, J., Boehme, R., Kelly, W., and Huber, G. The effect of pulmonary edema on antibacterial defenses of the lung. *J. Lab. Clin. Med.* 82:634, 1973.

109. Lang, D., and Noren, B. Cytomegaloviremia following congenital infection. *J. Pediatr.* 73:812, 1968.

110. Lau, W. K., Remington, J. S., and Young, L. Pneumocystis carinii pneumonia: Diagnosis by examination of pulmonary secretions. *J.A.M.A.* 236:2399, 1976.

111. Leigh, D. Bacteremia in patients receiving human cadaveric renal transplants. *J. Clin. Pathol.* 24:295, 1971.

112. Levin, S. The fungal skin test as a diagnostic hindrance. *J. Infect. Dis.* 122:343, 1974.

113. Levine, A., Seigel, S., Schreiber, A., Hauser, J., Preisler, H., Goldstein, I., Seidler, F., Simion, R., Perry, S., Bennett, J., and Henderson, E. Protected environments and prophylactic antibiotics. *N. Engl. J. Med.* 288:477, 1973.

114. Little, G. Clinical pharmacology of the anti-inflammatory steroids. *Clin. Pharmacol. Ther.* 2:615, 1961.

115. Liver Transplantation. *Lancet* 2:29, 1974.

116. London, W. T., Drew, J. S., Blumberg, B. S., Grossman, R. A., and Lyons, P. J. Association of graft survival with host response to hepatitis B infection in patients with kidney transplants. *N. Engl. J. Med.* 296:241, 1977.

117. Lopez, C., Simmons, R., Mauer, S., Najarian, J., Good, R., and Gentry, S. Association of renal allograft rejection with virus infections. *Am. J. Med.* 56:280, 1974.

118. Lopez, C., Simmons, R., Park, B., Najarian, J., and Good, R. Cell-mediated and humoral immune responses of renal transplant recipients with cytomegalovirus infections. *Clin. Exp. Immunol.* 16:565, 1974.

119. Luby, J., Burnett, W., Hull, A., Ware, A., Shrey, J., and Peters, P. Relationship between cytomegalovirus and hepatic function abnormalities in the period after renal transplant. *J. Infect. Dis.* 129:511, 1974.

120. Mahony, J., Tambyah, J., Dalton, V., and Wolfenden, W. Pontomedullary listeriosis in renal allograft recipient. *Br. Med. J.* 1:705, 1974.

121. Manz, H., Dinsdale, H., and Morrin, P. Progressive multifocal leukoencephalopathy after renal transplant. *Ann. Intern. Med.* 75:77, 1971.

122. Martin, D. Urinary tract infection in clinical renal transplantation. *Arch. Surg.* 99:474, 1969.

123. McCormick, W. F., Schochet, S. S., Sarles, H. E., and Calverley, J. R. Progressive multifocal leukoencephalopathy in renal transplant recipients. *Arch. Intern. Med.* 136:829, 1976.

124. Medoff, G., Kunz, L., and Weinberg, A. Listeriosis in humans: An evaluation. *J. Infect. Dis.* 123:247, 1971.

125. Meuwissen, H. J. Bone marrow transplantation in immunosuppressed or congenitally immune deficient patients. *Transplant. Proc.* 5:1291, 1973.

126. Monaco, A. P. Kidney transplantation. *Behring Inst. Mitt.* 51:135, 1972.

127. Montgomerie, J., Barrett, F., and Williams, T. Infectious complications in cardiac transplant patients. *Transplant. Proc.* 5:1239, 1973.

128. Montgomerie, J., Croxson, M., Becroft, D., Doak, P., and North, J. Herpes-simplex-virus infection after renal transplantation. *Lancet* 2:867, 1969.

129. Montgomerie, J., Doak, P., Taylor, D., and North, J. *Klebsiella* in faecal flora of renal-transplant patients. *Lancet* 2:787, 1970.

130. Moore, T., and Hume, D. The period and nature of hazard in clinical renal transplantation. I. The hazard to patient survival. *Ann. Surg.* 170:1, 1969.

131. Murphy, J. F., McDonald, F. D., Dawson, M., Reiter, A., Turcotte, J., and Fekety, F. R. Factors affecting the frequency of infection in renal transplant recipients. *Arch. Intern. Med.* 136:670, 1976.

132. Murphy, S., Drash, A., and Donnelly, W. Disseminated coccidioidomycosis associated with immunosuppression therapy following renal transplant. *Pediatrics* 48:144, 1971.

133. Murray, J. E., Merrill, J. P., Harrison, J. H., Wilson, R. E., and Dammin, G. J. Prolonged survival of human-kidney homografts by immunosuppressive drug therapy. *N. Engl. J. Med.* 268:1315, 1963.

134. Myerowitz, R., Medeiros, A., and O'Brian, T. Bacterial infection in renal homotransplant recipients. *Am. J. Med.* 53:308, 1972.

135. Myerowitz, R. L., Stadler, H., Oxaman, M. N., Levin, M. J., Moore, M., Leith, J. D., Gantz, N. M., Pellegrini, J., and Hierholzer, J. C. Fatal disseminated adenovirus infection in a renal transplant recipient. *Am. J. Med.* 59:591, 1975.

136. Nagington, J. Cytomegalovirus antibody production in renal transplant patients. *J. Hyg.* (Camb). 69:645, 1971.

137. Nagington, J., Cossart, Y. E., and Cohen, B. J. Reactivation of hepatitis B after transplantation operations. *Lancet* 1:558, 1977.
138. Neff, T., and Hudgle, D. Miliary tuberculosis in a renal transplant recipient. *Am. Rev. Resp. Dis.* 108:677, 1973.
139. Neiman, P. E., Reeves, W., Ray, G., Flournoy, N., Lerner, K. G., Sale, G. E., and Thomas, E. D. A prospective analysis of interstitial pneumonia and opportunistic viral infection among recipients of allogeneic bone marrow grafts. *J. Infect. Dis.* 136:754, 1977.
140. Neiman, P., Wasserman, P., Wentworth, B., Kao, G., Lerner, K., Storb, R., Buckner, C., Clift, R., Fefer, A., Fass, L., Glucksberg, H., and Thomas, E. Interstitial pneumonia and cytomegalovirus infection as complications of human marrow transplantation. *Transplantation* 5:478, 1973.
141. Nirmul, G., Glabman, S., Haemov, M., Ceiter, E., and Burrows, L. *Listeria monocytogenes* meningitis during immunosuppression. *N. Engl. J. Med.* 285:1323, 1971.
142. Oliver, W. A. Tuberculosis in renal transplant patients. *Med. J. Aust.* 1:828, 1976.
143. Pappagianis, D. Unpublished data, 1971.
144. Pattison, C., Maynard, J., Berquist, K., and Webster, H. Serological and epidemiological studies of hepatitis B in haemodialysis units. *Lancet* 2:172, 1973.
145. Pien, F. D., Smith, T. F., Anderson, C. F., Webel, M. L., and Taswell, H. Herpesviruses in renal transplant patients. *Transplantation* 16:489, 1973.
146. Pirofsky, B., Beaulieu, R., Bardana, E., and August, A. Antithymocyte antiserum effects in man. *Am. J. Med.* 56:290, 1974.
147. Pirson, Y., Alexandri, G. P. J., and van Ypersele de Strihou, C. Long-term effect of HB$_s$ antigenemia on patient survival after renal transplantation. *N. Engl. J. Med.* 296:194, 1977.
148. Platt, B., Rosenblatt, M., and Koppel, M. Cryptococcosis in renal transplant recipients. *Clin. Res.* 18:182, 1973.
149. Pletka, P., Cohen, S., Hulme, B., Kenyon, J., Owen, K., Thompson, A., Snell, M., Mowbray, J., Porter, K., Leigh, D., and Peart, W. Cadaveric renal transplants. *Lancet* 1:1, 1969.
150. Post, C., Fakoughi, T., Dutz, W., Bandarizadeh, B., and Kohout, E. Prophylaxis of epidemic infantile pneumocystosis with a 20 : 1 sulfadoxine and pyrimethamine combination. *Curr. Ther. Res.* 13:273, 1971.
151. Prout, G., Hume, D., Lee, H., and Williams, G. Some urological aspects of 93 consecutive renal homotransplants in modified recipients. *J. Urol.* 97:409, 1967.
152. Puritilo, D., Meyers, W., and Connor, D. Fatal strongyloidiasis in immunosuppressed patients. *Am. J. Med.* 56:488, 1974.
153. Rand, K. H., Pollard, R. B., and Merigan, T. C. Increased pulmonary superinfections in cardiac-transplant patients undergoing primary cytomegalovirus infection. *N. Engl. J. Med.* 298:951, 1978.
154. Reinarz, J., Pierce, A., Mays, B., and Sanford, J. The potential role of inhalation equipment in nosocomial pulmonary infection. *J. Clin. Invest.* 44:831, 1965.
155. Remington, J. Toxoplasmosis in the adult. *Bull. N.Y. Acad. Med.,* Second Series 50 (Suppl. 2):211, 1974.
156. Remington, J., and Anderson, S. Pneumocystis and fungal infection in patients with malignancies. *Int. J. Radiat. Oncol. Biol. Phys.* 1:313, 1976.
157. Remington, J., Gaines, J., and Gilmer, M. Demonstration of *Candida* precipitins in human sera by counter-immunoelectrophoresis. *Lancet* 1:413, 1972.
158. Reynolds, E., Walls, K., and Pfeiffer, R. Generalized toxoplasmosis following renal transplantation: Report of a case. *Arch. Intern. Med.* 118:401, 1966.
159. Rifkind, D. The activation of varicella-zoster virus infections by immunosuppressive therapy. *J. Lab. Clin. Med.* 68:463, 1966.
160. Rifkind, D., Faris, T., and Hill, R. *Pneumocystis carinii* pneumonia: Studies on the diagnosis and treatment. *Ann. Intern. Med.* 65:943, 1966.
161. Rifkind, D., Goodman, N., and Hill, R. The clinical significance of cytomegalovirus infection in renal transplant recipients. *Ann. Intern. Med.* 66:1116, 1967.
162. Rifkind, D., Marchioro, R., Schneck, S., and Hill, R. Systemic fungal infections complicating renal transplantation and immunosuppressive therapy. *Am. J. Med.* 43:28, 1967.
163. Rifkind, D., Starzl, R., Marchioro, T., Waddell, W., Rowlands, D., and Hill, R. Transplantation pneumonia. *J.A.M.A.* 189:114, 1964.
164. Rogers, W., and Nelson, B. Strongyloidiasis and malignant lymphoma. *J.A.M.A.* 195:685, 1966.
165. Ruskin, J. Pneumocystis. In Remington, J., and Klein, J. (Eds.), *Infections of the Fetus and Newborn.* Philadelphia: W. B. Saunders, 1976, pp. 691–746.
166. Ruskin, J., and Remington, J. S. Toxoplasmosis in the compromised host. *Ann. Intern. Med.* 84:193, 1976.
167. Ryning, F. W., McLeod, R., Maddox, J. C., Hunt, S., and Remington, J. S. Probable

transmission of *Toxoplasma gondii* by organ transplantation. *Ann. Intern. Med.,* in press.

168. Rytel, M., and Balay, J. Impaired production of interferon in lymphocytes from immunosuppressed patients. *J. Infect. Dis.* 127: 445, 1973.

169. Rytel, M., and Kilbourne, E. The influence of cortisone on experimental viral infection. VII: Suppression by cortisone of interferon formation in mice injected with Newcastle disease virus. *J. Exp. Med.* 123:767, 1966.

170. Schimpff, S. C., Greene, W. H., Young, V. M., Fortner, C. L., Lipsan, L., Cusack, N., Block, L. B., and Wiernik, P. H. Infection prevention in acute nonlymphocytic leukemia. *Ann. Intern. Med.* 82:351, 1975.

171. Schneck, S. Neuropathological features of organ transplantation. *J. Neuropathol. Exp. Neurol.* 24:415, 1965.

172. Schröter, G. P., Bakshandeh, K., Husberg, B. S., and Weil, R. Coccidioidomycosis and renal transplantation. *Transplantation* 23: 485, 1977.

173. Schröter, G. P., Hoelscher, M., Putnam, C. W., Kendrick, A., Porter, K. A., and Starzl, T. E. Fungus infections after liver transplantation. *Ann. Surg.* 186:115, 1977.

174. Schröter, G. P., Hoelscher, M., Putnam, C. W., Porter, K. A., Hansbrough, J. F., and Starzl, T. E. Infections complicating orthotopic liver transplantation. *Arch. Surg.* 111: 1337, 1976.

175. Schröter, G. P., and Weil, R. *Listeria monocytogenes* infection after renal transplantation. *Arch. Intern. Med.* 137:1395, 1977.

176. Seelig, M. Mechanisms by which antibiotics increase the incidence and severity of candidiasis and alter the immunological defenses. *Bacteriol. Rev.* 30:442, 1966.

177. Sheldon, W., and Bauer, H. The role of predisposing factors in experimental fungus infections. *Lab. Invest.* 11:1184, 1962.

178. Shelp, W., Wen, S., and Weinstein, A. Ureteropelvic obstruction caused by *Candida* pyelitis in homotransplanted kidney. *Arch. Intern. Med.* 117:401, 1966.

179. Shons, A. R., Simmons, R. L., Kjellstrand, C. M., Buselmeier, T. J., and Najarian, J. S. Renal transplantation in patients with Australia antigenemia. *Am. J. Surg.* 128:699, 1974.

180. Silva, J., Hoeksema, N., and Fekety, F. Transient defects in phagocytic functions during cardiopulmonary bypass. *J. Thorac. Cardiovasc. Surg.* 67(Suppl. 2):175, 1974.

181. Simmons, R., Kjellstrand, C., and Najarian, J. Sepsis following Kidney Transplantation. In Hardy, J. D. (Ed.), *Critical Surgical Illness.* Philadelphia: W. B. Saunders, 1971, p. 559.

182. Simmons, R., Weil, R., Tallent, M., Kjellstrand, C., and Najarian, J. Do mild infections trigger the rejection of renal allografts? *Transplant. Proc.* 2:419, 1970.

183. Slapak, M., Lee, H., and Hume, D. Transplant lung—a new syndrome. *Br. Med. J.* 1: 80, 1968.

184. Slapak, M., Lee, H., and Hume, D. "Transplant Lung" and Lung Complications in Renal Transplantation. In Dausset, J., Hamburger, J., and Mathe, G. (Eds.). *Advance in Transplantation.* Baltimore: Williams & Wilkins, 1968, p. 769.

185. Solberg, C., Matsen, J., Vesley, D., Wheeler, D., Good, R., and Meuwissen, H. Laminar airflow protection in bone marrow transplantation. *Appl. Microbiol.* 21:209, 1971.

186. Solberg, C., Meuwissen, H., Needhams, R., Good, R., and Matsen, J. Infectious complications in bone marrow transplant patients. *Br. Med. J.* 1:18, 1971.

187. Spencer, E., and Anderson, H. Clinically evident, non-terminal infections with herpesviruses and the wart virus in immunosuppressed renal allograft recipients. *Br. Med. J.* 2:251, 1970.

188. Starr, J., Calafiore, D., and Casey, H. Experience with human cytomegalovirus complement-fixing antigen. *Am. J. Epidemiol.* 36:507, 1967.

189. Starzl, T. Unpublished data, 1974.

190. Starzl, T. E., with the assistance of Putnam, C. W. *Experience in Hepatic Transplantation.* Philadelphia: W. B. Saunders, 1969, p. 329.

191. Starzl, T., Groth, C., Brettschneider, L., Penn, I., Fulginiti, V., Moon, J., Blanchard, H., Martin, A., and Porter, K. Long-term survival after renal transplantation in humans. *Ann. Surg.* 168:392, 1968.

192. Starzl, T., Porter, K. A., Putnam, C. W., Schröter, G. P. J., Halgrimson, C. G., Weil, R., III, Hoelscher, M., and Reid, H. A. S. Orthotopic liver transplantation in 93 patients. *Surg. Gynecol. Obstet.* 142:487, 1976.

193. Starzl, T., and Putnam, C. Chronic immunosuppression, Australia antigenemia, and hepatitis. *Transplant. Proc.* 4:685, 1972.

194. Steere, A. C., Aisner, J., Anderson, R. L., Bennett, J. V., and Schimpff, S. C. The Predictive Value of Nose Cultures in the Diagnosis of Aspergillosis (Abstract No. 207). In Program and Abstracts of the 15th Interscience Conference on Antimicrobial Agents and Chemotherapy, September 1975, Washington, D.C. Washington, D.C.: American Society for Microbiology, 1975.

195. Steiness, I., and Shinhoj, P. Hepatitis associated antigen: Elimination from a dialysis

unit and persistence in renal transplant recipients. *Acta Pathol. Microbiol. Scand.* [*B*]. 79:721, 1971.

196. Stevens, K., Newell, R., and Bergstrom, L. Mucormycosis in a patient receiving azathioprine. *Arch. Otolaryngol.* 96:250, 1972.

197. Stinson, E. B., Breber, C. P., Griepp, R. B., Clark, D. A., Shumway, N. E., and Remington, J. S. Infectious complications after cardiac transplantation in man. *Ann. Intern. Med.* 74:22, 1971.

198. Strauch, B., Siegel, N., Andrews, L., and Miller, G. Oropharyngeal excretion of Epstein-Barr virus by renal transplant recipients and other patients treated with immunosuppressive drugs. *Lancet* 1:234, 1974.

199. Subramanian, V., Lowman, J. T., and Gans, H. Effect of extracorporeal circulation on reticuloendothelial function. *Arch. Surg.* 97:330, 1968.

200. Swenson, R., Kountz, S., Blank, N., and Merigan, T. Successful renal allograft in a patient with pulmonary cryptococcus. *Arch. Intern. Med.* 124:502, 1969.

201. Taschdjian, C., Kozinin, P., Cuesta, M., and Toni, E. Serodiagnosis of candidal infections. *Am. J. Clin. Pathol.* 57:195, 1972.

202. Tilney, N., Collins, J., and Wilson, R. Hemorrhagic pancreatitis. *N. Engl. J. Med.* 274:1051, 1966.

203. Turcotte, J. Infection and renal transplantation. *Surg. Clin. North Am.* 52:1501, 1972.

204. Uranga, V., Simmons, R., Kjellstrand, C., Buselmeier, T., and Najarian, J. Pathogenesis of "transplant lung." *Ann. Surg.* 178:573, 1973.

205. Vietzke, W., Gelderman, A., Grimley, P., and Valsamis, M. Toxoplasmosis complicating malignancy. *Cancer* 21:816, 1968.

206. Waldram, R., Kemp, A., Williams, R., and Calne, R. Bile secretion following liver transplantation in man. *Gut* 14:819, 1973.

207. Wang, N., Huang, S., and Thurlbeck, W. Combined *Pneumocystis carinii* and cytomegalovirus infection. *Arch. Pathol.* 90:529, 1970.

208. Watanabe, J., Chinchinian, H., Weitz, C., and McIlvaine, S. *Pneumocystis carinii* pneumonia in a family. *J.A.M.A.* 193:685, 1965.

209. Watson, G. W., Fuller, T. J., Elms, J., and Klug, R. M. *Listeria cerebritis. Arch. Intern. Med.* 138:83, 1978.

210. Weinstein, L., and Chang, T. The chemotherapy of viral infection. *N. Engl. J. Med.* 289:725, 1973.

211. Weisse, K., and Wedler, E. Ulser das vorkommen der sogenannten *Pneumocystis carinii. Klin. Wochenschr.* 32:270, 1954.

212. Weissman, G., and Thomas, C. Studies on lysosomes II. *J. Clin. Invest.* 42:661, 1963.

213. Weller, T. Cytomegaloviruses: The difficult years. *J. Infect. Dis.* 122:532, 1970.

214. Wildevuur, C., and Benfield, J. A review of 23 lung transplantations by 20 surgeons. *Ann. Thorac. Surg.* 9:489, 1970.

215. Winn, W. Coccidioidomycosis and amphotericin B. *Med. Clin. North Am.* 47:1131, 1963.

216. Winston, D. J., Meyer, D. V., Gale, R. P., Young, L. S., and the U.C.L.A. Bone Marrow Transplant Team. Further experience with infections in bone marrow transplant recipients. *Transplant. Proc.* 10:247, 1978.

217. Woodruff, M., Robsin, J., Nolan, B., and MacDonald, M. Renal transplantation in man. *Lancet* 1:6, 1969.

218. Worthington, M., and Baron, S. Effectiveness of an interferon stimulator in immunosuppressed mice. *Proc. Soc. Exp. Biol. Med.* 136:349, 1971.

219. Wyhinny, G., Apple, D., Guastella, F., and Vygantas, C. Adult cytomegalic inclusion retinitis. *Am. J. Ophthalmol.* 76:733, 1973.

220. Yates, J., and Holland, J. A controlled study of isolation and endogenous microbial suppression in acute myelocytic leukemia patients. *Cancer* 32:1490, 1973.

221. Young, N., Kwong-Chung, K., and Freeman, J. Subcutaneous abscess caused by *Phoma* sp. resembling *Pyrenochaeta romeroi. Am. J. Clin. Pathol.* 59:810, 1973.

222. Yu, D., Clements, P., Paulus, H., Peter, J., Levy, J., and Barnett, E. Human lymphocyte subpopulations: Effect of corticosteroids. *J. Clin. Invest.* 53:565, 1974.

28

Other Procedure-Related Infections

*Robert A. Weinstein and
Lowell S. Young*

With his yards of entrails, miles of vascular network, dozens of extravascular spaces, and several organ systems, any patient is a candidate for a staggering array of diagnostic and therapeutic procedures. Although many of these procedures provide information that is essential for sophisticated patient care, supplant more traumatic intervention, or are critical for life support, most procedures also bypass natural host defenses and place patients at increased risk of nosocomial infection. It is not surprising, then, that the introduction of any new procedure is often followed closely by case reports of procedure-associated infections. Occasionally, epidemiologic experiments of nature, in the form of nosocomial outbreaks, provide more detailed information on certain procedure-related hazards, and eventually such hazards may be subjected to prospective study. In this chapter, we discuss a variety of procedure-associated infections that have been highlighted by retrospective or prospective investigations and that have not been discussed elsewhere in this volume.

Because of the seemingly eclectic contents of this chapter, it is important to recognize from the outset that the procedures to be discussed have certain themes in common. First, all the procedures are exquisitely vulnerable to inexperienced operators, to breaks in aseptic technique, and to contaminated equipment or ineffective antiseptics. Second, various procedures involving many different sites have the bloodstream as a common site of infection, although, as will be seen, the risk of infection differs depending on whether the bloodstream contamination is transient or persistent as well as on host and organism-specific factors. Finally, many procedures bear the burden that the specific risks have not been defined sufficiently to justify certain preventive measures, such as the use of prophylactic antimicrobial therapy.

Infections from Diagnostic Procedures Involving the Vascular System

Phlebotomy

Phlebotomy is one of the oldest and certainly the commonest invasive procedure practiced in hospitals and clinics, and ever since the leech was replaced by the sterile hypodermic needle, blood-drawing has been regarded by most clinicians as totally safe and simple. In the 1940s, however, it became apparent that despite sterile needles, epidemic jaundice was being transmitted by the nonsterile syringes that were used commonly for phlebotomy. With a mock venous system and methylene blue as a marker, investigators showed that reflux occurred from the syringe into the test system when tourniquet pressure was released. By sterilizing syringes between uses, clinic workers abruptly halted the transmission of phlebotomy-associated hepatitis [41].

Historically, the next major risk of phlebotomy to be recognized was septic arthritis of the hip in neonates. In the early 1960s, it was noted that this complication occasionally followed five to nine days after femoral venipuncture. Localized suppuration at the puncture site and thrombosis of the femoral vein, both unusual findings with isolated septic arthritis, suggested a causal relationship between pyoarthritis and a preceding femoral venipuncture. Isolation of staphylococci from the infected joints suggested that either the operator or the inguinal skin of the infant was the source of contamination [2]. Since it is common to strike the femoral head during femoral venipuncture in neonates (which denotes that the joint capsule has been entered), femoral "sticks" demand the same aseptic conditions used for arthrocentesis, rather than the more lax conditions under which venipuncture is frequently performed. In light of the severe disability that may follow septic arthritis, many pediatricians now condemn the use of femoral venipuncture and recommend at least ten other sites for pediatric phlebotomy.

The most recent innovation in blood-drawing —the popular and ingeniously simple evacuated collection tube—has streamlined blood collection, but unfortunately, it has also reintroduced the reflux, or backflow hazard, that was first recognized in the 1940s. Because commercial evacuated tubes are not sterilized routinely, they may be a source of hospital-acquired sepsis. One hospital recently traced an outbreak of five cases of "primary" *Serratia* bacteremia to contaminated commercial vacuum tubes used for blood collection. This outbreak prompted a detailed study of the backflow phenomenon, and it was shown that reflux may occur not only when the tourniquet is released (after active flow of blood into the tube has ceased), but also when the tube is tilted upward, when blood touches the stopper, when pressure on the end of the tube compresses the stopper, or when a "short draw" occurs due to insufficient vacuum [25]. While practices that might increase the risk of backflow are proscribed in the package insert that accompanies many commercial vacuum tubes, such inserts are not always seen by those responsible for blood-drawing, and many of the recommendations, particularly those concerning the positioning of patients for phlebotomy, are difficult to observe.

Even when a sterile syringe is used to draw blood, backflow during serial inoculation of vacuum tubes and blood culture bottles can result in cross-contamination and false-positive blood cultures. Although potentially avoidable, such serial inoculation is a convenient and common practice, particularly when blood is obtained from pediatric patients for hemogram and culture, and it has resulted in two reported false "outbreaks" of bacteremia [23]. Although none of the patients was affected directly, false-positive cultures put them at risk of unwarranted antibiotic therapy.

Over 500 million commercial evacuated blood-collection tubes are used annually in the United States and Canada. The feasibilities of requiring that these tubes be sterile and of developing a system that prevents backflow are under investigation. (Even if the evacuated tubes were sterile, the preservative and diagnostic reagents present in many tubes pose an additional, albeit probably minimal, risk that has not been fully evaluated.) Until the problem of backflow is returned to the shelf with the leeches, health workers should be aware of the hazard, particularly when investigating the source of a "primary" bacteremia and when ordering blood tests on patients with increased susceptibility to infection.

Cardiac Catheterization
Serious local and systemic infections may result from cardiac catheterization procedures, particularly when contaminated instruments or ineffective antiseptics (e.g., dilute aqueous benzalkonium chloride) are used inadvertently or when breaks in technique occur in the cardiac catheterization laboratory. During the period from January 1970 to August 1973, a total of 22 cardiac catheterization "site" infections were reported to the National Nosocomial Infections Study (NNIS); this number yields an overall incidence of 2 per 100,000 discharges on medical and pediatric services. More than half of these infections were due to staphylococci and gram-negative bacteria.

The incidence of systemic infections following cardiac catheterization is not known. Up to 50 percent of patients undergoing cardiac catheterization develop an increase in temperature of more than 34°F (1°C) within 24 hours after catheterization. Their fever, however, seems directly associated with the use of angiocardiographic contrast material, rather than with infection [39]. In fact, bacterial endocarditis has been reported very rarely in large series evaluating the complications of cardiac catheterization, and individual examples may have been due to concurrent infection that was initially undetected.

Transient bacteremia during cardiac catheterization has been observed to occur in 4 to 18 percent of patients. In the studies reporting such an incidence, however, blood cultures were obtained from the intravascular catheter or from the vessel from which the catheter had been removed; it is therefore possible that some of the isolates represented contamination of the external part of the catheter or the site of insertion and that bacteremia was actually less frequent. In a study designed to assess this possibility, blood for culture was obtained by standard techniques from a vein distant from the site of catheter manipulation [39]. Venous blood cultures of 106 patients, the majority of whom had valvular heart disease, were ob-

tained in this manner during cardiac catheterization and all were sterile. Three of 38 samples that were drawn through the catheter that was placed in the heart or aorta during the procedure grew diphtheroids or microaerophilic streptococci. It was concluded that contamination of the "hub" end of the catheter with normal skin flora led to an overestimation of the incidence of bacteremia. Removal of organisms by lung "filtration" may also have accounted in part for the failure to isolate organisms from distal sites. In either case, it is clear that some contamination of the catheterization cutdown field had occurred. With rigorous application of strict aseptic technique and adoption of the working principle that cardiac catheterization is a surgical procedure, catheterization-associated infection should be very infrequent, and systemic antibiotic prophylaxis does not appear justified.

Indwelling Arterial Catheters
Indwelling arterial catheters are being used with increasing frequency in patients whose precarious cardiovascular status necessitates pressure monitoring or repeated blood-gas determinations. Even though they provide information that is essential for sophisticated patient care and eliminate the need for potentially traumatic repeated arterial punctures, such catheters also provide a continuing portal of entry for microbial invasion of the bloodstream.

The infectious complications of the use of arterial catheters have been studied most extensively in neonates. In different centers, the incidence of colonization of indwelling umbilical artery catheters varies from 6 to 60 percent [3,27,36]. Unexpectedly, however, the incidence of colonization fails to increase with duration of catheterization, which suggests that catheters become contaminated initially or soon after insertion through the umbilical stump, an area that is heavily colonized and impossible to sterilize completely by local or systemic antibiotics. Indeed, the same organisms usually are isolated from both the cord and catheter in any individual patient. The most frequent contaminants are staphylococci, streptococci, and gram-negative bacilli, particularly *Pseudomonas, Proteus, Escherichia coli,* and *Klebsiella.*

The clinical significance of umbilical catheter colonization is difficult to assess, because the incidence of sepsis in most studies has been low. When serial prospective blood cultures have been obtained from catheterized neonates, however, transient catheter-related bacteremia has been noted. In a prospective study of temporary (two to four hours) umbilical catheterization for exchange transfusion, investigators showed a 60 percent incidence of catheter contamination and a 10 percent incidence of transient bacteremia due to *Staphylococcus epidermidis* (and, in one case, *Proteus*) that occurred four to six hours after transfusion; this study suggests that the risk from umbilical catheterization may be greatest during the insertion and removal of catheters [1]. In this study and others, prophylactic systemic antibiotics failed to reduce the incidence of catheter contamination or bacteremia. At present, antibiotic prophylaxis does not appear to be beneficial during umbilical catheterization; instead, attention should be focused on meticulous cord preparation and care.

In adults, the rate of bacterial colonization of indwelling arterial catheters and the risk of associated sepsis have not been studied extensively. Gardner and co-workers [20] recently demonstrated positive arterial catheter-tip cultures in 4 percent of 200 patients exposed to radial artery catheterization (the preferred site in adults). The source of these organisms was not evaluated, and no direct relationship with patient disease was established, but the incidence of colonization of radial catheters (in contrast to umbilical catheters) did appear to be related to longer durations of catheterization.

Breaks in aseptic technique may create a greatly increased risk of arterial catheter contamination and sepsis, as was highlighted by a recent outbreak of *Flavobacterium* bacteremia [43]. In the affected hospital, the sterile, heparinized, glass syringes used for clearing arterial lines and for withdrawing arterial blood samples were submerged routinely in ice for a few minutes before use. The ice machine in the hospital's intensive-care unit was contaminated with *Flavobacterium* (an organism that can survive and grow at temperatures as low as $-38°C$), and contamination of in-use phlebotomy syringes with this ice resulted in 14 cases of *Flavobacterium* sepsis. Control of the outbreak depended on improved aseptic technique, that is, on discontinuing the practice of cooling syringes in ice before blood withdrawal and of reinjecting blood to clear the catheter system.

Other measures that may help to reduce the risk of sepsis associated with arterial catheters include inserting the catheters under aseptic conditions by a gloved operator; avoiding cannulation of arteries that lie below areas of heavy skin colonization, such as the inguinal fold; applying antimicrobial ointment and sterile dressings to the catheter-skin junctions daily; treating arterial catheters and stopcocks as sterile fields to be manipulated as little as possible and only after hand-washing; placing sterile caps on stopcock portholes; changing arterial infusion fluid and tubing every 24 hours; and using arterial catheters only when absolutely necessary and then removing them as soon as possible.

Transducers

Pressure-monitoring devices (transducers or gauges connected to a closed space by a length of fluid-filled tubing) are being used with increasing frequency for monitoring cardiovascular and cerebrospinal fluid (CSF) pressures of critically ill patients. These devices can provide a portal of entry for microbial invasion of the blood or CSF. Although such devices frequently are used in the setting of arterial cannulation or cardiac catheterization, we feel that the threat posed by monitoring devices is so prominent and so frequently overlooked that a separate section on transducer-related infection is warranted.

Although many hospital personnel assume that a protective pressure gradient exists between patients and transducers, contaminated monitoring devices have been the source of nosocomial infection in several recent outbreaks of gram-negative bacteremia, candidemia, and dialysis-associated hepatitis [48]. As in infusion-related sepsis, any organism that can survive in the fluid used in the monitoring system is capable of causing monitoring-related infection. *Pseudomonas* species and members of the tribe Klebsielleae (*Klebsiella, Enterobacter,* and *Serratia*) have caused the reported bacteremias. The *Pseudomonas* species—*P. cepacia* and *P. acidovorans*—that were implicated in three outbreaks may reflect a weighting of experience toward unusual epidemics that are more readily recognized and evaluated. Pathogens such as *P. cepacia,* however, may have selective advantages in the hospital environment, because of their ability to grow with minimal nutrients and to resist commonly used disinfectants, such as dilute aqueous benzalkonium chloride.

In the outbreaks that we investigated, pressure-monitoring devices were contaminated most frequently by an index patient. Just as organisms from a contaminated transducer may migrate (or be flushed) through fluid-filled monitoring lines to infect a patient, organisms in the bloodstream of a patient with preexisting bacteremia or viremia may migrate (or be refluxed) through the lines to contaminate a transducer. If the transducer is not sterilized after use, cross-infection can result.

Although we do not know how often personnel fail to sterilize transducers between uses, there are several reasons to believe that this is a relatively common error. First, many hospital personnel, failing to recognize that transducers may be a source of infection, are loath to subject such expensive and relatively delicate instruments to adequate cleaning efforts. Second, transducers cannot withstand autoclaving, and heavy patient loads frequently may not allow time for the more lengthy gas or chemical sterilization procedures that these devices require. Finally, even when an attempt at proper care is made, the many "nooks and crannies" in the traditional dome-and-diaphragm transducer may hamper cleaning and sterilizing efforts.

Once transducers are sterilized for use, the many manipulations involved in using a monitoring system make extrinsic contamination of the equipment possible, and the frequent use of unsterile mercury manometers for calibrating sterile transducers makes contamination likely. Other potential vehicles for transducer contamination include cleaning solutions and intravenous fluids and medications, particularly those in multidose vials [46].

So far, only during outbreak situations—particularly when cases have been caused by uncommon or uniquely marked, and thus easily traced, pathogens—has it been possible to incriminate contaminated monitoring devices as a source of infection. For reasons outlined above, however, we suspect that transducer contamination is relatively common and that monitoring-related infections have been occurring sporadically since transducers were introduced into clinical medicine. As increasing use of invasive procedures places a large population at risk of monitoring-related infection and as awareness of this problem increases, such sporadic cases and the means for preventing them should receive more attention. In each hospital, guidelines need to be established for the care of transducers and for surveillance and management of monitoring-related infection. Transducers must be sterilized by appropriate means between uses. Strict aseptic techniques should be followed when setting up, calibrating, and using monitoring systems. Monitoring tubing, fluid, and monitoring devices should be changed at regular intervals for each monitored patient. Ongoing surveillance of transducer-related infection in patients undergoing cardiovascular monitoring, as well as obtaining periodic cultures from transducers and the fluid in monitoring lines, will help each hospital assess the adequacy of its monitoring practices and sterilization procedures.

Efforts are under way to improve the ease of transducer sterilization and to simplify the aseptic use of monitoring systems [47]. More recent innovations include miniature extravascular transducers that are built into the tips of standard Luer-Lok fittings and thus can be attached directly to monitoring lines, obviating the need for cumbersome domes; however, when sterilizing these miniature transducers, care must be taken to insure that the area between the transducer and the Luer fitting is thoroughly cleaned and comes into full contact with the sterilizing medium. Second, sterile disposable "chamber domes," which have a thin membrane that abuts the transducer diaphragm and which keeps the monitoring fluid within a sterile disposable circuit, could potentially eliminate the need for transducer sterilization; however, the viability of this recent innovation depends on the chamber dome not being reused and on the thin membrane reliably maintaining its integrity throughout a monitoring period. Any breaks in this membrane large enough for passage of endotoxin, viruses, or bacteria could permit contamination to enter the sterile monitoring circuit. Clinical investigations of these new domes and thorough study of the situations that could lead to breaks in the dome diaphragm are needed. Finally, inexpensive, disposable, pressure-monitor, "isolating" devices are available, but they allow only mean pressure readings, usually on a gauge-type manometer.

Transfusion-Associated Infections

This section will cover transfusion-associated infections other than hepatitis and cytomegalovirus infections, which are discussed elsewhere (see Part II, Chapters 24 and 27).

Blood Transfusion and Bacteremia

The first case reports of transfusion-related sepsis appeared in the 1940s and 1950s and involved shock syndromes produced by transfusion of cold-stored blood contaminated with psychrophilic organisms, such as *Achromobacter* and some *Pseudomonas* species. Prospective microbiologic studies soon followed these reports and documented a contamination rate of 1 to 6 percent in banked blood [24]. The majority of contaminants were normal skin flora, presumably introduced with fragments of donor skin cored out during phlebotomy. Such contaminants were usually present in extremely low concentrations (several logarithmic factors below the level of 10^6 to 10^8 organisms per milliliter of blood associated with transfusion sepsis), and further multiplication of organisms during storage seemed unlikely, because of the long lag phase produced by refrigeration and because of the antibacterial action of blood. Indeed, retrospective studies failed to document any clinical illness associated with the transfusion of blood that contained low level contamination with skin flora [6].

Today, as in 1940, the most common organisms associated with transfusion sepsis are gram-negative bacilli, particularly those able to survive and grow at 4°C (39°F). With the sterile, disposal, closed systems used at present for blood collection, with good collection technique, and with the prompt use of dated, refrigerated, banked blood, however, problems with blood transfusions should be minimal. When an episode of transfusion-associated sepsis does occur, it is important to search for breakdowns in technique or a contaminated common source (e.g., collection sets, disinfectants, and anticoagulants) that could put other patients at risk (also see Part I, Chapter 8). Furthermore, the possibility of transfusion-associated sepsis should be investigated in any case of febrile transfusion reaction.

Blood Transfusion and Parasitemia

The increased use of blood transfusions and the increased travel to countries where malaria is endemic have led recently to an increased occurrence of transfusion-related malaria. It is estimated that during the period between 1911 and 1950, about 350 cases of transfusion-associated malaria were reported worldwide, but during the period 1950 to 1972, the number of reported cases exceeded 2000 [7]. In the United States, 45 cases of transfusion-induced malaria were reported in the years 1958 to 1972 inclusive, of which 35 occurred between 1967 and 1972. This increase has been linked to imported cases of malaria, in that over 50 percent of the implicated donors had a history of recent military service in Southeast Asia [17].

Based on worldwide incidence data, *Plasmodium malariae* appears to be the most common cause of transfusion-associated malaria, accounting for almost 50 percent of cases. *P. vivax* and *P. falciparum* are second and third in worldwide incidence, respectively. This ordering probably reflects the fact that although *P. malariae* infection may persist in an asymptomatic donor for many years, the longevity of *P. vivax* malaria in man rarely exceeds three years and that of *P. falciparum* rarely a year. Hence, there is greater chance for an asymptomatic donor infected with *P. malariae* to escape detection and become the source of an infected transfusion. Of note in the United States, however, has been the recent relative increase in the percentage of cases due to the "malignant" species, *P. falciparum*. The majority of these cases have been traced to donors who were infected in Southeast Asia, where antimicrobial-resistant strains of falciparum malaria are prevalent.

Recommended guidelines for the selection of blood donors to prevent transmission of malaria were adopted by the American Association of Blood Banks in 1970 [17]. Prospective donors who have a definite history of malaria or who are immigrants or visitors from an endemic area are permanently rejected. Donors who have traveled to an endemic area but who have remained free of symptoms and have not taken antimalarial drugs are acceptable six months after their return to the United States; travelers to an endemic area who have taken antimalarials must have remained symptom-free for two years after discontinuation of drug therapy. Because platelet and leukocyte preparations also have been incriminated in the transmission of malaria, the above guidelines must be applied to potential donors of any formed elements of blood.

Although a recent decline in the incidence of malaria in the United States has been attributed to the termination of military involvement in Southeast Asia, the continuing exposure of millions of international travelers still makes this problem one to be considered in blood-banking centers. Current recommendations for blood banking will likely screen out most potentially infected donors, but for those donors where screening fails, a high index of suspicion about the recipient's disease is the best approach to rapid diagnosis and treatment of transfusion-associated malaria. The diagnosis should be considered in any patient who has received formed blood elements and who develops a fever for which no cause is determined by routine cultures. (Serologic methods are now available that accurately diagnose malaria, but they are not practical for screening donors or for rapidly diagnosing serious infection.)

Chagas' disease, or American trypanosomiasis, is prevalent through South and Central America, and there is a high potential for bloodborne transmission, because some infected individuals may become asymptomatic but still have persistent parasitemia for 10 to 30 years. Although the infectivity of blood contaminated with this parasite declines after ten days of storage, this frequently is not a useful method for preventing transmission. Fortunately, however, carriers of Chagas' disease can be detected by complement-fixation tests. In some areas of South America, 15 percent of potential blood donors are positive, and when blood from these donors has been used for transfusions, up to 25 percent of the recipients have developed clinical Chagas' disease. Thus, serologic screening has become mandatory for the acceptance of blood donors in many South American countries.

Toxoplasmosis is a disease that is receiving increasing clinical attention, particularly as a cause of opportunistic infection in patients with impaired host defenses. A large portion of the general population, perhaps one-half of adults, has specific antibodies for *Toxoplasma gondii*. In one prospective survey of thalassemic patients who were frequently transfused, subclinical toxoplasmosis was detected at a rate comparable to that seen in a control group, and this was felt to be evidence against the transmission of toxoplasmosis by transfusion [26]. In another study, however, patients treated for acute leukemia developed toxoplasmosis following leukocyte transfusions from donors with chronic myelogenous leukemia; serologic data retrospectively obtained from donors revealed elevated anti-*Toxoplasma* antibody titers [42]. This inferential evidence for transfusion-associated toxoplasmosis is supported by the findings that the disease can be transmitted between animals by transfusion, that *Toxoplasma* organisms retain their viability in stored blood for up to 50 days, and that organisms can be recovered from the blood buffy-coat layers of patients with toxoplasmosis. Because it seems likely that toxoplasmosis can be transmitted if large concentrations of leukocytes are transfused, it has been recommended that blood from donors with high anti-*Toxoplasma* antibody titers not be used for leukocyte transfusion, particularly since the host defenses of the recipients usually are severely compromised.

Platelet Transfusion

The incidence of bacterial contamination of platelet concentrates has been a source of controversy. While many investigators have reported no contamination, others have consistently found bacterial contaminants in 1 to 6 percent of concentrates [8]. Because it is now recommended that platelets be stored at room temperature (rather than at 4°C) to increase in vivo half-life, there is justifiable concern over the true incidence of "intrinsic" contamination and the possible proliferation of contaminants during storage. It seems reasonable to assume that platelet concentrates are as susceptible to contamination during collection as is blood, which is routinely found to have a 1 to 6 percent incidence of low-level contamination (see above). Moreover, platelet concentrates, unlike blood, have no protective antibacterial activity, and platelet transfusions are frequently obtained by pooling the contributions of several donors, which further increases the risk of contamination. Despite this seemingly grim picture, the majority of bacterial contaminants isolated from platelet concentrates have been normal skin flora, such as *Staphylococcus epidermidis* and diphtheroids, and they have been present in extremely low concentrations (less than 500 organisms per milliliter). Even in the highly susceptible patient populations that normally receive platelet transfusions, such contaminants have failed to produce any documented adverse reactions [13].

Although meticulous blood-banking techniques and the widespread use of closed collection systems have made platelet transfusion relatively safe, two recent outbreaks emphasize the possibility of sporadic, significant contamination of platelets. The first outbreak involved seven cases of *Salmonella choleraesuis* sepsis that were traced to platelet transfusions from a blood donor with clinically inapparent salmonellal osteomyelitis and intermittent asymptomatic bacteremia [37]. (As an interesting aside, a long incubation period in this outbreak —that is, a mean interval of nine days between the transfusion with contaminated platelets and the signs of sepsis—was caused by coincidental administration of antibiotics at the time of platelet transfusion in several cases, and this

initially delayed recognition of platelets as the vehicle of infection.) The second outbreak involved two cases of transfusion-induced *Enterobacter cloacae* sepsis [8]. An investigation prompted by the occurrence of these cases revealed that 20 percent of the platelet pools prepared in the affected hospital were contaminated. Although the majority of the contaminants were "nonpathogens" and present only in low concentrations, 6 of 258 platelet pools were shown to harbor *Enterobacter cloacae*. Despite extensive efforts, the source of these unusual contaminants was not discovered.

Albumin Infusion

Because of faith in commercial manufacturing practices and because of the extremely low incidence of reactions to albumin infusion, most physicians consider commercial human serum albumin to be a completely safe product. A recent nationwide outbreak of albumin-related *Pseudomonas cepacia* sepsis, however, emphasized that any commercial product, particularly any blood component, is susceptible to contamination [44]. The outbreak involved four lots of commercial 25% normal human serum albumin. One of the lots had an estimated 1 percent contamination rate and resulted in at least seven cases of albumin-associated sepsis in one Maryland hospital; the other three lots caused isolated cases of albumin-related disease in patients in four other states. The organisms most likely gained access to the albumin vials during a hand-filling procedure.

In addition to emphasizing the risk of infection associated with the infusion of a non-formed blood component, it is worthwhile noting that the albumin outbreak points up several general problems in the detection and evaluation of low-frequency contamination of commercial products. First, nosocomial infections caused by low-frequency contaminants may be difficult to distinguish from endemic problems in any one institution. In the Maryland hospital, the infusion-related infections became apparent only because of the enormous quantity of albumin that was used in the hospital. Second, since commercial products are usually prepared and sterilized in bulk lots, it is important to be able to trace the distribution of individual suspect lots. Although the Maryland hospital did not routinely record information on albumin distribution and use, an alert physician fortuitously noted the lot number and brand of albumin used in one case of suspected infusion-related sepsis. Third, sterility of an infusion product cannot be ascertained by visual inspection. Despite *P. cepacia* concentrations of 10^6 to 10^8 organisms per milliliters, the contaminated albumin was completely clear. Finally, when present in low frequency, some contaminants can be missed by the sampling schemes currently used for product quality control, and endotoxin may escape terminal filtration and be missed by currently used pyrogen tests. Although commercial albumin has been remarkably safe, the threat of contamination is clearly still present. To facilitate the monitoring of albumin-related reactions, many hospitals now distribute this product through their blood banks.

Albumin-transmitted hepatitis is discussed elsewhere (see Part II, Chapter 24).

Infection Hazards Associated with Anesthesia

As noted in previous chapters, severe bacterial infections have been well documented in association with the use of contaminated equipment for local or spinal anesthesia or the use of contaminated anesthesia machines for delivery of general anesthesia. An additional well-recognized infectious complication of general anesthesia unrelated to the use of contaminated equipment is aspiration pneumonia attributable either to the passage of an endotracheal tube or to postoperative difficulties.

Aspiration of stomach contents into the lungs during or following obstetric anesthesia was first described by Mendelson [32], who found the incidence of this complication to be 0.15 percent during the preantibiotic era. In about two-thirds of these cases, aspiration was reported as having definitely occurred in the delivery room, but in the remainder, the complication went unrecognized until later. A common clinical pattern was that two to five hours after vomiting and aspiration, a dramatic onset of cyanosis, tachycardia, and shock was noted.

More recent investigations have shown a surprisingly high incidence of aspiration associated with general anesthesia. In one ingenious study, Evans blue dye was placed in the stomach preoperatively to be used as a "marker" for chemical aspiration; following anesthesia, the dye was sought by bronchoscopy [12]. Of 300 patients observed in this manner, 25 percent vomited, and aspiration was documented in 16 percent of the overall group. Interestingly, aspiration was "silent" and unnoticed by the entire operating team in one-half of those patients who did aspirate (an overall rate of 8 percent), and there were no obvious clues to the time of occurrence. No incidence of pneumonia was reported in this series, but it seems that in normal patients, the aspirated inoculum is usually cleared without sequelae. Patients who have significant retention of gastric contents and preexisting pulmonary disease may be at much higher risk of developing a chemical aspiration pneumonitis and subsequent bacterial infection.

Despite these studies documenting intraoperative aspiration, it seems likely that postoperative aspiration accounts for the majority of aspiration pneumonias associated with general surgery. Surgical procedures involving the upper abdomen, thorax, or the upper gastrointestinal tract have been the operations most commonly associated with aspiration pneumonia. Although the insertion of a nasogastric tube is felt to reduce the incidence of aspiration during anesthesia, more than half the cases of postoperative aspiration occur in patients whose nasogastric tubes have been left in place, and a quarter of cases of postoperative aspiration pneumonia have also been associated with tracheostomy. It is difficult to interpret these data, however, since the more seriously ill and aspiration-prone patients have tracheostomies or nasogastric tubes left in place. Moreover, there are no rate-specific incidence data on aspiration pneumonia based on the denominator population of patients who have postoperative nasogastric tubes or tracheostomies.

The upper respiratory and gastrointestinal passages are colonized by vast numbers of aerobic and anaerobic organisms, and a mixture of both types of organisms is usually found when specimens from a patient with aspiration pneumonia are cultured appropriately. Among the aerobic organisms, gram-negative bacilli are now encountered more frequently than staphylococci in hospitalized patients. Penicillin is commonly used in the initial therapy for aspiration pneumonia, but an added compound with activity against gram-negative organisms would seem preferable. Use of antimicrobial agents with broader coverage of anaerobic organisms has been advocated, but there is no convincing evidence of the clinical superiority of such agents over the penicillins in therapy of aspiration pneumonia. The prophylactic use of antibiotics and steroids is of unproved value. Therapeutically, the administration of corticosteroids may be of value, but it usually is carried out too late to minimize the chemical inflammatory reaction that is the hallmark of early aspiration.

Measures to prevent anesthesia-associated aspiration have included prolonged preoperative fasting, adequate sedation, attention to problems during anesthesia, insertion of a nasogastric tube before anesthesia, and careful monitoring of the patient in the early period postoperatively. Such principles can be readily applied to elective surgical intervention, but it is obvious that a greater risk of aspiration follows emergency procedures. Thus, while it is certainly desirable to reduce gastric contents by passing a nasogastric tube, multiple unsuccessful attempts at passage may trigger the regurgitation that was initially feared. One approach to the emergency situation is to pass an endotracheal tube with an inflatable balloon under topical anesthesia with the patient awake and to attempt later to empty the stomach.

Endotracheal Intubation
Aside from aspiration, another potential hazard of anesthesia may be the occurrence of bacteremia secondary to the passage of an endotracheal tube. The organisms isolated from the blood usually are α-hemolytic streptococci, both aerobic and anaerobic diphtheroids, and other anaerobic organisms that normally colonize the upper respiratory tract. There may, however, be a higher incidence of such bacteremia following the nasotracheal route of intubation (16 percent in one series) than follow-

ing the less traumatic orotracheal route [5]. Although there is no information on the incidence of infections associated with transient bacteremia, the types of organisms that have been isolated in studies of anesthesia-associated bacteremia suggest that short courses of relatively low doses of penicillin (which would presumably not predispose to bacterial superinfection) may be effective in preventing significant bacteremia. Since such courses of penicillin are given to patients with rheumatic valvular disease who are undergoing other forms of trauma to the oral mucosa (e.g., dental extractions), they should be considered for the same type of patient about to receive general anesthesia.

Infections of the Central Nervous System: Reservoirs and Shunts
Serious infection can complicate the insertion or prolonged use of two very important neurosurgical devices: the Ommaya-type subcutaneous reservoir, which is used for administering intrathecal therapy for fungal or neoplastic meningitis, and the ventricular shunt, which is used for decompression of hydrocephalus.

Complications have been observed frequently following the insertion or chronic usage of subcutaneous intraventricular reservoirs. In one series involving 21 reservoirs, nine patients developed CSF bacterial infections as a result of reservoir usage or insertion, and complications associated with 17 reservoirs in 12 patients either necessitated reservoir removal or prevented their later use for intrathecal therapy [15]. *Staphylococcus epidermidis, Corynebacterium acnes,* and α-hemolytic streptococci were the major causes of the reservoir infections, and this predominance of normal skin flora suggests that the bacteria gained access to the CSF during repeated percutaneous injections of antifungal or antineoplastic agents into the reservoir. Therapy of the bacterial superinfection usually is given systemically, because the efficacy of antimicrobials added to the reservoir, either for prophylaxis or for treatment of superinfection, has not been established. Furthermore, although in one study 80 percent of the patients who completed the treatment course were cured by systemic antimicrobial therapy alone [15], we still feel that infected spinal fluid devices should be removed.

The use of the valved (Spitz-Holter type) catheters for the treatment of hydrocephalus (i.e., to shunt CSF from the lateral ventricle of the brain to the superior vena cava, the right atrium, or the peritoneum) has also been complicated by a high incidence of infections. In a number of series, the overall incidence of shunt infections has ranged from 6 to 23 percent, with a median of about 14 percent [30]. Most of these infections are caused by *S. aureus* or *S. epidermidis* and occur within two weeks to two months after surgery, which stresses the importance of intraoperative and perioperative shunt contamination in the pathogenesis of shunt infection. The equal risk of infection in patients with ventriculoatrial and ventriculoperitoneal shunts suggests that transient bacteremia is a less likely cause of such infections, since ventriculoperitoneal shunts are not exposed to the bloodstream [40].

Patients with infected ventricular shunts have several different clinical presentations. Some display a markedly toxic course with persistent pyrexia, progressive anemia, splenomegaly, and repeatedly positive blood cultures. Others have a chronic, indolent course, and considerable clinical suspicion may be necessary before appropriate steps are undertaken. In certain cases, the clinical pattern may be related to the bacteriologic characteristics of the infection. Only about one-third of infected shunts, for example, exhibit visible wound infection and necrosis, but when these occur, they are important signs of underlying infection, usually with *S. aureus*. In contrast to cases with obvious local inflammation, *S. epidermidis* is found in the great majority of other cases, and this organism is most frequently associated with bacteremic infections.

The antimicrobial treatment of the shunt infections that complicate hydrocephalus is usually unsatisfactory unless the shunt is removed. Although less than 10 percent of patients have their infection eradicated by systemic antimicrobial therapy alone, small numbers of patients have been treated with combinations of systemic and intraventricular antibiotics, and the addition of the latter appears to improve cure rates. Repeated administration of intraventricular antibiotics has its own complications, however, and when infection is widespread, the treatment of choice appears to be the administration of appropriate systemic antibiotics and the complete removal of the shunt to a new site. Preferably, some time should elapse between the removal of the infected shunt and the insertion of a new one. Despite this discouraging picture, it should be recognized that many of the antibiotics that were used to treat shunt infections in the past have been supplanted by newer agents that may prove to be more efficacious against this highly refractory infectious complication. In addition, the epidemiologic characteristics of shunt infections (e.g., perioperative acquisition of organisms) and the narrow spectrum of shunt pathogens suggest that the use of prophylactic antimicrobials at the time of shunt surgery may prove beneficial. Although one controlled study of relatively low-dose oxacillin prophylaxis failed to show that antibiotics had a significant protective effect [49], studies using larger doses of this or other drugs administered in such a way that high levels in the spinal fluid are attained at the time of surgery may be more successful.

Transient Bacteremia from Nonvascular Procedures

The occurrence of transient bacteremia associated with relatively noninvasive manipulation of colonized mucosa is well recognized. Such bacteremia usually lasts no longer than 5 to 15 minutes, may shower at its peak 100 organisms per milliliter of blood (although the peak concentration is almost always much less), and is largely asymptomatic. Over 60 studies have reported on bacteremia following oral treatments alone [11]. In this section, we will discuss bacteremia following diagnostic gastrointestinal procedures, genitourinary instrumentation, and bronchoscopy; bacteremia following endotracheal intubation and invasive vascular procedures is covered earlier in this chapter.

Table 28-1. Characteristics of Transient Bacteremia Associated with Selected Procedures

Procedure[a]	Maximum incidence of bacteremia	Maximum concentration of organisms per milliliter	Maximum duration of bacteremia (minutes after procedure)	Predominant organisms isolated	Symptoms
Dental	90%	130	10	3 : 1 anaerobes to aerobes	None
Urologic	66%	—[b]	—	Enterococcus, *Klebsiella*	Fever (percentage not stated)
Colonoscopy	27%	—	30	Anaerobes	Fever (33%)
Liver biopsy	13%	60	15	*E. coli, Streptococcus pneumoniae*	None
Barium enema	11%	102	15	Enterococcus	None
Sigmoidoscopy	9.5%	51	15	Enterococcus	None

[a] Excludes case reports of symptomatic bacteremia following procedures such as esophagoscopy, rectal biopsy, small intestine biopsy, cholangioscopy, and fiber-optic bronchoscopy; references for table cited in text.
[b] Dash indicates data not reported.

Table 28-1 presents a summary of the characteristics of bacteremia associated with selected nonvascular procedures.

Gastrointestinal Procedures

Bacteremia has been reported as a sequel to a variety of gastrointestinal procedures, including sigmoidoscopy, colonoscopy, barium enema, esophagoscopy, and biopsy of mucosal masses. In one prospective study of sigmoidoscopy, transient asymptomatic bacteremia was noted in 19 of 200 procedures [28]. The majority of organisms isolated were enterococci, and bacteremia was observed more frequently five minutes after than one minute after the termination of the procedure. Of note in this study, serial blood cultures were obtained through an indwelling venous needle. Although this convenient approach may have distorted or amplified culture results and is thus open to some criticism, the temporal profile and magnitude of bacteremia, as well as the types of organisms isolated, are consistent with bacteremia arising from the site of instrumentation. Other investigators using similar methods, however, have found bacteremia to be a rare complication of their sigmoidoscopic examinations, and they have concluded that other factors, particularly

the experience of the sigmoidoscopist, need to be evaluated before routine antibiotic prophylaxis can be advocated for patients undergoing sigmoidoscopy [19].

In a study of colonoscopy, careful anaerobic culturing and subsequent hourly temperature evaluation of patients showed a 27 percent incidence of transient bacteremia during the procedure and a 33 percent incidence of postprocedure fever in patients who had been bacteremic [34]. The greater trauma of colonoscopy compared to sigmoidoscopy may be responsible for the greater incidence of bacteremia and the more marked clinical response. Host factors may also influence the incidence and outcome of procedure-related bacteremia. In this regard, it is noteworthy that rare cases of symptomatic barium-enema septicemia have been reported in patients with impaired host defenses (acute leukemia) and in patients with active inflammatory bowel disease.

Although the role of antibiotic prophylaxis for endoscopy procedures is not certain, other preventive measures—particularly careful disinfection of endoscopes and good aseptic technique—are of definite importance. The importance of such measures is highlighted by several anecdotal reports. In one report, two cases of

Pseudomonas sepsis in leukemic patients undergoing esophagoscopy with mucosal biopsy were traced to exogenous bacteria introduced at the time of biopsy. Cultures of the esophagoscope and of the endoscopy room revealed widespread contamination with enteric organisms, including *P. aeruginosa,* and it was shown that in the routine handling of the instruments, aseptic technique was ignored [21]. In a second report, a case of cholangitis with polymicrobial sepsis followed endoscopic, retrograde, cholangiopancreatography in a patient without biliary tract obstruction. Inadequate disinfection of endoscopy equipment was implicated as the source of infection [18]. In a third report, several cases of infection with an uncommon, non-*typhosa, Salmonella* species were traced to an ineffectively cleaned endoscope [20]. Although endoscopy instruments pass through fields that are already grossly contaminated, the nosocomial organisms that may potentially be introduced by the equipment may be more invasive, more resistant, or more contagious than the patient's own flora. Clearly, any instrument that comes in contact with mucosal membranes during a procedure requires a high level of disinfection.

Percutaneous liver biopsy, although an invasive procedure, is not generally considered to be associated with infection risk. Two recent studies, however, have documented incidences of bacteremia of 6 and 14 percent following liver biopsy. In the first study, bacteremia was detectable in patients for several hours after biopsy, and it was associated in at least one patient with signs of gram-negative sepsis, but it may not have been attributable directly to the biopsy in all the cases [31]. In the second study, however, the bacteremias were transient, lasted for only 15 to 20 minutes after biopsy, and were asymptomatic [29]. In this study, cultures of liver biopsy specimens were positive in 7 percent of patients, and patients with positive specimens had a significantly higher incidence of bacteremia (83 percent) than did patients whose specimens were sterile (8.4 percent), which suggests a direct relationship between biopsy and bacteremia. One explanation of this relationship is that the hepatic reticuloendothe-

lial cells that were in the process of "clearing" gut bacteria from the portal system were biopsied, resulting in a culture-positive biopsy specimen, a temporary defect in the bacterial clearance mechanisms of the biopsied area, and an associated transient bacteremia. The incidence and clinical significance of liver biopsy-associated bacteremia need further evaluation, as does an association noted in the second study mentioned above between liver biopsy and transient pneumococcal bacteremia in patients with cirrhosis. Antibiotic prophylaxis with liver biopsy is not warranted at present.

Urologic Instrumentation

An association among urethral instrumentation, fever, and bacteremia has been recognized for many years. In various studies, the incidence of bacteremia associated with urologic procedures has been 2 to 67 percent, with the greatest risks of bacteremia occurring in patients with pre-existing urinary tract infections, in patients undergoing transurethral resection of the prostate, and in patients with prostatitis that is evident on histologic section of biopsy specimens [45]. In 50 to 67 percent of patients who develop bacteremia after instrumentation, similar organisms are recovered from both preinstrumentation urine cultures and postinstrumentation blood cultures. The available evidence suggests that the sources of the other 33 to 50 percent of postinstrumentation bacteremias include occult prostatitis, the introduction of normal urethral flora (which perhaps explains the relatively large number of blood cultures that were positive for anaerobes in one study), and the contamination of equipment or irrigating fluids before or during instrumentation. It is apparent that careful evaluation for genitourinary tract infection before instrumentation, treatment of any infection, appropriate disinfection of equipment, and careful aseptic technique are mandatory. Moreover, because of the relatively frequent occurrence of enterococcal bacteremia after urologic instrumentation and because of the association of instrumentation with gram-negative sepsis as well as with infection at distal sites (e.g., joints), a brief pulse of systemic prophylactic antibiotics at the time of instrumentation may be warranted in high-risk patients, such as those with valvular heart disease, preexisting joint disease, or impaired host defenses [10].

Bronchoscopy

Although fever and bacteremia have been documented in patients after rigid-tube bronchoscopy [10], bacteremia has not yet been documented prospectively in patients undergoing flexible fiber-optic bronchoscopy. There is, however, one case report of fatal *Pseudomonas* bacteremia that was related to fiber-optic bronchoscopy in a patient with preexisting *Pseudomonas* bronchitis. Furthermore, in one series of 100 patients who were followed carefully after fiber-optic bronchoscopy, 16 developed fever, five developed transient parenchymal infiltrates, and one developed rapidly fatal pneumonia. Older patients (more than 60 years old) and those with abnormalities on bronchoscopy were at greatest risk of complications. With the exception of the one fatal pneumonitis, however, all complicating infections resolved without antibiotic therapy, and prospective culturing failed to demonstrate bacteremia in any of the 100 subjects [35].

Conclusions

Two overall conclusions can be drawn from the studies on procedure-related bacteremia cited above: the equipment used for the procedures should be adequately disinfected or sterilized before every use and proper aseptic technique should be employed by the operator. Beyond this, it is apparent that carefully planned, prospective, multicenter studies are needed to assess the incidence and clinical significance of procedure-related transient bacteremia, to determine which hosts are at risk of associated sepsis or infection at distal sites, to determine if specific risks for certain procedures can be sufficiently defined to justify preventive measures such as antibiotic prophylaxis, and to determine which prophylactic regimens would be most efficacious. Although such studies may not be available for some time, the procedures obviously will continue, and we have tried to note situations where it seems reasonable to "cover" patients. In this regard, it should be noted that for years, dental patients with valvular heart disease have received endocarditis prophylaxis, largely on an empiric basis [10].

Other Procedures Associated with Infections

Cystoscopy

In addition to the risk of bacteremia associated with cystoscopy, a significant risk of urinary tract infection is associated with this procedure. Several remarkably similar outbreaks have been reported in which the use of dilute, aqueous, quaternary ammonium compounds as a cystoscope disinfectant was associated with procedure-related urinary tract infections with *Pseudomonas* species, particular *P. cepacia* (also see Part 2, Chapter 14). In these outbreaks, the quaternary ammonium compounds either were ineffective in decontaminating the equipment or were themselves actually harboring viable bacteria while in use as disinfectants [16].

Although the risk of infection associated with the use of dilute, aqueous, quaternary ammonium compounds has been known for at least 20 years, many hospital personnel persist in using these compounds as antiseptics and disinfectants. Such use has most likely resulted in many outbreaks of nosocomial urinary tract infection, as well as outbreaks of nosocomial bacteremia and occasional outbreaks of nosocomial respiratory tract and wound infection. To help decrease the risk of nosocomial urinary tract infection following cystoscopy, it is important that the equipment be thoroughly cleaned and properly disinfected between uses.

Arthrocentesis and Thoracocentesis

Although septic arthritis is caused most commonly by hematogenous spread of organisms, sporadic cases of staphylococcal arthritis and, at times, gram-negative bacillary arthritis have followed several days after invasive joint manipulations. During the mid-1960s, CDC epidemiologists investigated a cluster of cases of staphylococcal arthritis in which the infections occurred one to seven days after outpatient arthrocentesis or intraarticular injection of steroids. Epidemiologic evidence suggested that the physician who had performed these procedures was a disseminator of the epidemic strain, and microbiologic investigation showed that areas of chronic dermatitis on the physician's hands harbored the epidemic organism. A similar cluster of cases of staphylococcal arthritis, in which the infections occurred five to six days after arthrographic examination of the knee joint and three to four days after knee surgery, was traced epidemiologically to the surgeon who had performed these procedures, who was a nasal carrier of staphylococci.

Other diagnostic "taps," such as thoracocentesis [4], have also been associated with nosocomial infections and emphasize the fact that all invasive procedures should be performed only under strict aseptic conditions, with careful skin preparation, by an appropriately "scrubbed and gloved" operator, and using sterile equipment. While the relative rarity of centesis-associated infections may be considered as testimony that good technique is generally employed in our hospitals and clinics, the lack of such infections also may be evidence of the capacity of the local tissue response to limit bacterial invasion in uncompromised hosts [14]. When procedures are performed in patients with compromised host defenses or on tissues (e.g., rheumatoid joints) that may have diminished ability to limit bacterial invasion, the risk of procedure-associated infections may be considerable, which emphasizes the need for continued vigilance.

Peritoneal Manipulation
Infectious complications of laparoscopy and amniocentesis are rare, presumably because of careful technique, sterile equipment, local host defense mechanisms, and the frequently healthy nature of the subjects. Peritoneal dialysis has also been surprisingly free of infectious complications; peritonitis occurred only seven times in one prospective study of 6000 consecutive dialyses [38]. Although the most frequent reason for peritonitis in this study was poor cannula care, one case of *Acinetobacter* peritonitis was traced to contamination of the dialysate when it was warmed in a water bath.

Interestingly, a recent outbreak of *Acinetobacter* peritonitis in another institution also was traced to the contamination of dialysate from a water bath with a high inoculum of this organism.

Aseptic peritonitis may also occur occasionally during peritoneal dialysis, presumably as a result of chemical contaminants. The differentiation between aseptic and bacterial dialysis-associated peritonitis is important, because treatment of the former requires temporary discontinuation of dialysis, whereas the latter is treated currently by continued dialysis with antibiotic-containing dialysate. In either case, the source of contamination must be sought.

Ophthalmologic Examination
Manipulation of the conjunctivas and cornea occurs during tonometry, instillation of eye drops, and manual ophthalmologic examination, and it can result in transmission of conjunctivitis and other eye infections. The infection most commonly transmitted is epidemic keratoconjunctivitis, a highly contagious, frequently iatrogenic disease, which usually is caused by adenovirus type 8 [22]. Transmission of the virus occurs via fomites, such as inadequately disinfected tonometers and contaminated eye droppers, as well as by indirect person-to-person spread on the hands of health workers. Similar modes of transmission have been implicated in outbreaks of other viral and bacterial eye infection. Proper care of equipment and conscientious hand-washing between patient contacts is remarkably effective in halting the transmission of such diseases.

Barium Enema
In addition to transient bacteremia, patients undergoing barium enema are at risk of two other infectious complications. First, infants may aspirate barium when faulty technique produces excessive retrograde flow of contrast material. Second, if the enema bag or tip is not replaced or is not adequately disinfected between uses or if the barium is contaminated, then the procedure may transmit enteric pathogens. This risk was highlighted by Meyers and Richards [33] when they demonstrated that

attenuated poliovirus can be transferred via contaminated barium enema. At present, the use of disposable enema bags, tubing, and enema tips has largely put an end, as it were, to such risks.

References

1. Anagnostakis, D., Kamba, A., Petrochilon, V., Arsen, A., and Matsaniotis, N. Risk of infection associated with umbilical vein catheterization. *J. Pediatr.* 86:759, 1975.
2. Asnes, R. S., and Arendar, G. M. Septic arthritis of the hip. *Pediatrics* 38:837, 1966.
3. Bard, H., Albert, G., Teasdale, F., Doray, B., and Martineau, B. Prophylactic antibiotics in chronic umbilical artery catheterization in respiratory distress syndrome. *Arch. Dis. Child.* 48:630, 1973.
4. Bayer, A. S., Nelson, S. C., Galpin, J. E., Chow, A. W., and Guze, L. B. Necrotizing pneumonia and empyema due to *Clostridium perfringens. Am. J. Med.* 59:851, 1975.
5. Berry, F. A., Blankenbaker, W. L., and Ball, C. G. A comparison of bacteremia occurring with nasotracheal and orotracheal intubation. *Anesth. Analg.* (Cleve.) 52:873, 1973.
6. Braude, A. I., Sanford, J. P., Bartlett, J. E., and Mallery, O. T. Effects and clinical significance of bacterial contaminants in transfused blood. *J. Lab. Clin. Med.* 39:902, 1952.
7. Bruce-Chwatt, L. J. Blood transfusion and tropical disease. *Trop. Dis. Bull.* 69:825, 1972.
8. Buchholtz, D. H., Young, V. M., Friedman, N. R., Reilly, J. A., and Mardiney, M. R. Bacterial proliferation in platelets stored at room temperature. *N. Engl. J. Med.* 285:429, 1971.
9. Chmel, H., and Armstrong, D. *Salmonella oslo*—A focal outbreak in a hospital. *Am. J. Med.* 60:203, 1976.
10. Committee on the Prevention of Rheumatic Fever and Bacterial Endocarditis. Prevention of bacterial endocarditis. *Circ.* 56(S):139A, 1977.
11. Crawford, J. J., Sconyers, J. R., Moriarty, J. D., King, R. C., and West, J. F. Bacteremia after tooth extractions studied with the aid of pre-reduced anaerobically sterilized culture media. *Appl. Microbiol.* 27:927, 1974.
12. Culver, G. A., Makel, H. P., and Beecher, H. K. Frequency of aspiration of gastric contents by the lungs during anesthesia and surgery. *Ann. Surg.* 133:289, 1951.
13. Cunningham, M., and Cash, J. D. Bacterial contamination of platelet concentrates stored at 20°C. *J. Clin. Pathol.* 26:401, 1973.
14. Dann, T. C. Routine skin preparation before injection—An unnecessary procedure. *Lancet* 2:96, 1969.
15. Diamond, R. D., and Bennett, J. E. A subcutaneous reservoir for intrathecal therapy of fungal meningitis. *N. Engl. J. Med.* 288:186, 1974.
16. Dixon, R. E., Kaslow, R. A., Mackel, D. C., Fulkerson, C. C., and Mallison, G. F. Aqueous quaternary ammonium antiseptics and disinfectants. Use and mis-use. *J.A.M.A.* 236:2415, 1976.
17. Dover, A. S., and Schultz, M. G. Transfusion-induced malaria. *Transfusion* 11:353, 1971.
18. Elson, C. O., Hattori, K., and Blackstone, M. O. Polymicrobial sepsis following endoscopic retrograde cholangiopancreatography. *Gastroenterology* 69:507, 1975.
19. Engeling, E. R., Eng, B. F., Sullivan-Sigler, N., Bartlett, J. G., and Gorbach, S. L. Bacteremia after sigmoidoscopy: another view. *Ann. Intern. Med.* 85:77, 1976.
20. Gardner, R. M., Schwartz, R., Wong, H. C., and Burke, J. P. Percutaneous indwelling radial-artery catheters for monitoring cardiovascular function. *N. Engl. J. Med.* 290:1227, 1974.
21. Greene, W. H., Moody, M., Hartley, R., Effman, E., Aisner, J., Young, V. M., and Wienik, P. H. Esophagoscopy as a source of *P. aeruginosa* sepsis in patients with acute leukemia: the need for sterilization of endoscopes. *Gastroenterology* 67:912, 1974.
22. Hendley, J. O. Epidemic keratoconjunctivitis and hand washing. *N. Engl. J. Med.* 289:1368, 1973.
23. Hoffman, P. C., Arnow, P. M., Goldmann, D. A., Parrott, P. L., Stamm, W. E., and McGowan, J. E. False-positive blood cultures. Association with nonsterile blood collection tubes. *J.A.M.A.* 236:2073, 1976.
24. James, J. D. Bacterial contamination of preserved blood. *Vox Sang.* 4:177, 1959.
25. Katz, L., Johnson, D. L., Neufeld, P. D., and Gupta, K. G. Evacuated blood-collection tubes—The backflow hazard. *Can. Med. Assoc. J.* 113:208, 1975.
26. Kimball, A. C., Kean, B. H., and Kellner, A. The risk of transmitting toxoplasmosis by blood transfusion. *Transfusion* 5:447, 1965.
27. Krauss, A. N., Albert, R. F., and Kannan, M. M. Contamination of umbilical catheters in the newborn infant. *J. Pediatr.* 77:965, 1970.
28. LeFrock, J. L., Ellis, C. A., Turchik, J. B., and Weinstein, L. Transient bacteremia associated with sigmoidoscopy. *N. Engl. J. Med.* 289:467, 1973.
29. LeFrock, J. L., Ellis, C. A., Turchik, J. B., Zawacki, J. K., and Weinstein, L. Transient

bacteremia associated with percutaneous liver biopsy. *J. Infest. Dis.* 131(Suppl.):104, 1975.

30. Luthardt, T. Bacterial infections in ventriculo-auricular shunt systems. *Dev. Med. Child Neurol.* [*Suppl.*] 12:105, 1970.

31. McCloskey, R. V., Gold, M., and Weser, E. Bacteremia after liver biopsy. *Arch. Intern. Med.* 132:213, 1973.

32. Mendelson, C. L. The aspiration of stomach contents into the lungs during obstetric anesthesia. *Am. J. Obstet. Gynecol.* 52:191, 1946.

33. Meyers, P. H., and Richards, M. Transmission of polio virus vaccine by contaminated barium enema with resultant antibody rise. *Am. J. Roentgenol. Radium Ther. Nucl. Med.* 91:864, 1964.

34. Pelican, G., Hentges, D., and Butt, J. H. Bacteremia during colonoscopy. *Gastrointest. Endosc.* 22:233, 1976.

35. Pereira, W., Kovnat, D. M., Khan, M. A., Iacovino, J. R., Spivack, M. L., and Snider, G. L. Fever and pneumonia after flexible fiberoptic bronchoscopy. *Am. Rev. Respir. Dis.* 112:59, 1975.

36. Powers, W. F., and Tooley, W. H. Contamination of umbilical vessel catheters. *Pediatrics* 48:470, 1971.

37. Rhame, F. S., Root, R. K., MacLowry, J. D., Dadisman, T. A., and Bennett, J. V. *Salmonella* septicemia from platelet transfusions. *Ann. Intern. Med.* 78:633, 1973.

38. Rubin, J., Oreoponlos, D. G., Lio, T. T., Matthews, R., and deVeber, G. A. Management of peritonitis and bowel perforation during chronic peritoneal dialysis. *Nephron* 16:220, 1976.

39. Sande, M. A., Levinson, M. E., Lukas, D. S., and Kaye, D. Bacteremia associated with cardiac catheterization. *N. Engl. J. Med.* 281:1104, 1969.

40. Schoenbaum, S. C., Gardner, P., and Shillito, J. Infections of cerebrospinal fluid shunts. *J. Infect. Dis.* 131:543, 1975.

41. Sherwood, P. M. An outbreak of syringe-transmitted hepatitis with jaundice in hospitalized diabetic patients. *Ann. Intern. Med.* 33:380, 1950.

42. Siegel, S. E., Lunde, M. N., Gelderman, A., Halterman, R. H., Brown, J. A., Levine, A. S., and Graw, R. G., Jr. Transmission of toxoplasmosis by leukocyte transfusion. *Blood* 37:388, 1971.

43. Stamm, W. E., Colella, J. J., Anderson, R. L., and Dixon, R. E. Indwelling arterial catheters as a source of nosocomial bacteremia. *N. Engl. J. Med.* 292:1099, 1975.

44. Steere, A. C., Tenney, J. H., Mackel, D. C., Snyder, M. J., Polakavetz, S., Dunne, M. E., and Dixon, R. E. *Pseudomonas* species bacteremia caused by contaminated normal human serum albumin. *J. Infect. Dis.* 135:729, 1977.

45. Sullivan, N. M., Sutter, V. L., Carter, W. T., Attebery, H. R., and Finegold, S. M. Bacteremia after genitourinary tract manipulation. *Appl. Microbiol.* 23:1101, 1972.

46. Walton, J. R., Shapiro, B. A., and Harrison, R. A. *Serratia* bacteremia from mean arterial pressure monitors. *Anesthesiology* 43:113, 1975.

47. Weinstein, R. A. The design of pressure monitoring devices. *Med. Instrum.* 10:287, 1976.

48. Weinstein, R. A., Stamm, W. E., Kramer, L., and Corey, L. Pressure monitoring devices—Overlooked source of nosocomial infection. *J.A.M.A.* 236:936, 1976.

49. Weiss, S. R., and Raskind, R. Further experience with the ventriculoperitoneal shunt. *Int. Surg.* 53:300, 1970.

29

Gram-Negative Rod Bacteremia

Allen C. Steere, Walter E. Stamm,
Stanley M. Martin, and John V. Bennett

The organisms included in studies of gram-negative rod bacteremia have varied. Many authors have excluded certain gram-negative rod organisms, whereas others have included enterococci, which are gram-positive organisms. In accord with most reviews, we restrict the scope of this chapter to aerobic, rod-shaped, gram-negative bacteria that commonly cause nosocomial infections; *Salmonella, Shigella, Brucella, Yersinia,* anaerobic gram-negative rods, and enterococci are excluded.

"Primary" bacteremias are those without a clinically evident, underlying site of infection that is responsible for the bloodstream organisms. "Secondary" bacteremias are those that are bacteriologically, temporally, and clinically related to a recognized infection at another site within the patient. Bacteremias resulting from contaminated intravenous (IV) fluids (see Part II, Chapter 26) are considered primary bacteremias, whereas those resulting from certain complications of IV cannulation (e.g., cellulitis and purulent thrombophlebitis; see Part II, Chapter 25) are considered secondary bacteremias. Difficulties in classification arise either when a clinically evident infection at another site has not been cultured, or when cultures from it are negative. In such circumstances, the location of the underlying site of infection, the potentially confounding influence of antibiotic therapy, and the identity and antibacterial susceptibility of the bacteremic organisms can be used to judge whether a bacteremic episode is "primary" or "secondary." The consistency of inter-hospital surveillance of secondary bacteremias can be improved, however, by requiring culture-study documentation of underlying sites of infection. Such a requirement has been imposed on participants in Center for Disease Control (CDC) surveillance programs.

Primary bacteremias with clinical onset during hospitalization are considered nosocomial. Secondary bacteremias are considered nosocomial when the underlying site of infection is (1) nosocomial or (2) community-acquired where the clinical onset of bacteremia occurs more than 24 hours after admission. All other bacteremias are considered community-acquired.

Bacteremia may occur without clinical symptoms. The CDC surveillance data presented in this chapter, however, include only nosocomial, gram-negative rod bacteremias that were judged to be clinically significant.

Surveillance data were obtained from the National Nosocomial Infections Study (NNIS) and the Comprehensive Hospital Infections Project (CHIP) for the period 1970 through 1973. About 3100 patients with clinically significant, nosocomial, gram-negative rod bacteremia, from whom 3334 bacterial isolates were obtained, were reported from all participating hospitals. To avoid bias, a nine-month interval has been excluded in 1970–1971, during which a nationwide epidemic of gram-negative rod bacteremia caused by contaminated infusion fluid occurred (see Part II, Chapter 26).

Diagnostic Criteria
Clinical
The symptoms of gram-negative bacteremia usually begin abruptly with the onset of shaking chills and a temperature elevation of 101°F to 105°F (38.3°C to 40.5°C). Nausea, vomiting, diarrhea, and prostration may also occur. In elderly, debilitated patients or in infants, the symptoms may be nonspecific and may include hypothermia, increasing confusion, or lethargy. If septic shock develops, then tachycardia, tachypnea, mental obtundation, hypotension, and oliguria may occur. Early in endotoxic shock, the extremities may be warm, but they later become cool and pale. Organ hypoperfusion caused by extreme arteriolar constriction and venous pooling of blood is the most important consequence of septic shock. In severe cases, death may result from heart failure with pulmonary edema, cardiac arrhythmias, respiratory insufficiency, or disseminated intravascular coagulation.

The laboratory data on septic shock may vary greatly. Early in the course, the white blood cell count often shows a leukopenia, but in 6 to 12 hours, the white cell count frequently climbs to 15,000 to 30,000 cells per cubic

millimeter. Initially, tachypnea results in a low carbon dioxide tension (Pco_2) with resulting respiratory alkalosis, but, as shock develops, the oxygen tension (Po_2) drops, often below 70 mm. Hg, with resultant marked anoxia. As lacticacidemia increases, metabolic acidosis develops. Hemodynamic measurements usually show a high peripheral resistance, a low central venous pressure, a low cardiac output, and a slow circulation time. If heart failure develops, the central venous pressure becomes elevated.

Microbiologic
For rapid diagnosis, intraleukocytic forms may occasionally be seen in peripheral blood smears, but examination of the buffy coat is more likely to be rewarding [4,21]. Although these examinations may be helpful in making a rapid diagnosis, these procedures are usually not revealing, and a positive blood culture containing an organism of the appropriate identity (see above) is required to diagnose gram-negative rod bacteremia securely.

The *Limulus* amebocyte lysate test is the most sensitive known assay for the detection of endotoxin. Early reports suggested two clinical uses for the test: (1) a positive *Limulus* test may help confirm the diagnosis of gram-negative bacteremia if blood cultures are negative, and (2) the mortality rates were twice as high in patients with positive blood cultures and positive *Limulus* tests compared to patients in whom only one of the tests was positive [13]. Subsequent investigators, however, have been unable to confirm the validity of either statement, and they have pointed out that the test is not specific for endotoxin; proteins and polynucleotides may also cause a positive reaction. In one study, patients with gram-negative bacteremia and patients without infections were equally likely to have positive *Limulus* tests [22]. Nevertheless, with better standardization of the lysate, the test may have some applicability in quantitating endotoxin levels in circumstances where one suspects its presence.

Specimens
Collection
Before blood culture specimens are taken, the skin of the patient and the rubber bung of the

blood-culturing apparatus must be properly prepared. Tincture of iodine (1 to 2% iodine in 70% alcohol) is an excellent antiseptic for this purpose. After a two-minute exposure and collection of blood for culture, the tincture of iodine should be removed from the skin with 70% alcohol to avoid the possibility of skin burns. Either 70% alcohol alone or an iodophor may be used.

Bacteremia can be intermittent in certain patients (e.g., those with subacute bacterial endocarditis), and multiple blood cultures obtained at widely separated time intervals may increase the likelihood of isolating the causative organisms. However, antibiotic therapy should be rapidly instituted in patients with acute clinical manifestations of bacteremia. Three blood culture specimens taken within minutes of each other are advised, since the institution of antibiotic therapy should not be unduly delayed. For adult patients, 10 ml. of blood should be collected for each culture. Collection of lesser volumes may be associated with a lower recovery rate. In pediatric patients, 1 to 5 ml. should be collected for each culture. In order to reduce the normal bactericidal activity present in serum, blood should be inoculated into culture media in a proportion of 1 ml. of blood per 10 ml. or more of broth. Sodium polyanetholsulfonate (SPS), which is present as an anticoagulant in many blood-culture media, also inhibits the bactericidal activity in serum.

When blood is collected with a syringe, the original needle should not be used to inject blood into culture media, since this practice may introduce contaminants. A new sterile needle should be attached to the syringe. Blood from the same venipuncture is sometimes used for blood culture studies as well as other purposes. When this is done, blood for culture should be obtained first, because retrograde contamination of blood-collection equipment can occur from nonsterile vacuum tubes (see Part II, Chapter 28).

Most commercially available nutrient broths —such as trypticase-soy, Columbia,* or brain-

heart infusion media—can be successfully used for culturing blood. Because such liquid media are usually bottled under vacuum with carbon dioxide and contain SPS, they are satisfactory for culturing anaerobes as well as aerobes. Hospitals should not use thioglycolate fluid as their only culture medium, because this will result in lower isolation rates for aerobic and facultatively anaerobic organisms. (See Part II, Chapter 17, for special considerations involving the collection of blood cultures for diagnosis of infections of cardiac prostheses.)

Processing

Blood culture specimens should be incubated at least seven days at 35°C (95°F) to permit the growth of strict aerobes such as *Pseudomonas* species. One bottle of each set of three cultures should be vented by aseptically inserting a sterile, cotton-plugged needle through the bottle's rubber stopper. Addition of penicillinase to the culture media may improve the rate of recovery of organisms from patients who are being treated with penicillinase-sensitive antibiotics. SPS, which is present in most commercial media, will inhibit the activity of aminoglycosides and polymyxins.

Cultures should be macroscopically examined each day for evidence of turbidity, hemolysis, or gas production. Any culture suspected of having growth should have a Gram stain and subculture performed. A variety of regimens for performing Gram stains and subcultures on macroscopically negative culture bottles have been recommended. In many laboratories, Gram stains and subcultures are routinely performed at 48 hours, five days, and seven days. Many workers have shown that by using daily subcultures and Gram stains, about one-third of all positive cultures are detected at least 24 hours before there is macroscopic evidence of growth.

All positive cultures should be identified as to genus and species, and antibiotic susceptibility tests should be performed. In addition, subcultures of all blood isolates should be kept for one month or longer in the event that further testing or typing is required. Assistance in the identification of unusual organisms may be

* Names of manufacturers and trade names are provided for identification only and inclusion does not imply endorsement by the Public Health Service or the U.S. Department of Health, Education, and Welfare.

obtained from state public health laboratories.

Incidence and Mortality of Nosocomial Infections

Probably because of the advancing age of hospitalized patients, the introduction of antibiotics, medical advances that prolong the lives of debilitated patients, and the increasing use of catheters, respirators, and other devices and procedures that may predispose to infection, the incidence of gram-negative bacteremia has increased over the past 40 years. The average incidence of gram-negative bacteremia in selected studies from university and large municipal hospitals reported in the medical literature

Table 29-1. Incidence and Mortality of Gram-Negative Bacteremia in Selected Studies, 1935 to 1970

Year(s)	Hospital, author(s)	Incidence per 1000	Percent mortality	Mortality definition		
				Unstated criteria	Bacteremia and death on same admission	Deaths attributed to bacteremia
1935	Boston City, Finland [9]	1.1	58%		X	
1950–59	Boston City, Finland [9]	5.5	40%		X	
	Univ. of Minnesota, Weil and Spink [23]	—	40%		X	
	Univ. of Illinois, McCabe and Jackson [16]	3.9	42%	X		
	Univ. of Minnesota, DuPont and Spink [7]	4.9	37%		X	
	Los Angeles County, Weil et al. [24]	2.8	35%	X		
Mean values, 1950–59		4.3	39%			
1960–65	Boston City, Finland [9]	7.1	42%		X	
	Stanford, Fried and Vosti [10]	2.8	36%	X		
	Parkland, Hodgin and Sanford [12]	—	45%	X		
	Johns Hopkins, Lewis and Fekety [14]	6.2	24%	X		
	Univ. of Minnesota, DuPont and Spink [7]	6.0	51%		X	
	Univ. of Cincinnati, Altemeier et al. [2]	—	52%	X		
Mean values, 1960–65		5.5	42%			
1965–70	Georgetown, Martin et al. [15]	—	32%			X
	Boston City, McGowan et al. [19]	13	37%		X	
	VAH, Nashville, Bryant et al. [5]	—	29%	X		
	Univ. of Minnesota, DuPont and Spink [7]	8.1	57%		X	
	Brigham, Myerowitz et al. [20]	10.7	25%			X
Mean values, 1965–70		10.6	36%			
Mean values, 1950–70		6.5	39%			

since 1950 was 6.5 cases per 1000 admissions, with a range of 2.8 to 13 per 1000 admissions (Table 29-1).

A number of factors make the comparison of rates from different studies very difficult to interpret: organisms included as "gram-negative rods" differ; some rates are based on the number of isolates, some on infectious episodes, and others on the number of patients with bacteremia; community-acquired infections are included in some studies; the definitions used for nosocomial and community-acquired bacteremias are often unstated, and they vary when stated; a stipulation that the isolates be associated with clinically significant disease is often omitted; and the frequency of blood culturing and the type of bacteriologic techniques vary from study to study.

Surveillance data from university hospitals in the CDC studies reveal an incidence of 2.4 patients with clinically significant, nosocomial, gram-negative rod bacteremias (as defined above) per 1000 discharges. The category of hospital is importantly related to the incidence of bacteremia (Table 29-2). University, federal, and municipal hospitals have substantially higher rates than community hospitals, but the last category accounts for more than one-half of all admissions. The overall incidence in hospitals from all categories, including community hospitals, was 1.2 cases per 1000 admissions.

The annual number of cases in the United States can be estimated from CDC rates for each category of hospital (see Table 29-2), which yield an overall estimate of about 39,000 cases per year. If the difference between the average for published rates and the rate for university hospitals in CDC's surveillance programs (6.5 and 2.4 per 1000 admissions, respectively) is attributed solely to underreporting in the latter category, and if the rates for all hospital categories are adjusted upward by this factor, then about 100,000 cases—which correspond to an overall rate of about 3 per 1000 admissions—would be expected annually. We believe, however, that these are inflated estimates and that the true annual number of cases probably lies between 40,000 and 50,000.

Published studies generally show that an underlying site of infection cannot be found in about 30 percent of all cases, whereas about 66 percent of the bacteremias in CDC surveillance data are not attributed to underlying sites. CDC's surveillance system requests that secondary bacteremias be reported only when an underlying site is involved in a clinically significant infection and an organism(s) is cultured from the underlying site that matches the blood isolate(s). Anatomic sites judged to be the portal of entry, in the absence of clinically significant infections at that site, are not included in tabulations of secondary bacteremia.

In 13 published studies undertaken since 1950, the average overall case-fatality ratio was about 40 percent (see Table 29-1). Most studies, however, have not reported whether the patient's death was caused by the bacteremia or the patient's underlying disease. Probably only 25 to 30 percent of patients with gram-negative bacteremia die because of the infection.

Endotoxic shock occurs in about a third of patients who experience gram-negative bacteremia. The mortality in patients with endotoxic shock is about 80 percent, and in those without shock, the rate is about 32 percent.

Polymicrobial bacteremia involving one or

Table 29-2. Estimated National Magnitude of Nosocomial Gram-Negative Rod Bacteremias

Hospital type	Estimated admissions in 1972[a]	Rate per 1000[b]	Estimated cases in 1972
University	7,194,000	2.4	17,266
Federal	1,683,000	1.9	3164
Municipal	7,788,000	1.5	11,526
Community (300 beds or more)	5,280,000	0.6	3326
Community (less than 300 beds)	11,055,000	0.4	3869
Totals and overall rate	33,000,000	1.2	39,151

[a] Based on random sample from American Hospital Association Guide for 1972 [3].
[b] Number of patients with clinically significant, nosocomial, gram-negative rod bacteremia (as defined in text) per 1000 admissions.
Data from National Nosocomial Infections Study, 1970 through 1973, excluding a nine-month interval in 1970–1971 (see Part II, Chapter 26).

more gram-negative pathogens represents 6 to 10 percent of all recognized bacteremias, and it often originates from infections in the gastrointestinal tract or in patients with hematologic or solid malignancies. Mortality in patients with polymicrobial bacteremia increases with the severity of the underlying disease, and, in most series, the mortality rate exceeds that associated with bacteremia due to a single type of organism.

Pathogens

Although *Escherichia coli* is the most common pathogen causing nosocomial gram-negative bacteremia, members of the tribe Klebsielleae (*Klebsiella, Enterobacter,* and *Serratia*) are also frequently isolated (Table 29-3). Several recent studies have demonstrated an increase in the proportion of bacteremias due to tribe Klebsielleae organisms, and in some hospitals, individual members of this tribe now exceed *E. coli* as the most common cause of gram-negative bacteremia. An increase in bacteremia due to gram-negative anaerobic organisms has also been noted in recent studies; this increase may be explained at least partially by the improved anaerobic culture methods now used in many hospitals.

*Table 29-3. Organisms Causing Nosocomial Gram-Negative Rod Bacteremias**

Primary bacteremia		Secondary bacteremia	
Agent	Percent	Agent	Percent
E. coli	29%	*E. coli*	35%
Klebsiella	22%	*Pseudomonas*	20%
Pseudomonas	18%	*Klebsiella*	17%
Enterobacter	11%	*Proteus*	11%
Proteus	8%	*Enterobacter*	9%
Serratia	6%	*Serratia*	6%
Acinetobacter	3%	Other	2%
Citrobacter	1%		
Other	2%		
Total percentages	100%		100%
Total isolates	2177		1157

* Surveillance data from NNIS for 1970 through 1973 excluding a nine-month interval in 1970–1971 (see Part II, Chapter 26).

The profile of microorganisms isolated from primary and secondary nosocomial bacteremias differs in a few respects (see Table 29-3). *E. coli* is the most frequent microorganism isolated in both types of bacteremia, but it occurs more frequently in secondary bacteremias. In contrast, *Klebsiella* is a more frequent cause of primary than of secondary bacteremia. Unusual gram-negative organisms—such as *Acinetobacter, Citrobacter, Flavobacterium,* and *Pseudomonas* species other than *aeruginosa*—are relatively more important in primary bacteremias, but none of these is a frequent cause of nosocomial bacteremia.

Although overall mortality rates for bacteremia caused by each gram-negative organism can be calculated, such rates are strongly influenced by host factors. McCabe and Jackson [17] were the first to demonstrate that pathogen-specific differences in mortality rates could be explained by the severity of the host's underlying disease (i.e., rapidly fatal, ultimately fatal, or nonfatal). Similar results were later confirmed by others. Several studies, including ours, have described an increased mortality rate for patients with *Pseudomonas* bacteremia even after the patient's underlying disease has been taken into account. Bryant and co-workers [5] reported a 33 percent mortality attributable to *Pseudomonas* bacteremia in patients with nonfatal underlying illness.

The pathogens isolated from blood cultures of patients with secondary bacteremia are presented in Table 29-4 according to the underlying infected site from which they derived. *E. coli* is the most common pathogen in bacteremias deriving from urinary tract infections, cutaneous infections other than burns, and surgical wound infections. *Pseudomonas* predominates in bacteremias deriving from respiratory and burn infections, and *Klebsiella* is most prominent in phlebitis. The profiles of organisms involved in secondary bacteremias that derive from underlying sites of infection in the urinary and respiratory tracts are generally not influenced by the presence or absence of catheterization or respiratory therapy, respectively. However, miscellaneous gram-negative rods accounted for a greater proportion of infections that were not procedure-associated, and *Serra-*

Table 29-4. Pathogens Causing Secondary Bacteremia: Percentage Distribution by Site from which the Bacteremia Derived*

Pathogen	Urinary tract		Respiratory tract		Cutaneous		Surgical wound	Phlebitis	Other
	Catheter-associated	Not catheter-associated	IPPB-associated	Not IPPB-associated	Burns	Other			
E. coli	46.5%	49.0%	16.3%	17.8%	9.7%	33.3%	33.1%	11.1%	43.1%
Klebsiella	13.6%	13.1%	16.3%	22.4%	6.5%	16.7%	14.5%	33.3%	22.6%
Enterobacter	5.2%	4.2%	16.3%	10.3%	9.7%	5.6%	13.4%	17.5%	7.3%
Proteus	13.1%	12.7%	7.0%	7.9%	6.5%	16.7%	12.2%	7.9%	12.4%
Pseudomonas	15.5%	13.5%	30.2%	32.2%	41.9%	25.0%	19.8%	20.6%	10.9%
Serratia	5.2%	5.8%	13.9%	7.0%	16.1%	0.0%	5.2%	6.3%	1.5%
	0.9%	1.5%	0.0%	2.3%	9.7%	2.8%	1.7%	3.2%	2.2%
Totals	100.0%	99.8%	100.0%	99.9%	100.1%	100.1%	99.9%	99.9%	100.0%
Percentage of blood isolates deriving from site	18.4%	22.2%	3.6%	18.1%	2.7%	3.1%	14.8%	5.4%	11.6%
Totals	40.6%		21.7%		5.8%		14.8%	5.4%	11.6%

* Surveillance data from NNIS for 1970 through 1973. Data encompass 1157 isolates from nosocomial secondary bacteremias (see text).

tia was more common in bacteremias deriving from infections associated with intermittent positive-pressure breathing (IPPB) machines than in bacteremias deriving from other respiratory infections.

Host Factors Predisposing to Infection
Age and Sex
Gram-negative bacteremia occurs in all age groups, but attack rates are highest in neonates and the elderly.

Neonatal gram-negative bacterial septicemia is usually included in reviews of neonatal sepsis, but it has rarely been separately reported. Table 29-5 presents data abstracted from those few studies that contained sufficient information to permit an analysis of neonatal gram-negative rod bacteremias. About half of all neonatal sepsis is caused by gram-negative rods. Incidence rates vary enormously from study to study, and thus the overall incidence cannot be reliably assessed. These rates seem heavily influenced by the proportion of premature infants included in each study. Only about 10 percent of all live births are premature, but a far greater proportion of premature births are associated with cases of neonatal sepsis; the incidence of gram-negative rod bacteremias appears to be several times higher in premature infants. When compared to pathogens causing adult gram-negative rod bacteremia, *E. coli* appears to be a more frequent cause of neonatal cases, *Klebsiella* is less common, and the remaining pathogens are remarkably similar in frequency. Neonatal sepsis is fatal in 30 to 45 percent of cases, and the mortality rate may be higher in premature infants. After this high-risk period, the percentage of patients dying from gram-negative bacteremia remains at about 25 percent until the fourth decade. The highest case-fatality ratios (about 60 percent) are observed in patients over 60.

From birth to age 19 and over age 50, a greater proportion of those who develop gram-negative bacteremia are males. From age 20 to 50, however, a greater proportion are females. This age-sex distribution has been explained by the increased incidence of urinary tract infections in women during the child-bearing years and by an increased incidence of urinary tract infections in older men when prostatic hypertrophy is common.

Presence of Underlying Disease
Gram-negative bacteremia is more common in patients with chronic renal disease, cirrhosis, diabetes mellitus, both solid and hematologic malignancies, and collagen-vascular diseases. All these diseases are associated with a compromised host immune system and a subsequently increased risk of infection. Gram-negative bacteremia is also more common in infants born to mothers with premature rupture of the membranes.

McCabe and Jackson [17] devised a three-category system for classifying the severity of the underlying disease. According to their system, patients who were expected to die during the same hospitalization in which the bacteremia occurred were classified as having a "rapidly fatal" disease; patients with an underlying disease in remission from which they were expected to die within four years (e.g., systemic lupus erythematosus, leukemia, or carcinoma) were classified as having an "ultimately fatal" disease; and patients with an underlying illness from which they were not expected to die were classified as having a "nonfatal" disease. The mortality from gram-negative bacteremia is about 84 percent with underlying "rapidly fatal" diseases, 48 percent with "ultimately fatal" diseases, and about 16 percent with "nonfatal" diseases.

Sources of Infection
Primary Bacteremia
In about 20 percent of patients, a portal of entry for the infectious agent cannot be determined; most of such infections are thought to derive from unrecognized sources within the patient, especially the gastrointestinal tract. Such primary bacteremias tend to occur in patients with impaired defense mechanisms (see above).

Additional sources of bacteria that cause primary bacteremia are IV cannulation (when local infectious complications are absent; see Part II, Chapter 25), IV infusions (Part II,

Table 29-5. Neonatal Sepsis and Gram-Negative Rod Bacteremia

Study	Years	Total sepsis cases	Percent premature	Cases per 1000 live births	Percent of all sepsis cases	Gram-negative rod bacteremias Percent caused by						
						E. coli	Klebsiella[a]	Pseudomonas	Serratia[b]	Proteus	Other gram-negative rods	Total
New York Hospital, McCracken and Shinefield [18]	1952–1964	71	50%	0.5	48%	48%	15%	15%	6%	13%	2%	99%
Yale New Haven Medical Center, Gluck et al. [11]	1957–1965	117	43%	1.4	75%	48%	31%	17%	4%	0	0	100%
Baltimore City Hospital, Buetow et al. [6]	1959–1963	158	100%	35.1	65%	25%	17%	23%	18%	9%	8%	100%
Boston City Hospital, Eickhoff et al. [8]	1961–1963	28	—	1.7	32%	66%	22%	0	0	0	13%	101%
Louisville General Hospital, Alojipan and Andrews [1]	1964–1972	50	24%	1.3	48%	54%	29%	8%	4%	4%	0	99%
Averages of reported values		—	—	—	54%	48%	23%	13%	6%	5%	5%	—

a Includes organisms designated "Klebsiella-Enterobacter," "K-E," and "Klebsiella-Aerobacter."
b Includes organisms designated "Paracolon."

Chapter 26), transfusion of contaminated blood and blood products (Part II, Chapter 28), monitoring transducers (Part II, Chapter 28), and other devices such as prostheses and arterial catheters (Part II, Chapter 17). Also, all "sterile" devices and infusions have a potential for intrinsic (i.e., manufacturer-derived) contamination.

Secondary Bacteremia

The underlying sites of infection most often associated with secondary gram-negative rod bacteremia (see Table 29-4) are the urinary tract (41 percent), the respiratory tract (22 percent), surgical wounds (15 percent), cutaneous sites (6 percent), and phlebitis (5 percent). All other sites constitute about 12 percent of the total, and these mainly consist of gastrointestinal and genital sites.

Secondary bacteremias deriving from the urinary tract were associated with catheterization of the urinary tract in 45 percent of instances, while those deriving from respiratory infections were associated with the use of IPPB in 17 percent of instances. If bacteremias from phlebitis and surgical infections are also considered to be procedure-associated infections, then about 40 percent of all nosocomial secondary bacteremias are procedure-associated. This, however, is a minimal estimate, because data on other procedures that may be associated with bacteremia from urinary and respiratory sites (e.g., cystoscopies, tracheostomies, and the like) have not been included.

The risk of secondary bacteremia from a gram-negative rod infection in different underlying sites is variable (Table 29-6). The underlying site of infection that is most likely to result in secondary bacteremia is the respiratory tract; cutaneous, urinary tract, and surgical wound sites of infection, in descending order of importance, are associated with lesser risks. The higher risk of bacteremia with respiratory infections is partly artifactual, since the identity of bloodstream isolates is often used as a means of establishing the causative agent in clinically recognized respiratory infections (see Part II, Chapter 15). The invasiveness of pathogens found at different sites, the differences in the effectiveness of defense mech-

Table 29-6. Risk of Secondary Nosocomial Bacteremias from Underlying Infections with Gram-Negative Rods

Underlying site of infection	Rate of Gram-Negative Rod Infection		Risk of secondary bacteremia
	In underlying site (per 10,000 discharges)[a]	In blood, deriving from underlying site (per 10,000 discharges)[b]	
Respiratory tract	30.9	0.77	2.5%
Cutaneous	9.1	0.19	2.1%
Urinary tract	117.4	1.40	1.2%
Surgical wound	48.4	0.51	1.1%

[a] From summary data of the National Nosocomial Infections Study (NNIS) for 1970 through 1972.
[b] From NNIS data, 1970 through 1973.

anisms at different sites in preventing the ingress of organisms to the bloodstream, and other host factors associated with infections in different sites doubtlessly underlie some of these observed differences.

Control Measures

Primary Bacteremia

The prevention of infections deriving from extrinsic sources and IV cannulation is covered in other chapters in this text. Prevention of bacteremias in immunologically compromised hosts has generally been disappointing. However, vaccines, hyperimmune globulin (Part II, Chapter 19), white blood cell infusions, and protective isolation of susceptible patients have been tried. Prophylactic antimicrobial agents have been used in an attempt to eradicate autogenous gastrointestinal flora of highly susceptible patients when periods of enhanced susceptibility are expected to be short. Such prophylactic use of antibiotics, however, should ideally be coupled with protective isolation to reduce the chance that the patient will acquire multiple-drug-resistant, exogenous, nosocomial organisms from food, water, air, and contact with hospital personnel. Some clinicians have resorted to microbiologic monitoring of the endogenous flora of susceptible patients in an attempt to provide early clues to the identity of organisms that may produce subsequent bacteremias.

Secondary Bacteremias

Measures directed toward the prevention of infections in underlying sites hold a greater potential for effective prevention of bacteremia, since nearly half of these bacteremic infections are procedure-associated. The risks and expected benefits from any procedure in a hospitalized patient should be carefully assessed. Unnecessary procedures should not be undertaken, even though they may be simple and may appear to be associated with a low risk of infection. When clearly indicated procedures must be undertaken, established infection control practices should be implemented. This objective seems best accomplished by special teams of skilled persons for urinary catheterization, IV infusion, and respiratory therapy.

Appropriate antibiotic use is also important. Antibiotic susceptibility patterns of organisms vary from site to site and from hospital to hospital, and each hospital should develop its own norms in order to guide appropriate initial therapy for nosocomial bacteremias as well as for infections in underlying sites. After culture and antibacterial sensitivity results become available, the choice of antibiotics should be reconsidered.

Effective treatment of infections in underlying sites, including surgical procedures for the drainage of abscesses and the removal of obstructions, is important in reducing the risk of secondary bacteremia from the underlying infection.

Indiscriminate use of antibiotics contributes to the likelihood of developing underlying infections and consequently increases the risk of secondary bacteremias. Antibiotics select and permit the proliferation of resistant organisms from a patient's endogenous flora, enhance the ability of exogenous resistant strains to colonize the patient, and stimulate the development of resistance in gram-negative rods, whether exogenous or endogenous. Given appropriate antibiotic exposure, these effects conspire to allow

pathogens to produce infections that are more difficult to eradicate from underlying sites and more difficult to treat successfully if secondary bacteremia develops. In addition, the mortality rates in gram-negative rod sepsis are importantly decreased by the use of appropriate antibiotics.

Epidemic Infections

Epidemics of bacteremia frequently result from epidemics of infections at other sites. Of 28 bacteremic outbreaks investigated by CDC, 18 were secondary bacteremic outbreaks that resulted from outbreaks of infections at other sites. In the ten outbreaks of primary bacteremia, nine were traced to contaminated IV solutions, IV catheters, or pressure transducers, while one was a "pseudoepidemic" traced to a contaminated antiseptic used to prepare skin for blood culture. Other pseudoepidemics have been caused by intrinsic contamination of blood culture media, contaminated penicillinase added to culture media, or improper laboratory techniques, including the transfer of organisms from culture to culture by improper function of contaminated equipment. Such pseudoepidemics should be suspected if multiple, sequential, blood cultures from different patients are positive for the same organism or if the positive culture results are not in accord with the patient's observed clinical course.

Cross-infection deriving from the bloodstream of patients with bacteremia is rare. However, reusable devices that come into direct or indirect contact with the vascular system (e.g., catheters and transducers) may become contaminated while in use in a bacteremic patient, and when they have been reused in another patient without proper sterilization, they have been responsible for cross-infections (see Part II, Chapters 17 and 28).

References

1. Alojipan, L. C., and Andrews, B. F. Neonatal sepsis—A survey of 8 years' experience at the Louisville General Hospital. *Clin. Pediatr.* (Phila.) 14:181, 1975.
2. Altemeier, W. A., Todd, J. C., and Wellford, W. I. Gram-negative septicemia: a growing threat. *Ann. Surg.* 166:228, 1967.

3. *American Hospital Association Guide for 1972.* Chicago: American Hospital Association, 1972.

4. Brooks, G. F., Pribble, A. H., and Beaty, H. N. Early diagnosis of bacteremia by buffy-coat examinations. *Arch. Intern. Med.* 132:673, 1973.

5. Bryant, R. E., Hood, A. F., Hood, C. E., and Koenig, M. C. Factors affecting mortality of gram-negative rod bacteremia. *Arch. Intern. Med.* 127:120, 1971.

6. Buetow, K. C., Klein, W., and Lane, R. B. Septicemia in premature infants. *Am. J. Dis. Child.* 110:29, 1965.

7. DuPont, H. L., and Spink, W. W. Infections due to gram-negative organisms, analysis of 860 patients. *Medicine* (Baltimore) 48:307, 1969.

8. Eickhoff, T. C., Klein, J. O., Daly, A. K., Ingall, D., and Finland, M. Neonatal sepsis and other infections due to Group B beta-hemolytic streptococci. *N. Engl. J. Med.* 271: 1221, 1964.

9. Finland, M. Changing ecology of bacterial infections related to antibiotic therapy. *J. Infect. Dis.* 122:419, 1970.

10. Fried, M. A., and Vosti, K. L. The importance of underlying disease in patients with gram-negative bacteremia. *Arch. Intern. Med.* 121:418, 1968.

11. Gluck, L., Wood, H. F., and Fousek, M. D. Septicemia of the newborn. *Pediatr. Clin. North Am.* 13:1131, 1966.

12. Hodgin, U. G., and Sanford, J. P. Gram-negative rod bacteremia. *Am. J. Med.* 39:952, 1965.

13. Levin, J., Poore, T. E., Young, N. S., Margolis, S., Zauber, N. P., Townes, A. S., and Bell, W. R. Gram-negative sepsis: detection of endotoxemia with the Limulus test. *Ann. Intern. Med.* 76:1, 1972.

14. Lewis, J., and Fekety, F. R. Gram-negative bacteremia. *Johns Hopkins Med. J.* 124:106, 1969.

15. Martin, C. M., Cuomo, A. J., Geraghty, M. J., Zager, J. R., and Mandes, T. C. Gram-negative rod bacteremia. *J. Infect. Dis.* 119:506, 1969.

16. McCabe, W. R., and Jackson, G. G. Gram-negative bacteremia. I. *Arch. Intern. Med.* 110:847, 1962.

17. McCabe, W. R., and Jackson, G. G. Gram-negative bacteremia. II. Clinical, laboratory, and therapeutic observations. *Arch. Intern. Med.* 110:856, 1962.

18. McCracken, G. H., and Shinefield, H. R. Changes in the pattern of neonatal septicemia and meningitis. *Am. J. Dis. Child.* 112:33, 1966.

19. McGowan, J. E., Barnes, M. W., and Finland, M. Host-pathogen-drug interactions in surgical patients with bacteremia. *Surg. Gynecol. Obstet.* 138:50, 1974.

20. Myerowitz, R. L., Medeiros, A. A., and O'Brien, T. F. Recent experience with bacillemia due to gram-negative organisms. *J. Infect. Dis.* 124:239, 1971.

21. Powers, D. L., and Mandell, G. L. Intraleukocytic bacteria in endocarditis patients. *J.A.M.A.* 227:312, 1974.

22. Stumacher, R. J., Koonat, M. J., and McCabe, W. R. Limitations of the usefulness of the Limulus assay for endotoxin. *N. Engl. J. Med.* 288:1261, 1973.

23. Weil, M. H., Shubin, H., and Biddle, M. Shock caused by gram-negative microorganisms, analysis of 169 cases. *Ann. Intern. Med.* 60:384, 1964.

24. Weil, M. H., and Spink, W. W. The shock syndrome associated with bacteremia due to gram-negative bacilli. *Arch. Intern. Med.* 101: 184, 1958.

Index

Index

Absorption of antibiotics, 209–
210
Acetic acid
nebulization regimen for disinfection, 267–268
prophylactic irrigation for urinary tract infections,
246–247
Achlorhydria predisposing to infectious gastroenteritis,
382
Achromobacter bacteremias associated with blood transfusions, 494
Acinetobacter peritonitis, 503
Actinomycotic wound infections,
305
Adenine arabinoside (ara-A) for
herpetic skin infections,
371–372
Adenovirus causing infections in
transplant patients, 468
Administrator, hospital, in control of infection, 33
Admitting department in infection control, 137–138
Aerobic gram-negative bacteria,
burn wound infections
due to, 351–352
Aerobic gram-negative rods
infections following total hip
replacement due to, 323
infections in transplant patients due to, 459–460
Aerobic streptococcal incisional
wound infections, 300–
302
Age predisposing to gram-negative rod bacteremia, 514,
515
Agent in chain of infection, 17–
20
Air
microbial contamination of, in
tuberculosis, prevention
of, 279–280
sampling of, for contamination, 164
Air-handling systems in operating rooms in infection
control, 132–133
Airborne organisms
bronchogenic spread of
pneumonia by, 262–264
removal of, 280

Airborne spread. *See also under*
specific pathogens
of incisional wound infections,
295, 296
of infection, 21–22
control of, in design of
ICU, 101
of nosocomial infections,
84
of organisms causing infection
following total hip re-
placement, 329
Albumin infusion, nosocomial
infections associated
with, 496–497
Amantadine hydrochloride in
prevention of transplant-
associated infections,
480
Amikacin
for gram-negative postpartum
endometritis, 402
for infections of intravascular
prostheses, 314
for pneumonia caused by
endogenous gram-nega-
tive bacilli, 276
for *Pseudomonas* burn wound
sepsis, 347
resistance of gram-negative
bacilli to, 201
for urinary tract infections,
246
Aminoglycosides
for aerobic streptococcal endometritis, 404
for aerobic streptococcal incisional wound infections,
301
for early deep infection following total hip replace-
ment, 328
for gram-negative postpartum
endometritis, 402
for pneumonia caused by endogenous gram-negative
bacilli, 276
for *Pseudomonas* burn wound
sepsis, 347
for puerperal endometritis,
401
resistance of gram-negative
bacilli to, 200–201
for urinary tract infections,
246

Amphotericin B
  for candidal burn wound infections, 350
  for mycotic burn wound infections, 351
  for pulmonary aspergillosis, 284
Ampicillin
  for aerobic streptococcal endometritis, 404
  for aerobic streptococcal incisional wound infections, 301
  for bacillary dysentery, 390
  for gram-negative postpartum endometritis, 402
  for meningitis, 412
  for meningococcal meningitis, 417
  for puerperal endometritis, 401
  for *Salmonella* gastroenteritis, 385
Anaerobes
  infections following total hip replacement due to, 323
  infections in transplant patients due to, 461
  specimens of, in diagnosis of infections following total hip replacement, 324
Anaerobic bacteria, burn wound infections due to, 351–352
Anaerobic streptococcal incisional wound infections, 302–303
Analytic epidemiology, 15–16
Anesthesia, infections associated with, 497–498
Antagonism and synergism between antibacterial drugs, 209
Antibacterial drugs, synergism and antagonism between, 209
Antibiotic sensitivity testing
  methods for, 154
  in microbiology laboratory, 154–159
  quality control for, 155–156
  selection of drugs for, 155
  selection of strains for, 154–155
  for typing of organisms by resistance, 156–157
  usefulness of, factors influencing, 157
  uses of, 157–159

Antibiotics. *See also specific drug*
  absorption of, 209–210
  bacteria resistant to, virulence of, 201
  for burn wound infections, 343–344
  in control of gram-negative rod bacteremia, 516, 517
  direct effect of, on host's defense mechanisms, 204–205
  excretion of, 209–210
  and host susceptibility to infections, 204–207
  inactivation of, 209–210
  indirect effect of, due to alteration of host's metabolic state, 205–206
  for infectious gastroenteritis, 383
  influence of, on host's microflora, 206–207
  for intravenous infusion-associated septicemia, 444–445
  for meningitis, 412
  and nosocomial infections, 195–221
  prophylactic, in prevention and control of nosocomial infections in newborn nursery, 108–109
    of infections following total hip replacement, 327
    of infections of intravascular prostheses, 317
    of meningitis, 414
    of puerperal endometritis, 400
  prophylaxis with, 211–216. *See also* Chemoprophylaxis antibiotic
  protein binding of, 209–210
  for puerperal endometritis, 401
  resistance to
    of bacteria in hospitals, 196–204
    of gram-negative bacilli, 200–201
    laboratory determination of, 203–204
    reversal of, 201–203
    of staphylococci, 197–200
  for shunt infections complicating hydrocephalus, 499
  for staphylococcal burn wound infections, 346
  for staphyloccal wound sepsis, 298

Antibiotics—*Continued*
  for streptococcal burn wound infections, 344–345
  for superficial staphylococcal infections, 364
  surveillance and control of, by pharmacy, 116
  tissue distribution of, 209–216
  for urinary tract infections, 246
  usage of
    control of, 216–217
    in hospitals, 196
Antigenic drift, 18
Antigenic shifts, major, 18
Antilymphocyte globulin for immunosuppression, infection associated with, 458–459
Antiseptics, contamination of, 116
Antispasmodic drugs in control of infectious gastroenteritis 384
Ara-A (adenine arabinoside) for herpetic skin infections, 371–372
Arterial catheters, indwelling, nosocomial infections associated with, 491–492
Arthrocentesis, bacteremia associated with, 502–503
Artificial immunity, definition of, 23
Aspergillosis, pulmonary, 283–284
Aspergillus
  burn wound infections due to, 351
  infections from
    associated with cardiac prostheses, 308, 317
    complicating heart transplant, 455
    in transplant patients, 472–473
Aspiration
  joint, in diagnosis of late deep infection following total hip replacement, 331
  of oropharyngeal bacteria, bronchogenous spread of pneumonia by, 261–262
  of stomach contents complicating anesthesia, 497
Atopic eczema predisposing patient to herpetic skin infections, 371
Attack rate, definition of, 57

Autoclaving for sterilization, 266

Autogenous infections
definition of, 12
spread of infection by, 20–21

Azathioprine for immunosuppression, infection associated with, 458, 459

Bacilli, gram-negative
aerobic
endogenous, pneumonia caused by, 273–276
exogenous, pneumonia caused by, 276–279
colonization of gastrointestinal tract by, due to antibiotic therapy, 206
incisional wound infections due to, 299–300
infections of intravascular prostheses due to, management of, 313–314
resistance of, to antibiotics, 200–203

Bacitracin for streptococcal skin infections, 369

Bacteremia
associated with catheterization, 245–246
and blood transfusion, 494
complicating incisional wound infections, 293
gram-negative rod, 507–518. *See also* Gram-negative rod bacteremia, nosocomial
invasive burn wound infections with, 340
secondary to intravenous cannula associated infections, 439
transient, from nonvascular procedures, 499–502

Bacteria
aerobic, gram-negative, postpartum endometritis due to, 401–402
anaerobic, burn wound infection due to, 352–353
antibiotic-resistant, virulence of, 201
causing infections in transplant patients, 459–461
colonization of respiratory tract by, due to antibiotic therapy, 206–209
gram-negative, aerobic, burn wound infection due to, 351–352

Bacteria—*Continued*
oropharyngeal, aspiration of, bronchogenic spread of pneumonia by, 261–262
resistance of, to antibiotics
in hospitals, 196–204
reversal of, 202–203

Bacterial endocarditis, chemoprophylaxis for, 214–215

Bacterial enzymes, role of, in incisional wound infections, 293

Bacterial meningitis, 409–418

Bacterial persistence, 210

Bactericidal versus bacteriostatic drugs, 208–209

Bacteriologic monitoring of patients on catheter drainage, 248

Bacteriophage typing of *Staphylococcus aureus,* 154

Bacteriostatic versus bactericidal drugs, 208–209

Bacteroides, infections due to, in transplant patients, 461

Bacteroides fragilis, postpartum endometritis due to, 402–403

Barium enema, bacteremia associated with, 503–504

Bathing, infant, in prevention of infection in newborn nursery, 111–112

Beds, isolation, 178–179

Benzathine penicillin for streptococcal skin infections, 369

Benzylpenicillin
for anaerobic streptococcal infections, 303
for pneumococcal pneumonia, 271–272
for streptococcal pneumonia, 273

Betadine. *See* Povidone-iodine

Biopsy
of capsule in diagnosis of late deep infection following total hip replacement, 331
of liver, bacteremia associated with, 501
specimens from, in diagnosis of infections following total hip replacement, 324

Biotyping of *Staphylococcus epidermidis,* 154

Bladder, colonization of, prevention of, 250–251

Blood
components of, routine sampling of, for contamination, 161–162
cultures of
in diagnosis of puerperal endometritis, 399
in evaluation of infections of cardiovascular prostheses, 310–312
precautions within isolation, 172, 176
transfusions of
and bacteremia, 494
cases on, legal aspects of, 181–183
nosocomial infections associated with, 494–497
and parasitemia, 494–495
in transmission of nosocomial infections, 83

Bone marrow, transplant of, nosocomial infections associated with, 456–457

Bowel surgery, chemoprophylaxis for, 215

Bronchogenous spread of bacteria, 261–264

Bronchoscopy, bacteremia associated with, 502

Bullous impetigo, 361, 362

Burn units in control of burn wound infections, 343

Burn wounds, nosocomial infections of, 335–353
from aerobic gram-negative bacteria, 351–352
from anaerobic bacteria, 352–353
antibiotic therapy for, 343–344
candidal, 349–350
clinical and microbiologic classification of, 338–340
versus community-acquired infections, 338
control measures for, 341–344
defects in immune response and, 341
incidence of, 335–336
invasive, 339–340
microbiologic specimens of, 340–341
mycotic, 350–351
nature of, 335–338
noninvasive, 339
pathogens in, 336–338
pseudomonas, 347–349
staphylococcal, 346–347
streptococcal, 344–346

Burns, chemoprophylaxis for, 215

Calculating rates in surveillance of nosocomial infections, 57–58
Candida
infections in transplant patients due to, 473–474
intravenous cannula-associated infections due to, 437, 438
intravenous infusion-associated infections due to, prevention of, 451
wound infections due to, 305
Candida albicans, burn wound infections due to, 349–350
Cannula, intravenous. *See* Intravenous cannula, nosocomial infections associated with
Caps in prevention of infection in newborn nursery, 110
Carbenicillin for meningitis, 412
Card system of isolation, 176–177
Cardiovascular prostheses, nosocomial infections of
classification of, 309
clinical aspects of, 312–315
diagnostic criteria for, 309–310
epidemiologic considerations in, 315–318
incidence of, 307–308
nature of, 307–310
pathogens causing, 308–309
predisposing factors for, 310
specimens of, 310–312
Carrier, definition of, 10
Case control studies
in analytic epidemiology, 15–16
in epidemiologic investigations, 73–77
Catheter
arterial, indwelling, nosocomial infections associated with, 491–492
sampling of, for contamination, 163
urinary, program for care of, 249–250
Catheterization
patients on, 248–249
urethral
indwelling, risks in, 244–245

Catheterization, urethral—
Continued
intermittent, use of, 247–248
risks in, 244–246
suprapubic, as alternative to, 248
urinary tract infections associated with, pathogens causing, 242
Cellulitis, streptococcal, 368
Central nervous system
infections of, 498–499
nosocomial infections of, 409–418, 498–499
Central Service Department in prevention and control of nosocomial infections, 123–126
Cephaloridine in prophylaxis for urinary tract infections, 246
Cephalosporins
for gram-negative postpartum endometritis, 402
for group-A β-hemolytic streptococcal endometritis, 405
for infections of intravascular prostheses, 313
for meningitis, 412
for pneumococcal pneumonia, 272
for pneumonia caused by endogenous gram-negative bacilli, 276
for postpartum endometritis due to *Peptostreptococcus* and *Peptococcus,* 404
for puerperal endometritis, 401
resistance of gram-negative bacilli to, 200
resistance of staphylococci to, 198
for staphylococcal pneumonia, 270
for staphylococcal wound sepsis, 298
for streptococcal burn wound infections, 344
for streptococcal pneumonia, 273
for superficial staphylococcal infections, 364
Cephalothin for aerobic streptococcal incisional wound infections, 301
Cesarean section, risk of puerperal endometritis associated with, 398

Chagas' disease, blood transfusion-related, 495
Chain of nosocomial infections, 17–24
agent in, 17–20
environment in, 24
host in, 22–24
transmission in, 20–22
Chemicals, liquid, in sterilization of equipment, 88
Chemoprophylaxis, antibiotic
for burn wound infections, 344
categories of, 212
contraindications to, 212
in control of infections in total hip replacement, 327
controversial use of, 212–214
for incisional wound infections, 297
indications for, 214–215
for infections of intravascular prostheses, 317
and nosocomial infection, 211–216
unnecessary effects of, 216
for urinary tract infections, 246
Chemotherapy
cases of failure of, 211
for infections of intravascular prostheses, 313
in prevention of microbial contamination in tuberculosis, 279
principles of, 208–211
for urinary tract infections, 246
Chlamydial nosocomial respiratory infections, 282
Chloramphenicol
for meningitis, 412
for postpartum endometritis due to *Bacteroides fragilis,* 402
resistance of gram-negative bacilli to, 200
resistance of staphylococci to, 198
for *Salmonella* gastroenteritis, 385
Citrobacter freundii, intravenous infusion-associated infections due to, 444
Clean-air systems
in control of infections following total hip replacement, 325–327, 329
medicolegal implications of, 188–190

Clean-core concept in surgical suite design, 129–130

Clean-contaminated wounds, 290

Cleaners, ultrasonic, for processing of supplies in Central Service Department, 124

Cleaning methods in operating rooms in infection control, 133–134

Clindamycin
for late deep infection following total hip replacement, 331
for pneumococcal pneumonia, 272
for postpartum endometritis, 402–404
for staphylococcal wound sepsis, 298
for streptococcal pneumonia, 273
for superficial staphylococcal infections, 364

Clinical isolates, identification and typing of, in microbiology laboratory, 149–154

Clinical laboratory, nosocomial infections and, 139–145

Closed-drainage methods, 250–252

Clostridium
antibiotic-resistant colitis due to, 206
burn wound infections due to, 352
infections due to, in transplant patients, 461
wound infections due to, 303–304

Clostridium perfringens, foodborne transmission of, 119
prevention of, 121

Cloxacillin in prevention of infection following total hip replacement, 327

Clustering, geographical, in epidemiologic investigation, 70

Coccidioides causing infections in transplant patients, 476–477

Codes and standards, medicolegal implications of, 190–191

Cohort programs in prevention of infection in newborn nursery, 110–111

Cohort study
in analytic epidemiology, 15–16
in epidemiologic investigation, 77

Colimycin for *Pseudomonas* burn wound sepsis, 347

Colistin for gastroenteritis due to *Escherichia coli,* 388

Colitis, pseudomembranous, due to antibiotic therapy, 206

Colon, effects of antibiotics on, altered host susceptibility due to, 205–206

Colonization
bladder, prevention of, 250–251
definition of, 10

Colonoscopy, bacteremia associated with, 500

Coma as contraindication to antimicrobial prophylaxis, 212

Common-vehicle spread
of infection, 21
of nosocomial infections, 83–84

Communicable disease, reporting of, 227–229

Community
and hospital, relationship between, 223–230
spread of nosocomial infections to, 224–225

Community-acquired infections
of incisional wounds, definition of, 288
spread of, in hospital, 224

Condom drainage as alternative to urethral catheterization, 248

Conjunctivitis, gonococcal, 377–378

Contact. *See also under specific pathogens*
direct and indirect, spread of infection by, 20–21
control of, in design of ICU, 101–102
in spread of nosocomial infections, 82–83

Contaminated wounds, 290

Contamination
definition of, 11
of intravenous fluids, 447–451
microbial, of air in tuberculosis, prevention of, 279–280

Control of nosocomial infections
clinical laboratory in, 6

Control of nosocomial infections—*Continued*
in and by personnel, 34–47
isolation procedures in, 6
in operating rooms, 131–134
program for, 4
responsibilities of hospital personnel in, 27-34
role of surveillance in, 53–54

Control groups, selection of, for epidemiologic investigations, 76–77

Copper sponges for disinfection, 267

Cord, care of, in prevention of infection in newborn nursery, 111–112

Corticosteroids for immunosuppression, infections associated with, 458

Corynebacterium acnes, infections associated with reservoirs and shunts due to, 498

Corynebacterium diphtheriae, wound infections due to, 303

Cruse and Foord study on incidence of surgical wound infection, 291

Cryptococcus causing infections in transplant patients, 474–475

Culture-swab-rinse technique for culturing disinfected equipment, 162

Cultures
blood
in diagnosis of puerperal endometritis, 399
in evaluation of infections of cardiovascular prostheses, 310–312
procedures for, in control of laboratory-acquired infections, 142–143
spore strip, to monitor sterilization in routine environmental sampling, 160–161

Curve, epidemic, in descriptive epidemiology, 14

Cutaneous infections, nosocomial, 355–380. *See also* Skin, nosocomial infections of

Cutdowns, purulent thrombophlebitis associated with, 434–435

Cyclophosphamide for immunosuppression, infections
associated with, 458, 459
Cystoscopy, bacteremia associated with, 502
Cytomegalovirus
control of, in and by hospital
personnel, 34–35
infections due to, nosocomial,
419–420
infections in transplant patients due to, 462–465
Cytotoxic drugs for immunosuppression, infection asso-
ciated with, 458, 459

Data
in epidemiologic investigation,
67, 71–72
in surveillance of nosocomial
infections, 54–57, 59–60
Debridement in control of burn
wound infections, 341–
342
Decontamination of supplies in
Central Service Depart-
ment, 124
Defense mechanisms against infection, 23
Descriptive epidemiology, 13–15
Devitalized tissue predisposing
to incisional wound in-
fections, 294
Diabetes mellitus predisposing to
superficial staphylococcal
infections, 363
Diarrhea in infectious gastroenteritis, 382
Dienes' typing of *Proteus mirabilis,* 154
Diphtheria
control of, in and by hospital
personnel, 35
surgical, 303
Diphtheroids, infections of intravascular prostheses due
to, management of, 313
Direct contact, spread of infection by, 20–21
Dirty wounds, 290
Discharge precautions in isolation, 172, 173, 175–176
Disinfectants, contamination of,
116
Disinfected equipment, periodic
sampling of, for contami-
nation, 162
Disinfection
in control of nosocomial infections, 84–85, 86

Disinfection—*Continued*
definition of, 265
for infection control in hemodialysis unit, 96
methods of, 266-267
of ventilatory equipment,
265–268
Dissemination, definition of, 10–
11
Dose of agent in chain of infection, 18
Drainage
urinary
condom, as alternative to
urethral catheterization,
248
systems for, 249–252
uterine, for puerperal endometritis, 401
Drift, antigenic, 18
Droplet spread of infection, 21
Drugs
antibacterial, synergism and
antagonism between, 209
bactericidal versus bacteriostatic, 208–209
cytotoxic, for immunosuppression, infection associated
with, 458, 459
dispensing and compounding
of, contamination during,
115–116
selection of, for antibiotic susceptibility testing, 155
Dry heat for sterilization of
equipment, 87
Dukes' drainage system, 250

Ecology of infection, 17
Eczema, atopic, predisposing
patient to herpetic skin
infections, 371
Education of personnel for infection control, 51
Encephalitis in transplant patient, 464
Endemic herpetic skin infections,
372–373
Endemic infections
of burn wounds, 345–350
general features of, 64
microbiology laboratory in
surveillance of, 147
nosocomial
incidence and nature of,
233–238
investigation of, 63–80
occurrence of, 12
pneumococcal pneumonia,
272

Endemic infections, noso-
comial—*Continued*
staphylococcal pneumonia,
prevention of, 270
ophthalmic *Neisseria gonorrhoeae,* 378
skin
herpetic, 372–373
streptococcal, 369
due to *Staphylococcus aureus,*
365–366
varicella-zoster, 375–376
Endocarditis
bacterial, chemoprophylaxis
for, 214–215
complicating cardiovascular
prostheses, 307–319
Penicillium, associated with
cardiac prostheses, 308
Endogenous infections, definition of, 12
Endogenous postpartum en-
dometritis from lower
genital tract flora, 401–
404
Endometritis, puerperal, 395–
407. *See also* Puerperal
endometritis
Endoscopy, bacteremia associated with, 500-501
Endotracheal intubation, nosocomial infections associ-
ated with, 498
Enema, barium, bacteremia associated with, 503–504
Engineering in control of nosocomial infections, 88
Enteric precautions in isolation,
172, 173, 174
Enterobacter
antibiograms for typing of,
157
bacteremia due to, 512, 513
contamination of intravenous
fluids from, 447–448, 449
drug resistance in, 200
infections from, associated
with platelet transfusions,
496
intravenous infusion-associated infections due to,
444
Enterococcus, infections of intravascular prostheses due
to, management of, 313
Enterocolitis
necrotizing
due to antibiotic therapy,
206
neonatal, 393

Enterocolitis—*Continued*
staphylococcal, 392–393
Entrance of organisms in chain
of infection, 22–23
Environment
in chain of infection, 24
inanimate
control measures, 88–90
disinfection of, 84–85, 86
related to nosocomial infections, 81–92
sterilization of, 85–88
surveillance of, 90–91
in transmission of noso-
comial infections, 82–84
for infection control
in burn wounds, 343
in hemodialysis unit, 97
in intravascular prostheses,
315–317
in outpatient department,
139
in puerperal endometritis
prevention, 400–401
in smallpox, 426
sampling of
microbiology laboratory in,
159, 160–162
routine, microbiology laboratory in, 147–148
surveillance of, 90–91
Enzymes, bacterial, role of, in
incisional wound infec-
tions, 293
Epidemic
curve in descriptive epidemiology, 14
definition of, 12
of intravenous infusion-associated septicemia, 447–448
Epidemic infections
of burn wounds, 345–350
of *Escherichia coli* gastrointestinal infections, 388–
389
general features of, 236–238
gram-negative rod bacteremia,
517
group-A β-hemolytic streptococcal endometritis, 405
investigation of. *See* Epidemiologic investigation
nosocomial
incidence and nature of,
233–238
investigation of, 63–80
pneumococcal pneumonia,
272
staphylococcal pneumonia,
270–271

Epidemic infections—*Continued*
ophthalmic *Neisseria gonorrhoeae,* 378
skin
herpetic, 373
streptococcal, 369–370
superficial, due to *Staphylococcus aureus,* 366–367
varicella-zoster, 376–377
Epidemiologic aspects
of foodborne disease, 118–
119
of hemodialysis, 94–95
Epidemiologic investigation,
63–80
administrative aspects of,
79–80
assessing initially available
information in, 66–68
characterizing cases of disease
by time, place, and
person in, 68–72
evaluating other hospital
practices in, 79
formulating tentative
hypotheses in, 72–73
geographical clustering in, 70
instituting and evaluating
control measure in, 78
principles of, 65
protocol for, in hospital,
65-79
refining hypotheses in, 73–78
responsibilities for dissemination of information in,
79
seeking additional cases in,
68
Epidemiologist, hospital
broader influence, 229
in control of infection, 32–33
Epidemiology
analytic, 15–16
definition of, 9
descriptive, 13–15
experimental, 16-17
general principles of, 81–82
of nosocomial infections,
9–25
Epidermal necrolysis, toxic, 362
Epstein-Barr virus causing infections in transplant
patients, 467
Equipment
care of, in prevention of infection in newborn nurs-
ery, 11
disinfected, periodic sampling
of, for contamination,
162

Equipment—*Continued*
hydrotherapy, in control of
burn wound infections,
343
for infection control in hemodialysis unit, 97
nebulization, role of, in spread
of pneumonia, 263–264,
265
in neonatal intensive-care
units, 112
specialized, in control of laboratory-acquired infec-
tions, 141–142
ventilatory, disinfection and
sterilization of, 265–268
Erythromycin
for aerobic streptococcal
endometritis, 404
for aerobic streptococcal incisional wound infec-
tions, 301
for anaerobic streptococcal
infections, 303
for group-A β-hemolytic
streptococcal endo-
metritis, 405
for pneumococcal pneumonia,
272
for postpartum endometritis
due to *Peptostreptococ-
cus* and *Peptococcus,* 404
for puerperal endometritis,
401
resistance of staphylococci to,
198
for staphylococcal wound
sepsis, 298
for streptococcal burn wound
infections, 344
for streptococcal pneumonia,
273
for streptococcal skin infections, 369
for superficial staphylococcal
infections, 364
Escherichia coli
bacteremia due to, 512, 513,
514
drug resistance in, 200
gastroenteritis due to, 387–
389
gastrointestinal infections
from, foodborne trans-
mission of, 119
infections from
in newborn nursery, 105,
106
in transplant patients, 459
isolates of, typing of, 152–153

Escherichia coli—Continued
  meningitis due to, 411, 412, 413
  pneumonia caused by, 275
  relative frequency of, 236
  in urinary tract infections, 241–242
Esophagoscopy, bacteremia associated with, 501
Ethylene oxide for sterilization, 266
  of equipment, 87–88
Excretion of antibiotics, 209–210
Excretions, discharge precautions for, 173, 175–176
Exogenous infections, definition of, 12
Experimental epidemiology, 16–17
Eyes
  examination of, bacteremia associated with, 503
  nosocomial infections of, 355–380
    classification of, 356–357
    control measures for, 358
    diagnostic criteria for, 357
    gonococcal, 377–378
    incidence of, 355, 356
    nature of, 355–357
    pathogens in, 355–356
    specimens of, collection and transport of, 357–358
    staphylococcal, 358–367
    streptococcal, 367–370

Federal health authorities, relationship of hospital to, regarding infection control, 225–227
Flavobacterium bacteremia associated with umbilical catheterization, 492
Flora
  of host, inactivation of antibiotics by, 210
  of lower genital tract, endogenous infections from, 401–404
Floor, sampling of, for contamination, 163–164
Fluids, intravenous, contamination of
  during manufacture, 447–448
  in use, 449–451
Food in transmission of nosocomial infections, 5, 83–84

Food-handling operations in control of nosocomial infections, 89
Food hygiene, in prevention of nosocomial infections, 120–121
Food services, nosocomial infections and, 117–123
  personal health and hygiene of personnel, in prevention, 121–122
Foodborne disease
  epidemiologic aspects of, 118–119
  transmission of, prevention of, 119–122
Foreign bodies
  as contraindication to antimicrobial prophylaxis, 212
  predisposing to incisional wound infections, 294
Formula, infant, routine sampling of, for contamination, 161
Fungi causing infections in transplant patients, 471–476

Gammaglobulin, hyperimmune anti-*Pseudomonas,* for *Pseudomonas* burn wound sepsis, 347
Gangrene, gas, in incisional wound infections, 303–304
Gantrisin. *See* Sulfisoxazole
Gastroenteritis
  infectious, nosocomial, 381–394
    control measures for, 383–385
    diagnostic criteria for, 382
    Escherichia coli in, 387–389
    incidence of, 382
    predisposing host factors for, 382–383
    salmonella, 385–387
    Shigella in, 389–391
    viral, 391–392
Gastrointestinal procedures, bacteremia associated with, 500–501
Gastrointestinal tract, colonization of, by gram-negative bacilli due to antibiotic therapy, 206

Genital tract, lower, flora of, endogenous infections from, 401–404
Gentamicin
  for gastroenteritis due to *Escherichia coli,* 388
  for gram-negative burn wound sepsis, 352
  for gram-negative postpartum endometritis, 402
  for infections of intravascular prostheses, 314
  for meningitis, 412
  for pneumonia caused by endogenous gram-negative bacilli, 276
  in prophylaxis for urinary tract infections, 246
  for *Pseudomonas* burn wound sepsis, 347
  resistance of gram-negative bacilli to, 200–201
  for urinary tract infections, 246
Gentamicin ointment
  for burn wound infections, 344
  for gram-negative burn wound sepsis, 352
German measles, 422–424
  control of, in and by hospital personnel, 40–41
Globulin
  antilymphocyte, for immunosuppression, infection associated with, 458–459
  immune serum
    for prevention of measles, 422
    for protection against hepatitis A, 35, 46
  zoster immune, in prevention of varicella-zoster infections, 375
Gloves
  in control of hepatitis, 429
  in control of infection in ICU, 102
  in prevention of infection in newborn nursery, 110
  in prevention of puerperal endometritis, 400
  punctured, as source of infection following total hip replacement, 328
Glutaraldehyde
  for disinfection, 85
  for sterilization, 266
Gonorrhea, ophthalmic infections due to, 377

Government health authorities, relationship of hospital to, regarding infection control, 225–227

Gowns
 in control of infection in ICU, 102
 in prevention of infection in newborn nursery, 110

Gram-negative aerobic bacteria burn wound infections due to, 351–352
 postpartum endometritis due to, 401–402

Gram-negative bacilli. *See* Bacilli, gram-negative

Gram-negative rod bacteremia control measures for, 516–517
 host factors predisposing to, 514, 515
 nosocomial, 507–518
  diagnostic criteria for, 508
  incidence and mortality of, 510–512
  pathogens in, 512–514
  sources of, 514, 516
  specimens of, 508–510

Gram-negative rods, aerobic, causing infections in transplant patient, 459–460

Gram-negative septicemia, common-vehicle spread of, 21

Group-A β-hemolytic streptococcus, postpartum endometritis due to, 404–406

Group-A *Streptococcus pyogenes*
 burn wound infections due to, 344–345
 M-typing of, 154

Group-B infections in newborn nursery, 105–106

Hand-washing
 in control
  of hepatitis, 429
  of infectious gastroenteritis, 383
  of nosocomial infections, 88–89
 in prevention
  of infection in newborn nursery, 110
  of puerperal endometritis, 400

Health
 of food service personnel in prevention of nosocomial infections, 121–122
 of nursery personnel in prevention and control of infection in newborn nursery, 109

Health services for hospital personnel, 47–51

Heart
 catheterization of, nosocomial infections associated with, 491
 surgery on, chemoprophylaxis for, 216
 transplant of, nosocomial infections associated with, 454–455

Heat
 dry, for sterilization of equipment, 87
 moist, for sterilization of equipment, 87

Helminths causing infections in transplant patients, 468–471

Hemodialysis unit, nosocomial, infections in, 93–99
 epidemiologic aspects of, 94–95
 methods of infection control in, 95–98

Hemophilus influenzae, antibiotic susceptibility testing for, 155

Hepatitis, 427–431
 control of, in, and by hospital personnel, 35–37
 control measures for, 428–430
 diagnosis of, 427–428
 etiology of, 427
 in newborn, 430–431
 nosocomial potential of, 427–431
 therapy of, 430
 in transplant patient, 464, 466–467
 viral, in hemodialysis unit, 93, 94

Hepatitis A
 common-vehicle spread of, 21
 contact spread of, 20
 control of, in, and by hospital personnel, 35
 diagnosis of, 427–428
 etiology of, 427
 in newborn, 431
 nosocomial infection potential of, 427

Hepatitis B virus (HBV)
 common-vehicle spread of, 21
 control of, in, and by hospital personnel, 35–37
 control measures for, 428–430
 diagnosis of, 427–428
 etiology of, 427
 in hemodialysis unit, 93, 94
 immunization against, passive and active, 98–99
 introduction and modes of transmission of, 94–95
 in newborn, 430–431
 nosocomial infection potential of, 427
 patients with, precautions for, 97–98
 precautions for, in clinical laboratory, 143–144
 transfusion–acquired, legal aspects of, 181–183

Herpes, control of, in and by hospital personnel, 37–38

Herpes simplex virus causing infections in transplant patients, 465

Herpes zoster infections, 374

Herpesvirus hominis, skin infections due to, 370–373

Hexachlorophene for superficial staphylococcal infections, dangers of, 364–365

High-efficiency particulate air-filtered (HEPA) systems for surgical suite, 132, 133

Hip
 replacement of, total, infections associated with, 321–333. *See also* Skeletal prostheses, nosocomial infections of
 surgery on, previous, predisposing to infections following total hip replacement, 324–325

Hospital(s)
 administrator of, in control of infection, 33
 antibiotic usage in, 196
 and community, relationship between, 223–230
 design of, in control of nosocomial infections, 88
 records of, containing diagnosis of nosocomial infections, medicolegal implications of, 192

Hospital(s)—*Continued*
  relationship of, to local, state, and federal health authorities regarding infection control, 225–227
  resistance of bacteria to antibiotics in, 196–204
  spread of community-acquired infection in, 224
  surveillance for nosocomial infections by, medicolegal implications of, 191–192
Hospital epidemiologist
  broader influence of, 229
  in control of infection, 32–33
Hospital personnel, 27–52
  control of infections in and by, 34–47
  health services for, 47–51
  immunization for, guidelines for, 46–47
  responsibilities of, in infection control of, 27–34
Host
  in chain of infection, 22–24
  defense mechanisms of, direct effect of antibiotics on, 204–205
  defenses of, impaired, as contraindication to antimicrobial prophylaxis, 212
  flora of
    inactivation of antibiotics by, 210
    suppression of, in severely compromised patients, antibiotic chemoprophylaxis in, 213–214
  response of, to infection, 23–24
  susceptibility of
    to infection, antibiotics and, 204–207
    to puerperal endometritis, 397–398
Housekeeping in control of nosocomial infections, 89
Human milk for infants in neonatal intensive-care units, 112–113
Hydrocephalus, shunt infections complicating, 499
Hydrotherapy equipment in control of burn wound infections, 343

Hygiene
  food, in prevention of nosocomial infections, 120–121
  of food service personnel in prevention of nosocomial infections, 121–122
  of laboratory personnel in control of laboratory-acquired infections, 142
Hyperalimentation in control of burn wound infections, 342–343
Hyperendemic infections, investigation of, 64
Hyperendemic occurrence of nosocomial infections, 12
Hyperimmune anti-*Pseudomonas* γ-globulin for *Pseudomonas* burn wound sepsis, 347

Ice and water, testing of, for contamination, 163
Idoxuridine for herpetic keratitis, 372
Immune response, defects in, and burn wound infections, 341
Immune serum globulin
  in control of hepatitis, 428–429
  for prevention of measles, 422
  for protection against hepatitis A, 35, 36
Immunity, artificial, definition of, 23
Immunization(s)
  against diphtheria, 35, 46
  against hepatitis, 429
  against hepatitis B virus, passive and active, 36, 46, 98–99
  for hospital personnel, guidelines, 46–47, 50
  against influenza, 38, 46
  against measles, 38–39, 46
  against mumps, 39, 46
  against pertussis, 39–40, 46
  against poliomyelitis, 40, 46
  against rubella, 40–41, 47
  against tetanus, 43, 47
  for prevention of measles, 421–422
  for prevention of rubella, 423–424
  against smallpox, 426
Immunoglobulin
  hepatitis B, in control of hepatitis, 429

Immunoglobulin—*Continued*
  zoster, uses of, 45, 47
Immunosuppression for transplants, nosocomial infections associated with, 457–459
Impetigo
  staphylococcal, 361
  streptococcal, 368
Inactivation of antibiotics, 209–210
Inanimate environment related to nosocomial infections, 81–92
Incidence and prevalence of nosocomial infections, 13
  definition of, 57
  estimation of, prevalence data for, 60–61
Incisional wounds
  classification of, 290
  infections in, 287–306
    acquired, 294–296
    actinomycotic, 305
    clostridial, 303–304
    complications of, 293
    control measures for, 296–297
    diphtheria as, 303
    factors predisposing to, 293–294
    gas gangrene in, 303–304
    gram-negative bacillary, 299–300
    incidence of, 290–292
    mycotic, 305
    pathogens of, 292–293
    sources and modes of acquisition of, 294–296
    staphylococcal, 297–299
    streptococcal, 300–302
    synergistic, 303
    tuberculous, 304–305
    viral, 305
  location of, predisposing to incisional wound infections, 294
Incubation period in descriptive epidemiology, 14
Index case in descriptive epidemiology, 14
Indirect contact, spread of infection by, 21
Indwelling catheters
  arterial, nosocomial infections associated with, 491–492
  risks in, 244–245
Infants. *See* Neonates

Infection Control Committee
activities and functions of,
28–29
composition of, 27–28
objectives of, methods for
accomplishing, 29–30
pitfalls of, 30
relationship of microbiology
laboratory to, 148
responsibilities of, 27–30,
117
Infection control nurse, 30–32
role of, in data collection for
surveillance, 55
Infections
autogenous, 20–21
community-acquired, spread
of, in hospital, 224
control of, relationship of
hospital to health authorities regarding, 225–227
data on, sources of, in surveillance, 56–57
definition of, 9–10
ecology of, 17
endemic
general features of, 234–
236
microbiology laboratory in
surveillance of, 147
epidemic, general features of,
236–238
host-susceptibility to, antibiotics and, 204–207
minimal data to collect about,
in surveillance, 55
nature of, establishing, in
epidemiologic investiga-
tion, 66
nonpreventable, definition of,
11–12
nosocomial, 3–7
preventable, definition of, 11
remote, predisposing to incisional wound infec-
tions, 294
subclinical, definition of, 10
surgical, 287–306. *See also*
Incisional wounds, infec-
tion in
transmission of. *See* Transmission of infection
urinary tract, 239–254. *See
also* Urinary tract
infections, nosocomial
Infectious gastroenteritis, 381–
394
Infectious hepatitis. *See* Hepatitis A
Infective dose, definition of, 18

Infectivity, period of, definition
of, 19–20
Influenza
control of, in and by hospital
personnel, 38
vaccine for, in prevention of
transplant-associated in-
fections, 480
viral, nosocomial, 281–282
Infusions
of albumin, nosocomial infections associated with,
496–497
intravenous, nosocomial infections associated with. *See*
Intravenous infusion,
nosocomial infections
associated with
Insects, control of, in control of
nosocomial infections, 90
Intensive-care unit (ICU), infections in, 99–104
Intermittent catheterization, use
of, 247–248
Intracellular bacteria causing
infections in transplant
patients, 460–461
Intravascular infections, clinical
aspects of, 312–315
Intravenous cannula, nosocomial
infections associated
with
clinical and microbiologic
criteria of, 438–439
control measures for, 440–
441
incidence of, 434–437
nature of, 433–438
microbiologic specimens of,
439–440
pathogens in, 437–438
Intravenous fluids, contamination of
during manufacture, 447–448
in use, 449–451
Intravenous infusion, nosocomial infections asso-
ciated with, 443–452
diagnostic criteria for, 445–
446
due to fluid contamination,
447–451
incidence of, 443–444
pathogens in, 444
specimen collection in, 446–
447
therapy of, 444–445
Intraventricular reservoirs, subcutaneous, infections
associated with, 498–499

Intubation, endotracheal,
nosocomial infections
associated with, 498
Invasive procedure, in control
of infection in ICU, 102–
103
Invasiveness, definition of, 18
Investigations of employee
nosocomial infections,
50–51
Iododeoxyuridine for corneal
lesions of smallpox, 426
Iodofor for burn wound infections, 344
Irrigation, prophylactic, for
urinary tract actions,
246
Isolates, clinical, identification
and typing of, 151–154
Isolation
beds for, 178–179
blood precautions in, 172, 176
card system of, 176–177
categories of, 171–176
in control of hepatitis, 429–
430
enteric precautions in, 172,
173, 174
facilities needed for, 178–179
orders for, 177–178
procedures for, 169–179
in control of nosocomial
infections, 6
in newborn nursery in prevention and control of
nosocomial infections,
108
protective, 172, 176
respiratory, 171–174
skin precautions in, 172–175
strategies for, 170–171
strict, 171, 172, 174
wound precautions in, 172–
175
Isoniazid in prevention of transplant-associated infec-
tions, 480
IV site infection, 438–439

Joint aspiration in diagnosis of
late deep infection fol-
lowing total hip replace-
ment, 331

Kanamycin
for gram-negative postpartum
endometritis, 402
for pneumonia caused by
endogenous gram-nega-
tive bacilli, 276

Kanamycin—*Continued*
in prophylaxis for urinary
tract infections, 246
for puerperal endometritis,
401
resistance of gram-negative
bacilli to, 200–201
resistance of staphylococci to,
198
Kidneys
effect of antibiotics on, altered
host susceptibility due to,
205
transplant of, nosocomial infections associated with,
454
Kitchen in control of nosocomial
infections, 89
Klebs-Löffler bacillus, wound
infections due to, 303
Klebsiella
bacteremia due to, 512, 513,
514
contamination of intravenous
fluids from, 449
drug resistance in, 200
drug-resistant, gastrointestinal
colonization by, 206
gastrointestinal infections
from
foodborne transmission of,
119
in newborn nursery, 107
infections due to, in transplant patients, 459–460
meningitis due to, 411, 412,
413, 414
pneumonia caused by, 275
relative frequency of, 236
serotyping of, 153–154
susceptibility data on, uses of,
158
urinary tract infections due
to, 243

Laboratory
clinical, nosocomial infections
and, 139–145
design of, in control of
laboratory-acquired in-
fections, 141
in determination of drug resistance, 203–204
infections acquired in, problem of, extent of, 139–
140
microbiology, 147–167. *See
also* Microbiology
laboratory

Laminar air-flow systems
medicolegal implications of,
188–190
in prevention of transplant-
associated infections,
481
for surgical suite, 133
Lassa fever, direct transmission
of, in ICU, control of,
101–102
Laundry in control of nosocomial infections, 89–90,
125–129
Legal aspects of nosocomial infections, 181–194. *See
also* Medicolegal impli-
cations of nosocomial in-
fections
Legionnaires' disease, 284
Lights, ultraviolet, in removal of
airborne organisms in
tuberculosis, 280
Limulus amebocyte test in detection of gram-negative
rod bacteremia, 508
Lincomycin
for aerobic streptococcal incisional wound infec-
tions, 301
for postpartum endometritis,
403–404
in prevention of infection
following total hip re-
placement, 327
for staphylococcal wound
sepsis, 298
for streptococcal burn wound
infections, 344
Linen packs for processing by
Central Service Depart-
ment, 124–125
Linens, processing of, in prevention of nosocomial
infections, 126–129
Liquid chemicals in sterilization
of equipment, 88
Listeria monocytogenes
infections due to, in transplant patients, 460–
461
meningitis due to, 416–417
Liver
biopsy of, bacteremia associated with, 501
effects of antibiotics on,
altered host susceptibility
due to, 205
transplant of, nosocomial infections associated with,
455–456

Lower respiratory tract. *See
Respiratory tract, lower,
infections of, nosocomial*
Lumbar puncture
in acquisition of meningitis,
412–413
technique for, in prevention
of meningitis, 414
Lungs
effects of antibiotics on,
altered host susceptibility
due to, 206
transplant of, nosocomial infections associated with,
457
Lyell's TEN, 362
Lymphadenitis complicating incisional wound infec-
tions, 293
Lymphangitis complicating incisional wound infec-
tions, 293
Lymphocytosis, atypical, in
transplant patient, 463
Lymphohematogenous spread of
pneumonia, 264

M-typing of group-A *Streptococcus pyogenes,* 154
Mafenide (Sulfamylon)
for burn wound infections,
344
for staphylococcal burn
wound infections, 347
Mafenide (Sulfamylon) cream,
for gram-negative burn
wound sepsis, 352
Maintenance in control of nosocomial infections, 88
Malaria, blood transfusion-
related, 494–495
Marrow, bone, transplant of,
nosocomial infections
associated with, 456–457
Masks in prevention
of infection in newborn
nursery, 110
of microbial contamination in
tuberculosis, 279–280
Mastitis, staphylococcal, 361,
362
Matched sample in selection of
control groups in epi-
demiologic investigation,
76
Measles, 421–422
control of, in and by hospital
personnel, 38–39
direct transmission of, in ICU,
control of, 101

Measles—*Continued*
droplet spread of, 21
German, 422–424
control of, in and by hospital personnel, 40–41
Mechanical ventilation in removal of airborne organisms in tuberculosis, 280
Media, selective survey, for culturing specimens in outbreak investigation, 159–160
Medical evaluation, preemployment, 49
Medical reevaluation and health maintenance for health personnel, 49–50
Medicines in transmission of nosocomial infections, 83
Medicolegal implications
of clean-air systems, 188–190
of codes and standards, 190–191
of hospital records containing diagnosis of nosocomial infections, 192
of hospital's furnishing defective products to patients, 192–193
of nosocomial infections, 181–194
for blood transfusion cases, 181–183
specific problems in, 188–193
for staphylococcal infection cases, 183–188
of surveillance for nosocomial infections, 191–192
Meningitis, nosocomial, 409–418
classification of, 409–410
diagnostic criteria for, 410–411
incidence of, 409
primary, pathogens causing, 415–417
secondary, pathogens causing, 411–415
specimens of, 411
Meningococcus, control of, in and by hospital personnel, 39
Methicillin
for early deep infection following total hip replacement, 328
in prevention of infection following total hip replacement, 327

Methicillin—*Continued*
resistance of staphylococci to, 198–199
laboratory determination of, 203–204
for staphylococcal burn wound infections, 346
for staphylococcal pneumonia, 270
Metronidazole for postpartum endometritis due to *B. fragilis,* 403
Microaerophilic streptococcal incisional wound infections, 302
Microbial contamination of air in tuberculosis, prevention of, 279–280
Microbiologic criteria for diagnosis of nosocomial respiratory infections, 259–261
Microbiologic study in epidemiologic investigations, 78
Microbiology laboratory, 147–167
administrative aspects of, 148–149
antibiotic susceptibility testing in, 154–159
in classification of burn wound infections, 338–340
in diagnosis
of bacterial meningitis, 410–411
of burn wound infections, 340–341
of gram-negative rod bacteremia, 508
of herpetic skin infections, 371
of infections following total hip replacement, 323–324
of infectious gastroenteritis, 382
of intravenous infusion-associated septicemia, 446
of ophthalmic *Neisseria gonorrhoeae* infections, 377
of puerperal endometritis, 398–399
of staphylococcal superficial infections, 362–363
of streptococcal skin infections, 368
of superficial infections, 357

Microbiology laboratory, in diagnosis—*Continued*
of varicella-zoster infections, 374–375
identification and typing of clinical isolates in, 149–154
records of, 149
in sampling and surveys, 159–164
as source of infection data in surveillance, 56
specimens for
from intravenous cannula-associated infections, 439–440
from surgical wound infections, 289
in surveillance and control of nosocomial infections, 147–148
Microflora of host, influence of antibiotic therapy on, 206–207
Milk, human, for infants in neonatal intensive-care units, 112–113
Moist heat for sterilization of equipment, 87
Monitoring
bacteriologic of patients on catheter drainage, 248
transvaginal, risk of puerperal endometritis associated with, 398
Mononucleosis, cytomegalovirus, in transplant patient, 463
Mouth, covering of, in prevention of microbial contamination in tuberculosis, 279
Mucor, burn wound infections due to, 351
Mumps, direct transmission of, in ICU, control of, 101
Mycobacterium, infections due to, in transplant patients, 461
Mycobacterium tuberculosis
airborne spread of, 279
laboratory acquired, control measures for, 141
Mycotic burn wound infections, 350–351
Mycotic wound infections, 305
Mystatin (Mycostatin) for candidal burn wound infections, 350

Nafcillin
    for staphylococcal burn
        wound infections, 346
    for staphylococcal pneumonia,
        270
    for superficial staphylococcal
        infections, 364
Nalidixic acid for bacillary
    dysentery, 390
Natural immunity, definition of,
    23
Nebulization equipment, role of,
    in spread of pneumonia,
    263–264, 265
Necrolysis, toxic epidermal,
    362
Necrotizing enterocolitis due to
    antibiotic therapy, 206
Needles, sampling of, for con-
    tamination, 163
Neisseria, antibiotic susceptibil-
    ity testing for, 155
Neisseria gonorrhoeae, reporting
    of, 229
Neisseria meningitidis, menin-
    gitis due to, 417
Neomycin
    for gastroenteritis due to
        Escherichia coli, 388
    resistance of gram-negative
        bacilli to, 200–201
    resistance of staphylococci to,
        198
Neomycin-polymyxin method of
    prophylactic irrigation
    for urinary tract infec-
    tions, 247
Neonatal Intensive-Care Units,
    special considerations
    involving, 112–113
Neonatal necrotizing entero-
    colitis, 393
Neonates
    bathing of, in prevention of
        infection in newborn
        nursery, 111–112
    formula for, routine sampling
        of, for contamination,
        161
    gram-negative rod bacteremia
        in, 514, 515
    hepatitis in, 430–431
    Listeria monocytogenes men-
        ingitis in, 416–417
    nursery for. *See* Newborn
        nursery
    premature, human milk for,
        112–113
    superficial staphylococcal in-
        fections in, 361–362

Nervous system, central, noso-
    comial infections of,
    409–418. *See also*
    Meningitis, nosocomial
Neurosurgical operations in
    acquisition of meningitis,
    413
Newborn nursery
    design of, in prevention and
        control of nosocomial
        infections, 107–108
    nosocomial infections in, 5,
        104–113
        classification of, 104–105
        incidence of, 105
        pathogens causing, 105–107
        patterns of, 107
        predisposing factors in, 104
        prevention and control
            measures for, 107–112
Nocardia causing infections in
    transplant patients, 476–
    477
Nonpreventable infection, defini-
    tion of, 11–12
Nose, covering of, in prevention
    of microbial contamina-
    tion in tuberculosis, 279
Nosocomial infections
    definition of, 11
    general features of, 234–238
    spectrum of occurrence of,
        12–13
NRC-USPHS study on incidence
    of surgical wound infec-
    tion, 290–291
Numerator in calculation of
    rates in surveillance, 57–
    58
Nursery, newborn. *See* Newborn
    nursery, nosocomial in-
    fections in
Nurses
    in control of infections, 33
    infection control, 30–32
        role of, in data collection
            for surveillance, 55
Nutrition in control of burn
    wound infections, 342–
    343

Operating room, 129–137
    clothing for, in infection con-
        trol, 135–136
    incisional wound infections
        acquired in, 294–296
    and nosocomial infections,
        129–137
    numbers of, in surgical suite,
        131

Operating room—*Continued*
    personnel of, in infection con-
        trol, 134–136
    size of, optimal, 131
    surfaces of, in infection con-
        trol, 131–132
Operations, scheduling of, in
    infection control, 134
Operative wounds, 287–306. *See
    also* Incisional wounds
Ophthalmic *Neisseria gonor-
    rhoeae* infections, 377–
    378
Ophthalmologic examination,
    bacteremia associated
    with, 503
Oral secretions, discharge pre-
    cautions for, 173, 175
Organisms, typing of, by resist-
    ances, antibiotic sensitiv-
    ity testing for, 156–157
Oropharyngeal bacteria, aspira-
    tion of, bronchogenous
    spread pneumonia by,
    261–262
Orthopedic surgery, chemopro-
    phylaxis for, 215–216
Outbreaks
    definition of, 12
    of nosocomial infections
        detection of, 147, 158
        surveys during microbiol-
            ogy laboratory in, 148
Outpatient departments in in-
    fection control, 138–139
Oxacillin for staphylococcal
    pneumonia, 270
Oxolinic acid for bacillary
    dysentery, 390

Papovavirus causing infections
    in transplant patients,
    467–468
Parasitemia and blood trans-
    fusion, 494–495
Parenteral fluid and equipment,
    sampling of, for con-
    tamination, 163
Pasteurization
    for disinfection, 266
    wet, in control of nosocomial
        infections, 85
Pathogenicity, definition of, 17
Pathogens involved in urinary
    tract infections, 241–242
Patients
    physical condition of, predis-
        posing to incisional
        wound infections, 294

Patients—*Continued*
protection of, for infection control in hemodialysis unit, 96
spacing of, in control of infection in ICU, 103
Pelvic surgery, chemoprophylaxis for, 215
Penicillin(s)
for aerobic streptococcal endometritis, 404
for aerobic streptococcal incisional wound infections, 301
benzathine, for streptococcal skin infections, 369
G
for anaerobic streptococcal infections, 303
for group-A β-hemolytic streptococcal endometritis, 405
for meningitis, 412
for pneumococcal pneumonia, 271–272
staphylococcal resistance to, 197–198
for streptococcal pneumonia, 273
for infections of intravascular prostheses, 313
for meningococcal meningitis, 417
for ophthalmic *Neisseria gonorrhoeae* infections, 378
for postpartum endometritis due to *Peptostreptococcus* and *Peptococcus,* 404
in prevention of infection following total hip replacement, 327
prophylactic, for burn wound infections, 344
in prophylaxis for urinary tract infections, 246
for puerperal endometritis, 401
resistance of gram-negative bacilli to, 200
for staphylococcal wound sepsis, 298
for streptococcal burn wound infections, 344
for superficial staphylococcal infections, 364
tolerance of *Staphylococcus aureus* to, 199–200
V for streptococcal skin infections, 369

Penicillium endocarditis associated with cardiac prostheses, 308
Pentamidine isethionate for *Pneumocystis carinii* pneumonia, 283
Peptococcus, postpartum endometritis due to, 403–404
Peptostreptococcus, postpartum endometritis due to, 403–404
Period of infection, definition of, 19–20
Periodic trends in descriptive epidemiology, 13
Peritoneal manipulation, bacteremia associated with, 503
Persistence, bacterial, 210
Person
characterizing disease by, in epidemiologic investigation, 70–71
in descriptive epidemiology, 15
Personnel
admitting-department, in infection control, 138
food service, health and hygiene of, in prevention of nosocomial infections, 121–122
hospital, 27–52. *See also* Hospital personnel
laboratory, hygiene of, in control of laboratory-acquired infections, 142
nursery, health of, in prevention and control of infection in newborn nursery, 109
operating room, in infection control, 134–136
outpatient department, in infection control, 138–139
protection of, for infection control in hemodialysis unit, 96–97
responsibilities of, for isolation, 178
Pertussis
community-acquired, spread of, in hospital, 224
control of, in and by hospital personnel, 39–40
Pharmacy
nosocomial infections and, 115–117
in transmission of nosocomial infections, 6

Pharyngitis, streptococcal, droplet spread of, 21
Phlebitis of IV site, 438
Phlebotomy, nosocomial infections associated with, 490–491
Phycomycetes
burn wound infections due to, 351
causing infections in transplant patients, 475–476
Physicians in control of infection, 33
Place
characterizing disease by, in epidemiologic investigation, 70
in descriptive epidemiology, 14–15
Plague, control of, in and by hospital personnel, 40
Plasma, zoster immune, uses of, 45, 47
Plasmids, resistance-transfer, in nosocomial infections, 18–19
Plasmodium, infections from, associated with blood transfusions, 494–495
Platelets, transfusions of, nosocomial infections associated with, 496
Pneumococcal pneumonia, 271–272
Pneumocystis carinii
causing infections in transplant patients, 469–471
infections due to, complicating renal transplants, 459
pneumonia due to, 282–283
Pneumonia
caused by endogenous, aerobic, gram-negative bacilli, 273–276
caused by exogenous, aerobic, gram-negative bacilli, 276–279
cytomegalovirus, in transplant patient, 463
nosocomial
diagnosis of, 257–261
pneumococcal, 271–272
Pneumocystis carinii, 282–283
sources and modes of acquisition of, 261–265
staphylococcal, 268–271
from *Streptococcus pyogenes,* 272–273

Pneumonia—*Continued*
 in tracheostomized patients,
  antibiotic chemoprophy-
  laxis in, 212–213
 transplantation, 464
Point prevalence, 60
Poliomyelitis, control of, in and
  by hospital personnel, 40
Polymyxin B for *Pseudomonas*
  burn wound sepsis, 347
Polymyxin-neomycin method of
  prophylactic irrigation
  for urinary tract infections, 247
Polyomavirus causing infections
  in transplant patients,
  467
Povidone-iodine (Betadine) for
  staphylococcal burn
  wound infections, 347
Povidone-iodine ointment for
  burn wound infections,
  344
Preemployment medical evaluation, 49
Premature infant, human milk
  for, 112–113
Pressure-monitoring devices,
  nosocomial infections
  associated with, 492–494
Prevalence
 definition of, 57, 60
 point, 60
Prevalence data, uses of, 60–61
Prevalence survey, 61
Preventable infection, definition
  of, 11
Prevention of nosocomial
  infections
 Central Service Department
  in, 123–126
 role of surveillance in, 54
Prophylactic irrigation for
  urinary tract infections,
  246
Prophylaxis
 antimicrobial, 211–216. *See
  also* Chemoprophylaxis,
  antibiotic
 postexposure and preexposure,
  against hepatitis B virus,
  98–99
 routine, in control of laboratory-acquired infec-
  tions, 142
Prospective intervention study in
  epidemiologic investigations, 77–78
Prospective study in analytic
  epidemiology, 15

Prostheses
 cardiac and vascular. *See*
  Cardiovascular pros-
  theses, nosocomial infections of
 skeletal. 321–333. *See also*
  Skeletal prostheses, nosocomial infections of
 valvular
  infections of, clinical
   aspects of, 312
  removal of, due to infection, 314–315
Protective isolation, 172, 176
Protein binding of antibiotics,
  209–210
Proteus
 drug resistance in, 200
 pneumonia caused by, 275–
  276
 relative frequency of, 236
 susceptibility data on, uses of,
  158
 urinary tract infections due
  to, 243
Proteus mirabilis, subtyping of,
  154
Protozoa causing infections in
  transplant patients, 468–
  471
Pseudomembranous colitis due
  to antibiotic therapy, 206
Pseudomonas
 bacteremias from
  associated with blood transfusions, 494
  associated with bronchoscopy, 502
  associated with cystoscopy,
   502
  associated with transducers,
   492–493
 drug resistance in, 200
 gastrointestinal infections
  from, in newborn nur-
  sery, 107
 infections of intravascular
  prostheses due to, man-
  agement of, 314
 infections from
  associated with esophagoscopy, 500–501
  associated with external
   arteriovenous shunts, 309
  associated with extracorporeal circulation,
   sources and spread of, 317
  associated with intracardiac
   prostheses, 314
 in transplant patients, 459

Pseudomonas—Continued
 intravenous infusion-associated infections due to,
  prevention of, 451
 pneumonia caused by, 278
 relative frequency of, 236
 susceptibility data on, uses of,
  158
 urinary tract infections due to,
  244
Pseudomonas aeruginosa
 antibiograms for typing of,
  157
 infections from, foodborne
  transmission of, 119
 intravenous infusion-associated infections due to,
  444
 pyocine typing of, 154
Pseudomonas thomasii, contamination of intravenous
  fluids from, 447–448
Puerperal endometritis, 395–407
 community-acquired versus
  nosocomial, 396
 control measures for, 400–401
 deficiencies in reporting of,
  395–396
 diagnostic criteria for, 398–
  399
 endogenous, from lower
  genital tract flora, 401–
  404
 incidence of, 395
 mechanisms of, 396–397
 nature of, 395–397
 predisposing host factors for,
  397–398
 specimens in, collection and
  transport of, 399–400
 streptococcal, 404–406
Pulmonary aspergillosis, 283–
  284
Pulmonary tuberculosis, 279–
  281
Purulent thrombophlebitis, 433–
  438. *See also* Thrombophlebitis, purulent
Pustulosis, staphylococcal, 361
Pyocine typing of *Pseudomonas
  aeruginosa*, 154
Pyrimethamine in prevention of
  transplant-associated infections, 480

Quality control
 for antibiotic susceptibility
  testing, 155–156
 in microbiology laboratory,
  152

R factors in resistance of gram-negative bacilli to antibiotics, 200–201

Radionuclide scintimetry in diagnosis of late deep infection following total hip replacement, 331

Random sample in selection of control groups in epidemiologic investigation, 76–77

Rates
  calculation of, in surveillance of nosocomial infections, 57–58
  definition of, in surveillance of nosocomial infections, 57

Records
  hospital, containing diagnosis of nosocomial infections, medicolegal implications of, 192
  keeping of, on operating room-related infections, 136
  of microbiologic laboratory, 149

Recovery areas of surgical suite, 130

Rectal examinations, limiting of, in prevention of puerperal endometritis, 400

Reporting of communicable diseases, 227–229

Reservoirs
  of infection, definition of, 19
  subcutaneous intraventricular, infections associated with, 498–499

Resistances, typing of organisms by, antibiotic sensitivity testing for, 156–157

Respiratory isolation, 171–172, 172–173, 174

Respiratory syncytial viruses, 282

Respiratory tract
  colonization of, by bacteria due to antibiotic therapy, 206–207
  lower, infections of, nosocomial, 255–286
  causative agents in, 256–257, 258, 259
  chlamydial, 282
  classification of, 255
  diagnostic criteria for, 257–261

Respiratory tract, lower, infections of, nosocomial—*Continued*
  disinfection and sterilization of ventilatory equipment in prevention of, 265–268
  due to endogenous, aerobic, gram-negative bacilli, 273–276
  due to exogenous, aerobic, gram-negative bacilli, 276–279
  incidence of, 255–256
  nature of, 255–257
  pneumococcal, 271–272
  Pneumocystis carinii pneumonia as, 282–283
  pulmonary aspergillosis as, 283–284
  pulmonary tuberculosis as, 279–281
  rickettsial, 282
  sources and modes of acquisition of, 261–265
  staphylococcal, 268–271
  streptococcal, 272–273
  susceptibility to, 261
  viral, 281–282

Retrospective study in analytic epidemiology, 15

Rhizopus, burn wound infections due to, 351

Rickettsial nosocomial respiratory infections, 282

Ritter's disease, 362

Rodents, control of, in control of nosocomial infections, 90

Rods, gram-negative aerobic, causing infections in transplant patients, 459–460

Roentgenography in diagnosis of late deep infection following total hip replacement, 331

Rotaviruses, gastroenteritis due to, 391–392

Rounds, ward, as source of infection data in surveillance, 56

Rubella, 422–424
  control of, in, and by hospital personnel, 40
  direct transmission of, in ICU, control of, 101

Safety officer for infection control in hemodialysis unit, 95

Salmonella
  foodborne transmission of, prevention of, 120–121
  gastroenteritis due to, 385–387
  infections from
    associated with endoscopy, 501
    associated with platelet transfusions, 496
    community-acquired, spread of, in hospital, 224
    foodborne transmission of, 118, 119
    septicemia from, in transplant patient, 461
    vectorborne spread of, 22

Salmonellosis
  airborne transmission of, 2
  common-vehicle spread of, 21
  control of, in, and by hospital personnel, 41

Sanitation in control of nosocomial infections, 90

"Scalded skin" syndrome, 362

Scientific value, inherent, of surveillance of nosocomial infections, 53

Scintimetry, radionuclide, in diagnosis of late deep infection following total hip replacement, 331

Scrub in infection control in operating room, 136

Seasonal trends in descriptive epidemiology, 13

Secondary transmission in descriptive epidemiology, 14

Secretions, oral, discharge precautions for, 173, 175

Secular trends in descriptive epidemiology, 13

Selective survey media for culturing specimens in outbreak investigation, 159–160

Septicemia
  catheter-caused, 436, 437
  complicating incisional wound infections, 293
  gram-negative, common-vehicle spread of, 21
  intravenous infusion-associated, 443

Serotyping of isolates, 153–154

Serratia
  bacteremia due to, 512–514
  contamination of intravenous fluids from, 449

Serratia—Continued
 intravenous infusion-associated infections due to,
  444
 pneumonia caused by, 278
 susceptibility data on, uses of,
  158
 urinary tract infections due to,
  243
Serum hepatitis. *See* Hepatitis B
Sex predisposing to gram-negative rod bacteremia, 514
Shifts, antigenic, major, 18
Shigellae
 drug resistance in, 200
 gastroenteritis due to, 389–
  391
 vectorborne transmission of,
  22
Shigellosis, control of, in and by
  hospital personnel, 41
Shunts, ventricular, infections
  associated with, 499
Sigmoidoscopy, bacteremia associated with, 500
Silver nitrate for burn wound
  infections, 344
Silver sulfadiazine cream
 for burn wound infections,
  344
 for gram-negative burn wound
  sepsis, 352
Skeletal prostheses, nosocomial
  infections of, 321–333
 classification of, 321–322
 control measures for, 325–327
 deep
  early, 327–330
  late, 330–333
 incidence of, 322, 323
 microbiologic diagnosis of,
  323–324
 pathogens in, 322–323
 predisposing factors for, 324–
  325
Skin
 nosocomial infections of,
  355–380
  classification of, 356–357
  collection and transport of
   specimens of, 357–358
  control measures for, 358
  diagnostic criteria for, 357
  from herpesvirus hominis,
   370–373
  incidence of, 355, 356
  nature of, 355–357
  pathogens causing, 355–356
  staphylococcal, 358–367
  streptococcal, 367–370

Skin, nosocomial infections of—
  Continued
  from varicella-zoster virus,
   373–377
  precautions for, in isolation,
   172, 173, 174–175
  preparation of, in infection
   control in operating
   room, 136
Smallpox, 424–427
 direct transmission of, in ICU,
  control of, 101
Sorting of supplies in Central
  Service Department, 124
Source of infection, definition of,
  19
Spatial separation of patients in
  control of infection in
  ICU, 103
Specificity in chain of infection,
  18
Specimens
 from anaerobes in diagnosis
  of infections following
  total hip replacement,
  324
 in bacterial meningitis, collection and transport of, 411
 biopsy, in diagnosis of infections following total hip
  replacement, 324
 collection and transport of,
  for processing by microbiology laboratory, 149–
  151
 in evaluation of infections of
  cardiovascular pros-
  theses, 310–312
 from gram-negative rod bacteremia, collection and
  processing of, 508–510
 from herpetic skin infections,
  collection and transport
  of, 371
 from intravenous cannula-
  associated infections, collection and culture of,
  439–440
 from intravenous infusion-
  associated septicemia,
  collection of, 446–447
 liquid, in diagnosis of infections following total hip
  replacement, 323–324
 microbiologic, from surgical
  wound infections, 289
 microscopic evaluation of,
  prior to processing in
  microbiology laboratory,
  150–151

Specimens—Continued
 from puerperal endometritis,
  collection and transport
  of, 399–400
 selection of, for processing by
  microbiology laboratory,
  149–151
 from staphylococcal superficial infections, collection and transport of, 363
 from streptococcal skin infections, collection and
  transport of, 368
 from superficial infections,
  collection and transport
  of, 357–358
 from varicella-zoster infections, collection, shipment, and storage of, 275
Spectinomycin, resistance of
  gram-negative bacilli to,
  200
Spinal cord injuries, intermittent
  catheterization for, 247–
  248
Sponges, copper, for disinfection, 267
Sporadic occurrence of nosocomial infections, 12
Spore strip cultures to monitor
  sterilization in routine
  environmental sampling,
  160–161
Staff. *See* Personnel
Staffing of personnel health
  services, 48
Standards and codes, medicolegal implications of,
  190–191
Staphylococcus
 airborne transmission of, 21
 control of, in, and by hospital
  personnel, 42
 enterocolitis due to, 392–393
 foodborne transmission of,
  prevention of, 121
 incisional wound infections
  due to, 297–299
 infections from
  associated with cardiovascular prostheses, 308–309
  associated with intravascular prostheses, man-
   agement of, 313
  associated with reservoirs
   and shunts, 498–499
  associated with valvular
   prostheses, 312–313
  legal aspects of, 183–188
  in newborn nursery, 105

Staphylococcus—Continued
  intravenous cannula-asso-
    ciated infections due to,
    437, 438, 439
  penicillin-resistant, 197–198
  nosocomial infections from,
    spread of, to community,
    224–225
  resistance of
    to antibiotics, 197–200, 202
    to methicillin, 198–199,
      203–204
  susceptibility data on, uses of,
    158
  transmission of, by linens,
    prevention of, 126
Staphylococcus aureus
  airborne spread of, in ward,
    296
  antibiotic typing of, 157
  burn wound infections due to,
    336–337, 346–347
  classification of, 363
  clinical manifestations of,
    361–362
  direct transmission of, in ICU,
    control of, 102
  endemic, 365–366
  enterocolitis due to, 392–393
  epidemic, 366–367
  infections following total hip
    replacement due to, 323
    antibiotics for, 328
    prophylaxis for, 327
  infections from, in new-
    born nursery, 105, 107
  meningitis due to, 411,
    413–414
  microbiologic diagnosis of,
    362–363
  penicillin tolerance of, 199–
    200
  predisposing host factors to,
    363–364
  relative frequency of, 236
  respiratory infections due to,
    268–271
  shedders of, causing infection
    following total hip re-
    placement, 329
  specimen of, collection and
    transport of, 363
  superficial infections due to,
    355–356, 358–367
  transmissibility of, 359–361
  treatment of, 364
Staphylococcus aureus, wound
    infections due to, 292
Staphylococcus epidermidis
  biotyping of, 154

*Staphylococcus epidermidis—
    Continued*
  infection following total hip
    replacement due to, 323,
    330–333
  infection following umbilical
    catheterization due to,
    492
State health authorities, relation-
    ship of hospital to, re-
    garding infection control,
    225–227
Sterile goods, storage of, in Cen-
    tral Service Department,
    125–126
Sterilization
  in control of nosocomial in-
    fections, 85–88
  definition of, 265
  for infection control in hemo-
    dialysis unit, 96
  methods of, 266
  spore strip cultures to mon-
    itor, in routine environ-
    mental sampling, 160–
    161
  of ventilatory equipment,
    265–268
Sterilizers, washer, for process-
    ing of supplies in Central
    Service Department, 124
Strains, selection of, for anti-
    biotic susceptibility test-
    ing, 154–155
Streptococcal infections in new-
    born nursery, 105–106
Streptococcus
  aerobic
    incisional wound infections
      due to, 300–302
    postpartum endometritis
      due to, 404
  anaerobic, incisional wound
    infections due to, 302–
    303
  control of, in and by hospital
    personnel, 42–43
  foodborne transmission of,
    prevention of, 121
  group-A β-hemolytic, post-
    partum endometritis due
    to, 404–406
  group-B, meningitis due to,
    415–416
  infections from
    complicating intravascular
      prostheses, management
      of, 313
    in newborn nursery, 105–
      106

Streptococcus, infections from—
    Continued
  transmitted by linens, pre-
    vention of, 126
  microaerophilic, incisional
    wound infections due to,
    302
  pharyngitis from, droplet
    spread of, 21
  skin infections due to, 367–
    370
  susceptibility data on, uses of,
    158
Streptococcus pneumoniae, men-
    ingitis due to, 411
Streptococcus pyogenes
  burn wound infections due to,
    336
  group-A
    burn wound infections due
      to, 344–346
    M-typing of, 154
    pneumonia due to, 272–273
Streptomycin
  for infections of intravascular
    prostheses, 313
  in prophylaxis for urinary
    tract infections, 246
  resistance of gram-negative
    bacilli to, 200
  resistance of staphylococci to,
    198
Strict isolation, 171, 172, 174
Strongyloides stercoralis causing
    infections in transplant
    patients, 469
Subclinical infection, definition
    of, 10
Sulfadiazine
  in prevention of transplant-
    associated infections, 480
  silver, cream
    for burn wound infections,
      344
    for gram-negative burn
      wound sepsis, 352
Sulfamethoxazole for *Pneumo-
    cystis carinii* pneumonia,
    283
Sulfamylon. *See* Mafenide
    (Sulfamylon)
Sulfisoxazole (Gantrisin) for
    meningococcal meningi-
    tis, 417
Sulfonamides, resistance of
    gram-negative bacilli to,
    200
Suprapubic catheter as alterna-
    tive to urethral catheter-
    ization, 248

Surgery
   chemoprophylaxis for, 215–216
   clean, as contraindication to antimicrobial prophylaxis, 212
Surgical diphtheria, 303
Surgical infections, 287–306.
   See also Incisional wounds, infection in
Surgical suite, environmental design of, 129–131
Surveillance
   of antibiotic use by pharmacy, 116
   in control of infection
      in hemodialysis unit, 95
      in ICU, 103
      in newborn nursery, 109
      in outpatient department, 138
   in control of infectious gastroenteritis, 384
   environmental, 90–91
   of nosocomial infections, 53–61
      analysis in, 58–59
      to augment control efforts, 53–54
      data collection in, 54–56
      definition of, 53
      efficiency of, prevalence for determining, 60
      elements of, 54–60
      interpretation in, 59
      medicolegal implications of, 191–192
      microbiology laboratory in, 147–148
      rate calculation in, 57–58
      to reinforce prevention practice, 54
      reporting data in, 59–60
      scientific value of, 53
      sources of infection data in, 56–57
      uses of, 53–54
   in prevention of foodborne infections, 122
Sutures predisposing patient to superficial staphylococcal infections, 363–364
Swabs in diagnosis of infections following total hip replacement, 323–324
Syncytial viruses, respiratory, 282
Synergism and antagonism between antibacterial drugs, 209
Syphilis, reporting of, 228

Tetanus
   in burn wound patient, 352
   control of, in and by hospital personnel, 43
Tetracycline
   for anaerobic streptococcal infections, 303
   for bacillary dysentery, 390
   for postpartum endometritis due to *Bacteroides fragilis,* 403
   resistance of gram-negative bacilli to, 200
   resistance of staphylococci to, 198
Thiabendazole in prevention of transplant-associated infections, 480
Thoracocentesis, bacteremia associated with, 502–503
Thrombophlebitis, purulent
   control measures for, 440–441
   incidence of, 434–437
   nature of, 433–438
   pathogens in, 437–438
Thrombosis
   of IV site, 438
   septic, complicating incisional wound infections, 293
Time
   characterizing disease by, in epidemiologic investigation, 69–70
   in descriptive epidemiology, 13–14
Tissue
   devitalized, predisposing to incisional wound infections, 294
   distribution of antibiotics in, 209–210
Tobramycin
   for infections of intravascular prostheses, 314
   for *Pseudomonas* burn wound sepsis, 347
   resistance of gram-negative bacilli to, 200–201
   for urinary tract infections, 246
Toxic epidermal necrolysis, 362
Toxoplasmosis
   blood transfusion-related, 495
   causing infections in transplant patients, 468–489
Tracheostomized patients, pneumonia in, antibiotic chemoprophylaxis in, 212–213

Training in control of laboratory-acquired infections, 141
Transabdominal specimens in diagnosis of puerperal endometritis, 399
Transducers, nosocomial infections associated with, 494–497
Transfer areas of surgical suite, 130–131
Transfusion-associated, 494–497
Transfusions
   of blood
      and bacteremia, 494
      cases on, legal aspects of, 181–183
      parasitemia, 494–495
   of platelets, nosocomial infections associated with, 496
Transmission
   in chain of infection, 20–22
   of nosocomial infections
      airborne, 84
      common-vehicle, 83–84
      contact, 82–83
      contamination food in, 5
      environmental, 82–84
      in nursery, 5
      operating room in, 6
      pharmacy in, 6
      vectorborne, 84
   secondary, in descriptive epidemiology, 14
Transplants, nosocomial infections associated with, 453–488
   of bone marrow, nosocomial infections associated with, 456–457
   classification of, 477
   diagnosis of, 477–479
   of heart, nosocomial infections associated with, 454–455
   immunosuppression and, 457–459
   of kidney, nosocomial infections associated with, 454
   of liver, nosocomial infections associated with, 455–456
   of lung, nosocomial infections associated with, 457
   organisms causing, 459–477
   prevention of, 480–481
   treatment of, 479–480
Transvaginal monitoring, risk of puerperal endometritis associated with, 398

Transvaginal specimens in diagnosis of puerperal endometritis, 399

Trimethoprim
  for *Pneumocystis carinii* pneumonia, 283
  resistance of gram-negative bacilli to, 200

Trimethoprim-sulfamethoxazole
  for bacillary dysentery, 390
  for *Salmonella* gastroenteritis, 385

Trypanosomiasis, American, blood transfusion-related, 495

Tuberculosis
  airborne transmission of, 21–22
  community-acquired, spread of, in hospital, 224
  control of, in and by hospital personnel, 43–45
  pulmonary, 279–281

Tuberculous infections of wounds, 304–305

Typing
  of clinical isolates by microbiology laboratory, 152–154
  of organisms by resistances, antibiotic sensitivity testing for, 156–157

Ultrasonic cleaners for processing of supplies in Central Service Department, 124

Ultraviolet lights
  in removal of airborne organisms in tuberculosis, 280
  use of, in operating rooms in infection control, 133

Umbilical cord, care of, in prevention of infection in newborn nursery, 111–112

Urethra, instrumentation of, bacteremia associated with, 501

Urethral catheters, alternatives to, 248

Urinary catheter, care of, 249–252

Urinary tract infections, nosocomial, 239–254
  catheterization and, 244–246
  classification of, 241
  community-acquired, incidence of, 240
  control measures in, 246–249

Urinary tract infections, nosocomial—*Continued*
  diagnostic criteria for, 240–241
  frequency of, 240
  nature of, 240–241
  pathogens involved in, 241–242
  transmission of, sources and modes of, 242–244

Urologic instrumentation, bacteremia associated with, 501–502

Uterine drainage for puerperal endometritis, 401

Vaccination. *See also* Immunization(s)
  against influenza, in prevention of transplant-associated infections, 480

Vaginal examinations, limiting of, in prevention of puerperal endometritis, 400

Valvular prostheses, 312, 314–315

Vancomycin
  for infections of intravascular prostheses, 313
  for staphylococcal pneumonia, 270
  for staphylococcal wound sepsis, 298
  for streptococcal burn wound infections, 344–345
  for superficial staphylococcal infections, 364

Varicella, direct transmission of, in ICU, control of, 101

Varicella-zoster
  causing infections in transplant patients, 465–466
  control of, in and by hospital personnel, 45
  infections due to, 373–377

Variola, 424–427

Vascular prostheses, infections of, 307–319. *See also* Cardiovascular prostheses, nosocomial infections of

Vascular system, diagnostic procedures involving, nosocomial infections from, 490–494

Vector control in control of nosocomial infections, 90

Vectorborne spread. *See also under specific pathogens*

Vectorborne spread—*Continued*
  of infection, 22
  of nosocomial infections, 84

Venereal diseases, reporting of, 228–229

Ventilation
  in control of nosocomial infections, 90
  mechanical, in removal of airborne organisms in tuberculosis, 280

Ventilatory equipment, disinfection and sterilization of, 265–268

Ventricular shunts, infections associated with, 499

Vibrio parahaemolyticus, foodborne transmission of, 119

Viral gastroenteritis, 391–392

Viral hepatitis. *See* Hepatitis

Viral infections
  acute, as contraindication to antimicrobial prophylaxis, 212
  community-acquired, spread of, in hospital, 224
  nosocomial, 419–432
  nosocomial respiratory, 281–282
  wound, 305

Virulence, definition of, 17–18

Viruses
  causing infections in transplant patient, 461–468
  hepatitis B, 93–99. *See also* Hepatitis B virus (HBV)

Visitors in control of infection in ICU, 103

Ward rounds as source of infection data in surveillance, 56

Washer-sterilizers for processing of supplies in Central Service Department, 124

Water
  and ice, testing of, for contamination, 163
  in transmission of nosocomial infections, 83–84

Wound precautions in isolation, 172, 173, 174–175

Wounds, incisional, infection in, 287–306. *See also* Incisional wounds, infection in

Yersinia enterocolitica infections, 393

Yersinia pestis organisms, vectorborne spread of, 22

Zoster immune globulin in prevention of varicella-zoster infections, 375

Zoster immune plasma, uses of, 45, 47

Zoster immunoglobulin, uses of, 45, 47

Zoster infections, 373–377